I0491313

Podrid's Real-World ECGs

A Master's Approach to the Art and Practice of Clinical ECG Interpretation

Volume 3 Conduction Abnormalities

Philip Podrid, MD

Professor of Medicine
Professor of Pharmacology and Experimental Therapeutics
Boston University School of Medicine

Lecturer in Medicine
Harvard Medical School
Boston, Massachusetts

Attending Physician
West Roxbury VA Hospital
West Roxbury, Massachusetts

Rajeev Malhotra, MD, MS

Instructor in Medicine
Cardiology Division
Massachusetts General Hospital
Harvard Medical School
Boston, Massachusetts

Rahul Kakkar, MD

Cardiology Fellow
Massachusetts General Hospital
Harvard Medical School
Boston, Massachusetts

Peter A. Noseworthy, MD

Cardiology Fellow
Massachusetts General Hospital
Harvard Medical School
Boston, Massachusetts

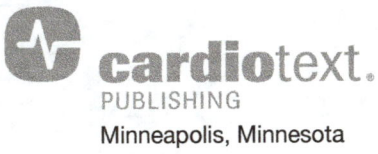

cardiotext.
PUBLISHING
Minneapolis, Minnesota

Cardiotext Publishing, LLC
3405 W. 44th Street
Minneapolis, Minnesota, 55410
USA
www.cardiotextpublishing.com

Any updates to this book may be found at:
www.cardiotextpublishing.com/titles/detail/9781935395010

Comments, inquiries, and requests for bulk sales can be directed to the publisher at:
info@cardiotextpublishing.com.

This book is intended for educational purposes and to further general scientific and medical knowledge, research, and understanding of the conditions and associated treatments discussed herein. This book is not intended to serve as and should not be relied upon as recommending or promoting any specific diagnosis or method of treatment for a particular condition or a particular patient. It is the reader's responsibility to determine the proper steps for diagnosis and the proper course of treatment for any condition or patient, including suitable and appropriate tests, medications or medical devices to be used for or in conjunction with any diagnosis or treatment.

Due to ongoing research, discoveries, modifications to medicines, equipment and devices, and changes in government regulations, the information contained in this book may not reflect the latest standards, developments, guidelines, regulations, products or devices in the field. Readers are responsible for keeping up to date with the latest developments and are urged to review the latest instructions and warnings for any medicine, equipment or medical device. Readers should consult with a specialist or contact the vendor of any medicine or medical device where appropriate.

Except for the publisher's website associated with this work, the publisher is not affiliated with and does not sponsor or endorse any websites, organizations or other sources of information referred to herein.

The publisher and the authors specifically disclaim any damage, liability, or loss incurred, directly or indirectly, from the use or application of any of the contents of this book.

Unless otherwise stated, all figures and tables in this book are used courtesy of the authors.

Cover design by Caitlin Crouchet Altobell and Elizabeth Edwards;
interior design by Elizabeth Edwards

A note on the format: The first printing of this book was in a landscape format bound on the short edge. Due to new printer requirements, and so that we may maintain the original landscape orientation, the binding is now on the long side.

Library of Congress Control Number: 201394965
ISBN: 978-1-935395-01-0

Printed in the United States of America   20 21 22 23 24 25 10 9 8 7 6 5 4 3 2 1

These workbooks are dedicated first to my wife Vivian and son Joshua, whose patience, tolerance, support, and love over the years have been limitless, exceptional, and inspirational. They are also dedicated to the many cardiology fellows, house staff, and medical students whom I have had the pleasure and honor of teaching over the past three decades and who have also taught me so very much.

Philip Podrid

To my wife Cindy and daughter Sapna, for all their love, support, and encouragement.

Rajeev Malhotra

To my darling daughters, Mia and Eila, whom I love to infinity.

Rahul Kakkar

For Katie and Jack

Peter A. Noseworthy

Contents

Foreword

The invention of the electrocardiogram (ECG) by Dr. Willem Einthoven, first reported in 1901, ranks as one of the all-time great discoveries in medicine. Einthoven's landmark achievement was duly recognized in 1924, when he was awarded the Nobel Prize in Medicine.

By the early 1940s, all of the components of the 12-lead ECG that we use today were in place. When I finished my cardiology training 50 years ago, the ECG was one of very few cardiodiagnostic tools available to us. As a result, we received an intensity of training in electrocardiography that is generally not encountered in many of today's cardiology fellowship programs, where the emphasis has shifted toward the newer high-tech diagnostic modalities. Yet the ECG remains a major pillar in the evaluation of disorders of the heart. In a patient with a cardiac arrhythmia, what diagnostic information does the treating physician want the most? Of course—the ECG. Although the medical world progresses rapidly and changes constantly, the body of knowledge surrounding the ECG is virtually timeless. What was true 50 years ago is largely true today, and will remain so 50 years from now.

This wonderful series of ECG workbooks, appropriately entitled "Real-World ECGs," by Dr. Philip Podrid and three outstanding young cardiologists from Massachusetts General Hospital—Dr. Rajeev Malhotra, Dr. Rahul Kakkar, and Dr. Peter Noseworthy—offers a splendid opportunity for self-education in electrocardiography (and a bit of fun at the same time). An esteemed academic cardiologist, Dr. Podrid has had a career-long interest in electrocardiography. Over many years he has collected and saved thousands of ECGs for teaching purposes, and it is a portion of his incredible collection that has been used to spawn these books.

There are scores of textbooks on electrocardiography, but what sets these volumes apart is that every ECG is tied directly to an actual clinical case. Each ECG is initially presented in a visually attractive and readable format accompanied by a clinical vignette. On the next page, the salient features of the ECGs are highlighted, dissected, and discussed in meticulous detail, followed by a summary of the patient's clinical problem and treatment, particularly as they relate to the ECG findings.

The first volume in this unique series covers electrocardiography basics. It is followed by five more volumes covering the entire spectrum of electrocardiography: myocardial abnormalities, conduction abnormalities, arrhythmias, narrow and wide complex tachycardias, and a sixth volume amalgamating a potpourri of paced rhythms, congenital abnormalities, and electrolyte disturbances. As I perused one of the workbooks, I truly enjoyed the experience. It is fun to try to guess the clinical problem from the ECG. In fact, on my teaching rounds, that is often exactly what I do. I will ask the trainee to present first just the ECG and with other trainees try to deduce from it what might be going on clinically. For example, in an adult with marked left ventricular hypertrophy and strain, one of three conditions is almost always present: severe aortic valve disease, hypertrophic cardiomyopathy, or hypertensive heart disease.

continues

These books should prove to be valuable for the teaching and learning of electrocardiography at all levels—from nursing and medical students to residents to cardiology fellows to practicing internists and cardiologists. They should be especially helpful for those seeking board certification or recertification in cardiovascular diseases, where knowledge of electrocardiography still is given a very high priority.

There is one further important dividend for those who utilize this series. In addition to the six workbooks, hundreds of other ECGs handled in a similar format are available online. From clinical diagnoses to interactive questions to patient management, realworldECGs.com offers ECG-centric clinical cases for the viewer to further master the art of ECG interpretation.

Anyone who reads these books and views the auxiliary electronic material cannot help but be impressed by the prodigious amount of work that went into their preparation. Drs. Podrid, Malhotra, Kakkar, and Noseworthy should be justifiably proud of the final results of their Herculean efforts. I am confident that other readers will find these books and their electronic supplement as informative and enjoyable as I did.

Roman W. DeSanctis, MD
Physician and Director of Clinical Cardiology, Emeritus
Massachusetts General Hospital
James and Evelyn Jenks and Paul Dudley White Professor of Medicine
Harvard Medical School

Foreword

The electrocardiogram (ECG) was born in the Netherlands at the beginning of the 20th century when physiologist Willem Einthoven made the first recording of the spread of electrical activity in the beating heart from the surface of the body in a living human being. Since then, the ECG has become the indispensable "workhorse" in the management of patients suspected to have a cardiac problem.

The reasons are obvious. An ECG can be obtained anywhere. A recording is easily and quickly made, noninvasive, inexpensive, reproducible, and patient-friendly. The ECG gives instantaneous diagnostic information, is essential in selecting appropriate management, and allows documentation of the effect of treatment in cases of acute and chronic cardiac ischemia, rhythm and conduction disturbances, structural changes in the cardiac chambers, electrolyte and metabolic disorders, medication effects, and monogenic ECG patterns indicating the likelihood of cardiac abnormalities. The ECG is also a valuable tool for epidemiologic studies and risk stratification of the cardiac patient.

In the 110 years during which the ECG has been in use, we have seen continual improvements in its value in light of information gleaned from other invasive and noninvasive diagnostic techniques, such as coronary angiography, intracardiac localization of abnormal impulse formation and conduction disturbances, echocardiography, MRI, and genetic evaluation. This means that not only does the novice health care professional need to be informed about all the information currently available from the ECG, but the more senior physician also needs to stay up-do-date with ever-evolving new developments.

Dr. Philip Podrid is known worldwide as an expert in electrocardiography. He is also a superb teacher. When you combine his input with beautiful ECGs, not surprisingly, you will have a series of "Real-World ECGs" that demonstrate the art and practice of clinical ECG interpretation as only a real master can. I hope that many readers will profit from this exceptional educational exercise.

Hein J. Wellens, MD
Professor of Cardiology
Cardiovascular Research Institute Maastricht
Maastricht, The Netherlands

Preface

The electrocardiogram (ECG) is one of the oldest technologies used in medicine and remains one of the most frequently obtained tests in the physician's office, outpatient clinic, emergency department, and hospital. ECGs continue to play an essential role in the diagnosis of many cardiac diseases and in the evaluation of symptoms believed to be of cardiac origin. The ECG is also important in the diagnosis of many noncardiac medical conditions.

Like any other skill in medicine, the art of ECG interpretation requires frequent review of the essentials of ECG analysis and continual practice in reading actual ECGs. However, many health care providers who wish to augment their expertise in the interpretation of ECGs and develop the skills necessary to understand the underlying mechanisms of ECG abnormalities have realized that the currently available resources do not adequately meet their needs.

Teaching in medical schools and house staff programs does not typically emphasize ECG analysis. Consequently, many physicians do not feel adequately trained in interpreting the ECG. The currently available textbooks used for teaching ECG analysis are based on pattern recognition and memorization rather than on understanding the fundamental electrophysiologic properties and clinical concepts that can be applied to an individual ECG tracing, regardless of its complexity. The physician is not, therefore, trained in the identification of important waveforms and subtle abnormalities.

The workbooks and website of *Podrid's Real-World* ECGs aim to fill the gap in ECG education. These unique teaching aids prepare students and health care providers of all levels for the spectrum of routine to challenging ECGs they will encounter in their own clinical practice by providing a broad and in-depth understanding of ECG analysis and diagnosis, including discussion of relevant electrophysiologic properties of the heart, associated case scenarios, and clinical management.

The Workbooks

Each of the six volumes in *Podrid's Real-World* ECGs teaches the art of ECG interpretation by careful analysis of specific examples and identification of important waveforms. Each ECG is taken from a real clinical case and incorporates a discussion of important diagnostic findings and essential associated electrophysiologic mechanisms, as well as critical clinical management decisions. The purpose of the series is to provide readers from all fields of medicine with a systematic approach to ECG interpretation using a concise, case-based format.

Volume 1 provides an essential introduction to the basics of ECG reading, outlining the approaches and tools that are utilized in the

continues

interpretation of all ECGs. This volume, the third in the series, discusses the mechanism, diagnosis, and treatment of atrioventricular (AV) and intraventricular conduction disturbances and enhanced AV conduction. The remaining volumes focus on other disease entities for which the ECG is useful:

- Atrial and ventricular hypertrophy, acute myocardial ischemia, acute and chronic myocardial infarction, and pericarditis
- Sinus, atrial, junctional, and ventricular arrhythmias
- Narrow and wide complex tachycardias and forms of aberration
- Recording methods and miscellaneous conditions, including pacemakers, electrolyte disorders, and acquired and congenital cardiac conditions

Each volume in the series starts with a didactic introduction that addresses the important ECG findings associated with each clinical category. This is followed by core illustrative case-based ECGs that lead the reader through identification of the important ECG findings associated with the specific abnormalities being discussed and provide information about the basic electrophysiologic mechanisms involved. This section is followed by a random assortment of topic-related ECGs and clinical scenarios to further enhance the student's skills at ECG analysis. Importantly, each case presentation is followed by an in-depth discussion of the ECG findings, with the important waveforms on the ECG highlighted.

The Website: realworldECGs.com

In addition to the didactic ECG cases found in the workbooks, the website (www.realworldECGs.com) offers easy access to a large, searchable repository of supplementary case-based ECGs. This ancillary material offers further practice in ECG interpretation using interactive case studies with Q&A that includes feedback and discussion about the important findings and clinical issues involved.

The benefit of a Web-based program is that many more ECGs can be presented and ECGs demonstrating specific abnormalities can be accessed quickly. In addition, the ECGs can be read using an approach that is similar to how they are analyzed in clinical practice—by identifying the waveforms important for diagnosis. Each of the relevant features is highlighted independently, providing a useful way to approach ECG reading.

This versatile Web-based program allows the user either to interpret ECGs in random fashion or to focus attention on a specific topic or ECG finding. This approach allows ECG interpretation to be performed in a way that is most effective for the user.

Philip Podrid, MD
Rajeev Malhotra, MD, MS
Rahul Kakkar, MD
Peter A. Noseworthy, MD

Introduction
Conduction Abnormalities

There are two general types of conduction abnormalities in the heart. Atrioventricular (AV) conduction abnormalities affect impulse transmission from the atria to the ventricles, while intraventricular conduction abnormalities affect impulse conduction through the ventricular myocardium.

Atrioventricular Conduction Abnormalities

AV conduction abnormalities may result from problems with impulse transmission through either the AV node or the His-Purkinje system. There are three types of AV conduction abnormalities: first-degree, second-degree, and third-degree block.

First-degree Atrioventricular Block

First-degree AV block is defined simply by a prolonged PR interval (*ie,* > 0.20 sec). However, the PR interval includes the P wave, representing atrial depolarization, and the PR segment, which represents conduction through the AV node and His-Purkinje system. With first-degree AV block, it is the PR segment that is prolonged as a result of slow conduction through either the AV node or the His-Purkinje system. This is usually the result of slowing of conduction through the AV node. Because the impulse does conduct from the atria to the ventricles, it is not accurate to refer to this as AV block; it is more appropriately termed prolonged or slow AV conduction.

Because the P wave is part of the PR interval, a very broad P wave, as seen in left atrial hypertrophy or abnormality, may cause the PR interval to be slightly prolonged while the PR segment is normal. It should be noted that AV nodal conduction velocity is variable and can change with heart rate as a result of change in autonomic inputs affecting AV nodal conduction velocity. Hence with sinus tachycardia there is enhancement of sympathetic tone and an increase in conduction velocity through the AV node; this results in a shortening of the PR interval. With enhanced parasympathetic tone, resulting in sinus bradycardia, there is prolongation of the PR interval due to a slowing of conduction through the AV node. However, there is no correction equation available to establish a rate-corrected PR interval. For example, a PR interval of 0.22 second is prolonged and by definition would be first-degree heart block. However, if the heart rate were 30 bpm, this PR interval would be appropriate for bradycardia. Likewise, a PR interval of 0.20 second, defined as normal, would probably be prolonged for a heart rate of 150 bpm.

Second-degree Atrioventricular Block

Second-degree AV block is identified by a pause in the RR interval due to an occasional nonconducted P wave. The PP intervals (*ie,* sinus or atrial impulses) are constant. The PR intervals may be normal or prolonged as first-degree AV block may be present along with second-degree AV block. There are two types of second-degree AV block as the block may be in either the AV node (Mobitz type I) or the His-Purkinje system (Mobitz type II).

Mobitz Type I Atrioventricular Block (Wenckebach)

Mobitz type I AV block (Wenckebach) results from a conduction abnormality within the AV node. In Wenckebach, progressive PR-interval prolongation results in a single nonconducted P wave and pause in the RR interval. The duration of the pause (the PP interval around the pause) is equal to two sinus intervals. After the pause, the PR interval shortens to the baseline PR interval. Hence the baseline interval is the PR interval of the complex immediately following the pause, and the PR interval after each pause should be the same. It may be normal or prolonged. There is only one nonconducted P wave each time, and hence there will be one more P wave than QRS complex. Therefore, Wenckebach is termed 3:2, 4:3, 5:4, etc. This results in a pattern of grouped beating. The pattern of block may be fixed (only 3:2, only 4:3, etc) or variable (periods of both 3:2 and 4:3, etc).

The basis of Mobitz type I AV block is that impulse generation within the AV node results from calcium currents (*ie*, a slow action potential). The slow action potential demonstrates changes in refractoriness and conduction velocity. Therefore, the rate of impulse conduction through the AV node is variable. AV nodal refractoriness and conduction velocity change as a result of various factors, including autonomic impulses, drugs, and electrolyte abnormalities. Because of changes in refractoriness, impulse velocity can change; that is, the ability of the AV node to conduct impulses is not all or none, as is

seen in the His-Purkinje system where impulse generation is the result of fast sodium currents (*ie*, the fast action potential). Therefore, the AV node demonstrates a property known as decremental conduction, (*ie*, conduction velocity through the AV node changes based on how rapidly the node is stimulated). In the absence of sympathetic stimulation, when the rate of impulse stimulation of the AV node increases, the impulse conduction velocity through it slows. This results in lengthening of the PR interval. Each successive atrial impulse reaches the AV node earlier, when it may be even more refractory. As a result, there is a progressive slowing of each subsequent impulse due to decremental AV nodal conduction, until the node finally fails to conduct the impulse because it has arrived at a time when it is absolutely refractory. As a result of blockade of impulse conduction within the AV node, there is no activation of the ventricle and no QRS impulse on the ECG. The increment of PR lengthening is greatest at the beginning of a Wenckebach cycle and may decrease progressively from one beat to the next. For example, the PR interval may lengthen from the baseline of 0.16 second, to 0.24 second, then to 0.28 second, and finally to 0.30 second. Since the PP interval is constant, this results in shortening of the RR interval. However, shortening of the RR interval may not be seen, especially if there is a long Wenckebach cycle length or if the underlying heart rate is fast. Hence this finding is not necessary to identify Wenckebach.

Although Wenckebach is seen most often in sinus rhythm, it may occur with an atrial rhythm, atrial tachycardia, or atrial flutter. Regardless of the underlying rhythm, there is a regular PP interval.

Wenckebach is most often benign and does not require any therapy. Importantly, if a failure of impulse conduction from atria to ventricles would develop (*ie,* complete heart block), the escape rhythm would be junctional. Junctional rhythms are generally reliable, predictable, and stable with regard to rate. In general, urgent pacemaker insertion is not required unless there are symptoms resulting from bradycardia.

Mobitz Type II Atrioventricular Block

With Mobitz type II AV block, there is an occasional nonconducted P wave, but when there is AV conduction the PR interval is constant (*ie,* the PR intervals before and after the pause are constant). There may be one or more nonconducted P waves; the occurrence of two or more nonconducted P waves is often called high-degree AV block. Mobitz type II block is failure of conduction within the His-Purkinje system. Since impulse generation within the His-Purkinje system results from the fast action potential mediated by a rapid influx of sodium currents, conduction through the His-Purkinje system is all or none; that is, it either conducts (always at the same rate) or does not conduct. Therefore, when there is AV conduction, the PR interval is always the same. Mobitz type II block has more serious implications because if there is a failure of AV conduction (*ie,* complete heart block), the escape rhythm will be ventricular. Ventricular escape rhythms are unreliable, unpredictable, and unstable with regard to rate. A temporary pacemaker should be inserted, even if there are no symptoms.

2:1 Atrioventricular Block

In 2:1 AV block, which is also a type of second-degree AV block, every other P wave is nonconducted. When the P wave is conducted, the PR interval is constant. 2:1 AV block may be Mobitz type I or II. The etiology can only be established if another pattern of AV conduction

is seen as a result of several sequentially conducted P waves. If there is progressive lengthening of the PR interval, then the 2:1 AV block is Mobitz type I. In contrast, if all the PR intervals are the same, then the 2:1 AV block is Mobitz type II. Alternatively, if complete heart block develops, the presence of an escape junctional rhythm indicates that the problem is within the AV node and hence the 2:1 AV block is Wenckebach. If there is an escape ventricular rhythm, the 2:1 AV block is within the His-Purkinje system and hence is Mobitz type II.

Third-degree Atrioventricular Block

Third-degree AV block (complete heart block) is manifest by the presence of AV dissociation; that is, there is no association between P waves and QRS complexes. Hence the PR intervals are variable and the variability has no pattern (unlike Mobitz type I, in which there is a pattern to the variability of the PR intervals, *ie,* progressive lengthening). In addition, the atrial rate is faster than the rate of the QRS complexes as the QRS complexes are the result of an escape rhythm. Complete heart block may be due to disease of the AV node or the His-Purkinje system (*ie,* infranodal); therefore, the escape rhythm may be junctional or ventricular. The origin of the escape rhythm is based on QRS morphology and not the rate of the escape rhythm.

Atrioventricular Dissociation

AV dissociation is identified by the absence of a relationship between the P wave and the QRS complex. Hence there are variable PR intervals that are random without any pattern to the variability. In contrast, there is variability of the PR intervals with Wenckebach, but there is a pattern with progressive PR interval lengthening. There are two causes for AV dissociation:

- Third-degree AV block, or complete heart block, in which there is no impulse conduction between the atria and ventricles. In this situation, the atrial rate is faster than the rate of the QRS complexes, which are the result of an escape rhythm. The location of the escape rhythm may be the junction (junctional escape) or the ventricle (ventricular escape). The location of the escape rhythm is not based on the rate of the escape rhythm but on the morphology of the QRS complexes. Although the teaching is that junctional escape rhythms have a rate of 50 to 60 bpm and ventricular escape rhythms have a rate of 20 to 30 bpm, the rate is influenced by autonomic tone and circulating catecholamines. Hence there may be an escape junctional rhythm at a rate of 30 bpm and an escape ventricular rhythm at a rate of 70 bpm.

- An accelerated junctional or ventricular rhythm may also present with AV dissociation. In this situation, the atrial rate is slower than the rate of the QRS complexes. The focus responsible for the accelerated rhythm (junction or ventricle) is based on the QRS complex morphology and not on the rate.

Isorhythmic Dissociation

Isorhythmic dissociation is a variation of AV dissociation. As noted, with complete heart block the atrial rate is faster than the rate of the QRS complexes, while with an accelerated rhythm the atrial rate is slower than the rate of the QRS complexes. However, if AV dissociation is present (*ie*, variable PR intervals), but the rate of the P waves and

QRS complexes is the same, the etiology for AV dissociation (*ie*, complete AV block or an accelerated lower focus) cannot be established. This is termed isorhythmic dissociation.

Ventriculophasic Arrhythmia

Ventriculophasic arrhythmia (*ie*, phasic changes in the sinus rate related to ventricular contraction) may be seen with 2:1 AV block or AV dissociation, particularly when there is complete heart block. Ventriculophasic arrhythmia is diagnosed when the sinus PP intervals are irregular with a repeating pattern (*ie*, the PP interval surrounding a QRS complex is slightly shorter than the PP interval without a QRS complex). This is termed ventriculophasic arrhythmia and is due to one of several causes:

- With ventricular contraction there is an increase in pulsatile sinus nodal artery blood flow that results in an increase in sinus node automaticity and hence the shorter PP interval.

- With ventricular contraction the stretch on the right atrium enhances sinus node automaticity.

- With ventricular contraction (and hence stroke volume) there are effects on the baroreceptors and, as a result, there are changes in vagal outputs that alter the sinus rate.

Intraventricular Conduction Abnormalities

Intraventricular conduction abnormalities may be due to one of three causes:

- Diffuse slowing of impulse conduction through the normal His-Purkinje system that innervates the ventricles (known as intraventricular conduction delay [IVCD])

- Block of conduction through either fascicle of the left bundle (left anterior or left posterior fascicle)
- Block of conduction within one of the bundle branches (right or left)

Impulse conduction of the ventricles for their activation or depolarization is via the His-Purkinje system, which originates at the distal portion of the AV node as a cylindric structure that contains many tracts; this is the bundle of His. This structure divides into two major bundles: a right bundle that innervates the right ventricle and a left bundle that innervates the left ventricle. As left ventricular muscle mass is far greater than right ventricular muscle mass, the left bundle divides into two major and one minor fascicles. The minor fascicle is the septal (intermediate or median) branch, which innervates the interventricular septum (the first part of the ventricle to depolarize in a left-to-right direction). Hence leads that are located laterally or in a right-to-left direction (ie, leads I, aVL, and V4-V6) often show a small septal Q wave (septal depolarization goes away from these leads), while lead V1, which is on the right side of the sternum, has a small septal R wave as the septal impulse goes toward this lead. The two major fascicles are the left anterior fascicle and the left posterior fascicle:

- The left anterior fascicle crosses the left ventricular outflow tract and terminates in the Purkinje system of the anterolateral wall of the left ventricle.
- The left posterior fascicle appears as an extension of the main bundle and fans out extensively posteriorly toward the papillary muscle and inferoposteriorly toward the free wall of the left ventricle.

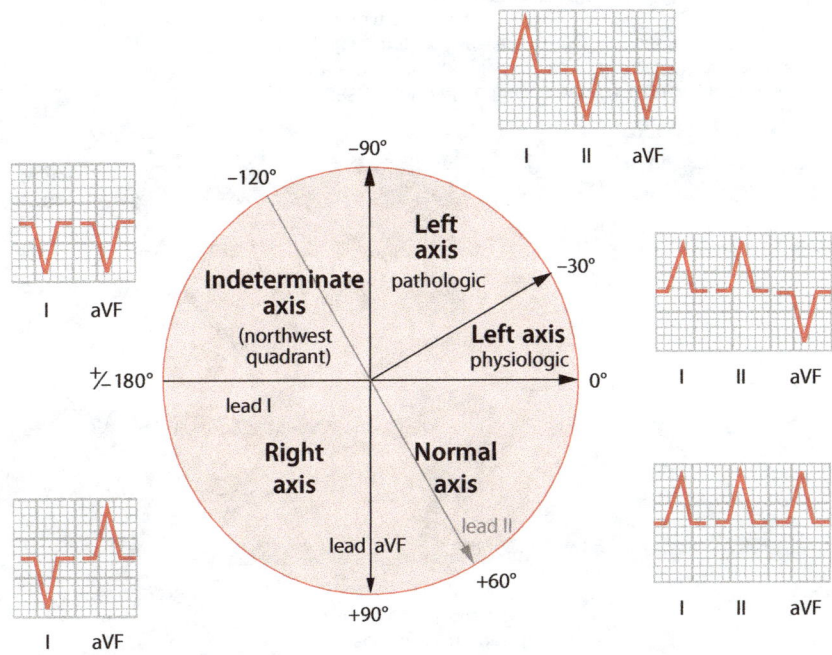

Figure 1. **The QRS axis in the frontal plane is determined by analyzing the direction of the QRS complex in the limb leads.** The heart is divided into four equal quadrants of 90° each (0° to +90°, +90° to +/-180°, 0° to −90° and −90° to +/-180°). The two leads that are perpendicular to each other and divide the heart in this fashion are leads I and aVF. Hence these two leads are looked at first. A normal axis is between 0° and +90° (positive QRS complex in leads I and aVF). A right axis, which is never normal, is between +90° and +180° (negative QRS complex in lead I and positive QRS complex in lead aVF). A left axis (ie, between 0° and −90° with a positive QRS complex in lead I and a negative QRS complex in lead aVF) may be physiologic (and hence normal) if it is between 0° and −30° or pathologic (and hence abnormal) if it is between −30° and −90°. This is established by looking at lead II, which is perpendicular to −30°. If the QRS complex is positive in lead II, the axis is physiologically leftward; if the QRS complex is negative in lead II, the axis is pathologically leftward.

Since the QRS complex is generated by the activation of the ventricular myocardium, abnormalities of intraventricular conduction affect the QRS complex (either axis or width). There are several types of intraventricular conduction abnormalities.

Fascicular Block

Fascicular block, which is due to impulse conduction block through one of the major fascicles of the left bundle (*ie,* left anterior or left posterior fascicle), causes an axis shift in the frontal plane (from normal to either the extreme left or right) (**FIGURE 1,** previous page). The QRS complex duration remains normal as intraventricular conduction is still via the His-Purkinje system. The normal activation sequence through the left ventricle without a fascicular block is associated with a normal axis, between 0° and +90° (positive QRS complex in leads I and aVF). An axis between 0° and −30° (positive QRS complex in leads I and II and negative QRS complex in lead aVF) is a physiologic left axis and is not a conduction abnormality; that is, it is not a left anterior fascicular block. A physiologic left axis may be seen with left ventricular hypertrophy or in normals.

Left Anterior Fascicular Block

With left anterior fascicular block, left ventricular activation is via the left posterior fascicle (**FIGURE 2**). Ventricular innervation originating from this fascicle results in an impulse that is directed superiorly and to the left. Hence a left anterior fascicular block is associated with an extreme or pathologic left axis that is between −30° and −90°. This produces a positive QRS complex in lead I and

a negative QRS complex in leads II and aVF. The QRS complexes in leads II and aVF have an rS morphology as ventricular activation remains normal. In contrast, an inferior wall myocardial infarction (MI), which may also result in a negative QRS complex in leads II and aVF, has a Qr morphology (**FIGURE 3**). The Q wave indicates that the initial electrical forces are directed away from the lead that is over this part of the myocardium, meaning that the tissue under the lead is infarcted. Hence it is important to distinguish between a left anterior fascicular block, which represents a conduction abnormality, and an

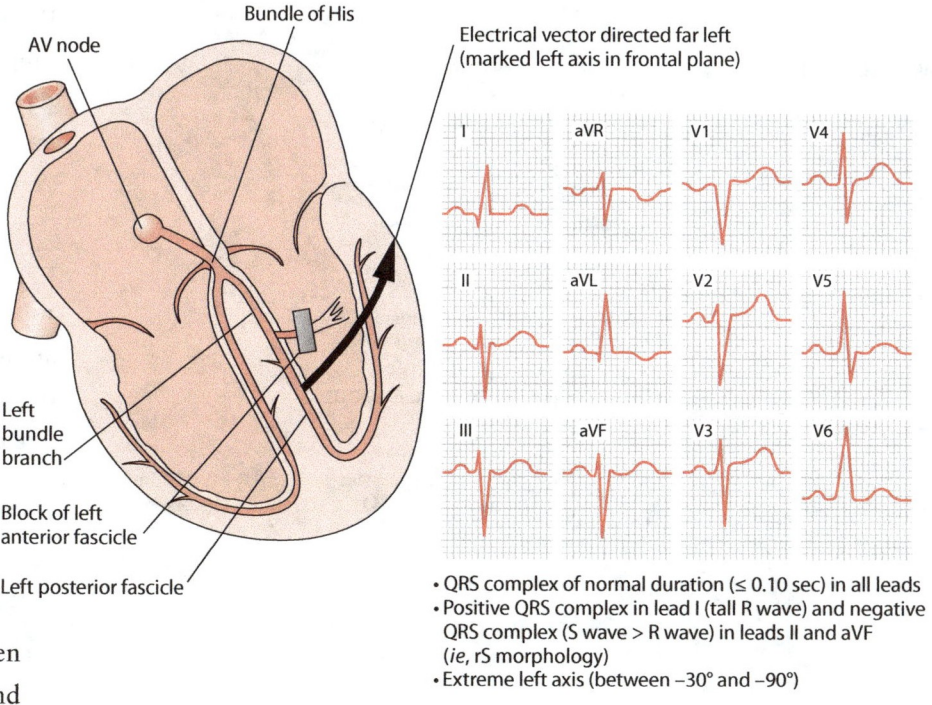

- QRS complex of normal duration (≤ 0.10 sec) in all leads
- Positive QRS complex in lead I (tall R wave) and negative QRS complex (S wave > R wave) in leads II and aVF (*ie,* rS morphology)
- Extreme left axis (between −30° and −90°)

Figure 2. Left anterior fascicular block.

Infarction	Conduction Abnormality
Qr morphology indicates an infarction pattern —When present in leads II, III, and aVF, represents inferior wall myocardial infarction —When present in leads I and aVL, represents lateral wall myocardial infarction	**rS morphology indicates a conduction abnormality** —When present in leads II, III, and aVF, represents left anterior fascicular block —When present in lead I (and aVL), represents left posterior fascicular block

Figure 3. Infarction versus conduction abnormality.

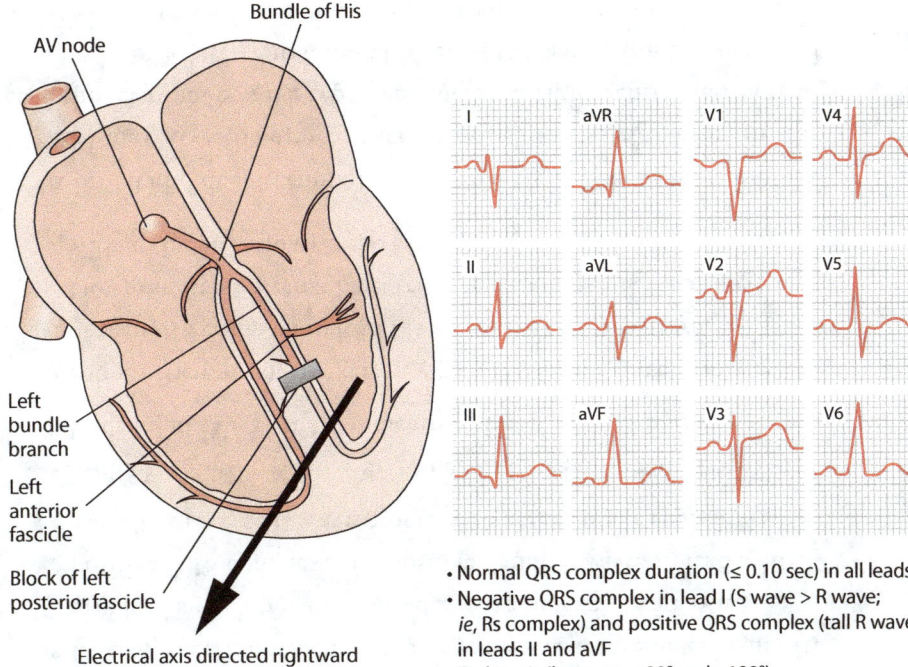

- Normal QRS complex duration (≤ 0.10 sec) in all leads
- Negative QRS complex in lead I (S wave > R wave; *ie*, Rs complex) and positive QRS complex (tall R wave) in leads II and aVF
- Right axis (between +90° and +180°)

Figure 4. Left posterior fascicular block.

inferior wall MI, which is not a conduction problem. Indeed, a left anterior fascicular block cannot be diagnosed in the presence of an inferior wall infarction pattern.

Left Posterior Fascicular Block

With a left posterior fascicular block, left ventricular activation is via the left anterior fascicle and the direction of impulse transmission is inferiorly and to the right (**FIGURE 4**). Hence a left posterior fascicular block results in a right axis (between +90° and +180°). There is a negative QRS complex in lead I and a positive QRS complex in leads II and aVF. The QRS complex has an rS morphology in lead I. In contrast, a lateral wall MI, which is not a conduction abnormality, will also be associated with a right axis (**FIGURE 3**). However, in this situation the QRS complex has a Qr morphology as the infarction results in the initial activation going away from the lateral wall and hence from left to right. There are several other causes for a right axis in addition to a lateral wall MI, and these must be considered before establishing the right axis as a left posterior fascicular block, which is a diagnosis of exclusion. Other causes for a right axis include:

- Right ventricular hypertrophy, which is diagnosed by the presence of a tall R wave in lead V1 and P pulmonale (right atrial hypertrophy or abnormality)

- Right–left arm lead switch, which is associated with negative P and T waves in leads I and aVL and positive P and T waves and a positive QRS complex in lead aVR

- Dextrocardia, in which there is a pattern that resembles right–left arm lead switch (*ie*, an inverted P wave in leads I and aVL, a positive QRS complex, and positive P and T waves in lead aVR), as well as reverse R-wave progression across the precordium

- Wolff-Parkinson-White syndrome, with negative delta waves in leads I and aVL that are indicative of a left lateral pathway

- A biventricular pacemaker, in which the initial waveform of the QRS complex in lead I is a Q wave or QS pattern. However, most often a biventricular pacemaker is associated with an indeterminate axis.

A broad and deep terminal S wave in a right bundle branch block (RBBB) may give the appearance of a right axis. However, in this case the terminal S wave represents delayed right ventricular activation and not a left ventricular force. In this situation the terminal S wave should be ignored and is not considered for axis determination.

Indeterminate Axis

An indeterminate axis with a supraventricular complex is defined as an axis that is between –90° and +/-180°. The QRS complex is negative in leads I and aVF. This may represent either a very extreme left axis or a very extreme right axis. In a human adult heart, it is unusual to see an indeterminate axis with a supraventricular QRS complex. There is no type of conduction pattern through the normal His-Purkinje system that will result in an indeterminate axis. Thus an indeterminate axis is the result of the simultaneous presence of two different abnormalities. For example, an indeterminate axis may be seen when there is right ventricular hypertrophy (which shifts the axis rightward) associated

with a left anterior fascicular block or an inferior wall MI (which shifts the axis leftward). An indeterminate axis may appear to be present if an old lateral and inferior wall MI is evident. However, in this case there are Q waves in leads I, II, III, and aVF and hence the axis shift is the result of an infarction. The presence of a lateral wall MI (which has a right axis) with a left anterior fascicular block (which has a left axis) or an inferior wall MI (which has a left axis) with a left posterior fascicular block (which has a right axis) will also have an indeterminate axis. However, in this case the negative QRS complex in either lead I (with a lateral wall MI) or lead aVF (inferior wall MI) is due to an infarction and not an axis shift. A right–left arm lead switch (which has a right axis) associated with either an inferior wall MI or a left anterior fascicular block (which has a left axis) will have an indeterminate axis. Lastly, the presence of a deep S wave due to an RBBB may give the appearance of a negative QRS complex in lead I, and the presence of a left anterior fascicular block will give the appearance of an indeterminate axis. In the presence of an RBBB the deep S wave in lead I is the result of terminal delay in right ventricular activation and is not considered as part of axis determination (which is the direction of impulse conduction within the left ventricle).

An indeterminate axis associated with a wide QRS complex may be seen with any situation in which there is direct ventricular myocardial activation, including a ventricular complex, a paced complex (especially biventricular pacing), or a preexcitation pattern, specifically Wolff-Parkinson-White.

Intraventricular Conduction Delay

An IVCD is a nonspecific QRS widening (QRS duration > 0.10 sec) without any specific bundle branch block pattern. Conduction is still via the entire His-Purkinje system, but it is slower than normal, accounting for the QRS widening. When the QRS complex is longer than 0.10 second but shorter than 0.12 second and has an RBBB pattern (*ie*, an RSR′ complex in lead V1), it is often called an incomplete RBBB. When the QRS complex is longer than 0.10 second but shorter than 0.12 second with a left bundle branch block (LBBB) pattern, it is often called in incomplete LBBB. However, the term incomplete bundle branch block is not accurate because conduction through the His-Purkinje system and bundle is all or none and will not be incomplete. Hence a more appropriate term is an IVCD to either the right

or left ventricle. As the activation of the ventricles is via the normal His-Purkinje system, abnormalities of the right or left ventricular myocardium can be diagnosed. This is in contrast to an LBBB or RBBB in which ventricular activation is not via the normal conduction system, but rather is via an abnormal pathway with direct myocardial activation. Hence abnormalities of the ventricular myocardium served by the particular bundle cannot be diagnosed.

A QRS complex duration exceeding 0.12 second is also termed an IVCD if there is no specific bundle branch block pattern present. IVCDs with QRS complexes that are very wide (> 0.18 sec) without a bundle branch block pattern may be seen with severe dilated cardiomyopathy or hyperkalemia. The only etiology for a QRS complex duration exceeding 0.24 second is hyperkalemia, which is a medical emergency that requires immediate therapy. In the absence of hyperkalemia, a bundle branch block, a ventricular complex, or a severe cardiomyopathy is not associated with a QRS complex that is this wide.

Bundle Branch Blocks

There may be failure of impulse conduction (complete block) through either the right or left bundle branch, resulting in delayed activation of the ventricular chamber served by that bundle.

Right Bundle Branch Block

An RBBB has the following characteristic morphology (**FIGURE 5**):

- The QRS complex duration is 0.12 second or longer due to delayed and slow activation of the right ventricle.

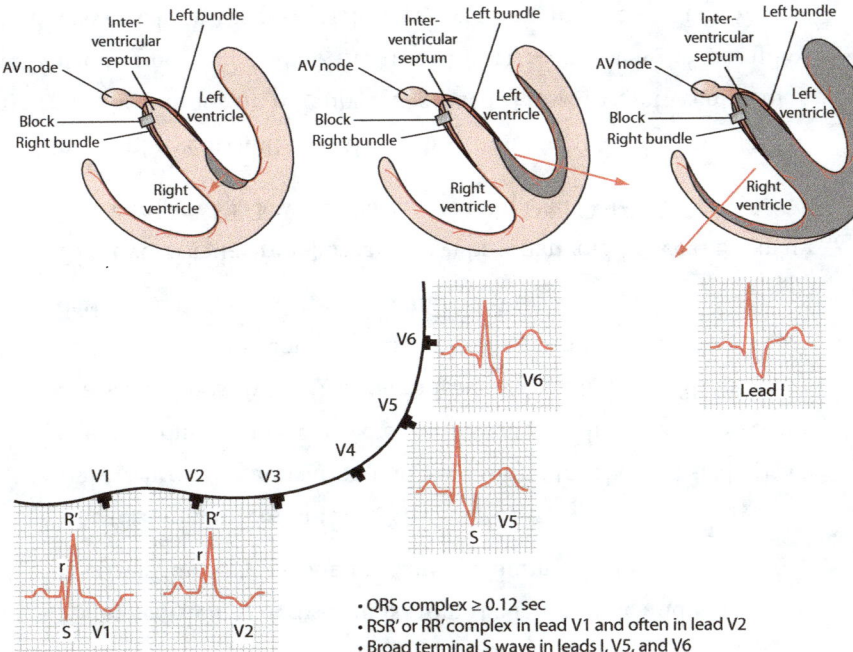

- QRS complex ≥ 0.12 sec
- RSR′ or RR′ complex in lead V1 and often in lead V2
- Broad terminal S wave in leads I, V5, and V6

Figure 5. **Complete right bundle branch block.**

- Right ventricular activation is from the left bundle and left ventricle, directly through the myocardium.

- The terminal forces of the QRS complex, representing delayed right ventricular activation and accounting for the widened QRS complex duration, are directed from left to right. Therefore, there is a second positive deflection in leads V1-V2 (*ie*, an RSR′, RR′, or only a broad R complex) and a broad terminal negative deflection or S wave in leads I and V5-V6.

- Right ventricular repolarization is abnormal and hence there may be secondary ST-T wave changes seen in leads V1-V3.

Since right ventricular activation is abnormal, right ventricular hypertrophy cannot be reliably recognized. However, left ventricular activation is normal and so the initial portion of the QRS complex or R wave, which represents left ventricular activation, is normal. Therefore, left ventricular abnormalities (*eg*, left ventricular hypertrophy, myocardial ischemia or infarction, pericarditis) can be recognized in the presence of an RBBB.

A left anterior fascicular block (extreme left axis) or left posterior fascicular block (right axis) may also be present. This is termed bifascicular block. However, it must be remembered that with an RBBB there is a broad terminal S wave in lead I that may give the appearance of a negative QRS complex in lead I and hence a right axis. The terminal S wave, which represents delayed right ventricular activation, should not be considered when determining the axis in the frontal plane as this is based on left ventricular activation.

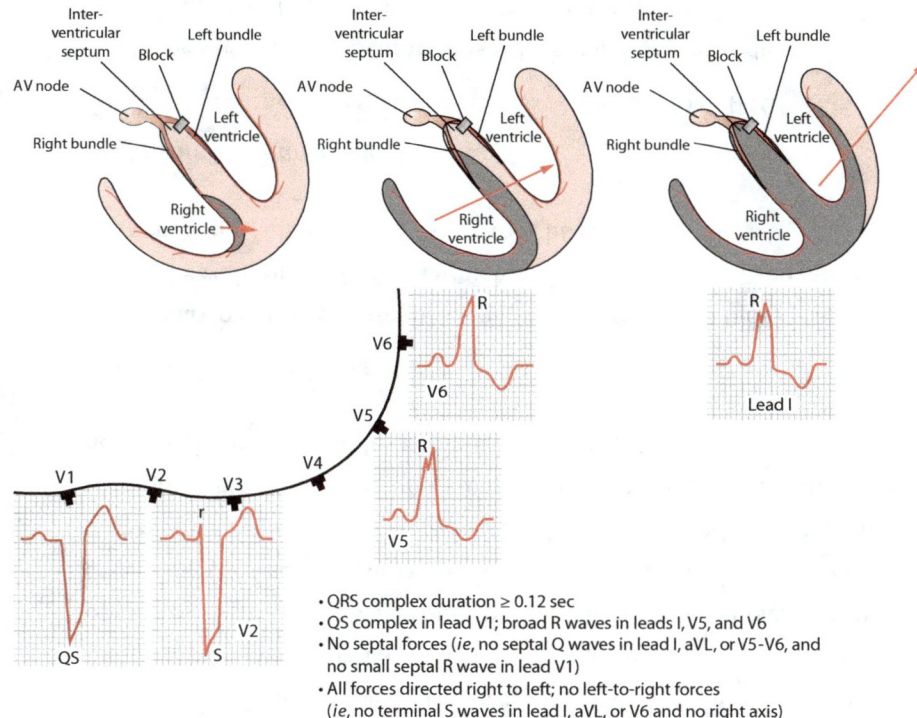

- QRS complex duration ≥ 0.12 sec
- QS complex in lead V1; broad R waves in leads I, V5, and V6
- No septal forces (*ie*, no septal Q waves in lead I, aVL, or V5-V6, and no small septal R wave in lead V1)
- All forces directed right to left; no left-to-right forces (*ie*, no terminal S waves in lead I, aVL, or V6 and no right axis)

Figure 6. Complete left bundle branch block.

An RBBB may be intermittent or rate-related, termed a functional bundle branch block. A rate-related RBBB may occur at any heart rate. Not uncommonly it resolves at a heart rate that is slower than the rate at which it develops. With a rate-related RBBB, the widening of the QRS complex occurs abruptly and resolves abruptly; it is not gradual. A QRS complex that has an RBBB morphology but a duration that is between 0.10 and 0.12 second has been called an incomplete RBBB but is actually an IVCD with conduction delay to the right ventricle.

Left Bundle Branch Block

An LBBB has the following characteristic morphology (FIGURE 6):

- The QRS complex duration is 0.12 second or longer due to delayed and slow activation of the left ventricle.

- Left ventricular activation is entirely from the right bundle and right ventricle and travels directly through the myocardium (hence prolonging the QRS complex duration).

- All ventricular forces are directed from right to left. Hence there is a broad, tall R wave in leads I, aVL, and V5-V6 (although a deep QS complex may be seen in leads V5-V6) and deep QS complexes in lead V1 and occasionally in lead V2. There should not be any ventricular forces directed from left to right. If there is an LBBB pattern present, but there are terminal S waves in leads I and V6, the etiology for the widened QRS complex is an IVCD.

- As an LBBB also involves the septal branch of the left bundle, there are no septal forces present; that is, small septal Q waves in leads I, aVL, and V5-V6 are not seen and there is no septal R wave in lead V1. If there is an LBBB pattern present in addition to septal forces, the etiology is an IVCD.

- Abnormal ventricular repolarization is associated with an LBBB, and hence there are typically diffuse secondary ST-T wave abnormalities.

- The QRS axis in the frontal plane may be normal or leftward. A left axis may represent abnormalities in the direction of impulse conduction through the left ventricular myocardium

(*eg,* due to the presence of fibrosis) and is not a left anterior fascicular block as both fascicles are blocked. A right axis should not be seen with an LBBB as all forces are directed from right to left.

Since left ventricular activation is abnormal (*ie,* bypassing the normal His-Purkinje system), abnormalities affecting the left ventricular myocardium (*eg,* left ventricular hypertrophy, myocardial ischemia and chronic infarction, pericarditis) cannot be recognized. However, an acute MI can be established with an LBBB (or any other situation in which there is direct myocardial activation, such as ventricular pacing, a ventricular complex, and likely a preexcited complex in Wolff-Parkinson-White pattern) using the Sgarbossa criteria:

- ST-segment elevation of 1 or 2 mm or more that is in the same direction (concordant) as the QRS complex in any lead

- ST-segment depression of 1 mm or more in any lead from V1 to V3

- ST-segment elevation of 5 mm or more that is discordant with the QRS complex (*ie,* associated with a QS or rS complex)

An LBBB may be intermittent or rate-related (functional bundle branch block). As with an intermittent RBBB, a rate-related LBBB may occur at any heart rate. Not uncommonly, it resolves at a heart rate that is slower than the rate at which it develops. With a rate-related LBBB, the widening of the QRS complex occurs abruptly and resolves abruptly; the widening is not gradual. When the QRS complex has an LBBB morphology but a duration of 0.10 to 0.12 second, it is often referred to as an incomplete LBBB. However, it is actually an IVCD. In this situation, left ventricular abnormalities and a left axis (left anterior fascicular block) or right axis (left posterior fascicular block) can be diagnosed because conduction is still via the normal His-Purkinje system, albeit slowed. As indicated, with an LBBB the normal His-Purkinje system is circumvented as left ventricular activation occurs via direct myocardial activation.

Trifascicular Block

Trifascicular block, or trifascicular disease, indicates conduction disease affecting both the right and left bundles. Because all three fascicles are affected, diagnosis of trifascicular disease requires evidence of conduction abnormalities in the right bundle, left anterior fascicle, and left posterior fascicle. This includes the following scenarios:

- Alternating RBBB and LBBB, which is also termed bi-bundle branch block

- RBBB with alternating left anterior and left posterior fascicular block

- Bifascicular disease (LBBB or RBBB with either a left anterior or left posterior fascicular block) with Mobitz type II second-degree AV block (with or without an associated first-degree AV block or prolonged AV conduction), which indicates disease of the His-Purkinje system

- Bifascicular disease with the development of complete heart block with an escape ventricular rhythm, which indicates disease of the His-Purkinje system

Trifascicular disease is not established by the finding of bifascicular disease (LBBB or RBBB with either a left anterior or left posterior fascicular block) and first-degree AV block (prolonged AV conduction) or the presence of second-degree AV block with 2:1 AV conduction. In

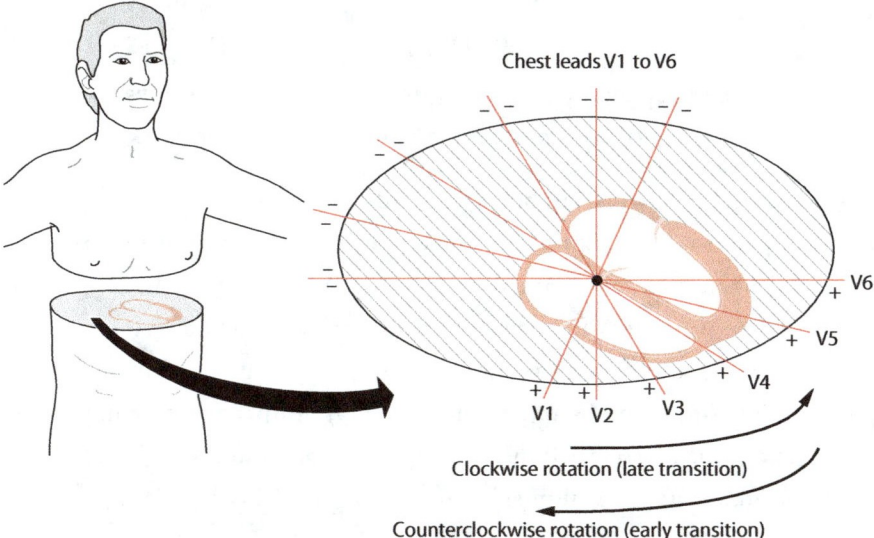

Chest leads V1 to V6

Clockwise rotation (late transition)

Counterclockwise rotation (early transition)

Figure 7. The QRS axis in the horizontal plane is determined by analyzing the direction of the QRS complex in the precordial leads. This is established by imagining the heart as viewed from under the diaphragm. With clockwise rotation, the left ventricular forces are seen later in the precordial leads. This presents with poor R-wave progression and late transition. With counterclockwise rotation, left ventricular forces develop earlier in the precordial leads. This presents with a tall R wave in lead V2, which is termed early transition.

these situations the AV conduction abnormality may be within either the AV node or the His-Purkinje system (in which case trifascicular disease cannot be definitively diagnosed). Trifascicular disease can only be established if there is evidence of a conduction abnormality within the remaining fascicle.

Axis in the Horizontal Plane

In addition to the axis in the frontal plane (*ie,* normal, right, left, indeterminate), there is also an axis in the horizontal plane of the heart. However, abnormalities in the axis of the horizontal plane are not the result of a conduction abnormality. The axis in the horizontal plane is established by imagining the heart as viewed from under the diaphragm (FIGURE 7). In this situation, the right ventricle is in front and the left ventricle is to the left. When there is an electrical rotation in a clockwise direction, right ventricular forces are still present in the lateral precordial leads, while the development of left ventricular forces is delayed. In this situation there is poor R-wave progression from leads V1-V3 or V4 and late transition (*ie,* the R wave does not develop an amplitude greater than the S wave until lead V5-V6) compared with the normal transition between leads V3-V4. The poor R-wave progression should not be confused with an anterior wall MI. When there is counterclockwise rotation, the left ventricular forces develop earlier and there is a tall R wave in lead V2 (*ie,* early transition). The tall R wave in lead V2 should not be confused with a posterior wall MI or right ventricular hypertrophy, in which there is a tall R wave in lead V1.

Enhanced Atrioventricular Conduction

In addition to slowing or block of AV conduction, AV conduction may be fast, due either to enhanced (accelerated) conduction through the AV node or to an accessory pathway (bypass tract) that bypasses the AV node (which is the site of slowest impulse conduction in the heart), serving as a second pathway for AV conduction from the atria to the ventricles. With enhanced AV conduction, the ECG shows a short (0.14 sec) PR interval at a normal rate (*ie,* < 100 bpm). It should be remembered that a short PR interval may also be seen with sinus tachycardia due to enhanced conduction through the AV node resulting from sympathetic stimulation.

There are two patterns for enhanced AV conduction due to a bypass tract. These patterns are also called preexcitation.

Wolff-Parkinson-White Pattern

Wolff-Parkinson-White pattern is due to an AV nodal bypass tract called the bundle of Kent, which is a direct connection between the atrial and ventricular myocardium, resulting in early ventricular myocardial activation that precedes activation via the AV node (*ie,* preexcitation). The QRS complex is widened as a result of the early, direct, and slow myocardial activation via the accessory pathway, which bypasses the normal AV node–His-Purkinje system. Thereafter there is normal ventricular activation via the AV node–His-Purkinje system. The QRS complex is, therefore, a fusion beat representing early but slow ventricular activation initiated via the accessory pathway and normal ventricular activation via the AV node–His-Purkinje system. As a result, the initial upstroke of the QRS complex is slowed due to direct myocardial activation. This is termed a delta wave, which produces a widening of the initial portion of the QRS complex, while the remainder of the QRS complex, due to activation via the His-Purkinje system, is narrow. The degree of aberration (delta wave width) is related to the balance between conduction through the AV node and accessory pathway, which is determined by AV nodal conduction because conduction through the accessory pathway is fixed (*ie*, it is all or none as it is Purkinje-like tissue). Hence if AV nodal conduction is slow, more of the initiation of ventricular activation is via the accessory pathway, resulting in a shorter PR interval and wider delta wave. If AV nodal conduction is fast, then less ventricular myocardial activation is via the accessory pathway and the PR interval is longer and the delta wave narrower. As the QRS complex in Wolff-Parkinson-White pattern is

a fusion complex, the degree of fusion may vary from one period of time to another, as changes in AV nodal conduction may occur in a variable and unpredictable fashion, in part related to changes in autonomic inputs into the AV node. Hence there may be variability in the PR interval and width of the QRS complex (*ie*, prominence of the delta wave). This is termed the concertina effect.

Lown-Ganong-Levine Pattern

Lown-Ganong-Levine pattern results from conduction via a bypass tract known as the bundle of James, which is a connection between the atrium and the bundle of His. Since the AV node is bypassed, the PR interval is short. However, ventricular activation is via the normal His-Purkinje system and, therefore, the QRS complex (morphology and duration) is normal. ■

A 76-year-old man with a history of hypertension presents for routine evaluation. On review, he admits to fatigue and a mild reduction in exercise capacity over the past year, but he is not functionally limited. He denies other symptomatology. On exam, he has a bradycardic but regular radial pulse. His carotid pulses are brisk and he has a soft S1, but S2 is normal. There is no S3 or S4. A soft, nonradiating early systolic murmur is heard best at the right upper sternal border. An ECG is obtained.

What does the ECG show?

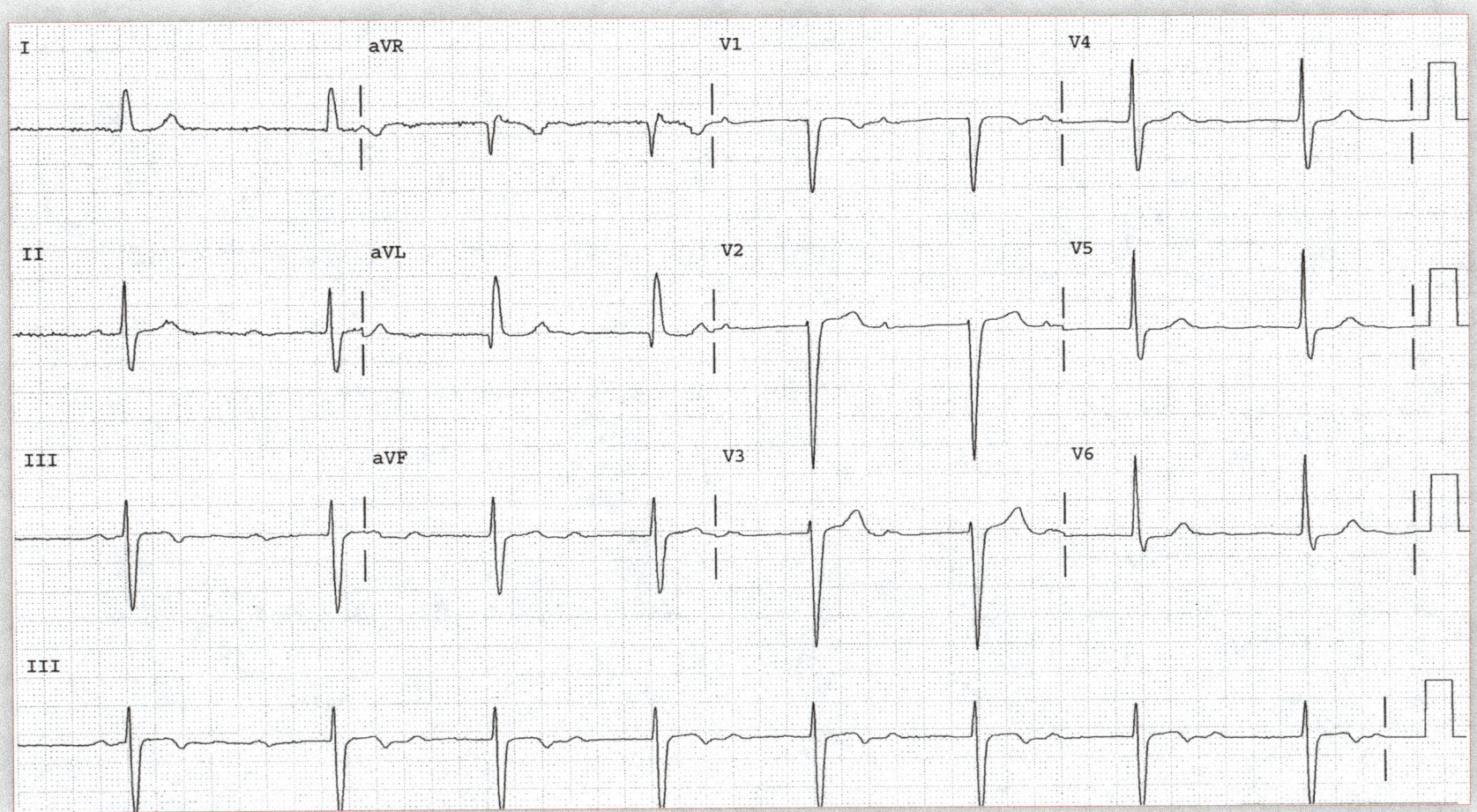

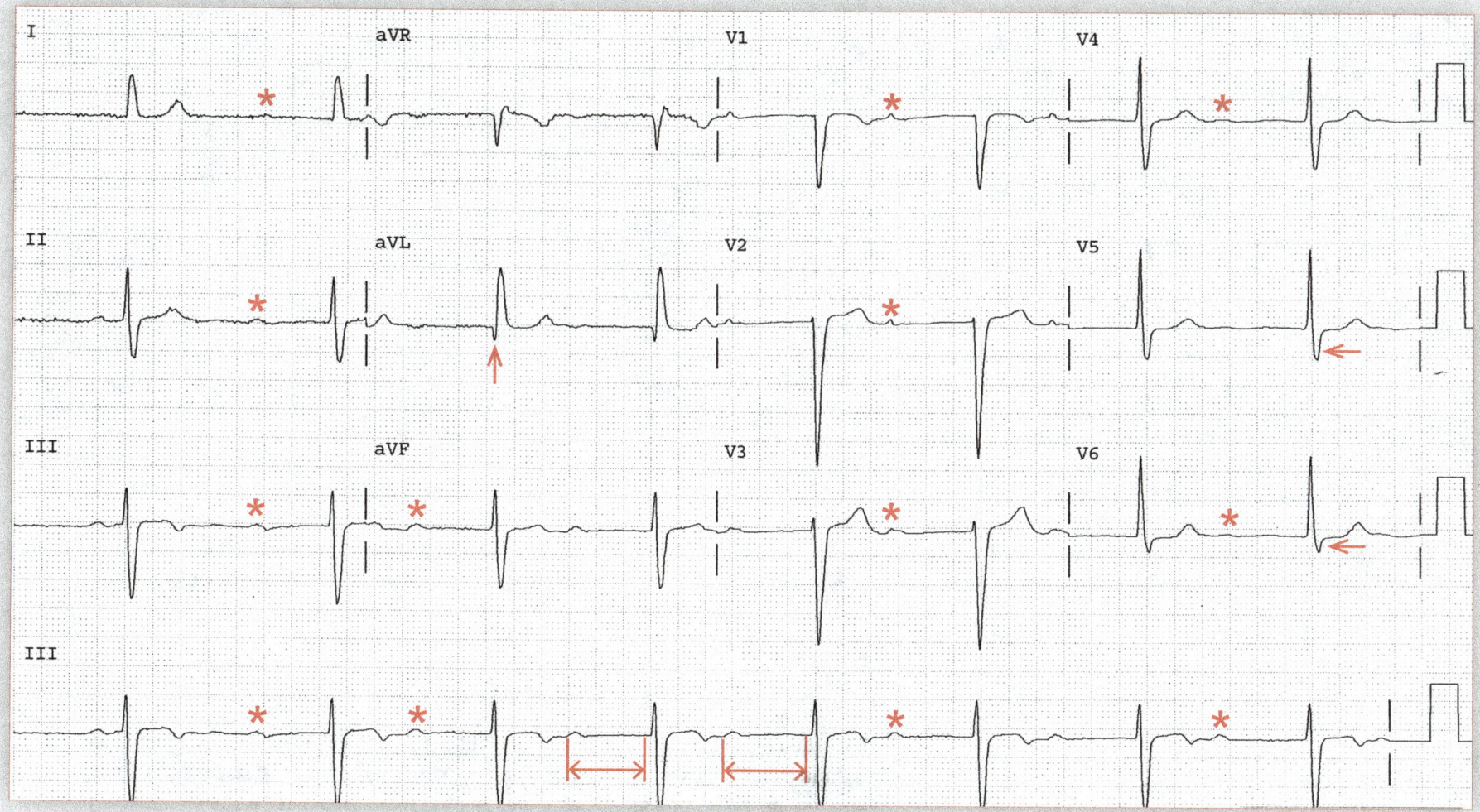

ECG 1 Analysis: Sinus bradycardia, first-degree AV block (prolonged AV conduction or AV conduction delay), intraventricular conduction delay

There is regular rhythm at a rate of 50 bpm. There is a P wave (*) before each QRS complex, with a stable but prolonged PR interval (0.60 sec) (↔). The P wave is positive in leads I, II, aVF, and V4-V6. Although the PR interval is long, it is constant and hence AV conduction is intact. Thus this is sinus bradycardia with first-degree AV block (or prolonged AV conduction).

The QRS complex duration is increased (0.12 sec). Although the morphology resembles that of a left bundle branch block (LBBB), there is a septal Q wave (↑) in lead aVL (due to left-to-right conduction across the septal myocardium) that cannot be present with an LBBB because the septal branch, which activates the septum, originates from the left bundle. In addition, there is a terminal S wave in leads V5-V6 (←), indicating left-to-right forces, which are also not seen with an LBBB (as all of the forces are directed right to left). Therefore, this is an intraventricular conduction delay (IVCD). Importantly, with an IVCD the impulse is conducted through the normal His-Purkinje system but conduction is slower than normal. Hence there is a normal activation

sequence of the left ventricular myocardium and abnormalities of the left ventricle can be diagnosed. With an LBBB there is no conduction through the left bundle and hence activation of the left ventricular myocardium bypasses the normal conduction system and is via an alternative pathway (*ie,* directly through the ventricular myocardium). Since the LV activation sequence is abnormal, abnormalities of the left ventricular myocardium cannot be reliably diagnosed. On this patient's ECG, the QRS axis is physiologically leftward, between 0° and −30° (positive QRS complex in leads I and II and negative QRS complex in lead aVF). The QT/QTc intervals are normal (480/440 msec and 440/400 msec when the prolonged QRS complex duration is considered).

The normal PR interval, measured from the onset of the P wave to the onset of QRS complex (either a Q wave or an R wave), ranges from 0.14 to 0.20 second and represents AV conduction (*ie,* the time for the impulse to be conducted from the atrium to the ventricle). The

continues

PR interval can be further divided into the P wave and the PR segment. The P wave includes conduction through the right and left atria. Conduction through these structures is via three separate bundles: Bachman's bundle courses along the posterosuperior aspect of the atria and conducts the impulse from the right to the left atrium, and two additional bundles (bundle of Thorel and bundle of Wenckebach) conduct the impulse from the sinus node to the AV node. The isoelectric PR segment represents conduction through the AV node and His-Purkinje system. As these are small structures, they do not generate enough electrical activity to be measured on the surface of the body; hence the PR segment is at baseline (*ie,* it is isoelectric).

A PR interval longer than 0.20 second defines first-degree AV block (or prolonged AV conduction), which may represent slowing of conduction anywhere along the conduction pathway from the AV node to the terminal portion of the Purkinje fibers. In the healthy heart, the most frequent site of conduction delay is the AV node, which is the part of the conduction system that manifests the slowest rate of conduction. As AV nodal conduction is affected by autonomic balance, the PR interval changes with heart rate. Sinus tachycardia, which is the result of enhanced sympathetic activity that increases AV nodal conduction velocity, is associated with a shortening of the PR interval while sinus bradycardia, which is the result of sympathetic withdrawal and an increase in vagal tone, is associated with a slowing of AV nodal conduction velocity and hence an increase in the PR interval.

This ECG, coupled with the description of a septuagenarian with physical exam findings consistent with aortic valve disease (sclerosis), may suggest Lev's disease (senile conduction system degeneration) as the etiology of a prolonged PR interval and IVCD. Idiopathic slowing of AV conduction in the elderly has been termed Lev's disease, attributed to the extension of mitral or aortic valve calcification into fibers of the conduction system. Idiopathic slowing of AV conduction in younger individuals has been termed Lenègre's disease, attributed to progressive sclerofibrotic degeneration of the conduction system that may be hereditary. Some cases that may be hereditary are autosomal dominant and associated with mutations in the cardiac sodium channel SCN5A. ◼

Core Case 2

A 58-year-old man is admitted to the hospital with an anterior wall myocardial infarction (MI), and an ECG is obtained (2A). He is treated

ECG 2A

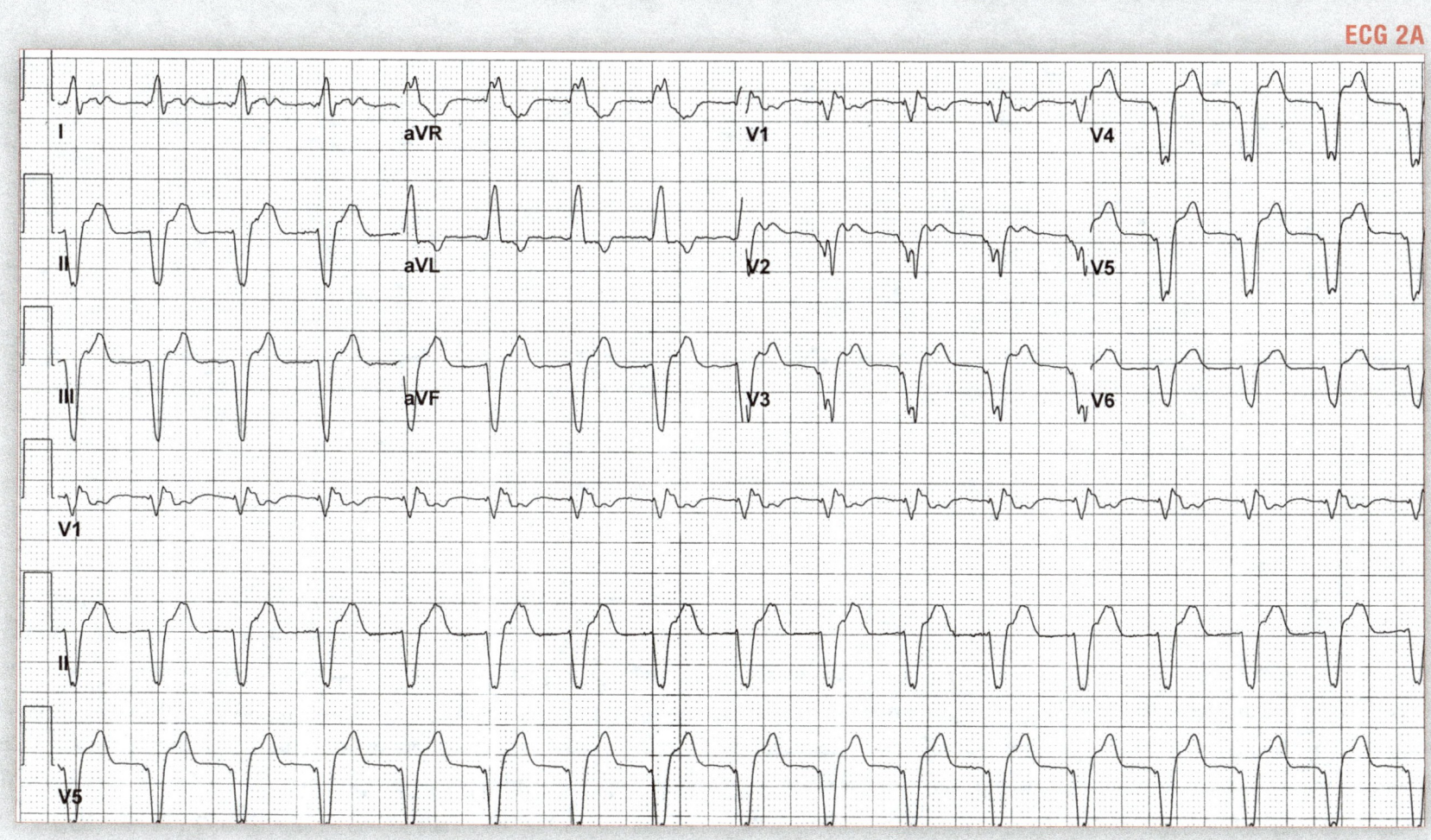

with thrombolysis without complication. Several
days later, he complains of palpitations and
feels diaphoretic. Another ECG (2B) is obtained.

What do the ECGs show?

ECG 2B

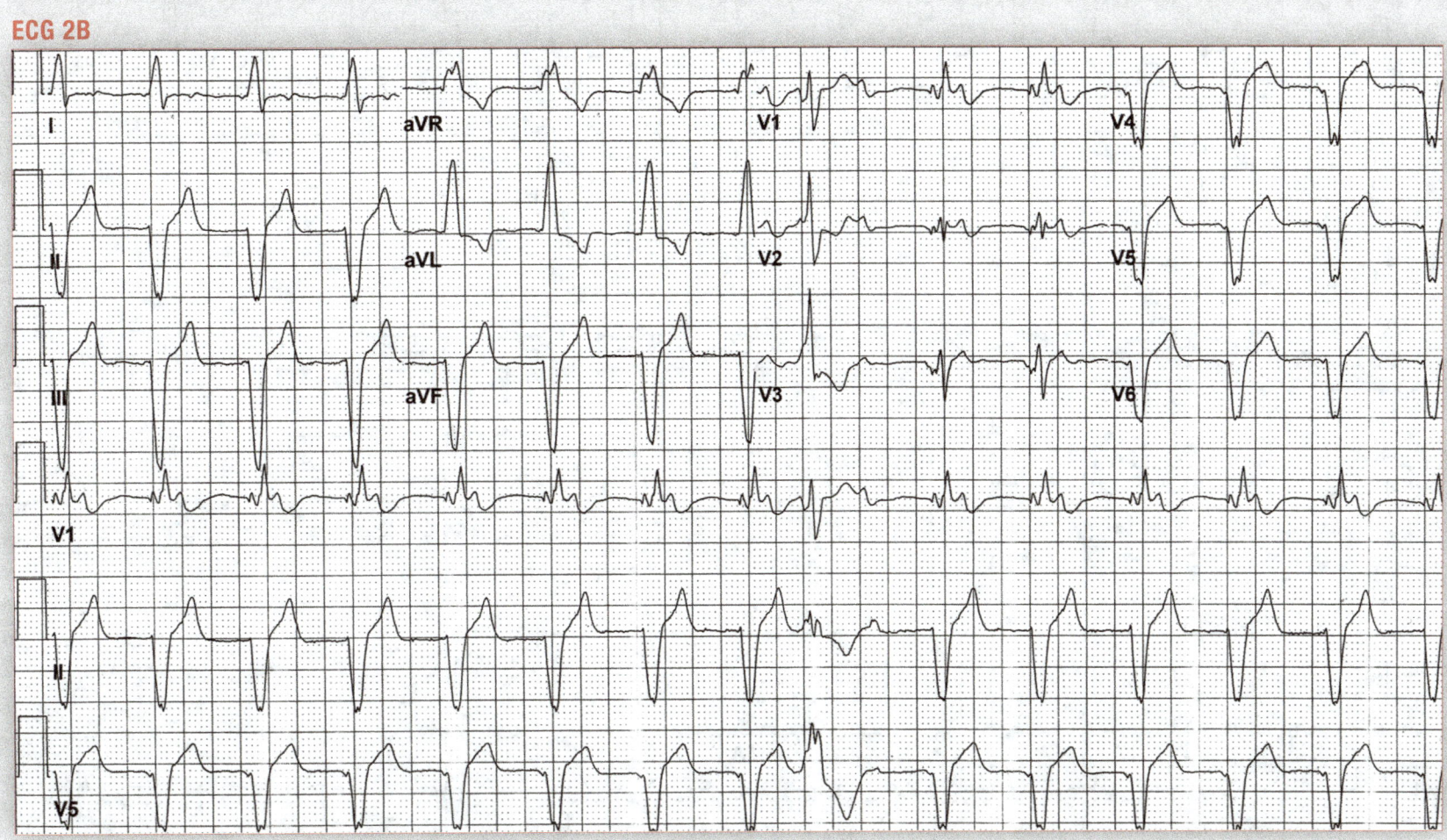

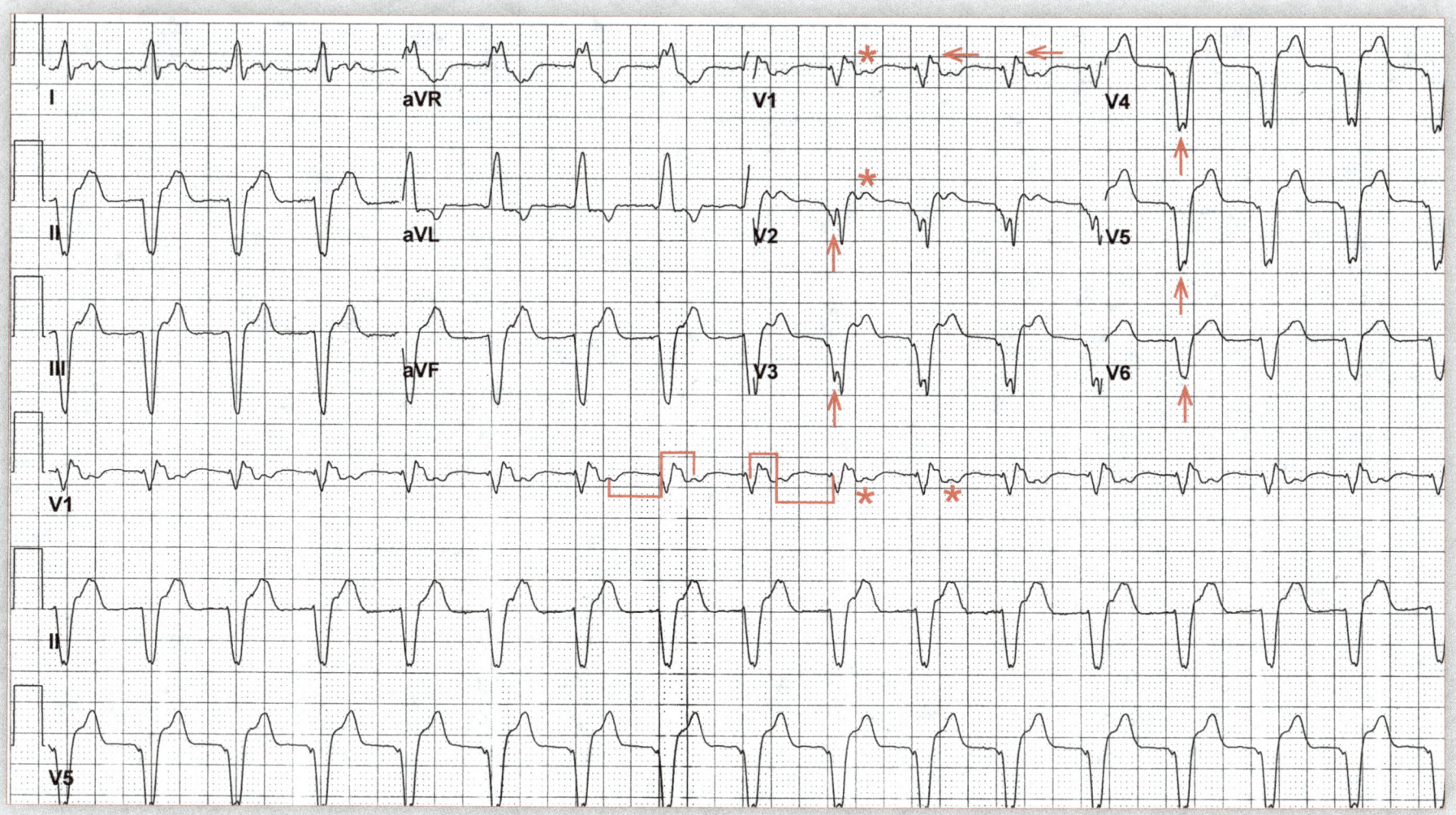

ECG 2A Analysis: Sinus tachycardia, first-degree AV block, intraventricular conduction delay (IVCD) to the right ventricle, left anterior fascicular block, anterior wall MI

In **ECG 2A** there is a regular rhythm at a rate of 100 bpm; hence this is tachycardia. The QRS interval is prolonged (0.16 sec). The morphology is not typical for either a left or a right bundle branch block. There is an RSR' morphology in lead V1 (←) but no broad terminal S wave in lead I. In addition, there is a QS morphology from leads V2 to V6, which suggests a left bundle branch block. Hence this is an intraventricular conduction delay (IVCD). The axis is extremely leftward, between −30° and −90° (positive QRS complex in lead I and negative QRS complex in leads II and aVF). An extreme left axis may be seen with an inferior wall myocardial infarction (MI) in which there are deep initial Q waves in leads II and aVF. In contrast, the QRS complexes in leads II and aVF have an rS morphology. This is characteristic of a left anterior fascicular block.

There are Q waves (↑) in leads V2-V6, diagnostic for an anterior wall MI. The QT/QTc intervals are prolonged (400/520 msec) but are normal when corrected for the prolonged QRS complex duration (320/410 msec). Although the P waves are not obvious, a suggestion of P waves can be seen after the QRS complexes, particularly in leads V1-V2 (*). The RP interval is short (0.20 sec, ⊓) and shorter than the PR interval (0.46 sec, ⊔). Therefore, this is termed short RP tachycardia. There are a number of etiologies for short RP tachycardia, including sinus tachycardia with first-degree AV block (prolonged AV conduction), atrial tachycardia, junctional tachycardia (with a retrograde P wave), atrial flutter with 2:1 AV block, AV reentrant tachycardia (associated with a preexcitation syndrome) or typical AV nodal reentrant tachycardia (AVNRT). Typical AVNRT does not usually manifest any P wave before or after the QRS complex. This is because the mechanism is a slow pathway to the ventricles and a fast pathway back to the atria, with simultaneous activation of the atria and ventricles. A variant of this is termed slow-slow (*ie*, the fast pathway conducting retrogradely back to the atria conducts relatively slowly).

continues

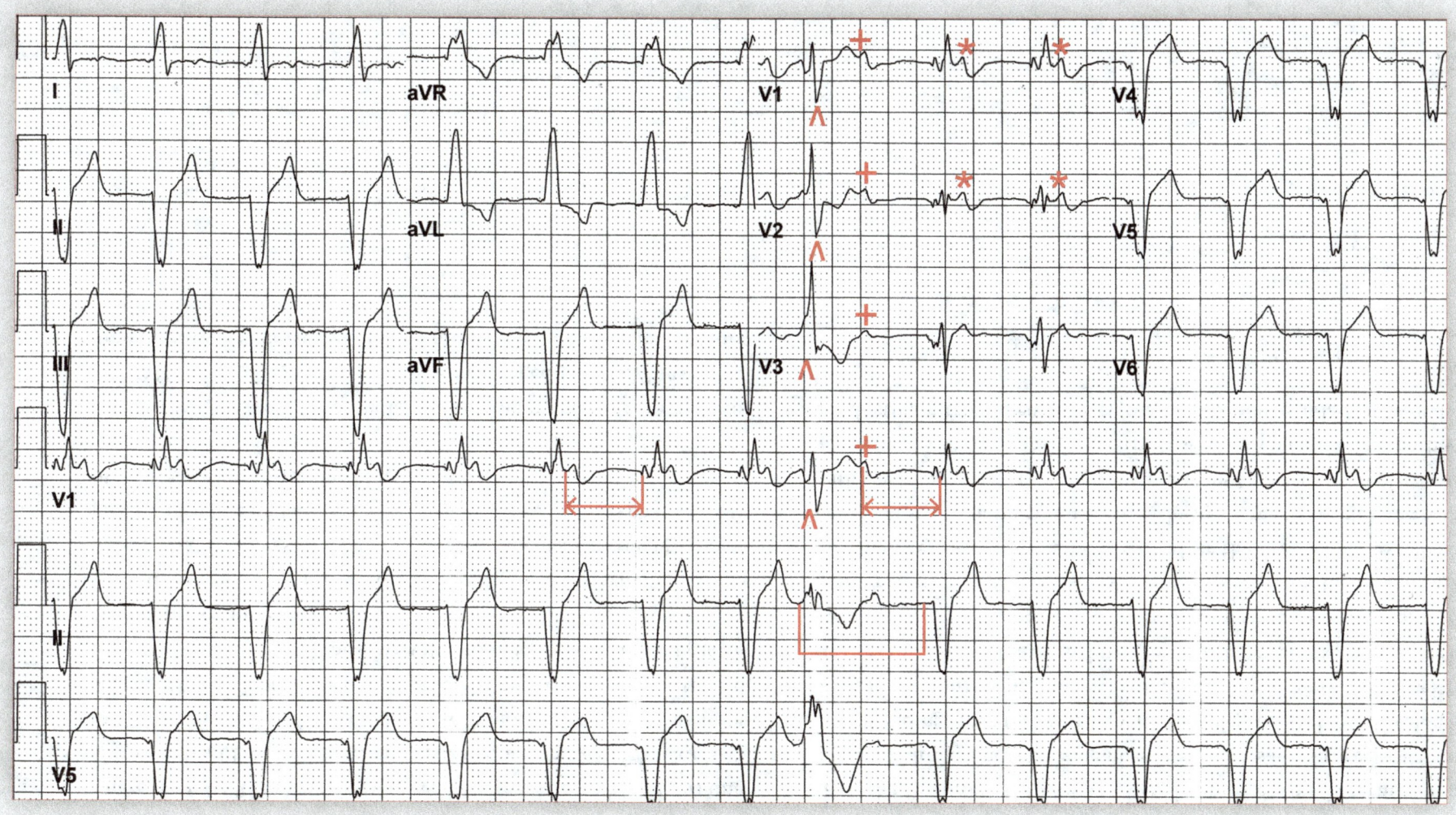

ECG 2B Analysis: Normal sinus rhythm, first-degree AV block, IVCD to the right ventricle, left anterior fascicular block, anterior wall MI, premature ventricular complex

In **ECG 2B**, the rhythm is regular at a rate of 86 bpm. The QRS complex morphology, duration, and axis are the same as those in **ECG 2A**. The QT/QTc intervals are also the same. Although the P waves are not obvious, there are waveforms (∗) seen at the end of the QRS complex (particularly in leads V1-V2), within the ST segment, that suggest a superimposed P wave. If these were superimposed P waves, the PR interval would be prolonged (0.54 sec) (↔). One premature complex can also be seen (^). It is wider than the other QRS complexes and has a different morphology. Hence it is a premature ventricular complex (PVC), and it aids in our assessment of the PR interval. After the PVC there is a pause (⊔). The P wave can be seen during the pause (+), and the measured PR interval is indeed 0.54 second (↔). Hence there is first-degree AV block (prolonged AV conduction). Using this PR interval, it can be seen that the ST-segment abnormality in both ECGs is in fact the P wave. In **ECG 2A**, the PR interval is slightly shorter (0.46 sec), perhaps due to the faster sinus rate. Thus the short RP tachycardia in **ECG 2A** is actually sinus tachycardia as the P waves are positive in leads I, II, aVF, and V4-V6.

The His bundle and the proximal bundle branches are generally resistant to ischemia given dual blood supply from both the AV nodal artery and the proximal septal perforator branches of the left anterior descending artery in most patients. However, in some patients, blood supply to the proximal bundle branches is not collateralized. In addition, infarction of the intraventricular septum can damage parts of the bundles, resulting in conduction abnormalities. In such cases, proximal left anterior descending artery occlusion results in ischemic injury and infarction of the septum and the conduction system, likely explaining the presence of a left anterior fascicular block associated with an anterior wall MI. The etiology of the prolonged PR interval is not clear; it may be due to slow conduction through the AV node or diffuse slowing of conduction through the His-Purkinje system, suggested by the presence of the IVCD as well as the anterior wall MI. ■

Core Case 3

A 24-year-old man presents to the emergency department with a complaint of palpitations that had occurred spontaneously while he was watching TV. The episode lasted for about 2 hours but terminated abruptly as he arrived at the hospital. He stated that he had

ECG 3A

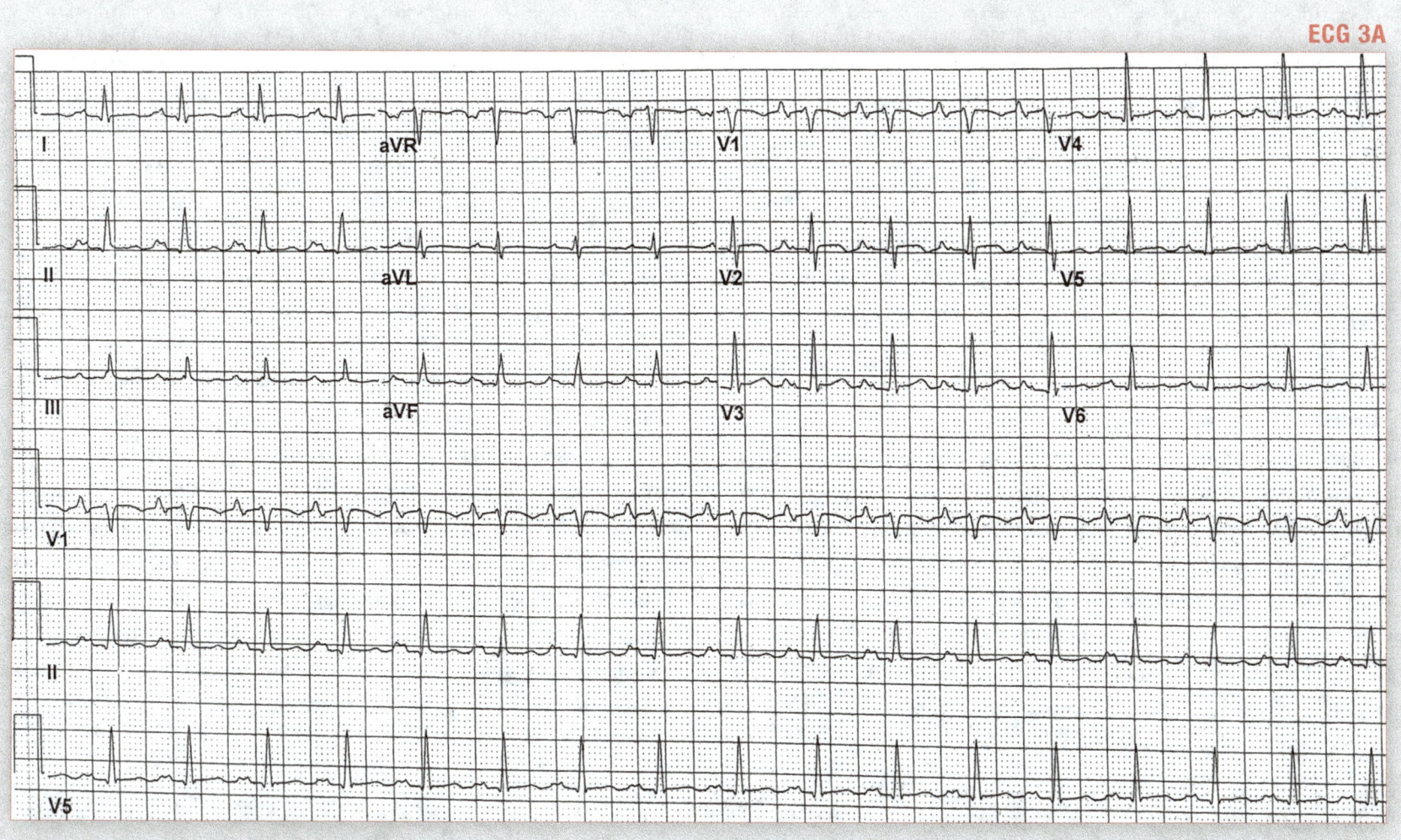

experienced occasional palpitations in the past, but they usually lasted less than 30 minutes and seemed to resolve with coughing. ECG 3A is the initial ECG. About 2 minutes, later, without any intervention, a second ECG (ECG 3B) is obtained.

What is the difference between the two ECGs?

What abnormality is suggested when both ECGs are considered?

What is the likely cause of the palpitations?

ECG 3B

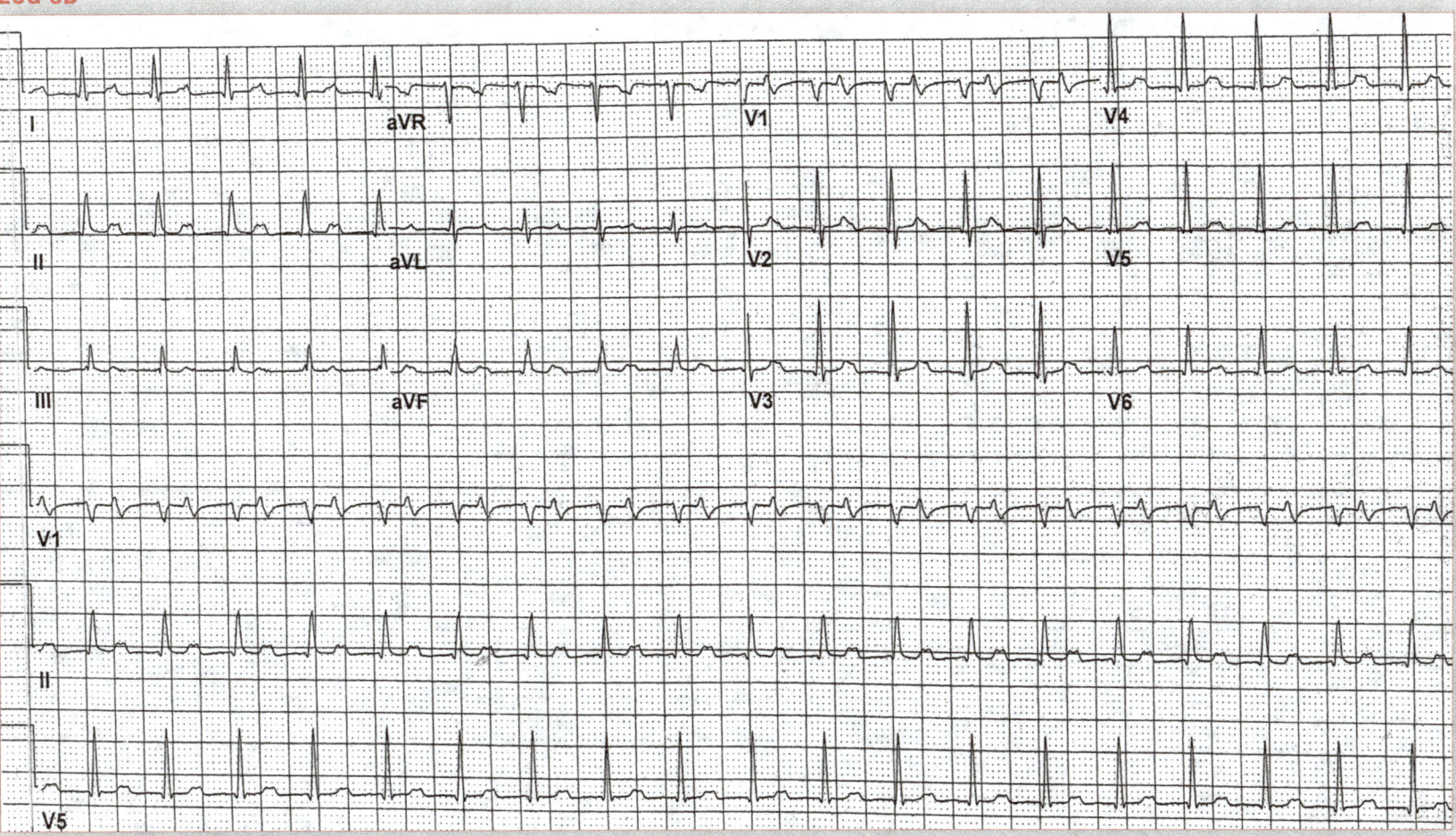

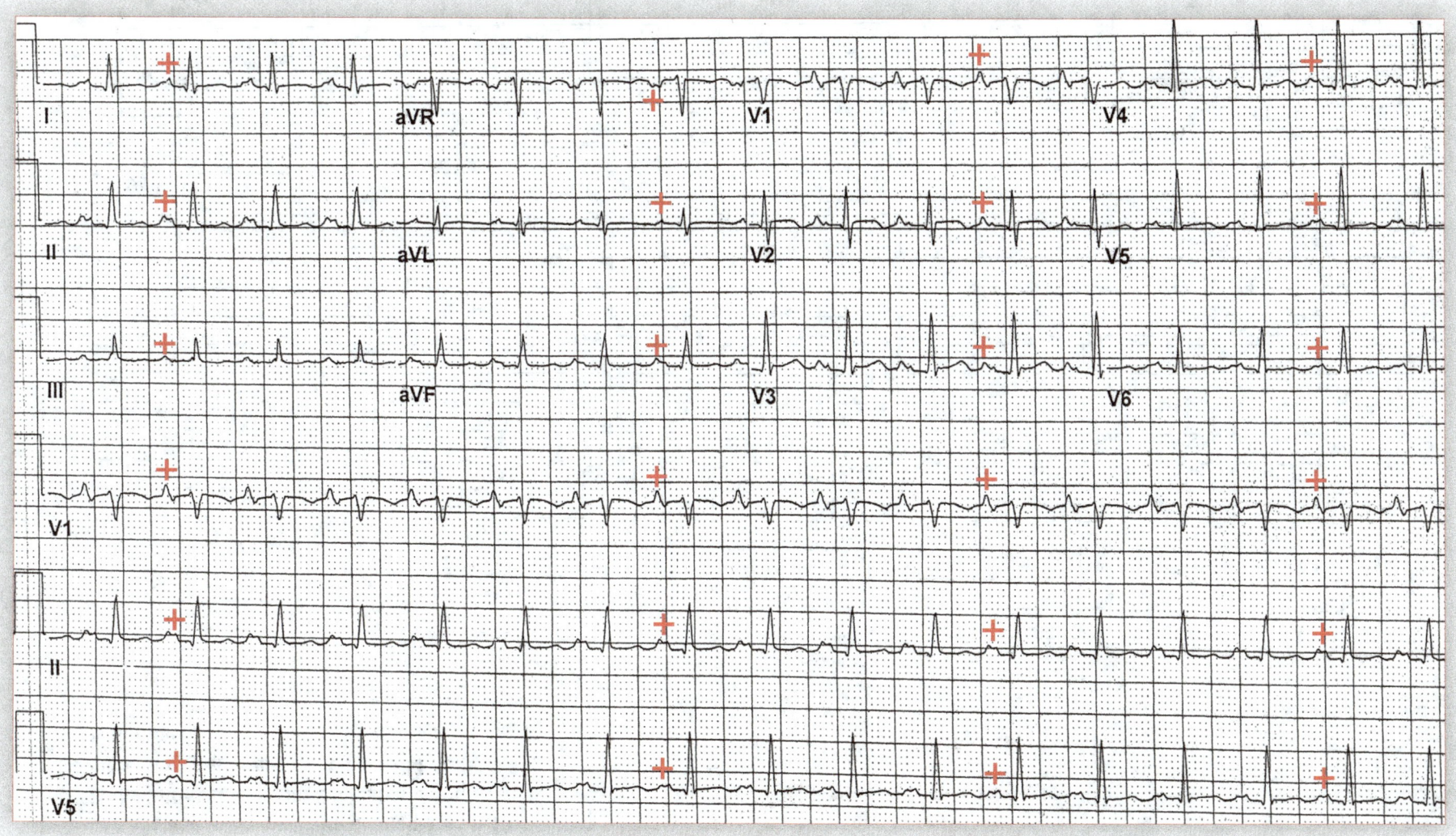

ECG 3A Analysis: Sinus tachycardia, left atrial hypertrophy (abnormality), early transition

In **ECG 3A**, there is a regular rhythm at rate of 110 bpm. There is a P wave (+) before each QRS complex with a stable PR interval (0.20 sec). The P wave is broad and notched, particularly in leads II, aVF, and V3-V6, consistent with left atrial hypertrophy (abnormality). The QRS complex duration is normal (0.08 sec), and there is a normal morphology, except for a tall R wave in lead V2, which is termed early transition or counterclockwise rotation. This is an axis shift in the horizontal plane. The axis is determined by imagining the heart as viewed from under the diaphragm; the right ventricle is in front and the left ventricle is lateral. With counterclockwise rotation the left ventricle is electrically shifted anteriorly and hence left ventricular forces occur early in the right precordial leads, producing a tall R wave in lead V2. The axis in the frontal plane is normal, between 0° and +90° (positive QRS complex in leads I and aVF). The QT/QTc intervals are normal (300/410 msec).

continues

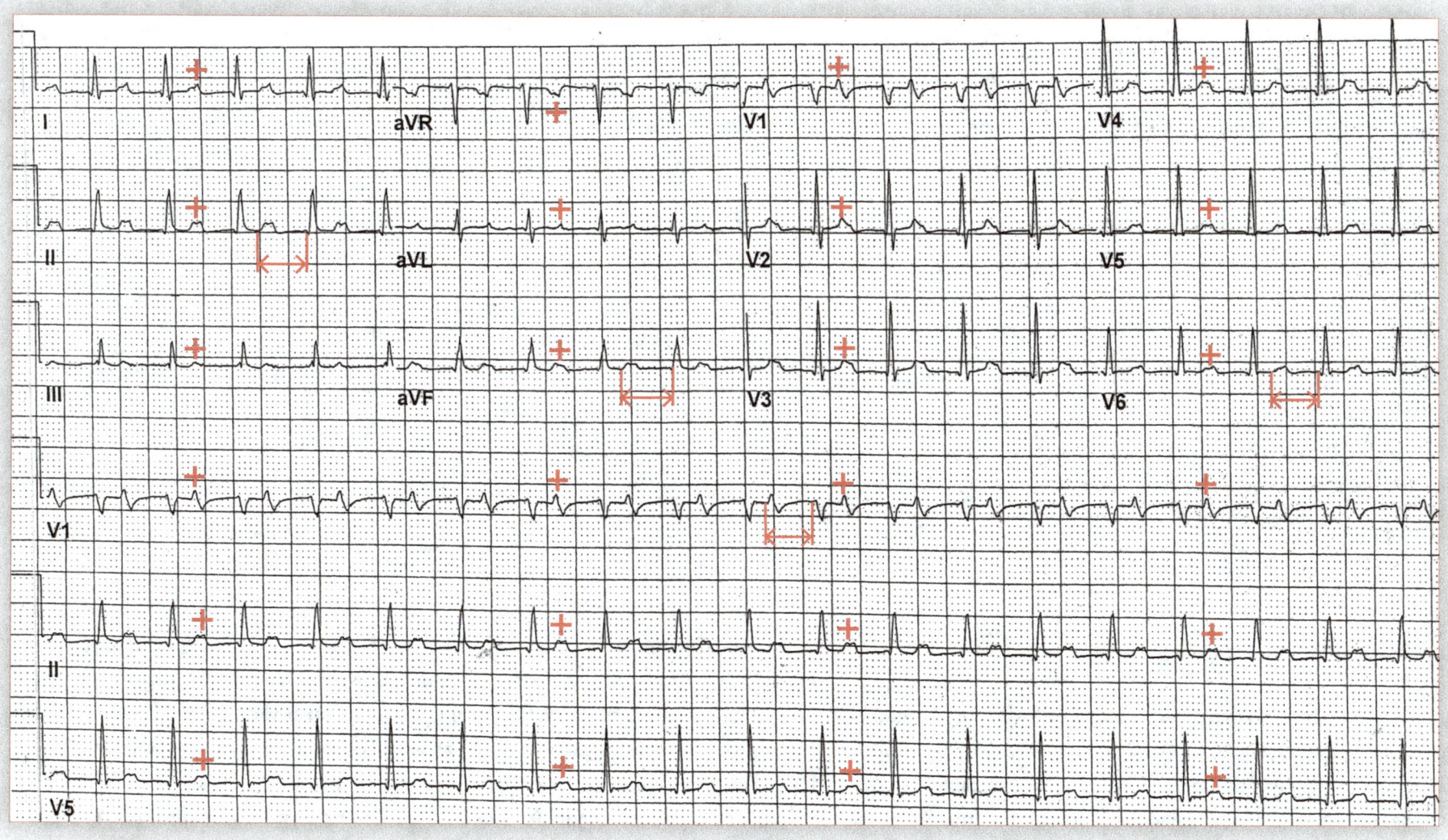

ECG 3B Analysis: Sinus tachycardia, first-degree AV block (prolonged AV conduction), dual AV nodal pathways, left atrial hypertrophy (abnormality), early transition

ECG **3B** was obtained 2 minutes after ECG **3A** without any intervention. There is a regular rhythm at a rate of 122 bpm. There is a P wave (+) before each QRS complex. The P wave might be mistaken for the T wave, especially in the limb leads, but the P wave is clearly distinct in leads aVL and V1. Also, this waveform is much narrower than a normal T wave and has a sharp upstroke and downstroke. The P wave in ECG **3B** has the same axis and morphology as the P wave in ECG **3A**. It is positive in leads I, II, aVF, and V4-V6 and there is a left atrial abnormality (hypertrophy). Although there is a stable PR interval, it is longer (0.34 sec) (↔) than what was seen in ECG **3A**. Hence this is sinus tachycardia with first-degree AV block (prolonged AV conduction). The QRS complex duration, morphology, and axis are the same as in ECG **3A**, as are the QT/QTc intervals.

Although ECG **3A** shows a normal PR interval, the PR interval in ECG **3B** is much longer, even though the sinus rate is also faster. The PR interval usually shortens when the sinus rate increases as a result of faster AV conduction due to sympathetic stimulation. However, in this case the PR interval is longer at a faster rate and shorter at a slower rate. The PR interval lengthening occurred abruptly in the absence of any intervention. The only situation during sinus rhythm in which this phenomenon can occur is with the presence of dual AV nodal pathways.

The presence of dual AV nodal pathways is the anatomic basis for atrioventricular nodal reentrant tachycardia (AVNRT). In order for AVNRT to occur, the following is required: One of the pathways conducts rapidly but has a long refractory period (*ie,* slow recovery). The second pathway conducts slowly but has a short refractory period (*ie,* fast

recovery). These two pathways are linked proximally in the atrial myocardium and distally at the distal part of the AV junction. During sinus rhythm, AV conduction is via the fast pathway. However, if a premature atrial complex occurs before the fast pathway has recovered, then the impulse is blocked in the fast pathway (unidirectional block) but is conducted to the ventricles via the slow pathway, which recovers more quickly. However, the PR interval will be much longer than the PR interval of the sinus complex. If the fast pathway has recovered by the time the impulse reaches the distal end of the circuit, the impulse can be conducted retrogradely by this fast pathway to activate the atrium in a retrograde direction at the same time the impulse travels antegradely to activate the ventricles. If the slow pathway has recovered by the time the impulse reaches the proximal part of the circuit, the impulse can reenter this pathway antegradely and then again conduct retrogradely through the fast pathway. This establishes a reentrant arrhythmia, known as AVNRT. This is termed slow-fast AVNRT, and in this situation no P wave is seen as there is simultaneous atrial and ventricular activation.

As the reentrant circuit is within the AV node, AVNRT can often be terminated by any intervention that alters the conduction characteristics of the AV nodal pathways. This includes enhancement of vagal tone, as with Valsalva, carotid sinus pressure, or coughing, which slows conduction primarily through the slow AV nodal pathway. The history from this patient is consistent with this arrhythmia, especially since there is evidence of dual AV nodal pathways. Adenosine, a calcium-channel blocker, or a β-blocker also alter AV nodal conduction and can be used to terminate this arrhythmia. ■

Notes

A 60-year-old woman with a prior inferior wall myocardial infarction (MI) is noted on routine exam to have an irregular pulse. She is otherwise asymptomatic. Her medications include a β-blocker, aspirin, and an angiotensin-converting enzyme inhibitor. An ECG is obtained.

What abnormalities are shown?

What is the cause of her irregular pulse?

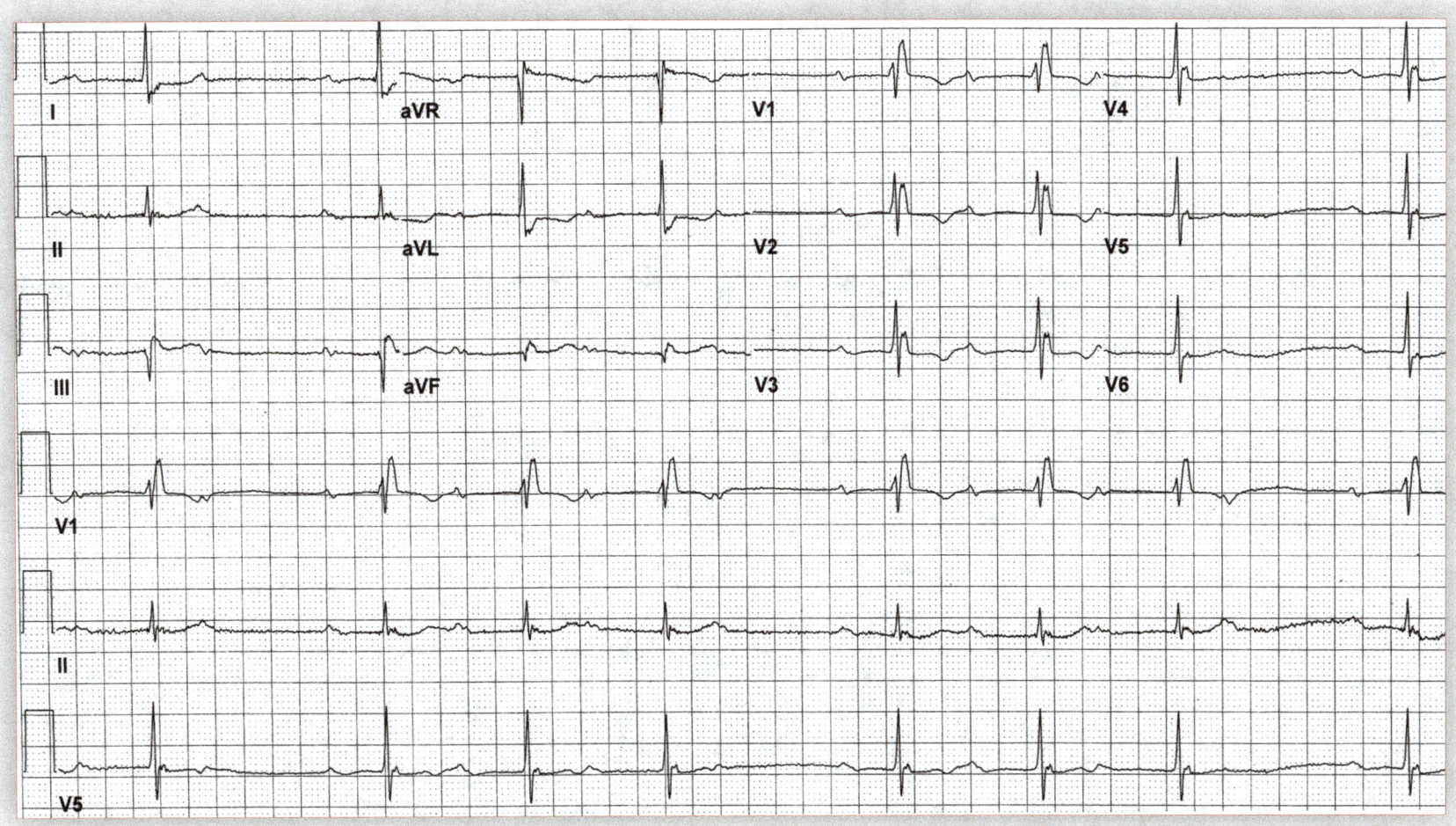

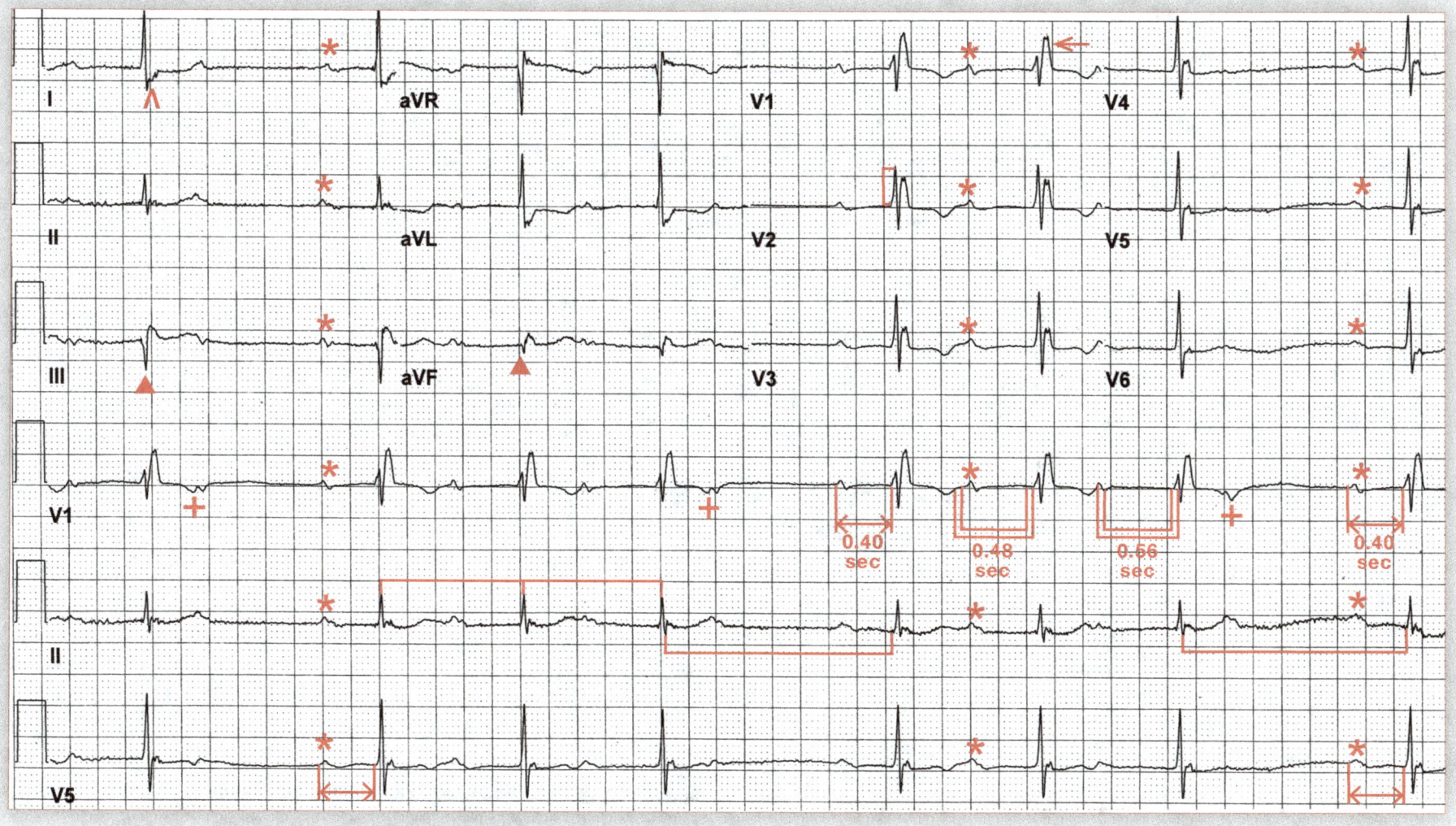

ECG 4 Analysis: Normal sinus rhythm, first-degree AV block
(prolonged AV conduction), Mobitz type I second-degree AV block (Wenckebach),
right bundle branch block, counterclockwise rotation, inferior wall MI

The rhythm is irregular, although there is a repeating pattern of long (⊔) and short (⊓) RR intervals. Therefore, the rhythm is regularly irregular at an average rate of 66 bpm. There are P waves (*) seen with a constant PP interval and a sinus rate of 84 bpm. The P waves are positive in leads I, II, aVF, and V4-V6. Hence this is a normal sinus rhythm. The QRS complexes are wide (0.14 sec) with an RSR′ morphology in lead V1 (←) and a broad terminal S wave in lead I (^). This is the pattern of a right bundle branch block. There is a tall R wave (R > S) in lead V2 ([ ), which is early transition, the result of counterclockwise rotation. This is determined by imagining the heart as viewed from under the diaphragm. With counterclockwise rotation, left ventricular forces are seen early in the precordial leads. There are Q waves in leads III and aVF (▲), consistent with a prior inferior wall myocardial infarction (MI). The QT/QTc intervals are normal (440/420 msec).

The ventricular rate is irregular, but there is a pattern to the irregularity. All of the short intervals are the same (⊓) and the long intervals (⊔), or pauses, are also the same. Therefore, the rhythm is regularly irregular and there is a pattern of grouped beating with three QRS complexes followed by a pause. The pause is the result of a nonconducted P wave (+). Hence there is second-degree AV block. The PR interval after each pause (↔) is the same (0.40 sec), and hence there is first-degree AV block (prolonged AV conduction). This represents the baseline PR interval. The PR intervals that follow (⊔) become progressively longer (0.48 and 0.56 sec). The third QRS complex of the group is followed by a nonconducted P wave (+), after which the PR interval shortens to its baseline (0.40 sec). This recurrent abnormality in AV conduction causes the appearance of "grouping" of the QRS complexes (so-called "grouped beating"); there is a pattern of 4:3 conduction (ie, four atrial beats for every three ventricular beats). This pattern is classified as second-degree AV block, Mobitz type I (Wenckebach). Second-degree AV block is identified by a pause in the RR interval due to a nonconducted P wave. With Wenckebach there is only one nonconducted P wave. Any pattern of block (eg, 2:1, 3:2, 4:3, etc) may occur depending on the AV nodal electrophysiologic properties and the degree of vagal tone. As a result the rhythm will be regularly irregular.

Second-degree AV block is subdivided into two types: Mobitz type I (or Wenckebach) and Mobitz type II. Mobitz type I is characterized by a progressive lengthening of the PR interval until a normally timed P wave is not followed by a QRS complex (ie, it is nonconducted). With PR interval prolongation, each successive atrial impulse reaches the AV node earlier, while it is still partially refractory. There is a progressive

continues

slowing of AV conduction of each subsequent impulse ("decremental" AV nodal conduction). Finally, the AV node fails to conduct completely if a sinus impulse arrives when it is absolutely refractory; the result is a lack of ventricular activation and the absence of a QRS complex.

Wenckebach is a conduction abnormality within the AV node. Since the electrophysiologic properties of the AV node are mediated by calcium currents (slow action potential), conduction through this structure is not all or none but can vary depending on changes in nodal electrophysiologic properties. Non-pathologic changes in the speed of AV conduction are usually due to changes in the node's refractory period. Entities that affect the refractory period include increases in parasympathetic vagal tone such as that seen in the pediatric population, during sleep, with gastrointestinal distress such as vomiting, and in well-conditioned people. An increase in the refractory period can be seen with an acute inferior wall MI, which is frequently accompanied by increased vagal discharge. Some pathologic conditions, such as sclerodegenerative disease and myocarditis, can result in Mobitz type I block. Many medications can alter AV node conduction as well, including digoxin, lithium, calcium-channel blockers, and β-blockers. It is possible that a β-blocker is the cause of Wenckebach in this patient. Wenckebach is predominantly a benign conduction abnormality that, if asymptomatic, does not require any therapy. ◼

A 55-year-old woman presents with several hours of nausea culminating in an episode of vomiting and chest pain that prompts activation of emergency medical services. On arrival to the emergency department, she appears pale, diaphoretic, and in moderate distress. Her vital signs are notable for tachycardia. Her physical exam reveals faint pulmonary rales, normal S1 with a widely but physiologically split S2, and an S3. No murmurs are noted. An ECG is performed.

What abnormalities are noted on the ECG, and what is the diagnosis?

What is the etiology of the conduction abnormalities?

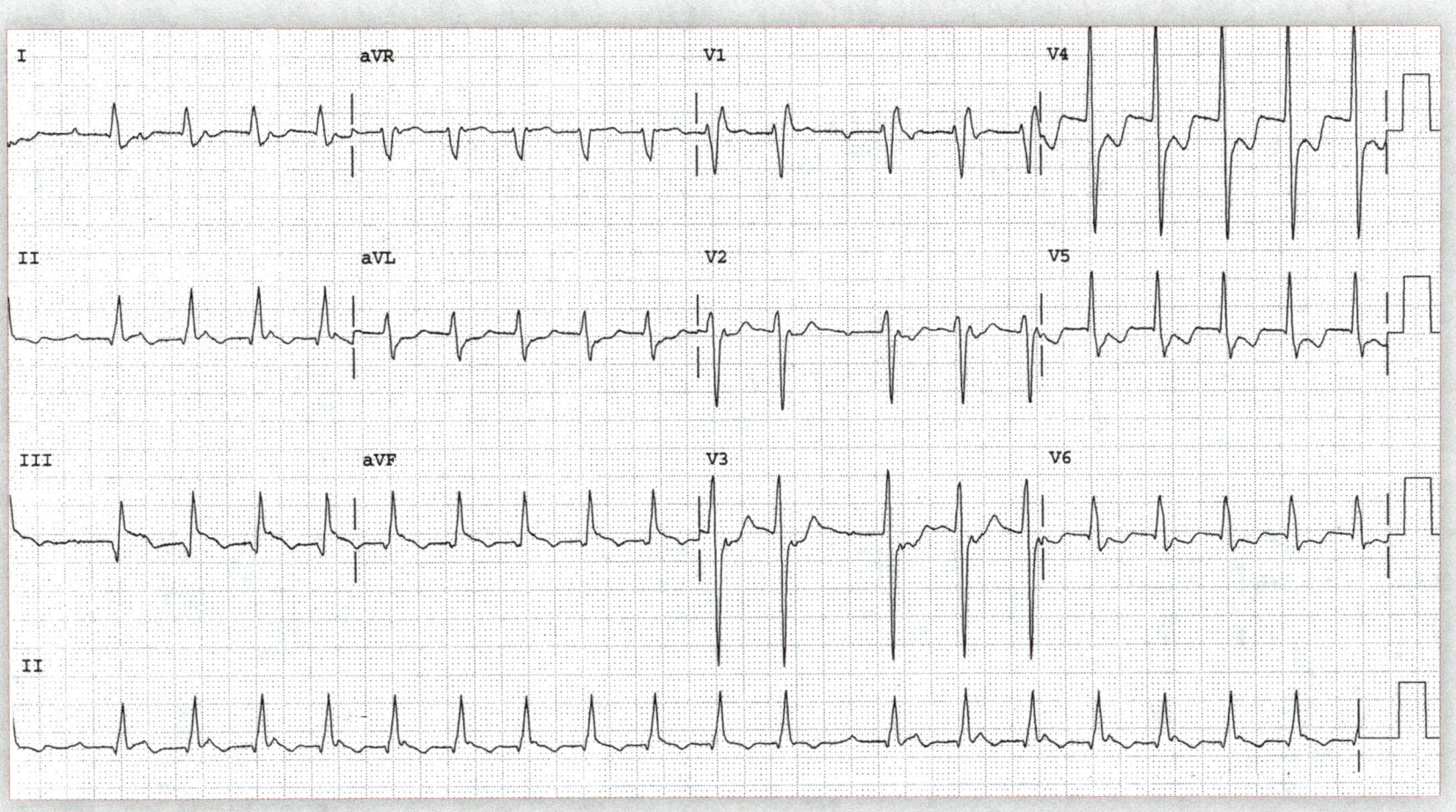

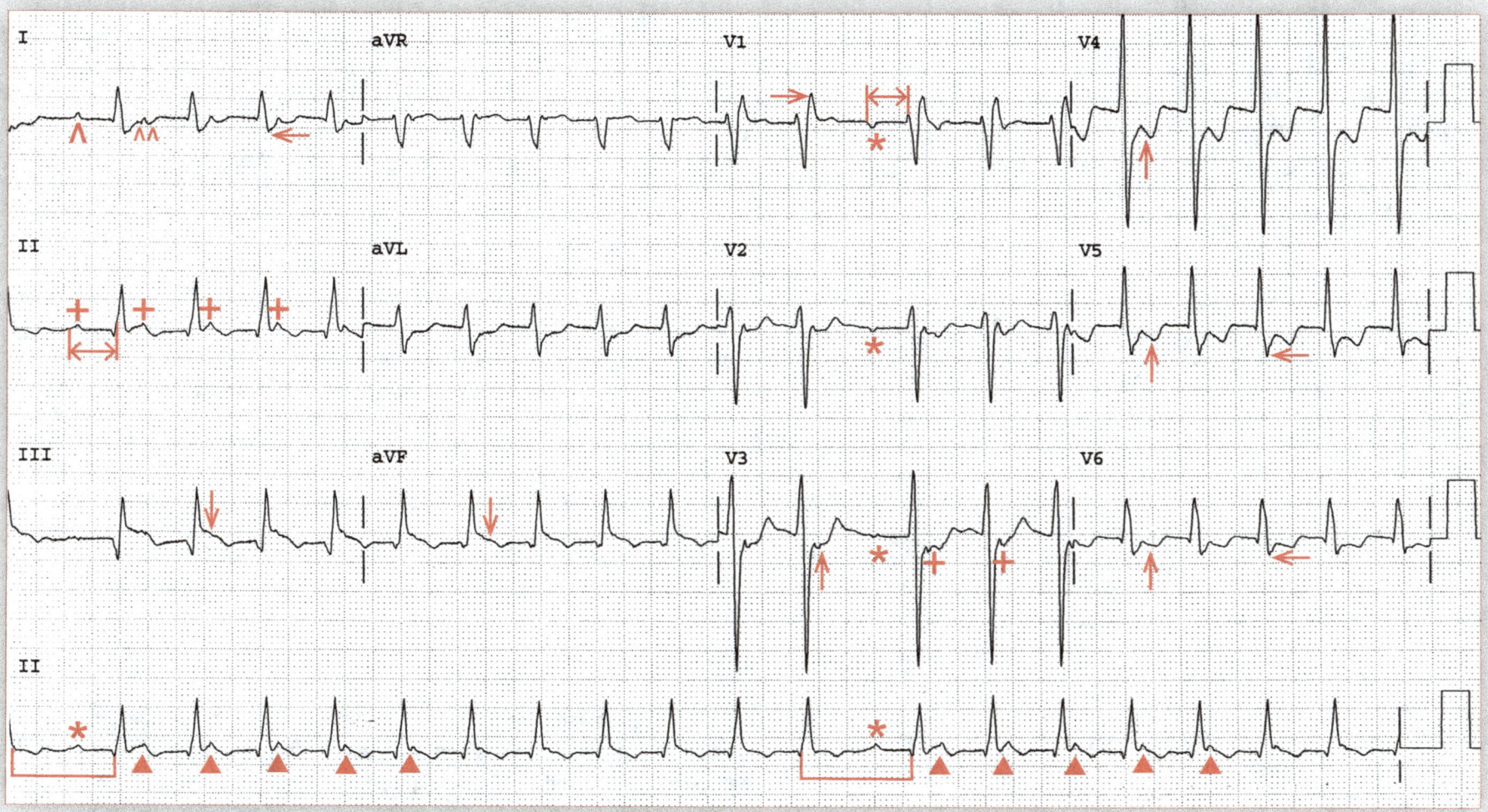

ECG 5 Analysis: Sinus tachycardia, first-degree AV block
(prolonged AV conduction), Mobitz type I second-degree AV block (Wenckebach),
right bundle branch block, acute inferior wall myocardial infarction

The rhythm is regularly irregular as a result of two pauses that have the same duration (⊔). P waves (*) can be seen during each pause, with a PR interval of 0.28 second after each pause (↔). Although other P waves are not immediately obvious, closer inspection of leads I, II, V2, and V3 reveals deflections consistent with P waves (+). Importantly, two sequential P waves (^,^^) can be seen in either lead I or II (surrounding the first QRS complex of the ECG), establishing the PP interval and an atrial rate of 122 bpm. The P wave is positive in leads I and II; hence this is likely sinus tachycardia.

Having established the PP interval, P waves with a constant PP interval can be seen in lead II beginning with the P wave after the pause at the beginning of the ECG. Over the course of the lead II rhythm strip, P waves (▲), which may be initially confused for T waves, are moving into the QRS complex, ultimately not being obvious because they are buried within the QRS complexes just prior to the second pause. Therefore, the change in the morphology of the terminal portion of the QRS complex (or actually within the ST segment) over the course of the lead II rhythm strip is the result of fusion between the P wave and the QRS complex; this waveform is not the T wave. This observation suggests that the PR interval is lengthening (rather than the QT interval shortening). Hence this is second-degree AV block, Mobitz type I (Wenckebach), with a long cycle. The long cycle length is the result of underlying sinus tachycardia, which results from enhanced sympathetic tone.

The QRS complex duration is increased (0.12 sec) and there is a normal axis, between 0° and +90° (positive QRS complex in leads I and aVF). There is a right bundle branch block morphology (RSR′ in lead V1 [→] and broad terminal S waves in leads I and V5-V6 [←]). The QRS axis is normal, between 0° and +90° (positive QRS complex in leads I and aVF). The QT/QTc intervals are slightly prolonged (320/460 msec) but are normal when corrected for the prolonged QRS complex duration (280/400 msec). There is ST-segment elevation (↓) in leads III and aVF, consistent with an acute inferior wall myocardial infarction (MI), and ST-T wave changes (↑) in leads V3-V6 that may be reciprocal (associated with the inferior wall MI).

continues

This patient is suffering from an acute inferior wall MI. The lack of a tall R wave in lead V1 or ST-T wave changes in leads V1-V3 argues against posterior left ventricular wall involvement. In terms of coronary anatomy, 80% to 85% of patients are "right dominant"; that is, the right coronary artery gives rise to the posterior descending and posterior left ventricular coronary arteries, which supply the inferior wall of the left ventricle as well as the inferior septum. About 10% of patients are "left dominant," with the left circumflex artery giving rise to these arteries, and 5% to 10% are co-dominant (with the posterior descending artery arising from either the right coronary artery or left circumflex artery, and the posterior left ventricular artery arising from the other). As the AV nodal artery is usually a proximal branch from the right coronary artery, AV conduction delay (manifesting as first- and second-degree AV block) is not likely to represent AV nodal ischemia. Moreover, the AV node generates a slow action potential, mediated by a calcium current, which is not energy dependent and hence does not depend on oxygen supply. The bundle branches usually receive blood supply from the septal perforators of the left anterior descending artery. Therefore, right bundle branch block in this patient is not likely to be due to the acute MI. Transient AV nodal conduction delay may be seen with an inferior wall MI due to resultant elevation in vagal tone as well as edema that may occur around the AV node. Therefore, AV nodal abnormalities are likely to be transient.

Note that despite elevated vagal tone and the presence of Wenckebach, this patient is tachycardic. This may be due to the presence of heart failure, which is evidenced on the physical exam. ■

A 73-year-old woman presents for her annual evaluation. She does not have a significant cardiac history. Her exam is normal. A routine ECG is performed.

What abnormality is noted?

What further management (if anything) is needed?

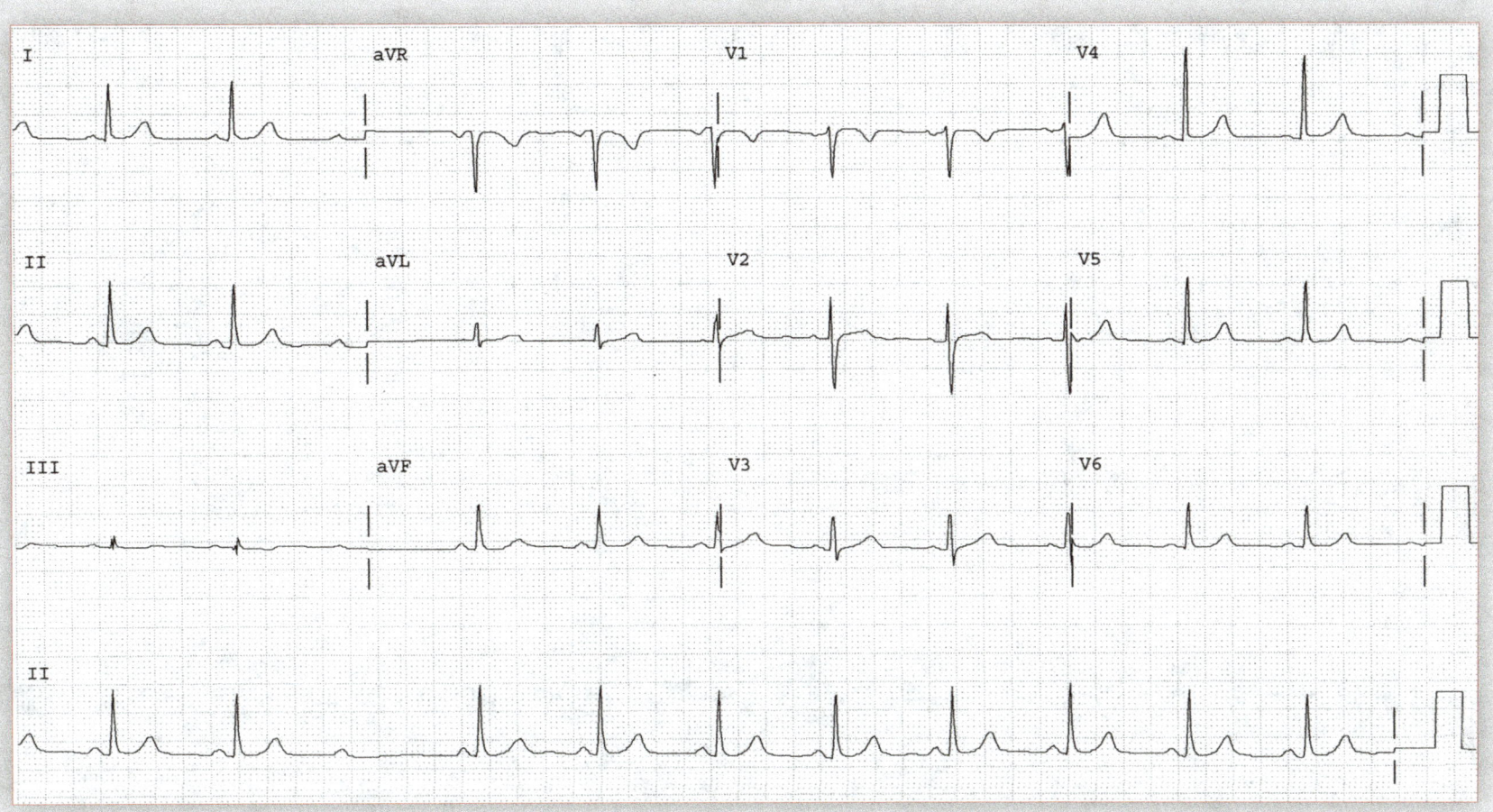

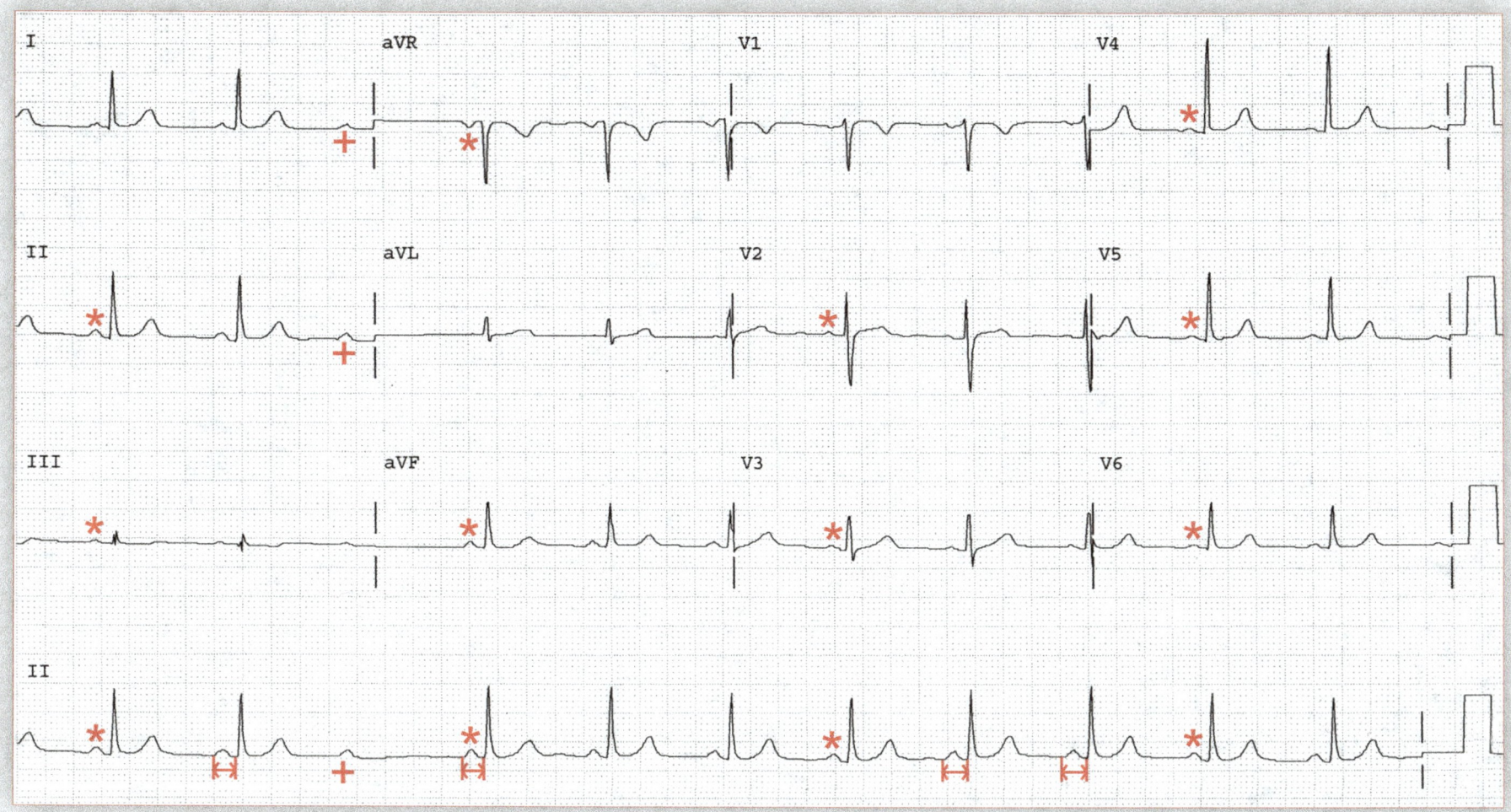

ECG 6 Analysis: Normal sinus rhythm, Mobitz type II second-degree AV block

There is a regular rhythm at a rate of 70 bpm. There is a P wave (∗) before each QRS complex. The P wave is positive in leads I, II, aVF, and V4-V6. Hence this is a normal sinus rhythm. The PR interval (↔) is stable at 0.16 second. Noted is a pause that results from a single on-time but nonconducted sinus P wave (+). An occasional nonconducted P wave is the hallmark of second-degree AV block. The QRS complex duration is normal (0.08 sec) and there is a normal morphology and axis, between 0° and +90° (positive QRS complex in leads I and aVF). The QT/QTc intervals are normal (400/430 msec).

The PR intervals are stable and hence the etiology for the pause or second-degree AV block is Mobitz type II. Mobitz type II block is characterized by an episodic and unpredictable failure of AV conduction. Mobitz type II block is due to blocked electrical conduction below the level of the AV node, within the bundle of His or bundle branches. Since the His-Purkinje system conducts in an "all or none" fashion (it either conducts with the same conduction velocity each time or fails to conduct any impulse), there is no change in the PR interval before or after the nonconducted P wave, in contrast to what is seen in Mobitz type I block. Therefore, failure of conduction represents underlying structural disease of the infranodal His-Purkinje system. In contrast, Mobitz type I AV block is a conduction abnormality within the AV node and is generally an exaggeration of AV nodal decremental

conduction; it typically does not represent underlying disease of the cardiac conduction system. In Mobitz type II block, there may be more than one successive nonconducted P wave, resulting in several P waves in a row without QRS complexes. This has often been termed "high-degree" AV block.

Both Mobitz type I and Mobitz type II block may progress to complete heart block. However, when Mobitz type II progresses to complete heart block, the escape rhythm is infra-Hisian (*ie*, ventricular), since the His-Purkinje system is diseased. Not uncommonly, the heart rate with a ventricular escape rhythm is slow and may be inadequate for systemic perfusion. The result may be "Stokes-Adams attacks" (unheralded syncope) and possibly sudden death. Therefore, even asymptomatic Mobitz type II block is a class IIA American Heart Association and American College of Cardiology recommendation for permanent pacemaker implantation. Therefore, pacemaker implantation should be considered in this patient.

In contrast, asymptomatic Mobitz type I block is not an indication for a pacemaker. In this situation the development of complete heart block is most often associated with an escape junctional rhythm, which is generally stable. ■

Notes

A 28-year-old man presents with a chief complaint of fatigue. He has no medical diagnoses and does not take medications. His family history is notable for his mother who has a pacemaker and his maternal uncles and grandfather who had heart failure of unclear etiology. He has two siblings in their 20s and 30s who have no medical issues. This patient's ECG is presented.

What abnormality is depicted?

What is the cause of this abnormality?

What further workup or therapy is indicated?

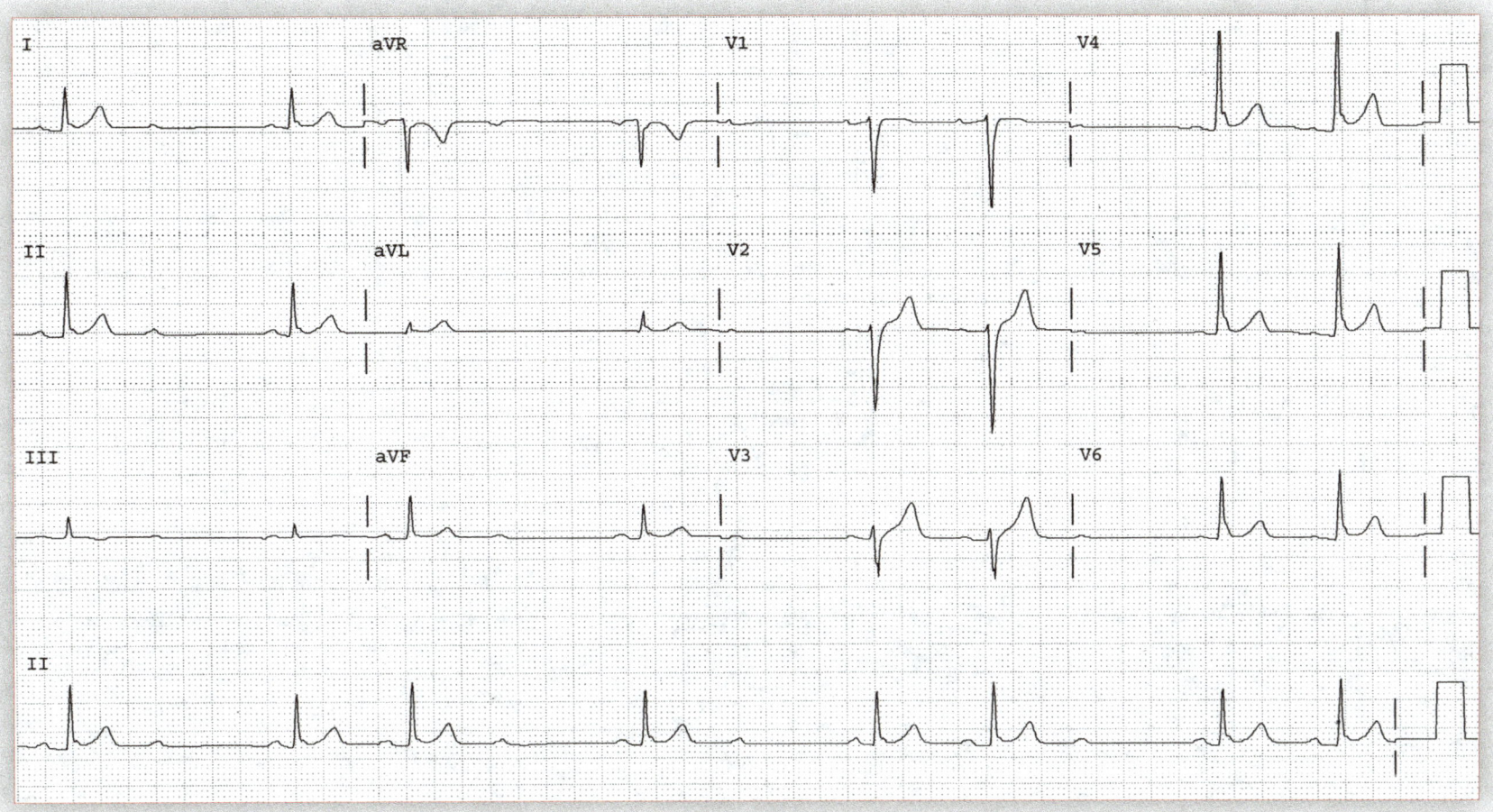

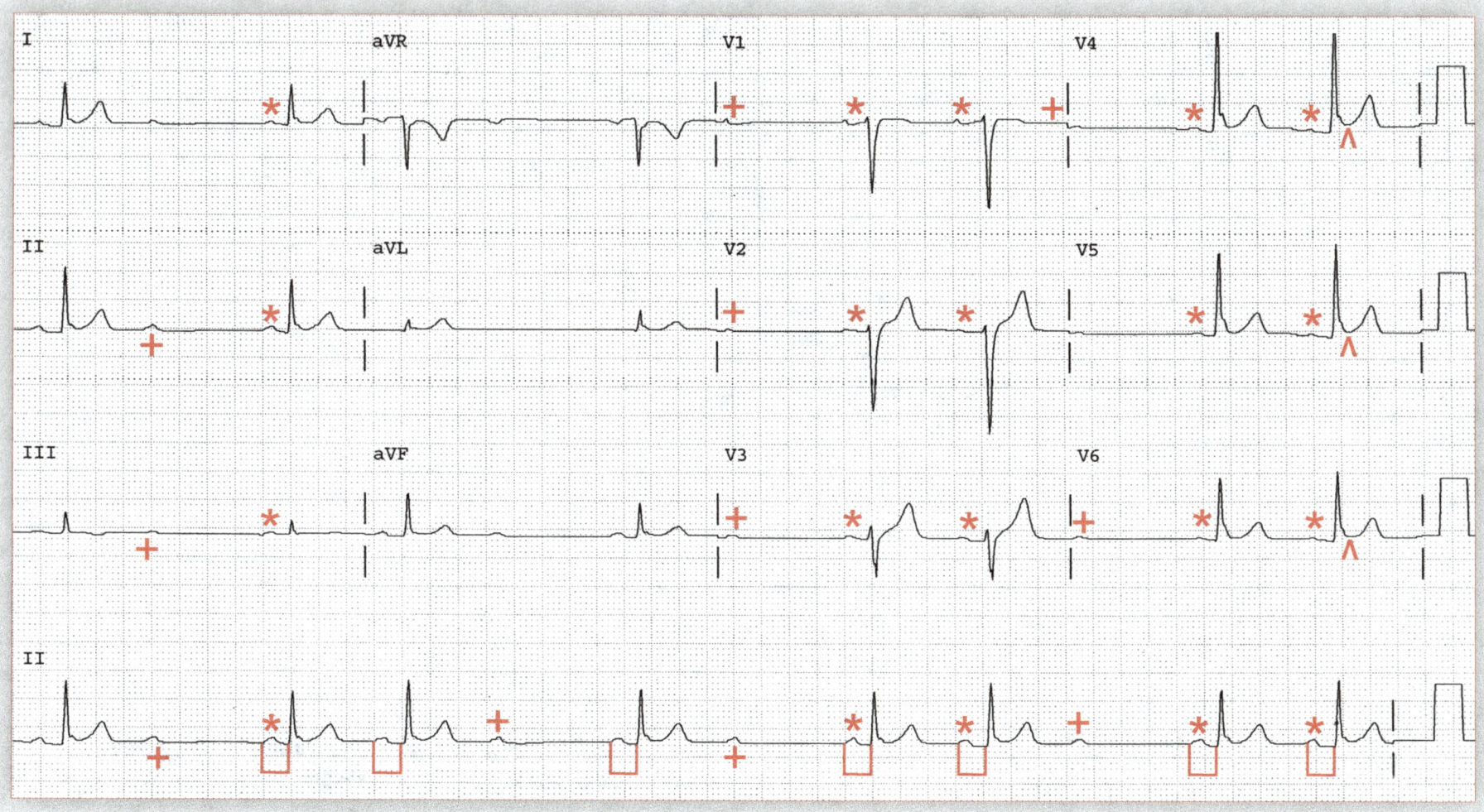

ECG 7 Analysis: Normal sinus rhythm, Mobitz type II second-degree AV block, early repolarization

There are regularly occurring P waves (*,+) at a constant rate of 74 bpm. The P waves are positive in leads I, II, aVF, and V4-V6. Hence there is an underlying sinus rhythm. Although each QRS complex is preceded by a P wave (*), there are a number of P waves without QRS complexes (+), resulting in frequent pauses in the ventricular rate (long RR intervals) as a result of on-time but nonconducted P waves (+). The PR interval of all the conducted beats is stable (⊔) (0.18 sec). The occurrence of an occasional nonconducted P wave defines second-degree AV block. Since all of the PR intervals are constant, this is Mobitz type II with a variable conduction pattern of 3:2 and 2:1 block. The QRS complex duration is normal. The axis is normal, between 0° and +90° (positive QRS complex in leads I and aVF). Slight J-point and ST-segment elevation (^) is noted in leads V4-V6; this is consistent with early repolarization, which is frequently seen in young individuals. The QT/QTc intervals are normal (380/340 msec).

This patient's fatigue is likely the result of his marked bradycardia from the frequent pauses. The rate is possibly slower at other times. His age and family history suggest a genetic cause for his conduction system disease. Some familial cardiomyopathies present initially with conduction system disease, including AV block. Permanent pacemaker implantation is warranted. As a familial cardiomyopathy is a very possible diagnosis, the patient will require close clinical surveillance as well as routine echocardiograms. In addition, ECG and echocardiographic surveillance should be considered for his siblings. Referral to a specialized center that performs genetic testing should be considered. ■

Notes

A 51-year-old man is admitted to the coronary care unit after suffering an acute non–ST-segment elevation myocardial infarction (NSTEMI). Coronary angiography documented 95% occlusion of the right coronary artery. He was treated with angioplasty and stenting, which was complicated by transient complete heart block requiring temporary transvenous pacing. On post-infarction day 2, the following ECG was obtained.

What abnormalities are depicted?

What is the appropriate management?

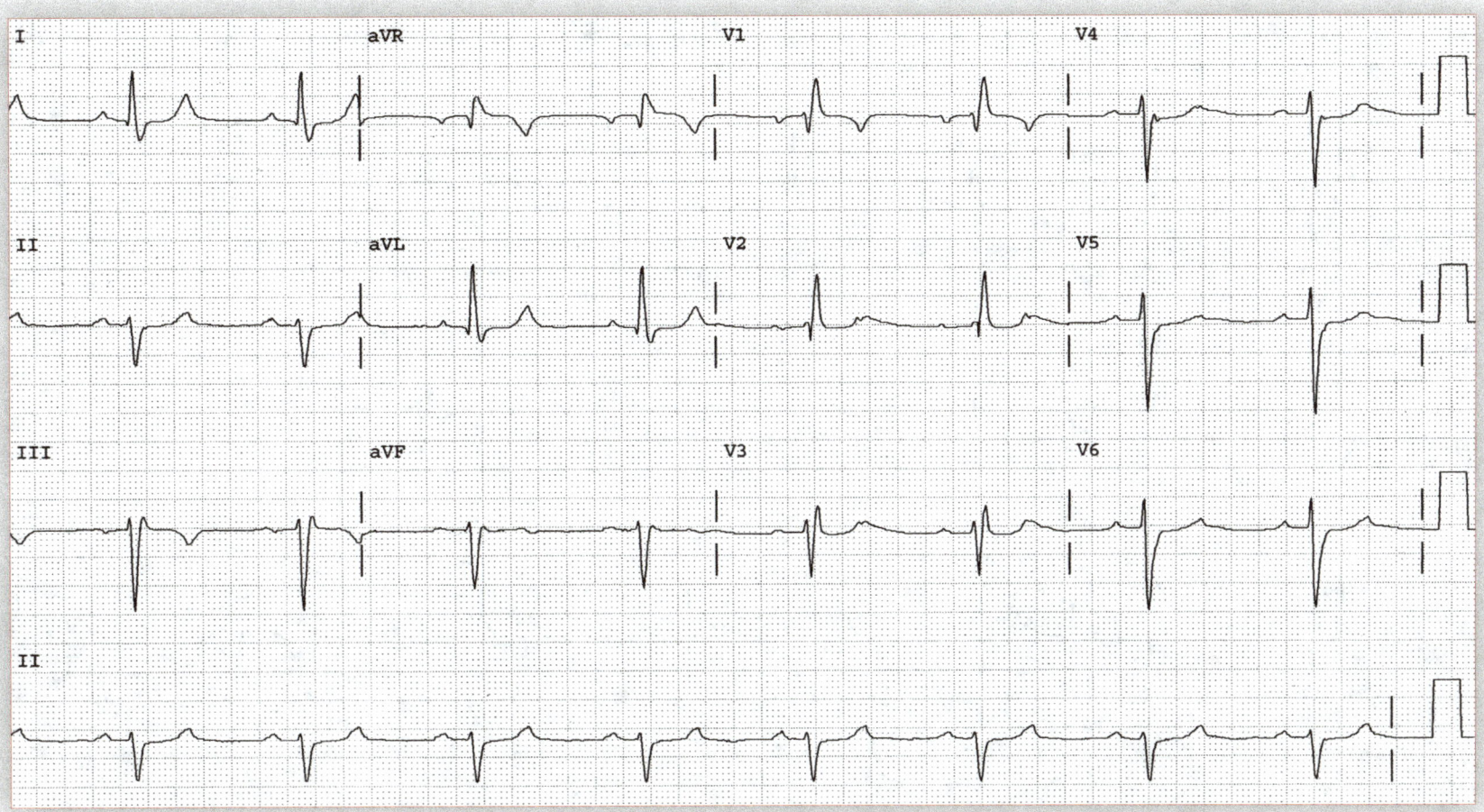

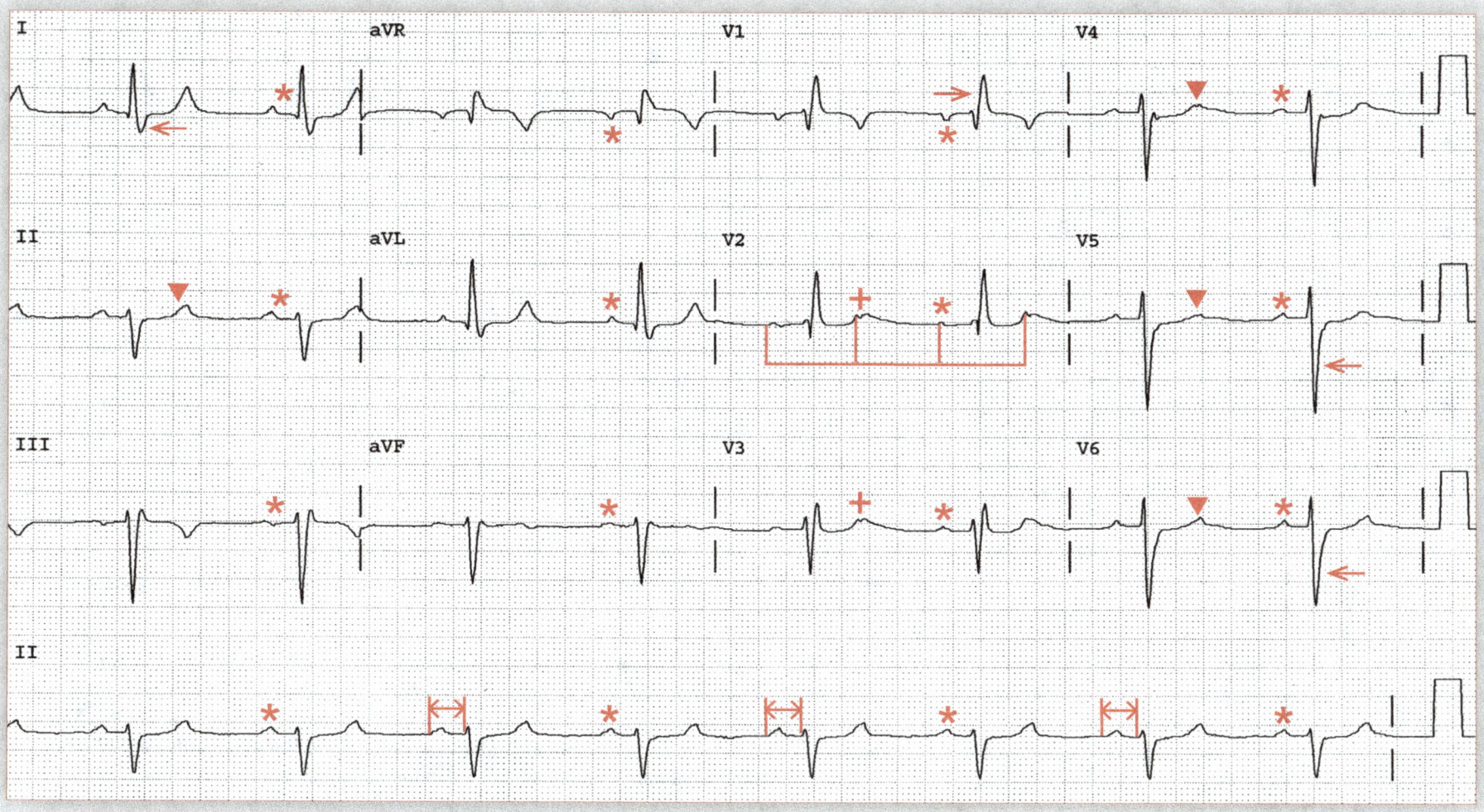

ECG 8 Analysis: Sinus tachycardia, first-degree AV block (prolonged AV conduction),
2:1 second-degree AV block, right bundle branch block, left anterior fascicular block,
poor R-wave progression and late transition (clockwise rotation)

There is a regular rhythm with a ventricular rate of 50 bpm. A P wave (*) can be seen before each QRS complex, and the PR interval (↔) is constant at 0.26 second (first-degree AV block or prolonged AV conduction). The P waves are positive in leads I, II, aVF, and V4-V6. The QRS complex duration is increased (0.16 sec), and there is a right bundle branch block pattern (RSR′ morphology in lead V1 [→] and a broad S wave in leads I and V5-V6 [←]). The axis is extremely leftward, between −30° and −90° (positive QRS complex in lead I and negative QRS complex in leads II and aVF). As there are no Q waves in leads II and aVF, but rather an rS morphology, the extreme left axis is the result of a left anterior fascicular block. The QT/QTc intervals are prolonged (520/470 msec), but they are normal when the prolonged QRS complex duration is considered (440/400 msec).

A second P wave (+) is present in the T wave (best seen in leads V2-V3), although there are also irregularities seen on the T waves in leads II and V4-V6 (▼), which are the result of superimposed P waves. The PP intervals (⊔) are regular. Hence the atrial rate is regular at 100 bpm. Therefore, there is sinus tachycardia with both first- and second-degree AV block with 2:1 AV conduction. The etiology (*ie*, Mobitz type I or II) cannot be established, even though other conduction system disease is present. While there is evidence of bifascicular disease (right bundle branch block and left anterior fascicular block), this does not necessarily establish Mobitz type II as the etiology. Moreover, the presence of first-degree AV block does not help establish the etiology; the prolonged PR interval may be due to slowing of conduction through the AV node or the remaining functioning fascicle (*ie*, left posterior fascicle). Importantly, this ECG does not show evidence of trifascicular block as the site of the first-degree AV block cannot be established even though there is evidence for bifascicular disease.

The QRS complexes in the precordium show poor R-wave progression and late transition. This is the result of a clockwise rotation of the electrical axis in the horizontal plane, determined by imagining the heart as viewed from under the diaphragm. With clockwise rotation, the left ventricular forces are seen late in the precordial leads.

As there is a right coronary artery lesion, the non–ST-segment elevation myocardial infarction involves the inferior wall. It is likely that the 2:1 AV block as well as the first-degree AV block are due to increased vagal tone or possibly edema of the AV node. Therefore, the AV conduction abnormalities are likely to be transient and will not require implantation of a permanent pacemaker. However, if this conduction abnormality persists and is symptomatic, permanent pacemaker

continues

insertion may be necessary. If no symptoms are present, it would be useful to establish the location of the block (*ie*, AV nodal or infra-Hisian) with an electrophysiologic study.

It is uncertain whether the bifascicular disease is preexistent or the result of the acute infarction. However, as the infarction involves the inferior wall, it is most likely that these conduction abnormalities were present before the acute event, since the right bundle receives its blood supply primarily from septal branches of the left anterior descending artery. Permanent pacemaker implantation in patients with evidence of bifascicular conduction block is not necessary.

Class I indications for pacemaker insertion after a myocardial infarction include:

- Third-degree AV block within or below the His-Purkinje system

- Persistent second-degree AV block in the His-Purkinje system with alternating bundle branch block

- Transient advanced second-degree infranodal AV block and associated bundle branch block (If the site of block is uncertain, an electrophysiologic study may be necessary.)

- Persistent and symptomatic second- or third-degree AV block

A 79-year-old woman presents with syncope. A neighbor answered her calls for help and found her lying on the floor of her apartment. Her medical history and current medications are unknown. She is bradycardic and hypotensive in the emergency department. On exam, she is quite somnolent but does move her extremities to vocal commands. Her lungs are clear and her cardiac exam is notable only for marked, regular bradycardia. An emergent ECG is obtained and you are asked to interpret it.

What is the diagnosis?

What treatment is indicated?

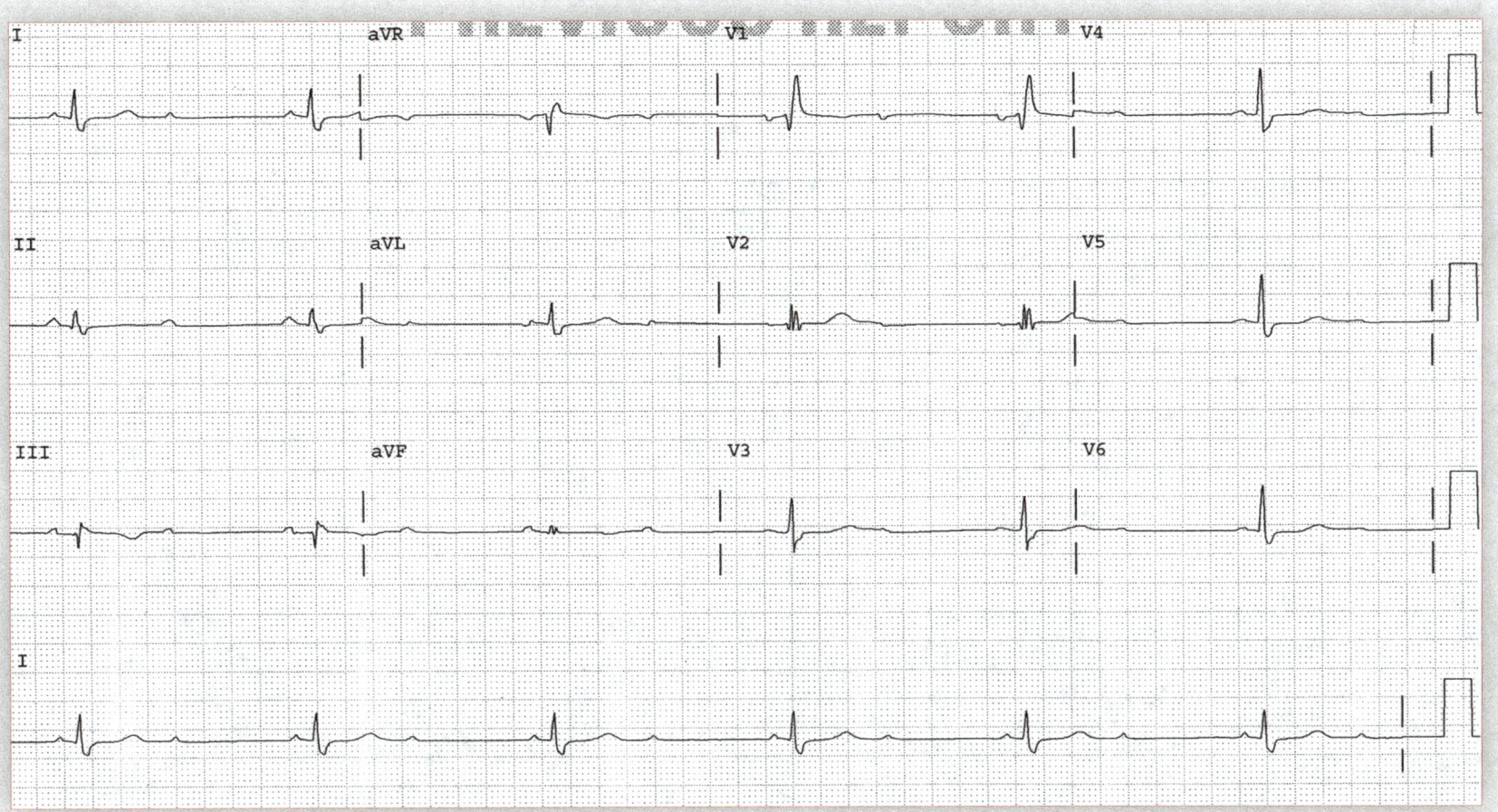

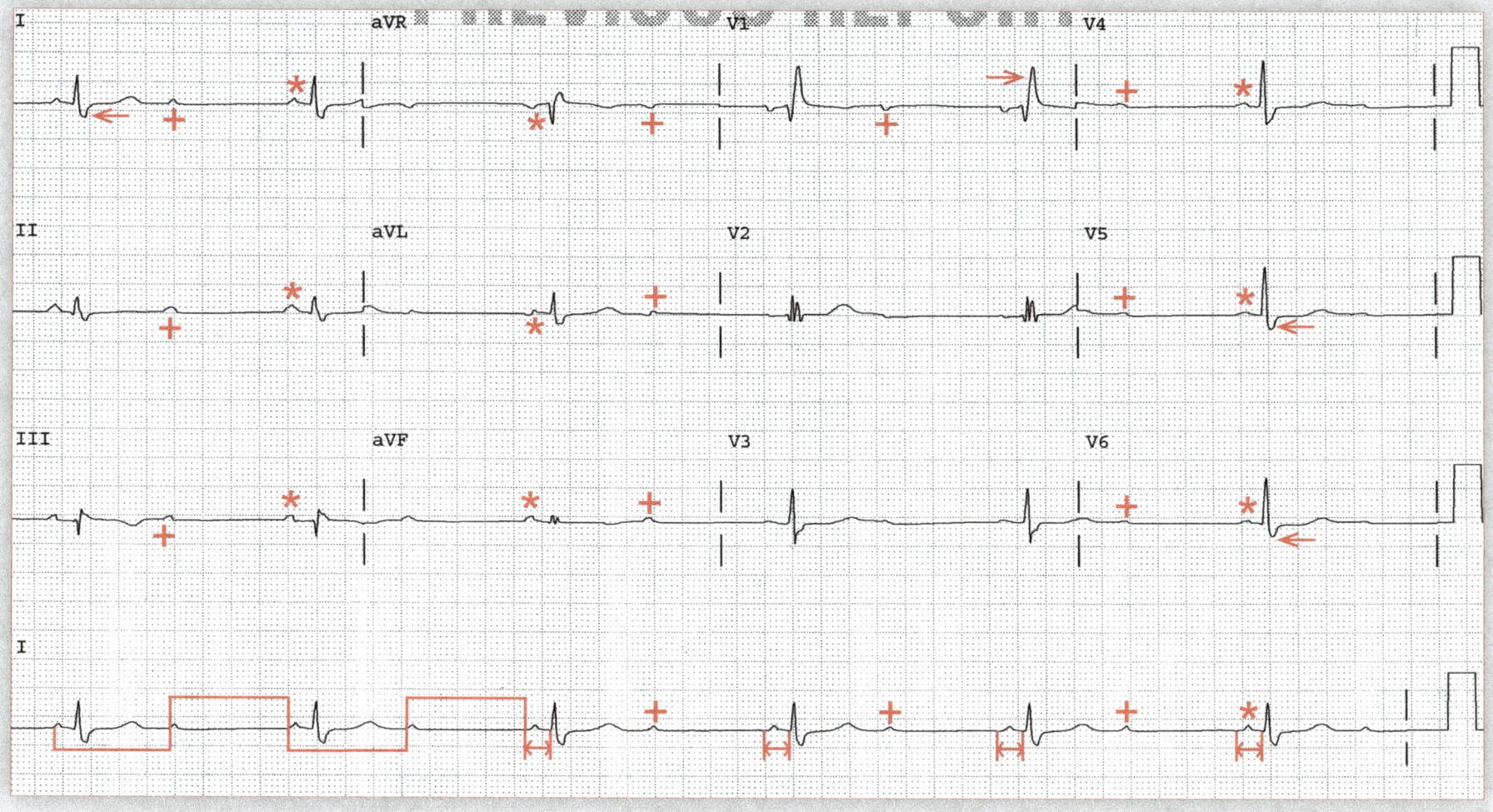

ECG 9 Analysis: Normal sinus rhythm, 2:1 second-degree
AV block, ventriculophasic sinus arrhythmia

There is a regular rhythm at a rate of 34 bpm. The QRS complex duration is increased (0.12 sec), and it has a right bundle branch morphology with an RSR′ morphology in lead V1 (→) and a broad terminal S wave in leads I and V5-V6 (←). The QRS axis is normal, between 0° and +90° (positive QRS complex in leads I and aVF). The QT/QTc intervals are normal (500/380 msec). There is a P wave (*) before each QRS complex with a stable PR interval (↔) of 0.16 second. A second, nonconducted P wave can be seen after each T wave (+). The P waves are positive in leads I, II, aVF, and V4-V6. Hence this is a normal sinus rhythm at a rate of 66 bpm. However, the PP interval is not completely regular and it can be seen that the PP interval surrounding the QRS complex (⊔) is slightly shorter (0.76 sec) than the PP interval when there is no intervening QRS complex (0.88 sec) (⊓). This is termed ventriculophasic sinus arrhythmia and it can be seen whenever 2:1 or complete AV block is present.

The etiology for ventriculophasic arrhythmia with a shortening of the PP interval surrounding the QRS complex is not certain. It has been suggested that ventricular contraction causes an increase in pulsatile blood flow through the sinus nodal artery that enhances the automaticity of the sinus node. Ventricular contraction also causes a stretch of the right atrium and of the sinus node that enhances nodal automaticity. Lastly, the occurrence of ventricular contraction and stroke volume results in activation of the baroreceptors in the carotid artery that affects sinus node automaticity.

Although the etiology of the 2:1 AV block (ie, Mobitz type I or II) cannot be established, this patient is hemodynamically unstable as a result of marked bradycardia and hence temporary transvenous pacing should be performed. If the 2:1 AV block is the result of Mobitz type II second-degree heart block (as established by some change in the conduction pattern or with electrophysiologic study demonstrating a prolonged HV interval with the conducted complexes in addition to A and H waves but no V wave associated with the nonconducted P wave, indicating block below the AV node within the His-Purkinje system) or if the 2:1 AV block is permanent, a permanent pacemaker would be indicated. A permanent pacemaker would also be indicated for Mobitz type I if the 2:1 block was frequent and associated with symptoms. With electrophysiologic study, Mobitz type I block would be associated with an A wave not followed by an H or V wave, indicating block in the AV node. ■

A 72-year-old woman with a history of myocardial infarction (MI) is seen by her cardiologist for a routine follow-up. When a slight irregularity is noted during carotid artery palpation, an ECG is obtained.

What is the cause for the physical exam finding noted by the physician?

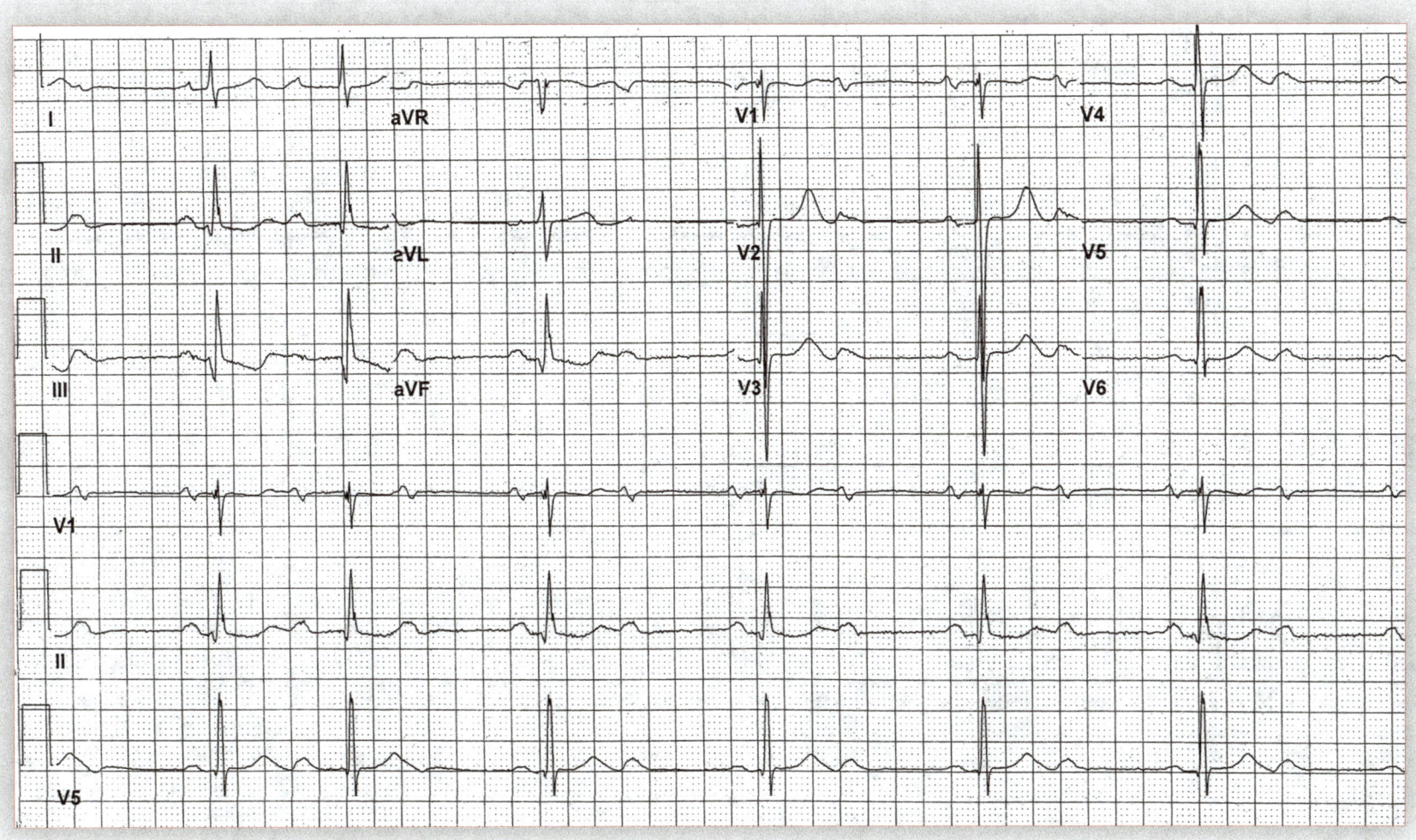

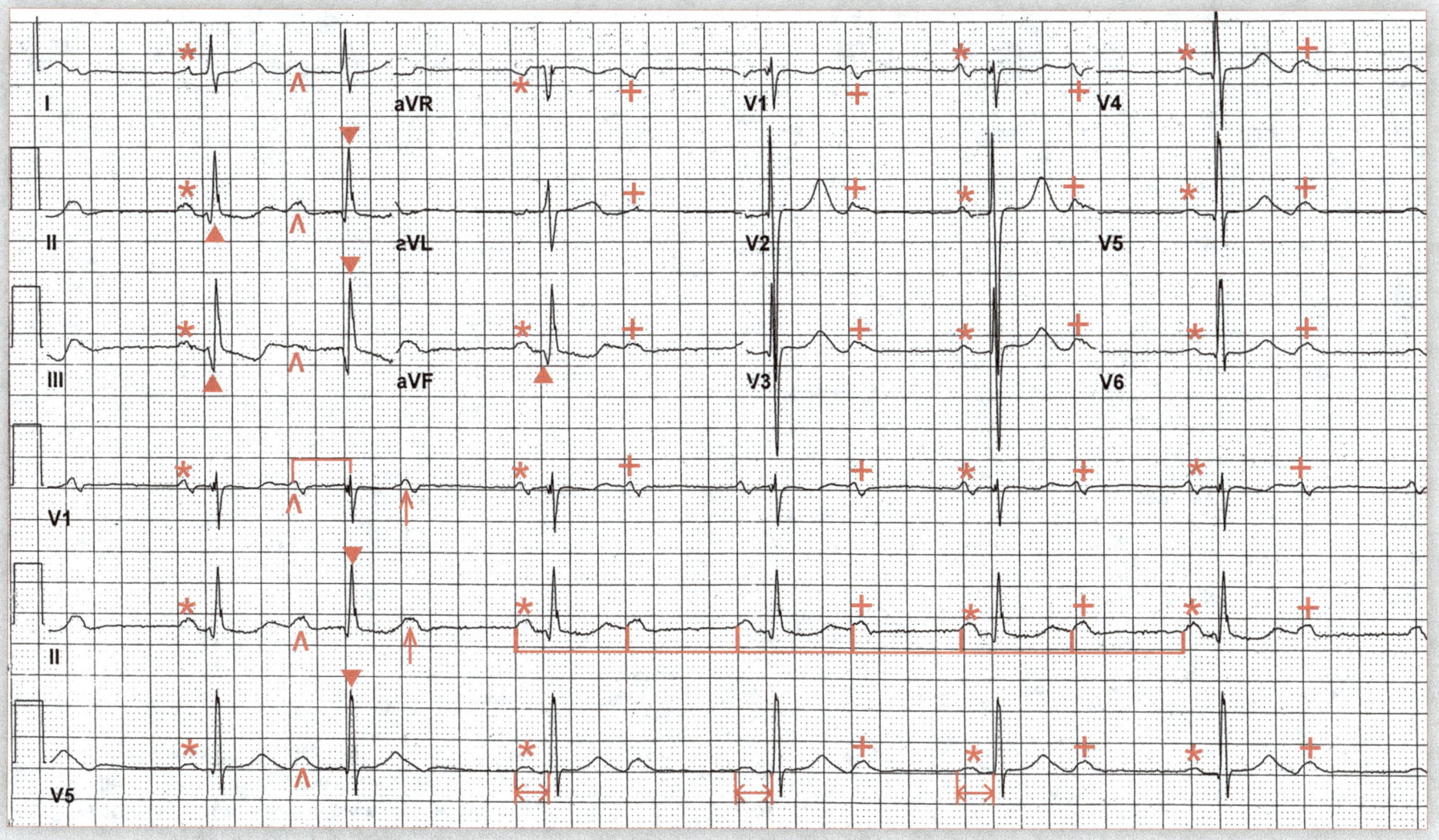

ECG 10 Analysis: Sinus rhythm, first-degree AV block (prolonged AV conduction), Mobitz type I second-degree AV block (Wenckebach) with 2:1 and 3:2 AV conduction, old inferior wall MI

The rhythm is regularly irregular as a result of one shorter RR interval (between the first and second QRS complexes). P waves (*) can be seen before each QRS complex. The PR interval (↔) is stable (0.26 sec); hence there is first-degree AV block (prolonged AV conduction). In addition, nonconducted P waves (+) can be seen after each QRS complex. The P waves are positive in leads I, II, aVF, and V4-V6. The PP interval is constant (⊔), and thus there is a normal sinus rhythm at a rate of 80 bpm. There is a pattern of 2:1 AV block with a stable ventricular rate of 40 bpm. However, it can be seen that the second QRS complex is early (▼) and it is preceded by a P wave (^). However, the PR interval (⊓) is longer (0.40 sec) than the baseline PR interval (0.26 sec) (↔). The on-time sinus P wave after the second QRS complex is nonconducted (↑). This is a pattern of Mobitz type I second-degree AV block (Wenckebach) with 3:2 AV conduction. Thereafter, there is a pattern of second-degree AV block with 2:1 conduction. Since there initially was Mobitz type I, the 2:1 AV conduction is also Mobitz type I.

The QRS complex duration is normal (0.08 sec) and there is a normal axis, between 0° and +90° (positive QRS complex in leads I and aVF). There are Q waves (▲) in the inferior leads II, III, and aVF, indicating an old inferior wall myocardial infarction (MI). The QT/QTc intervals are normal (520/424 msec).

As this patient is without symptoms, there is no reason for any therapy. The Wenckebach is the result of abnormalities in AV nodal conduction, possibly resulting from the old inferior wall MI. ■

An 18-year-old man with a history of an unspecified cardiomyopathy affecting only the men in his family presents to the emergency department with lightheadedness. He states that he has had on-and-off lightheadedness without frank syncope over the past month. Today, he noted its abrupt onset while having breakfast. The symptoms persisted long enough to cause concern. His review of systems is otherwise notable for an inability to keep up with his teammates on the track and field team over the past several months.

ECG 11A

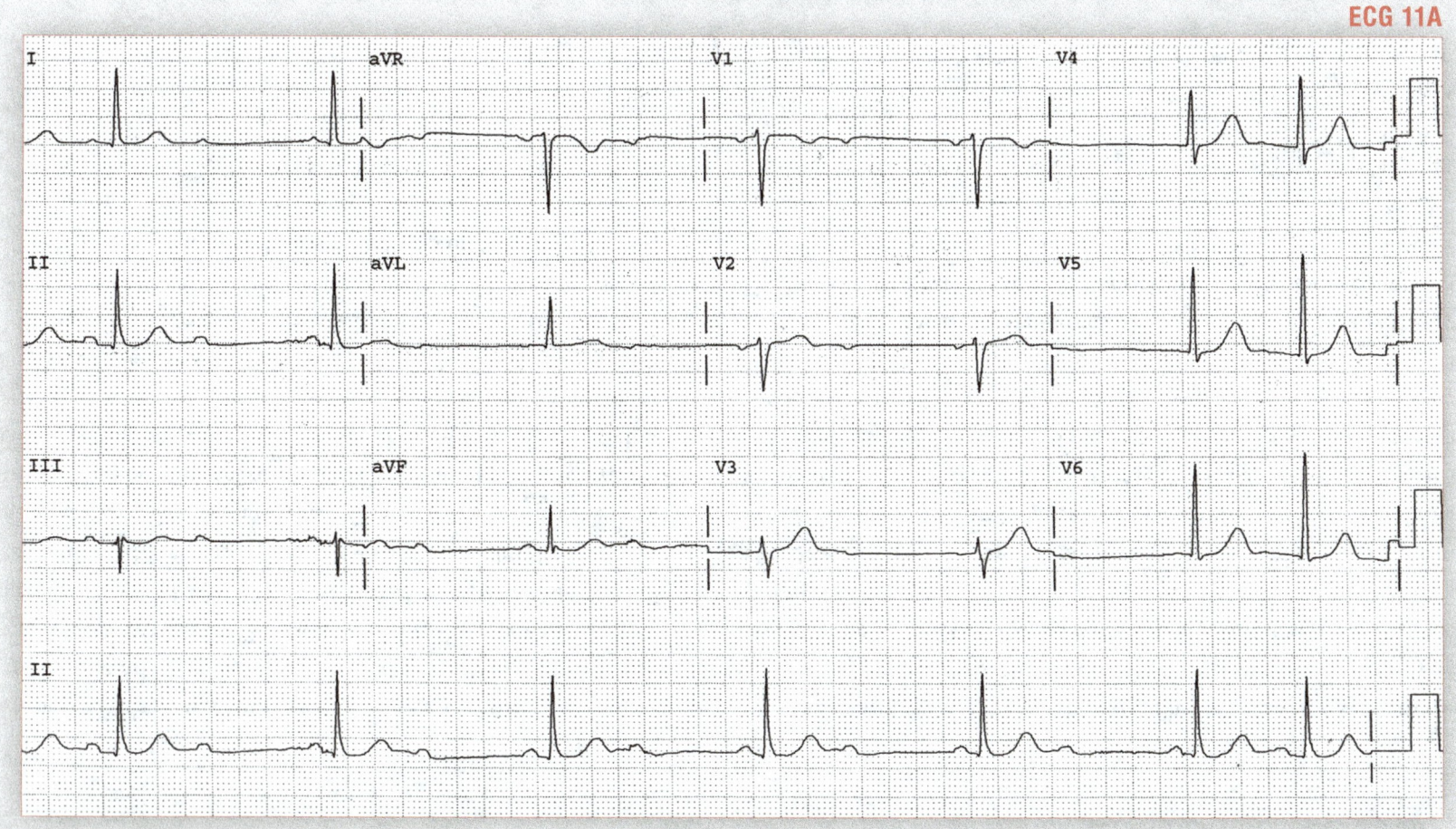

On exam, the man's vital signs include a radial pulse of 40 bpm and a blood pressure of 122/84 mm Hg. His overall appearance is normal. His head, ears, nose, and throat exam and neck exam are normal. His lung fields are clear. Jugular venous pressure is 5 cm H_2O. His cardiac exam displays a normal point of maximal impulse and normal cardiac sounds without a gallop or murmur. His abdominal, extremity, and neurologic exams are normal. An ECG is obtained (11A), and the man is admitted to the hospital. On the following day, a second ECG is obtained (11B).

What is the cause of the patient's symptoms?

What further workup is warranted?

What therapy is indicated?

ECG 11B

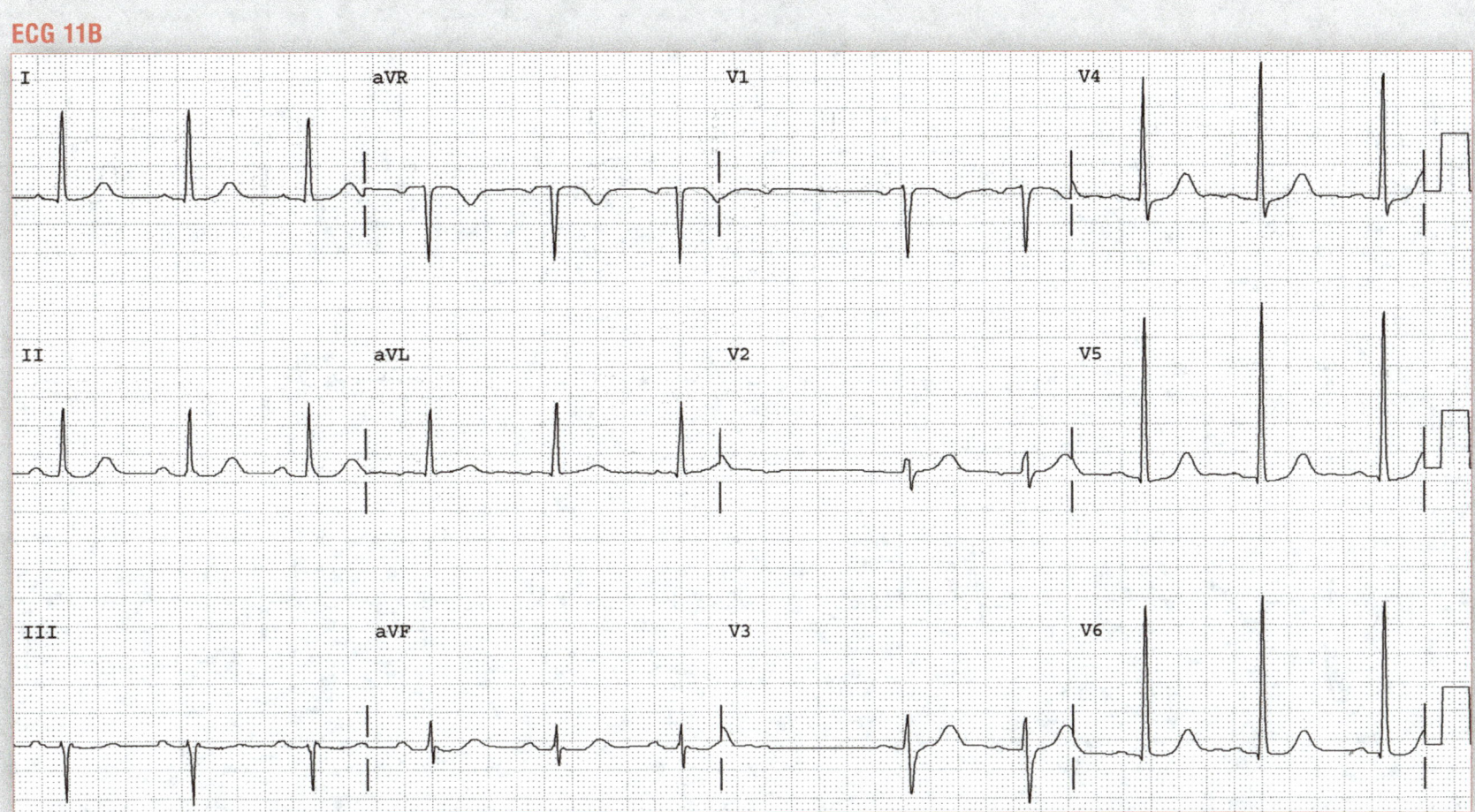

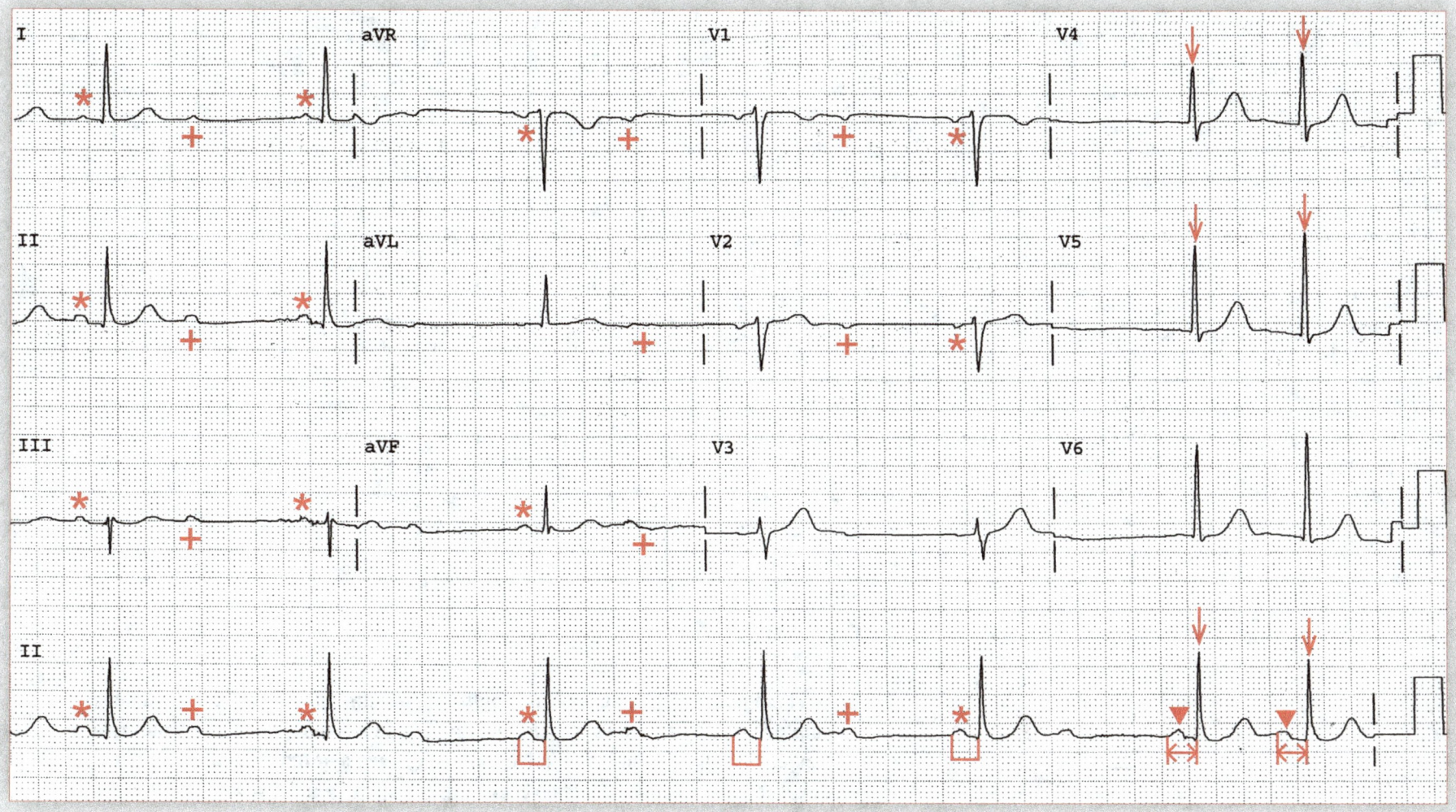

ECG 11A Analysis: Normal sinus rhythm, second-degree AV block with 2:1 AV conduction, Mobitz type II second-degree AV block

In **ECG 11A**, the ventricular rate is regular at 38 bpm; however, the last two QRS complexes (↓) are at a rate of 76 bpm. The QRS complex duration is normal (0.08 sec) with a normal morphology and axis, between 0° and +90° (positive QRS complex in leads I and aVF). The QT/QTc intervals are normal (440/350 msec). There are P waves (*/+) occurring at a regular interval at a rate of 76 bpm. The P waves are positive in leads I, II, aVF, and V4-V6; hence this is a normal sinus rhythm. There is a P wave (*) before each QRS complex. However, every other P wave is nonconducted (+) and there is a pattern of second-degree AV block with 2:1 AV conduction. The PR interval is stable at 0.20 second (⊔). Hence this can be either Mobitz type I or II. The last two QRS complexes (↓), at a rate of 76 bpm, have P waves (▼) before them and show intact AV conduction with a stable PR interval of 0.20 second (↔). Hence the 2:1 AV block is Mobitz type II as the two sequential complexes that are conducted have the same PR interval.

continues

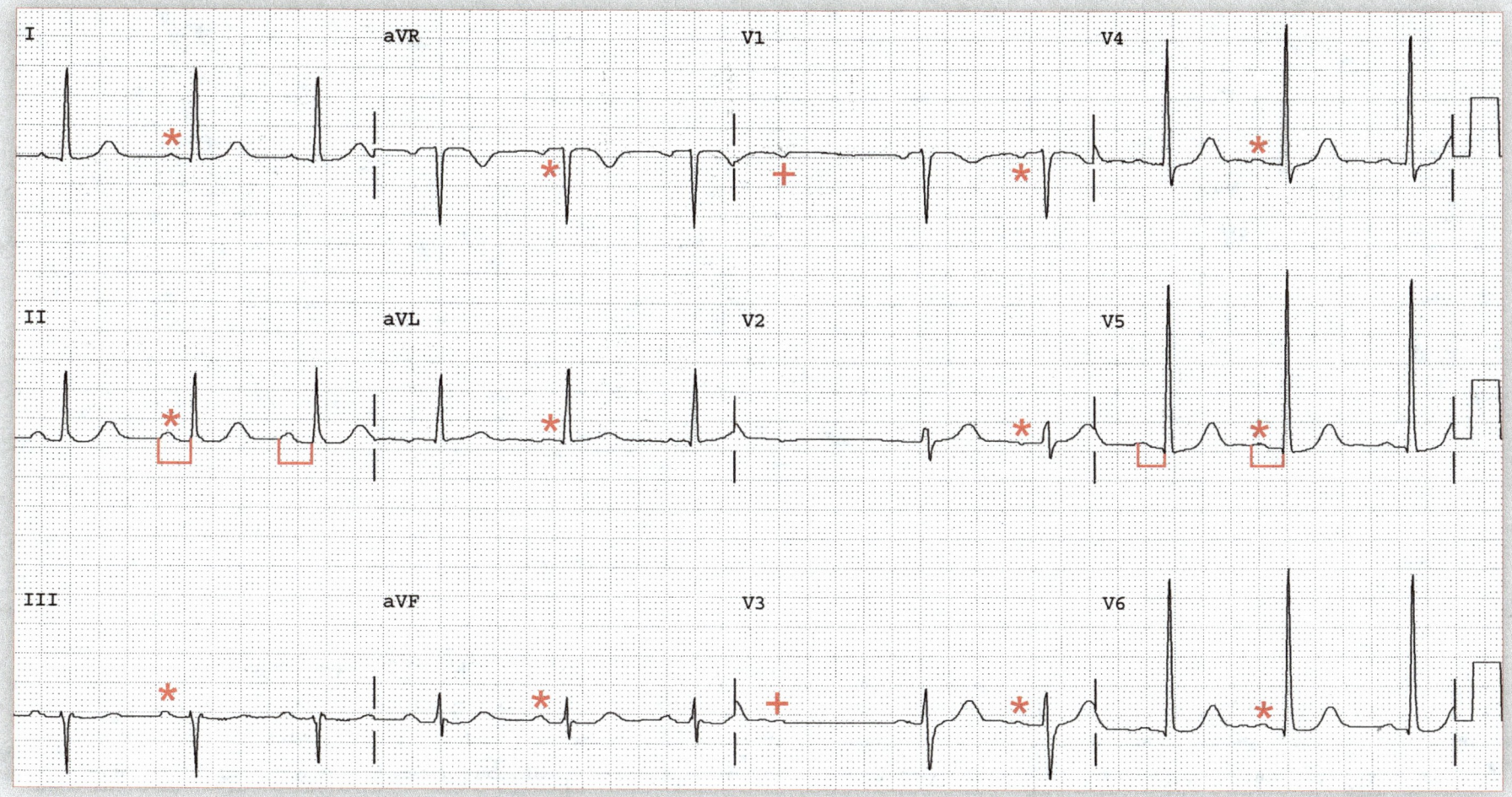

ECG 11B Analysis: Normal sinus rhythm, Mobitz type II second-degree AV block

ECG 11B is obtained the following day. The QRS duration, morphology, and axis are the same as in ECG 11A. Noted are a stable rhythm at a rate of 70 bpm and a P wave (*) before each QRS complex. The P wave is positive in leads I, II, aVF, and V4-V6. Hence this is a sinus rhythm. The PR intervals are stable at 0.20 second (⊔). There is one on-time sinus P wave (+) that is nonconducted. Hence this is second-degree AV block. As the PR intervals are constant, this is Mobitz type II block and confirms the presence of Mobitz type II block on ECG 11A.

It is likely that this patient is manifesting pathology attributable to a familial, X-linked conduction system disease. Although the patient does not have signs of global left ventricular dysfunction, an echocardiogram is warranted to confirm the physical exam findings. Pacemaker implantation is warranted based on Mobitz type II block that is symptomatic. ■

Core Case 12

A 48-year-old man with a recent anterior wall myocardial infarction treated with a stent presents for routine follow-up. He was placed on standard post-infarction medical therapy, and his recovery has been unremarkable. Echocardiography shows that left ventricular function has been preserved. He states that other than some mild fatigue, he feels well, can exercise without limitation, and is free of dyspnea and angina.

ECG 12A

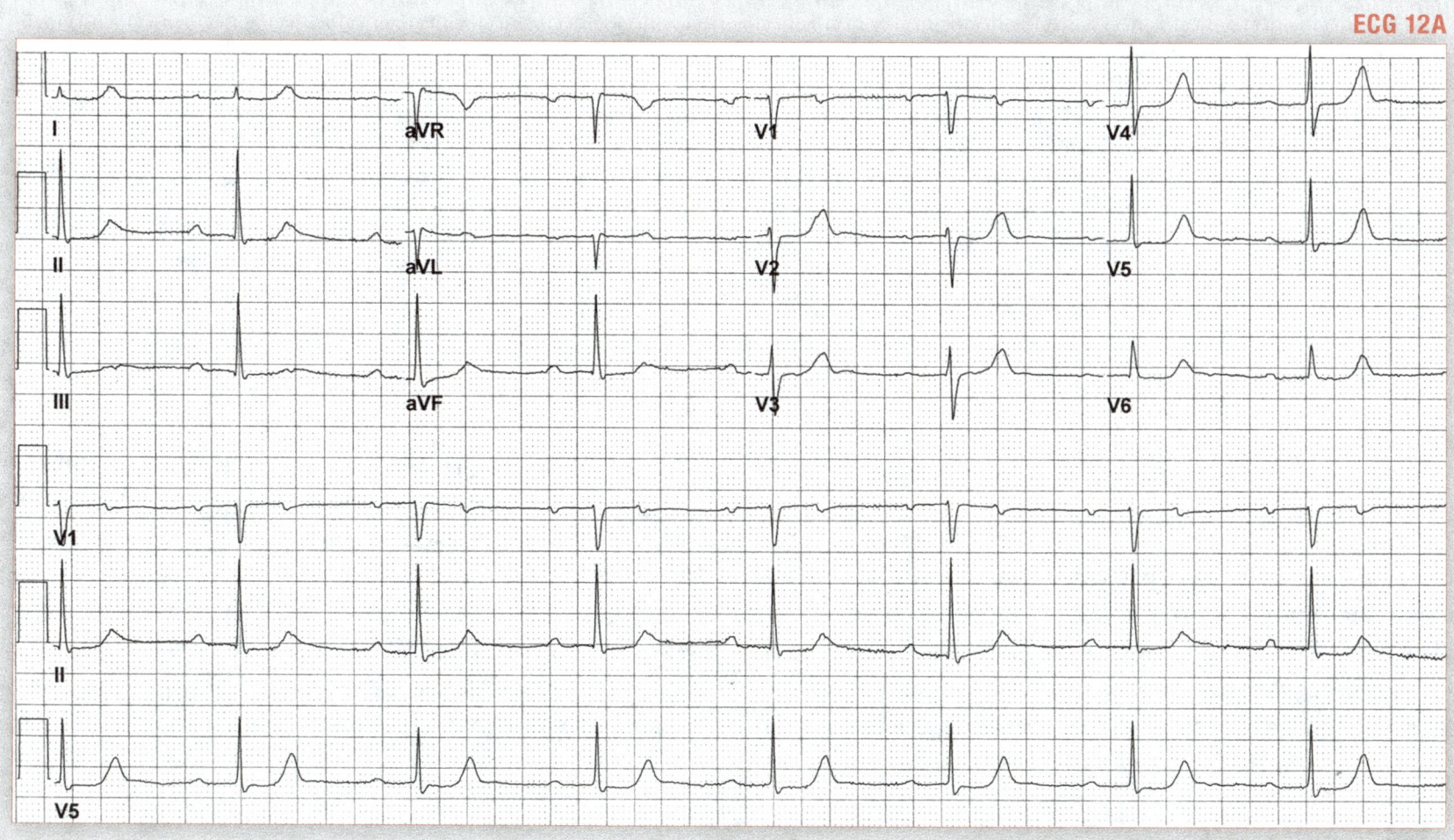

On review of systems, he notes symptoms consistent with erectile dysfunction since the event. His medical therapy includes dual antiplatelet therapy with aspirin and clopidogrel, a high-dose β-blocker, and a statin.

A routine ECG is obtained (12A). When the patient presents the following day to an urgent care clinic with complaints of fatigue and some lightheadedness, a second ECG is obtained (ECG 12B).

What abnormalities are notable, if any, on ECG 12A?

What abnormalities are notable on ECG 12B?

What is the likely cause?

ECG 12B

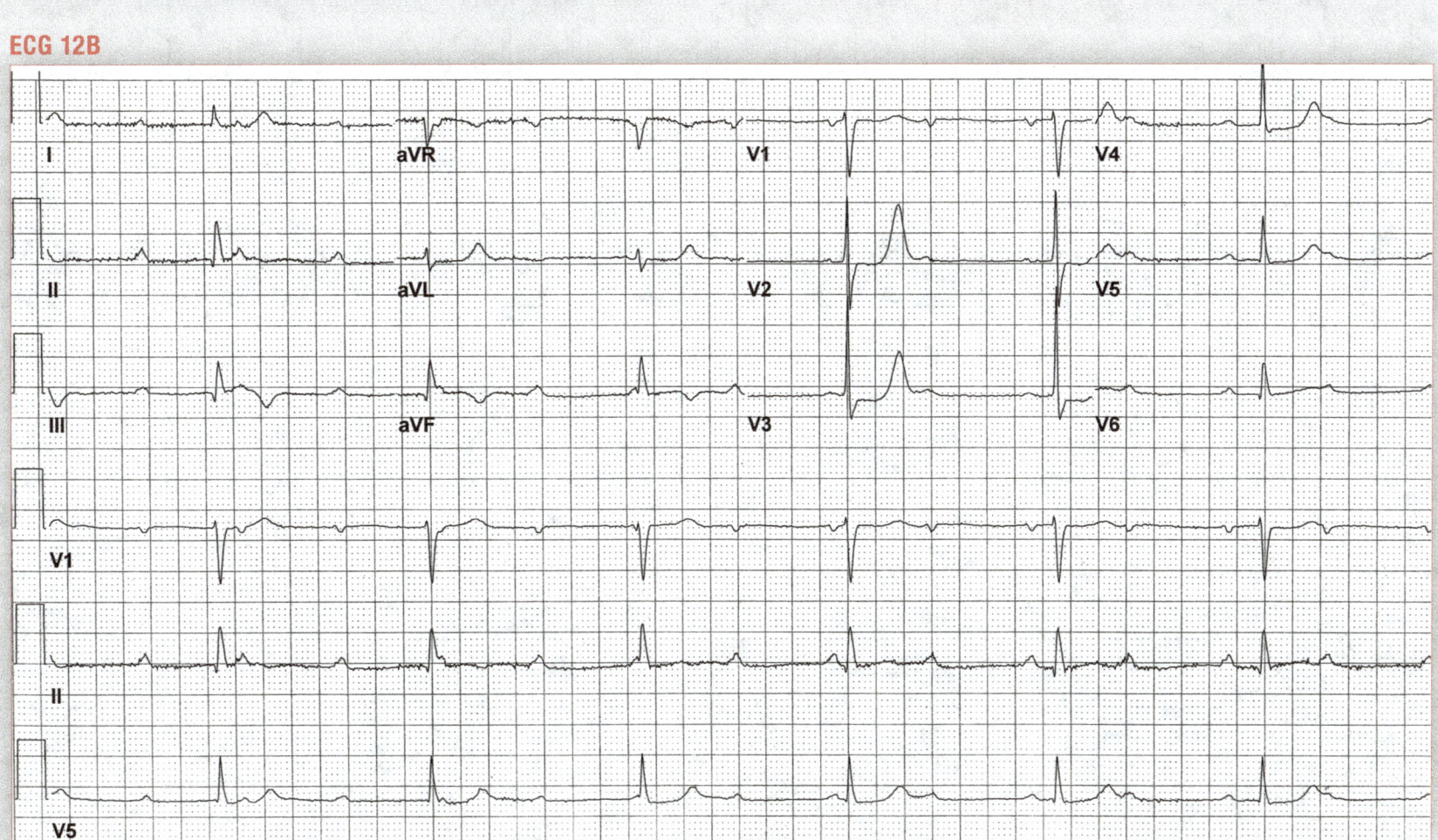

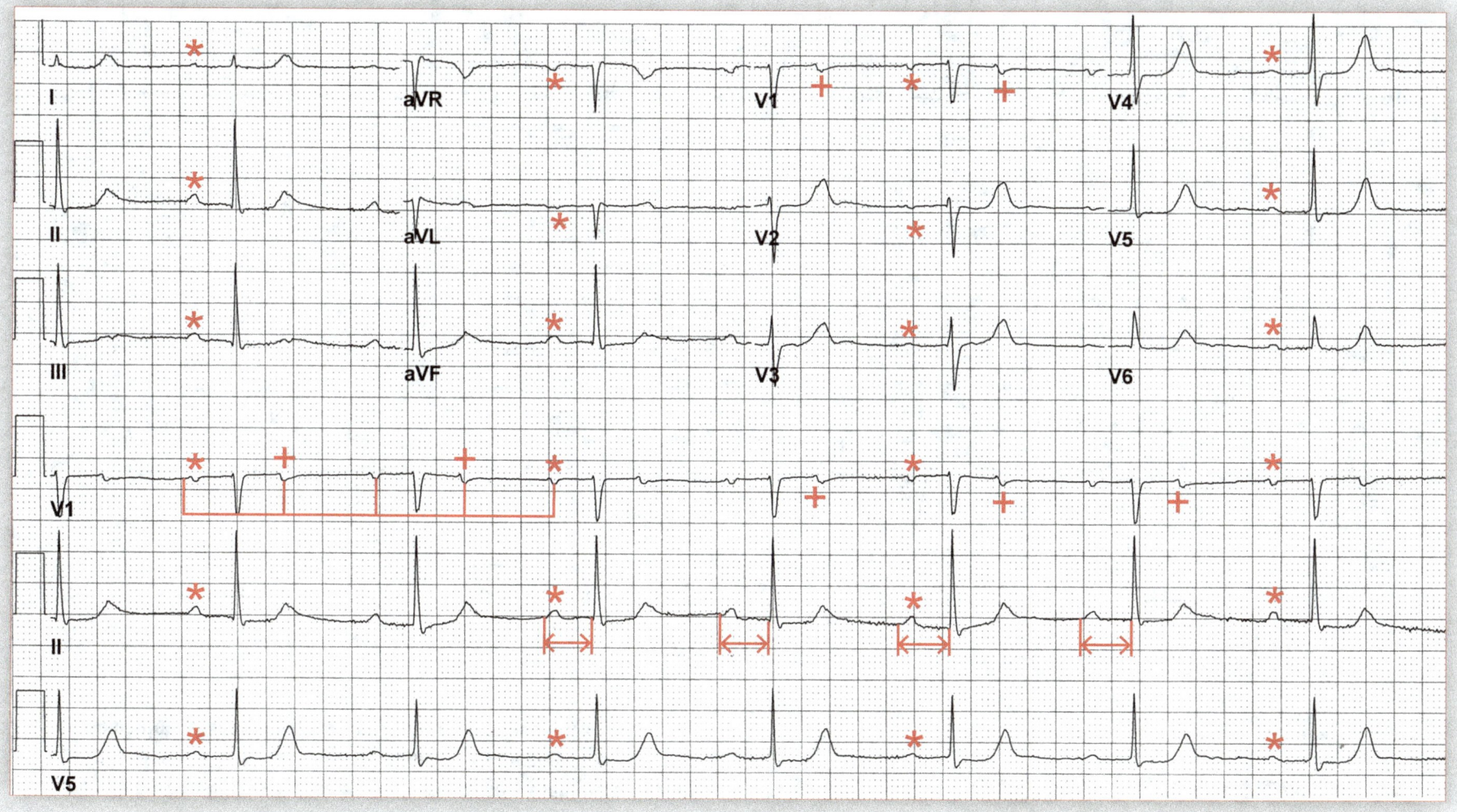

ECG 12A Analysis: Normal sinus rhythm, first-degree AV block, 2:1 second-degree AV block

ECG 12A shows is a regular rhythm at a rate of 48 bpm. There is a P wave (*) before each QRS complex with a stable PR interval (↔) (0.32 sec). The P wave is positive in leads I, II, aVF, and V4-V6. Hence there is a sinus rhythm with first-degree AV block (prolonged AV conduction). It is noted in lead V1 that there is a second P wave (+) that is nonconducted. The PP interval is constant (⊔), with an atrial rate of 96 bpm, and there is a pattern of 2:1 AV conduction. Hence there is a normal sinus rhythm with second-degree AV block and a pattern of 2:1 AV conduction in addition to first-degree AV block. This may be Mobitz type I or II. The QRS complex duration is normal (0.08 sec) and there is a normal morphology and axis, between 0° and +90° (positive QRS complex in leads I and aVF). The QT/QTc intervals are normal (490/435 msec).

continues

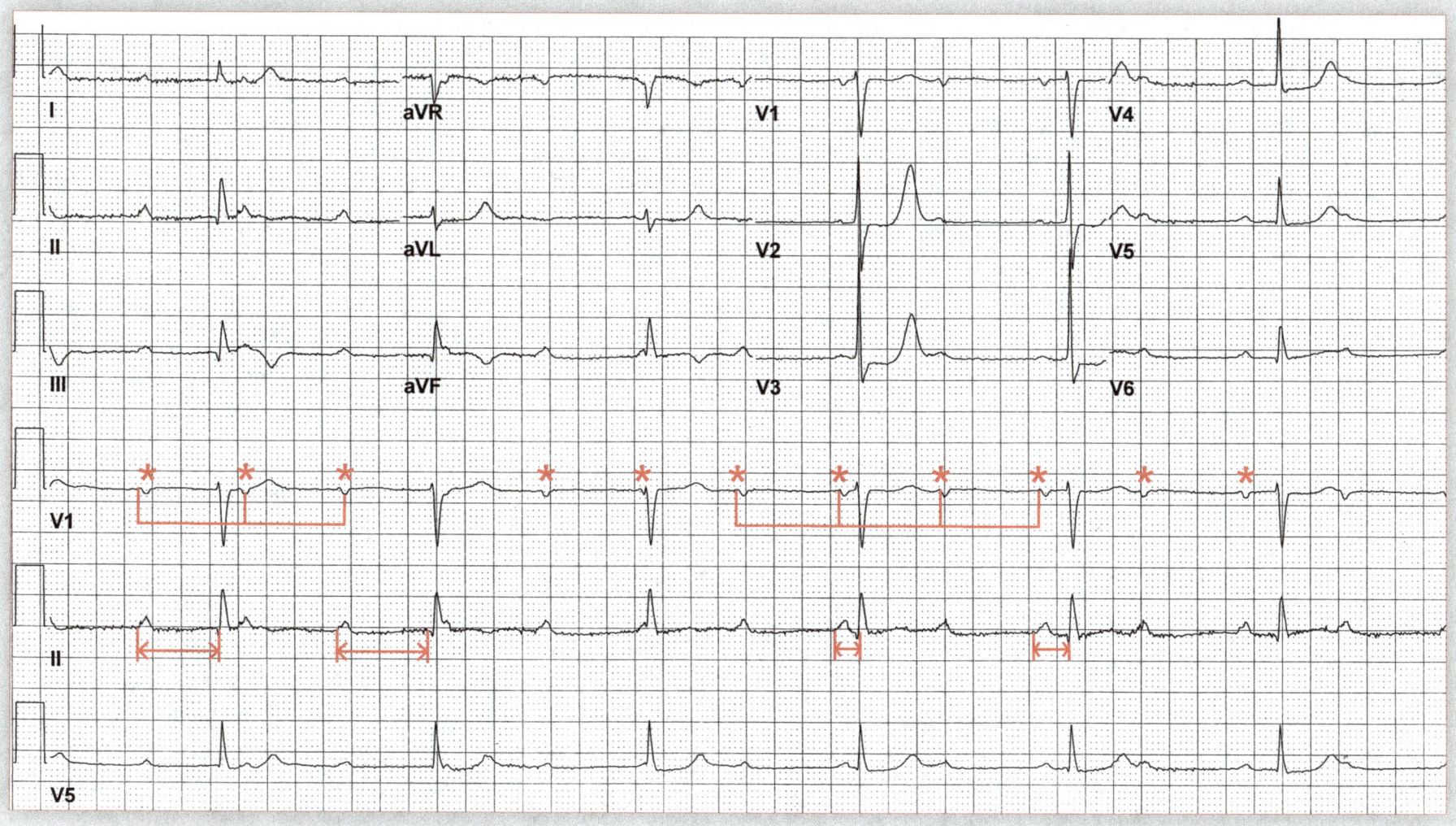

ECG 12B Analysis: Normal sinus rhythm, complete heart block with a junctional escape rhythm

ECG 12B shows regular QRS complexes at a rate of 40 bpm. The QRS complexes have a morphology, axis, and QT/QTc intervals that resemble those in **ECG 12A**. The atrial rate is regular (⊔) at 86 bpm, and the P waves (*) are positive in leads I, II, aVF, and V4-V6. Hence there is an underlying normal sinus rhythm. The PR interval (↔) is very variable, indicating AV dissociation. The presence of AV dissociation with an atrial rate that is faster than the ventricular rate indicates complete heart block. In contrast, an atrial rate that is slower than the ventricular rate would indicate an accelerated lower focus (*ie,* accelerated junctional or ventricular rhythm). The escape rhythm has a narrow QRS complex that is similar to the QRS complex in **ECG 12A**. Hence the escape rhythm is junctional. The escape rhythm is determined by the QRS morphology and not the heart rate. The fact that with the development of complete heart block the escape rhythm is junctional means that the 2:1 AV conduction seen in **ECG 12A** is Mobitz type I.

Complete heart block is manifest by AV dissociation (*ie,* there is no association between P waves and QRS complexes and the PR intervals are variable). The atrial rate is faster than the rate of the QRS complexes. The escape rhythm may be junctional or ventricular; the location of the escape rhythm is based on QRS morphology and not rate.

The patient is manifesting multiple symptoms of an excess β-blocker effect (fatigue, erectile dysfunction, and AV block). High doses of agents that prolong the normal, physiologic AV delay, such as digoxin, β-blockers, and calcium-channel blockers, may precipitate symptomatic AV block (second or third degree). The patient's infra-Hisian conduction system appears intact as he manifests a junctional escape rhythm when in complete heart block. Hospital admission for β-blocker washout and controlled re-institution of a low-dose β-blocker is a reasonable course of action at this time. ■

A 72-year-old homeless Korean War veteran is admitted to the Veterans Administration hospital with an episode of syncope. It is clear from his electronic record that he has obtained no medical care since his honorable discharge from the service. He is awake, alert, oriented, and conversant on admission. He denies any prodrome to the episode and is

ECG 13A

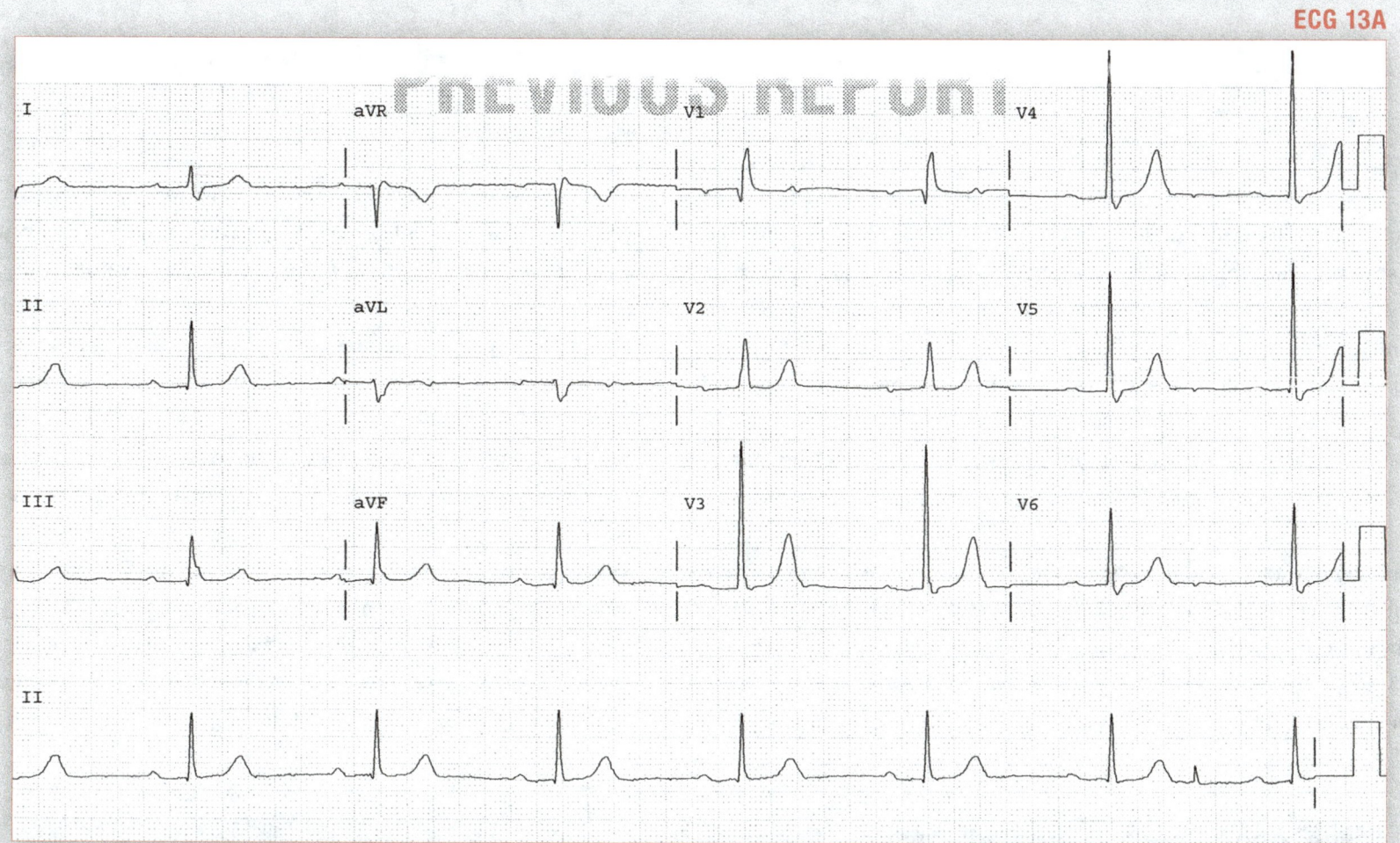

asymptomatic at present. His vital signs are notable for a heart rate of 42 bpm and a blood pressure of 170/90 mm Hg. An ECG is obtained (13A). The next morning, he has a witnessed episode of syncope. Again, no prodrome was evident, and he recovers consciousness spontaneously after a few seconds. The nurse quickly obtains an ECG (13B).

What abnormalities are depicted?

How does the ECG immediately after his syncopal event inform you of the mechanism and point to the necessary therapy?

ECG 13B

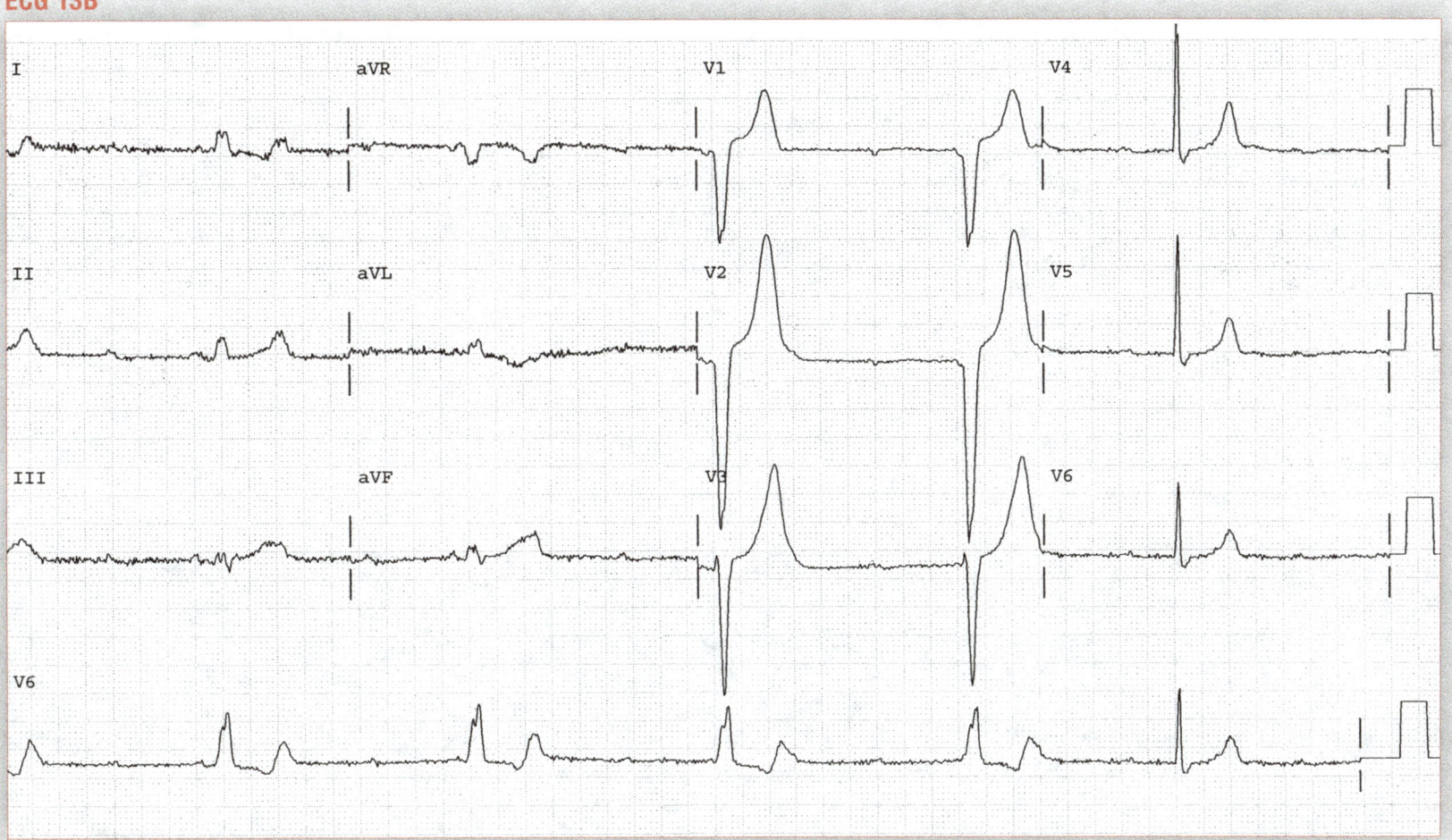

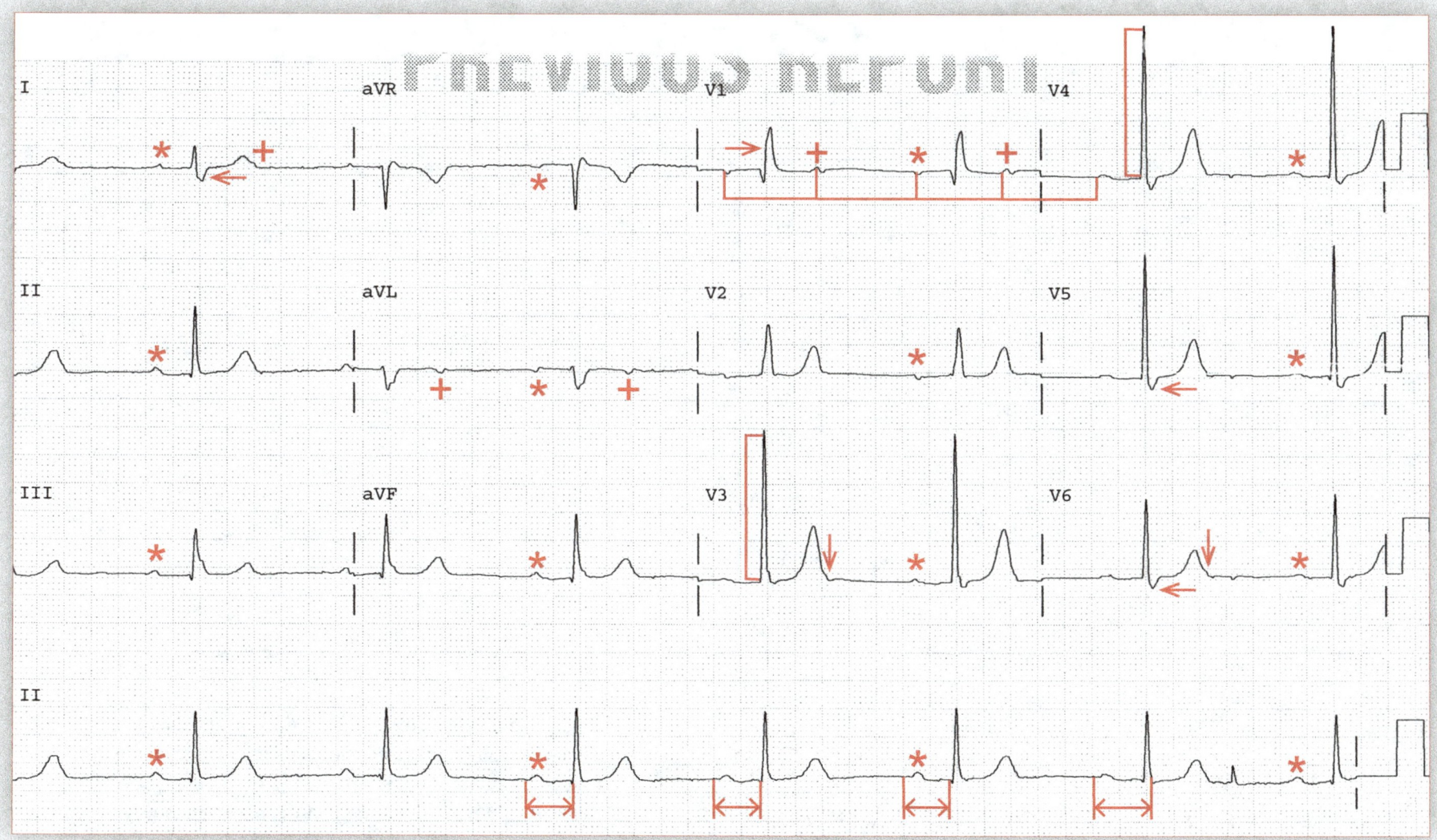

ECG 13A Analysis: Sinus bradycardia, first-degree AV block (prolonged AV conduction), second-degree AV block with 2:1 conduction, right bundle branch block, left ventricular hypertrophy

In **ECG 13A**, there is a regular rhythm at a ventricular rate of 42 bpm. There is a P wave (*) before each QRS complex with a stable PR interval of 0.32 second (↔) (*ie*, first-degree AV block or prolonged AV conduction). There is a second nonconducted, on-time sinus P wave (+), best seen in leads I (at the end of the T wave), aVL, and V1. T waves should be smooth in upstroke and downstroke. Any notching or bump on the T wave is suspicious for a superimposed P wave. This can be seen in leads V3 and V6 (↓), for example. The PP intervals are regular (⊔) at an atrial rate of 84 bpm. The P waves are positive in leads I, II, aVF, and V4-V6. Hence there is a sinus rhythm with first-degree AV block as well as second-degree AV block with 2:1 AV conduction. The QRS complexes are wide (0.14 sec) with a right bundle branch block pattern (RSR′ morphology in lead V1 [→] and broad S wave in leads I and V5-V6 [←]). The axis is normal, between 0° and +90° (positive QRS complex in leads I and aVF). The tall QRS amplitude in leads V3-V4 (27 mm) ([ ) meets the criteria for left ventricular hypertrophy (R-wave amplitude or S-wave depth in any precordial lead ≥ 25 mm). The QT/QTc intervals are normal (520/435 msec and 480/400 msec when the prolonged QRS complex duration is considered).

continues

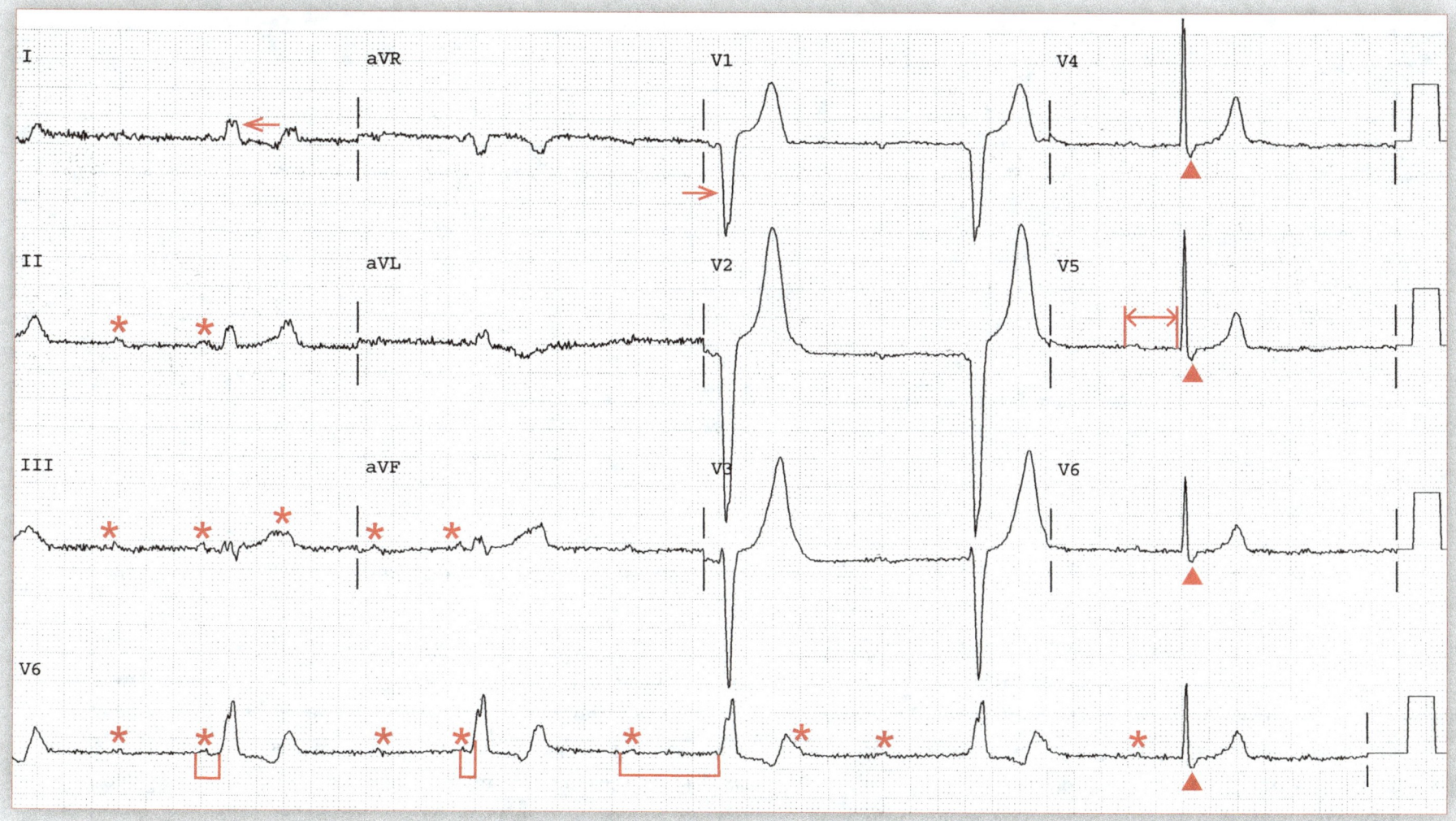

ECG 13B Analysis: Complete heart block with ventricular escape rhythm with a
left bundle branch block morphology and intermittent capture (AV conduction)

In **ECG 13B**, there is a regular rhythm at a rate of 42 bpm. There are regular P waves (*) at an atrial rate of 98 bpm. Some of the P waves are not obvious as they are within the QRS complex. However, when seen, the P waves are regular with a stable rate. The P waves are positive in leads I, II, aVF, and V4-V6. Hence there is an underlying sinus rhythm. The PR intervals are variable (⊔) and therefore dissociated from the QRS intervals (AV dissociation). An atrial rate that is faster than the ventricular rate with AV dissociation is diagnostic for complete or third-degree AV block. The QRS complexes are wide (0.16 sec) with a left bundle branch block morphology (*ie*, QS complex in lead V1 [→] and a tall R wave in lead I [←]). Moreover, the QRS complexes in **ECG 13B** are very different from those in **ECG 13A**, which have a right bundle branch block pattern. Therefore, the QRS complexes in this ECG are ventricular (*ie*, there is a ventricular escape rhythm). The last QRS complex (▲) is different and has a PR interval of 0.32 second (↔) and right bundle branch pattern, similar to the QRS complexes and PR intervals seen in **ECG 13A**; this complex is conducted. Therefore, this is complete heart block with an escape ventricular rhythm and intermittent capture. The presence of a ventricular escape rhythm means that the 2:1 AV conduction seen in **ECG 13A** is Mobitz type II and that the conduction abnormality is within the His-Purkinje system. Mobitz type II second-degree heart block as well as complete heart block with a clear relationship to symptoms of syncope is a definitive indication for permanent pacemaker implantation. ◼

Notes

A 52-year-old man is in the cardiac catheterization laboratory undergoing percutaneous coronary intervention for acute myocardial infarction. His presentation was typical, with marked substernal chest pressure and diaphoresis prompting activation of emergency medical services. Diagnosis and immediate catheterization laboratory referral were based on his history and the appearance of a left bundle branch block pattern on his index ECG; it was uncertain whether this pattern was new or predated his acute presentation. During the initial angioplasty of an occluded left anterior descending artery, the patient complains of severe lightheadedness. The ECG shown is representative of his rhythm at the time. His vital signs are notable for a heart rate of 46 bpm and a blood pressure of 88/46 mm Hg.

What abnormalities are depicted on the ECG?

What is the precise nature of the abnormality?

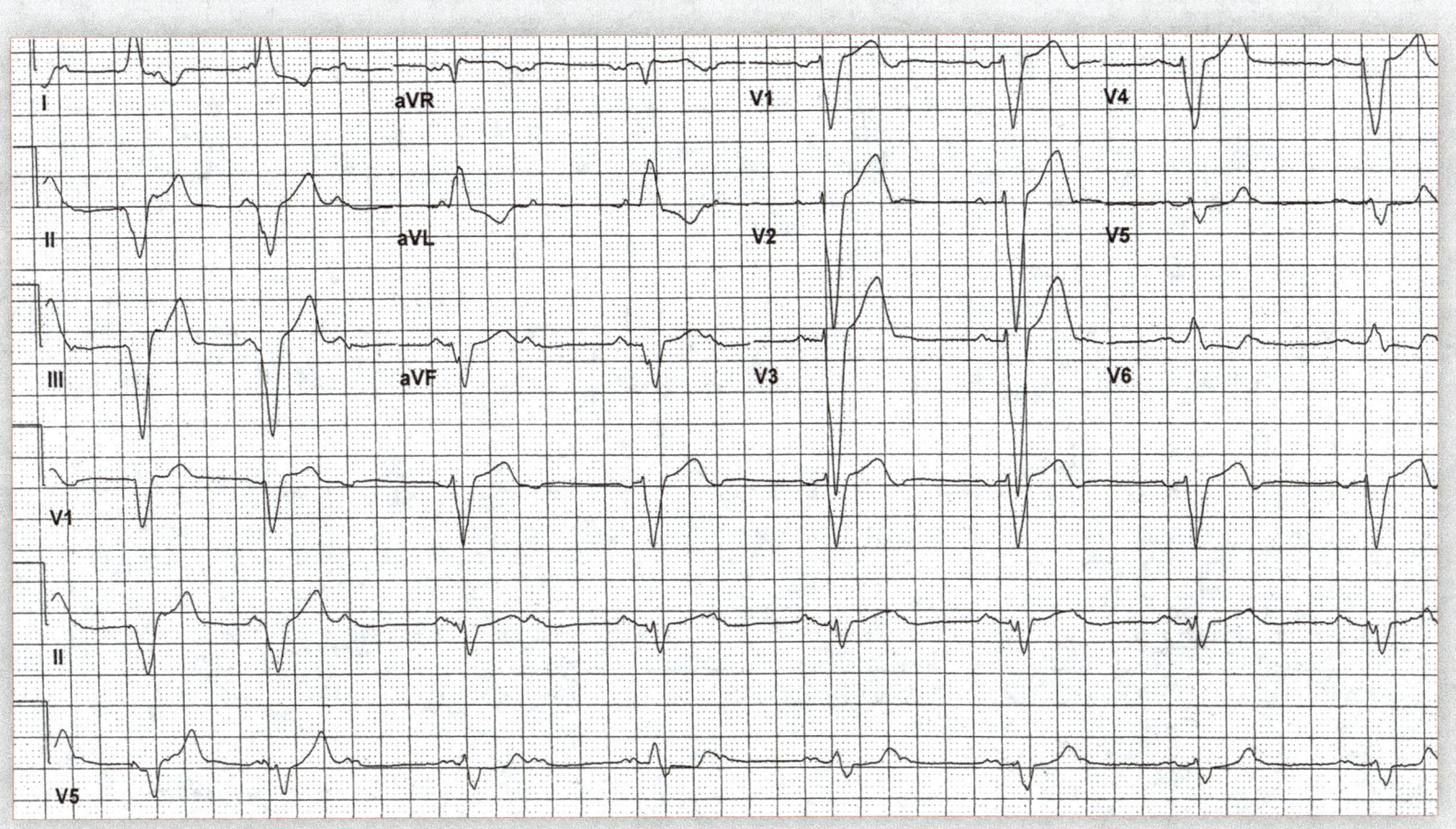

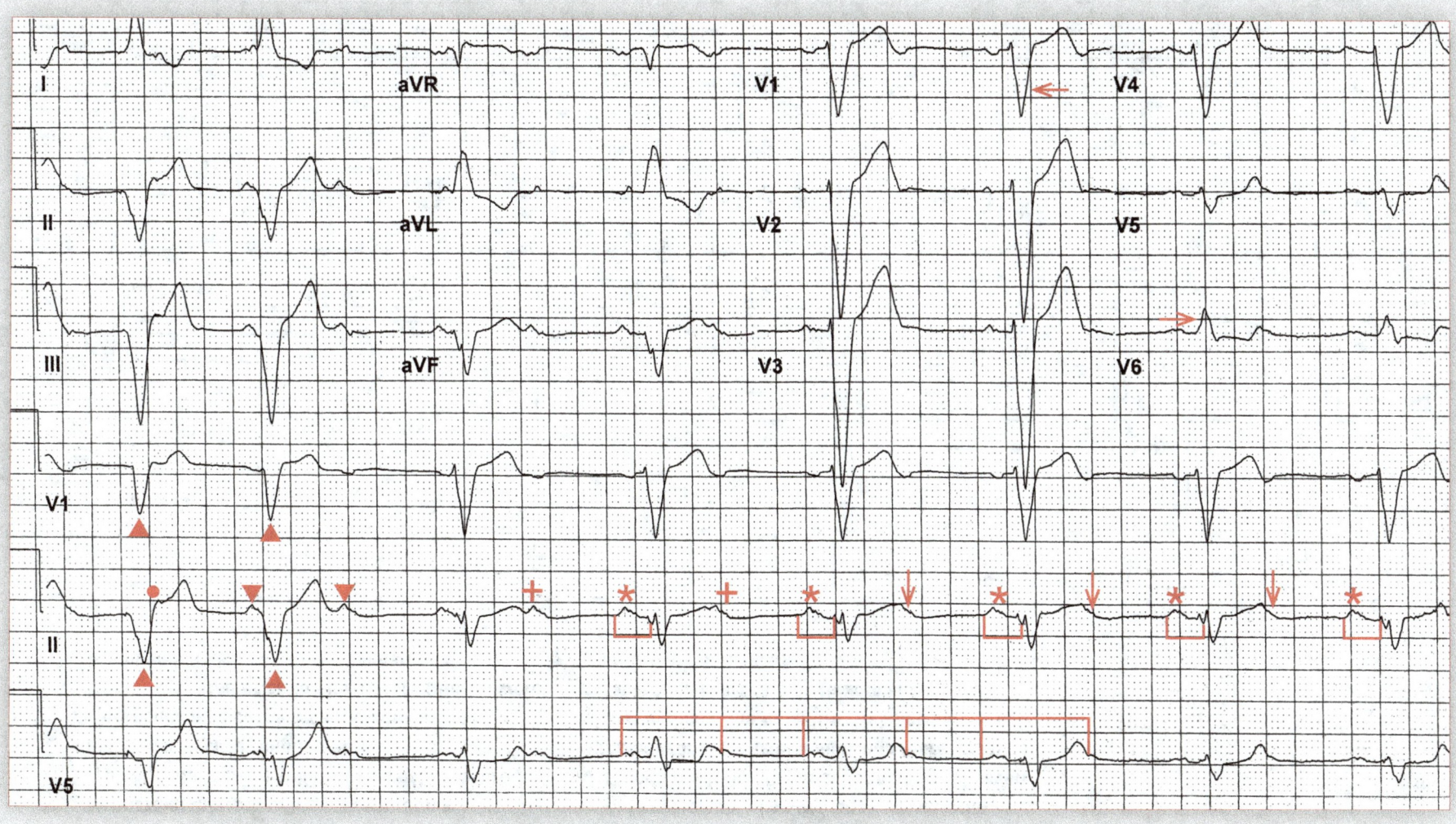

ECG 14 Analysis: Normal sinus rhythm, left bundle branch block, complete heart block with an escape ventricular rhythm, second-degree heart block with 2:1 conduction (2:1 AV block)

The first two QRS complexes (▲) have a rate of 64 bpm. Thereafter, the rhythm is regular at a ventricular rate of 46 bpm. There is a P wave (*) before each QRS complex with a stable PR interval (⊔) (0.16 sec). In addition, there is a second on-time P wave (+) after each QRS complex; these P waves are nonconducted. Occasionally this nonconducted P wave is seen at the end of the T wave, causing the downstroke of the T wave to have an irregular bump on it (↓). The PP intervals are regular (⊓), and the atrial rate is 92 bpm. The P waves are positive in leads I, II, aVF, and V4-V6. This is, therefore, a normal sinus rhythm with second-degree AV block and 2:1 AV conduction. The QRS complexes are wide (0.16 sec) and have a left bundle branch block pattern (deep S wave in lead V1 [←] and broad R wave in lead V6 [→]). The QT/QTc intervals are prolonged (520/460 msec) but are normal when the prolonged QRS complex duration is considered (440/390 msec).

The first two QRS complexes (▲) have a different morphology and rate (64 bpm). There are P waves noted (●,▼) at the same rate as the other P waves seen during 2:1 AV block (ie, 92 bpm). It can be seen that the morphology of the first QRS complex is slightly different than that of the second, as a result of a superimposed P wave at the end of the complex (●). However, there is no association between the P waves and the QRS complexes; hence AV dissociation is present. As the atrial rate is faster than the ventricular rate, this is a brief period of complete (third-degree) AV block with an escape ventricular rhythm. Following this there is second-degree heart block with 2:1 AV conduction that is the result of Mobitz type II due to block within the His-Purkinje system. This is established by the fact that with the development of complete AV block the escape rhythm is ventricular.

During an anterior wall myocardial infarction involving the septum, there may be significant injury to the infra-Hisian conduction system that can result in Mobitz type II second-degree AV block or complete AV block, the latter of which will be associated with a ventricular escape rhythm. When there is complete AV block, a temporary pacing electrode is often inserted for ventricular pacing. Although there may be some recovery of His-Purkinje conduction during the period after reperfusion, the fact that the patient has a left bundle branch block (which may be new or preexistent) that appears to be permanent would suggest that the septal damage is not reversible and the conduction abnormality within the His-Purkinje system will be permanent, requiring a permanent pacemaker. ■

Core Case 15

A 72-year-old man presents to an outpatient clinic for a routine physical exam. He has no complaints and does not admit to any previous cardiac problem. Except for an elevated blood pressure (170/90 mm Hg), his physical exam is normal. He is started on therapy with a β-blocker and hydrochlorothiazide. An ECG (15A) is obtained but not read.

ECG 15A

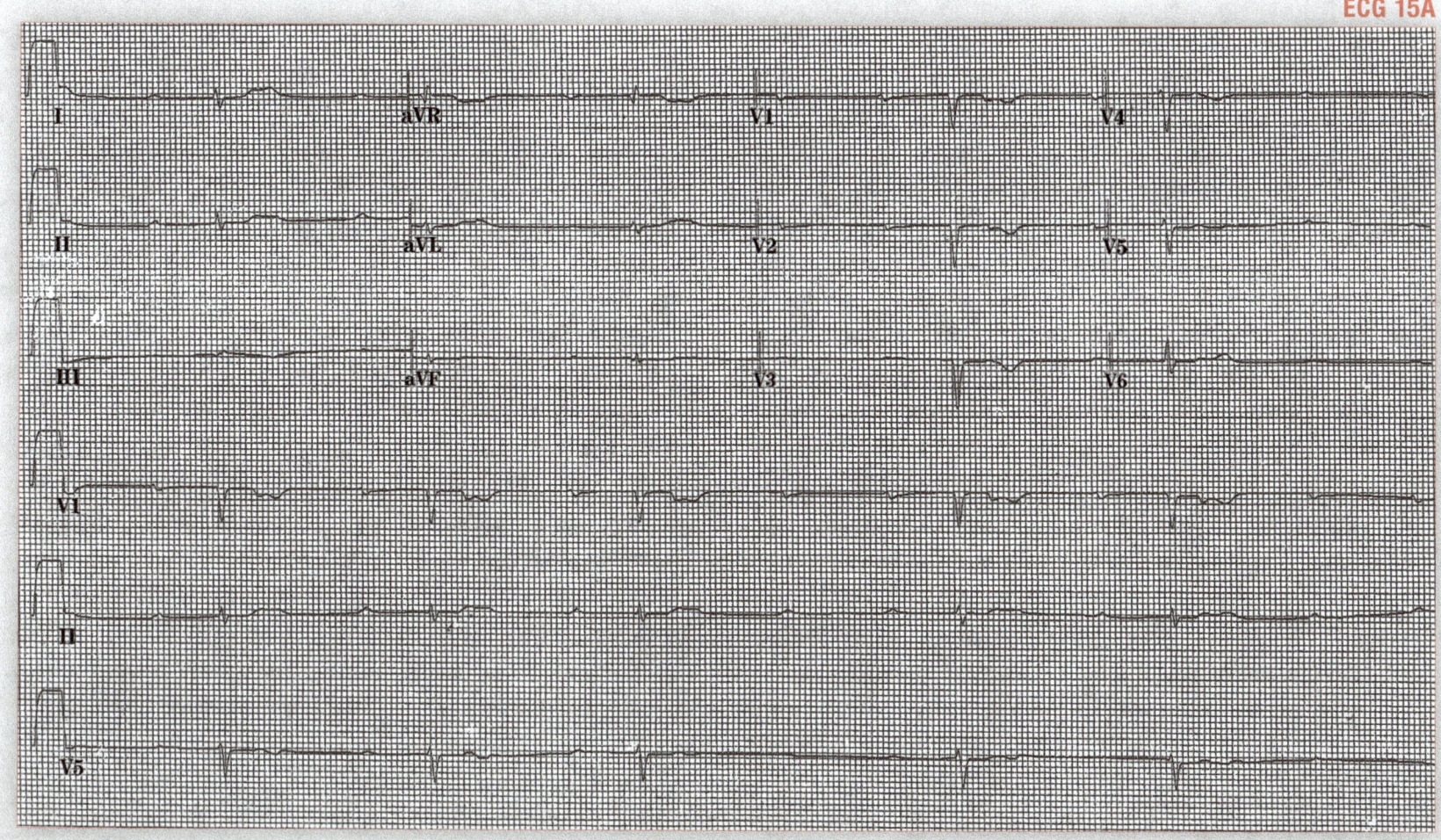

Two days later he presents to an emergency department with complaints of lightheadedness and a feeling that he might pass out, although he denies syncope. His physical exam is remarkable for a blood pressure of 140/80 mm Hg, although it appears to vary. His pulse rate is about 40 bpm. There are intermittent cannon A waves noted in his neck. An ECG (15B) is obtained.

What abnormalities can be seen on the ECGs?

Are the abnormalities related to each other?

Is there a relationship between the rhythm and the drug therapy that was prescribed?

ECG 15B

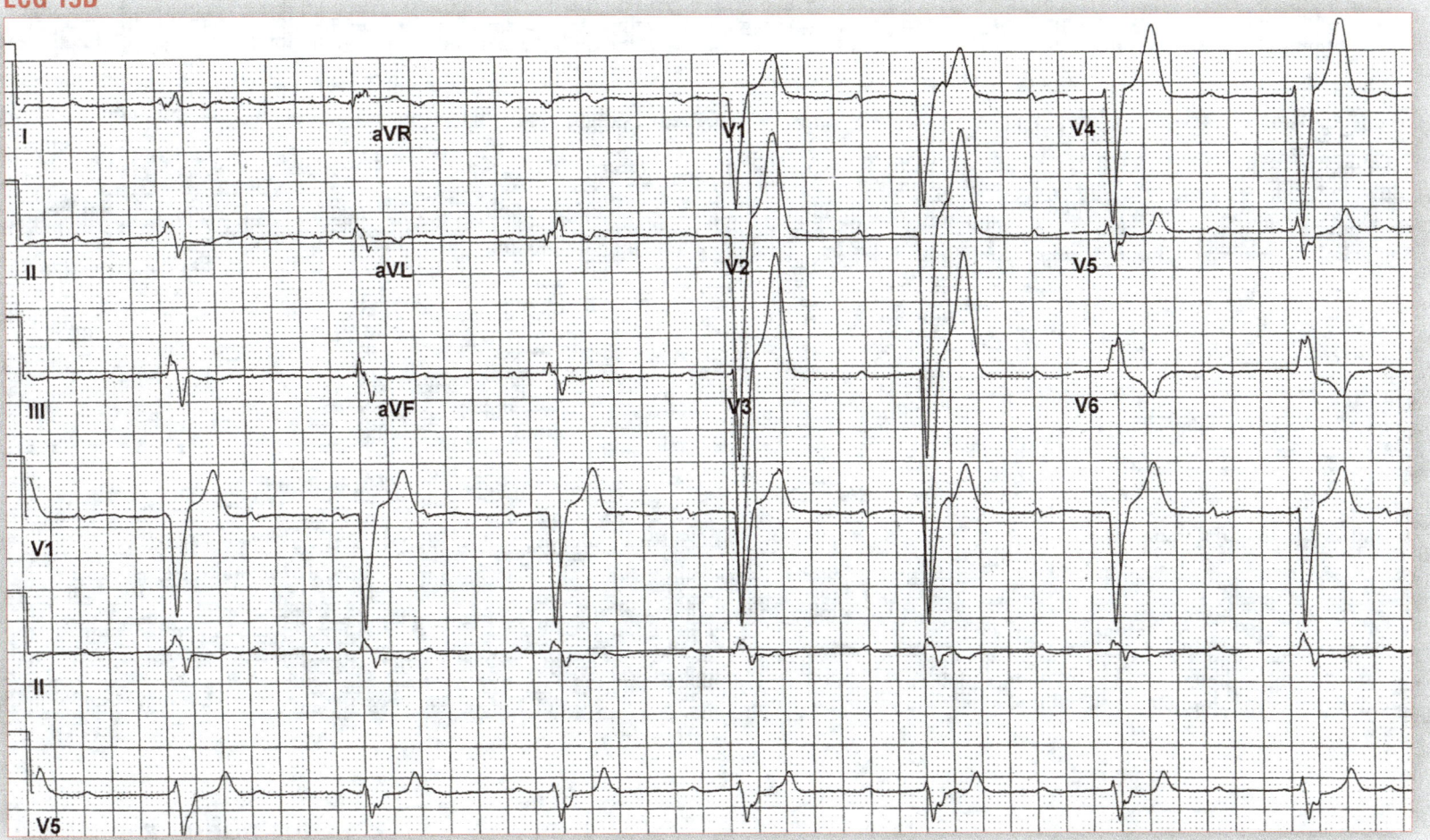

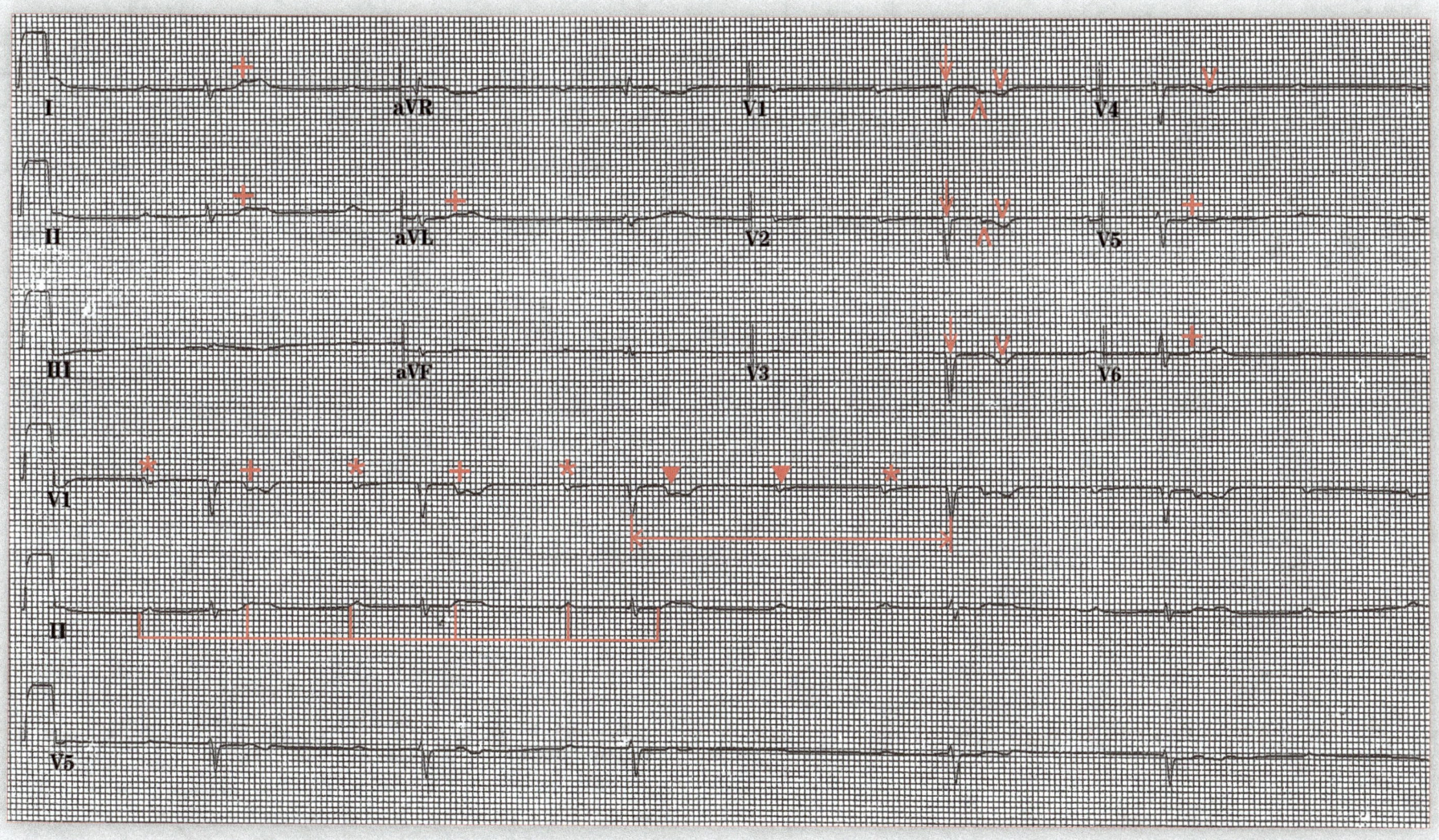

ECG 15A Analysis: Normal sinus rhythm, first-degree AV block
(prolonged AV conduction), Mobitz type II second-degree AV block,
high-grade AV block, old anterior wall myocardial infarction, low voltage

In **ECG 15A**, there is a regular rhythm with one long RR interval seen (↔). The ventricular rate is 42 bpm. There are P waves (*) before each QRS complex with a stable PR interval (0.48 sec), indicating first-degree AV block. A second P wave can be seen after each QRS complex (+); the P wave is within the T wave, best seen in leads V1-V2 (^). Normal T waves should be smooth in upstroke and downstroke. It can be seen that these T waves have a notching on the upstroke; this is apparent in leads I, II, aVL, and V6 (+). The PP intervals are constant (⊔), and the atrial rate is 84 bpm. Hence this is a normal sinus rhythm with first-degree AV block (prolonged AV conduction) and second-degree AV block with 2:1 AV conduction (or 2:1 AV block). There are two on-time but nonconducted P waves (▼) during the long RR interval (↔). With Mobitz type I there is only one nonconducted P wave at a time, while with Mobitz type II there may be more than one sequential nonconducted P wave. Hence this block is Mobitz type II, although it is often called high-grade AV block when more than one nonconducted P wave is seen.

The QRS complex duration is normal (0.08 sec), but there is low voltage (< 5 mm in each limb lead and < 10 mm in each precordial lead). The axis is probably normal, between 0° and +90°, although this is not certain as the QRS complex amplitude in lead aVF is very small. The QT/QTc intervals are normal (520/435 msec). There are QS complexes in leads V1-V3 (↓), consistent with an old anterior wall (anteroseptal) myocardial infarction (MI). The T waves are inverted in leads V1-V4 (∨); this is the result of the old MI.

continues

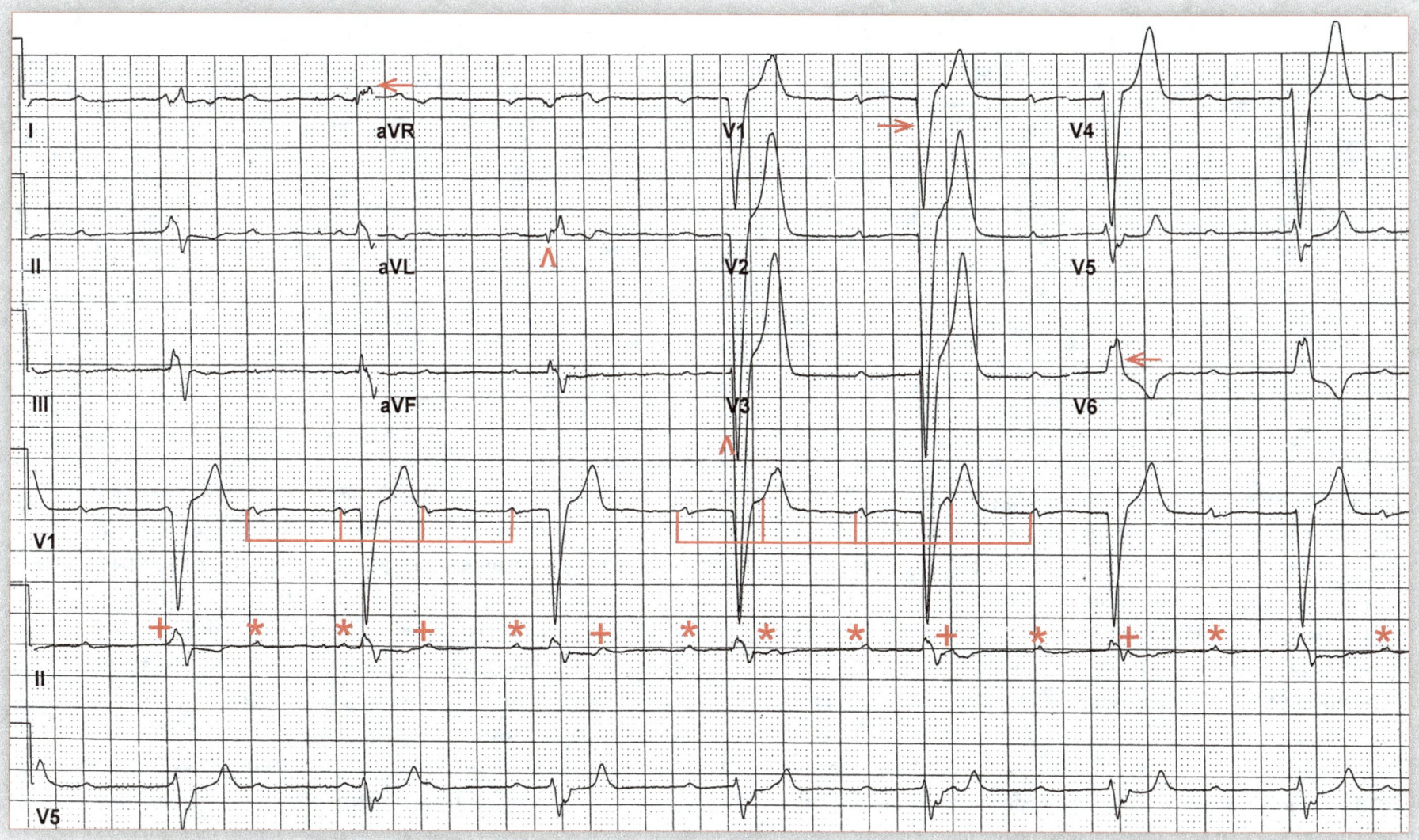

ECG 15B Analysis: Normal sinus rhythm,
complete heart block, escape ventricular rhythm

ECG 15B shows a regular rhythm at a rate of 46 bpm. P waves can be seen (*), although some of them are obscured by the QRS complex or are within T waves or ST segments (+). However, the PP interval (⊔) is constant and the atrial rate is 98 bpm. There is no relationship between the P waves and the QRS complex (*ie*, the PR intervals are variable). Hence this is a sinus rhythm with AV dissociation. As the atrial rate is faster than the ventricular rate, this is complete (third-degree) AV block. The QRS complex duration is increased (0.14 sec) and, although the QRS complexes have a morphology that resembles a left bundle branch block (LBBB; *ie*, QS complex in lead V1 [→] and a tall R wave in leads I and V6 [←]), the morphology is not typical of an LBBB as there is a Q wave in lead aVL (^) and a strange QRS morphology in leads II, III, and aVF with a prominent terminal S wave. Importantly, the QRS complex in ECG 15B is wider and has a different morphology than the conducted QRS complexes in ECG 15A. Hence this is a ventricular escape rhythm, confirming the fact that ECG 15A showed a Mobitz type II block with infranodal disease. Cannon A waves are seen with AV dissociation of any cause and are due to intermittent right atrial contraction against a closed tricuspid valve (*ie*, when the P wave resulting in atrial contraction is simultaneous to or slightly after the QRS complex, resulting in ventricular contraction).

Since Mobitz type II is due to a conduction abnormality that is infra-Hisian (below the AV node and within the Purkinje system), the occurrence of complete heart block will be associated with an escape ventricular rhythm, as the ventricular myocardium is the only remaining distal site from which an impulse can activate the ventricles. The development of complete heart block in this patient is the result of degenerative disease within the His-Purkinje system, and it may be the result of a previous anterior wall MI with the development of fibrosis of the interventricular septum. This conduction abnormality is not related to the medications that were prescribed; specifically, it is not due to the β-blocker. A β-blocker can cause complete heart block, but this is due to block of the AV node and hence would be associated with an escape junctional rhythm. The His-Purkinje system is not affected by β-blockade. The appropriate therapy for this patient is implantation of a permanent pacemaker. ■

Notes

A 68-year-old woman is brought to the hospital by emergency medical services after being found unresponsive at home. The time from loss of consciousness to presentation is unknown, but she began to regain consciousness en route to the hospital. She is not responding to commands but is moving her left side spontaneously. Her vital signs are notable for a pulse of 42 bpm and a blood pressure of 210/105 mm Hg. She is breathing spontaneously but has been intubated for airway protection. She is afebrile. An ECG is obtained.

What abnormalities are depicted?

What etiologic entity do these abnormalities suggest in this clinical scenario?

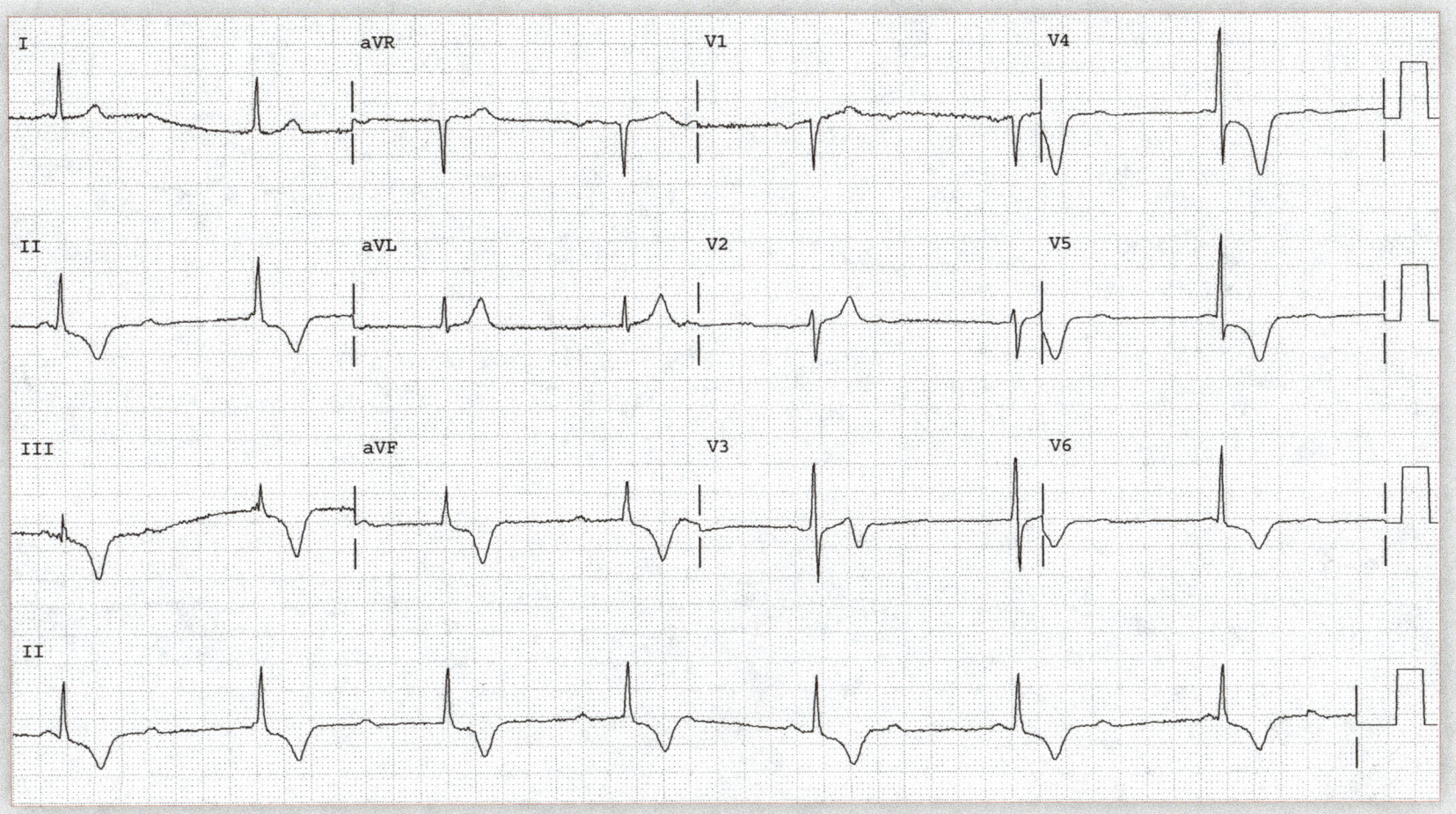

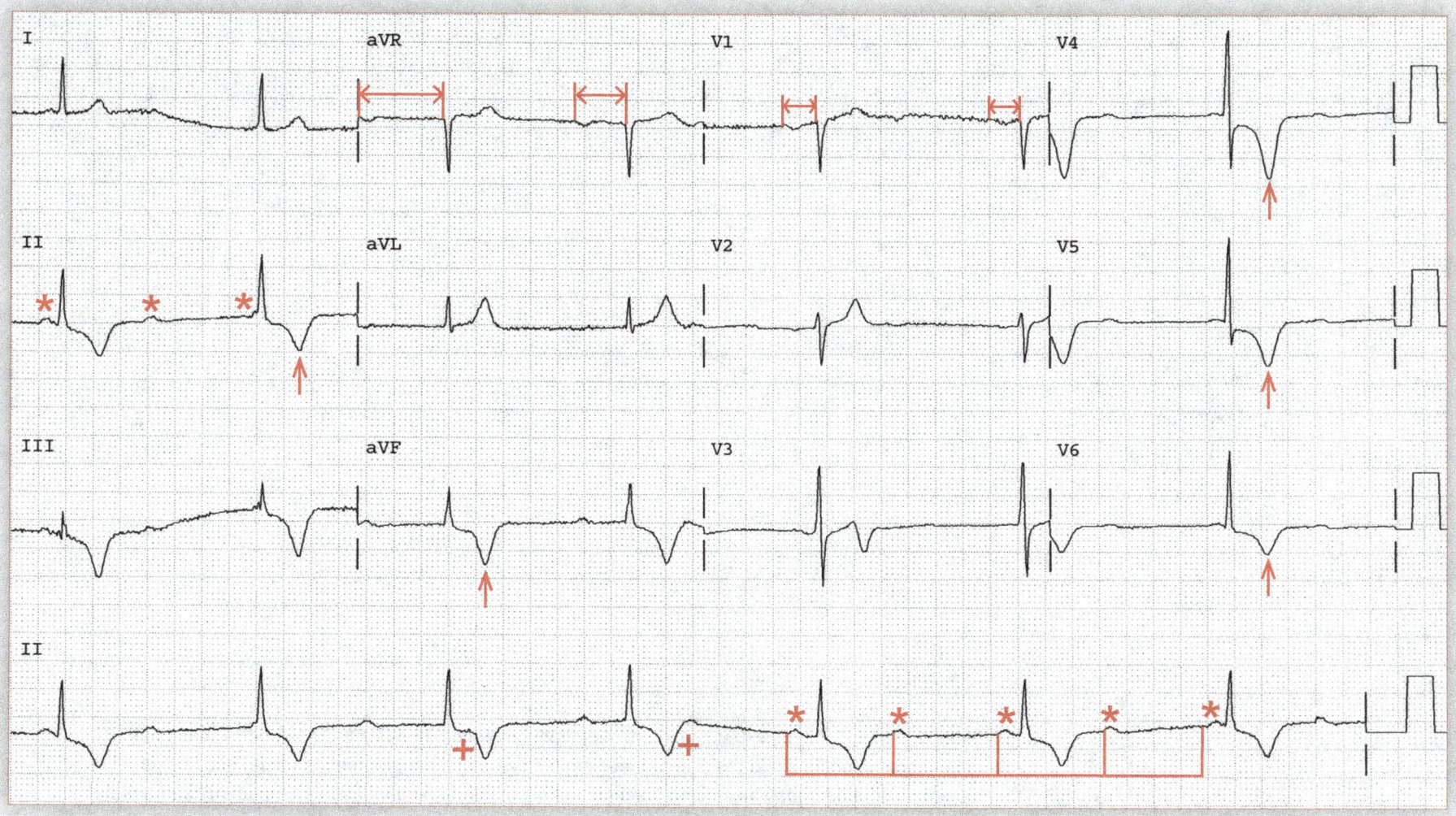

ECG 16 Analysis: Normal sinus rhythm, AV dissociation from third-degree
AV block, junctional escape rhythm, diffuse T-wave inversions

The heart rate is stable at 42 bpm. The P waves (*) are positive in leads I, II, aVF, and V4-V6. There is a stable PP interval (⊔), and the atrial rate is 76 bpm; hence this is a normal sinus rhythm. However, the PR intervals (↔) are not constant and there is no association between the P waves and the QRS complexes. Some of the P waves are superimposed on the T waves or on the beginning or end of the QRS complex and, therefore, are not obvious (+). However, when P waves are seen (*), they are on time. Hence this represents AV dissociation. As the atrial rate is faster than the rate of the QRS complexes, this is complete or third-degree AV block. The QRS complex has a normal duration (0.08 sec) and morphology. The axis is normal, between 0° and +90° (positive QRS complex in leads I and aVF). The QT/QTc intervals are normal (440/360 msec). The QRS complexes are, therefore, supraventricular and the escape rhythm is junctional.

AV dissociation may be subclassified based on etiology. AV dissociation may be due to an accelerated idioventricular rhythm or a junctional rhythm, in which a ventricular or junctional pacemaker is faster than the atrial rate. A ventricular or junctional etiology is based on the morphology of the QRS complex and not the rate. AV dissociation may also be due to complete (third-degree) AV block in which the atrial activity is not conducted to the ventricles and the atrial rate will be faster than the ventricular rate. In these cases, it is important to identify the origin of the "escape" rhythm (ie, junctional/AV nodal or ventricular). The origin of the escape rhythm is based on QRS morphology and not rate. Junctional escape rhythms may be at rates of less than 50 bpm, while a ventricular escape rhythm may have a rate of that exceeds 70 bpm.

continues

The QRS complex of an escape junctional rhythm will resemble the native QRS complex; the complex will be narrow if no baseline conduction disease is present, whereas it will be wide with a conduction delay if such a conduction abnormality was present prior to the development of complete AV block. The QRS complex of an escape ventricular rhythm will be wide and unusual in morphology (not resembling either a right or left bundle branch block), and it will not resemble the native QRS complex during intact AV conduction. In the ECG shown, the QRS complexes are narrow and, therefore, junctional in origin. A temporary pacemaker is not necessary unless there are symptoms from the bradycardia.

There are also T-wave abnormalities (inversions) in leads II, III, aVR (positive T waves are actually inverted in this lead), aVF, and V3-V6 (↑). T-wave inversions have a broad differential diagnosis, including subendocardial ischemia, myocardial infarction, cerebrovascular accidents (particularly hemorrhagic), left ventricular hypertrophy and hypertrophic cardiomyopathies, "memory" T waves (post-ventricular pacing), and idiopathic. Without a history or other ECG changes, they are considered to be nonspecific. Importantly, the T waves are asymmetric, which also suggests that they are nonspecific.

The clinical scenario in this case suggests that the T-wave inversions may be the result of a cerebrovascular accident. However, these are not cerebral T waves, which are usually markedly deeply inverted in all leads and associated with a long QT interval. Common ECG changes during acute stroke include a long QT interval, diffuse deep T-wave inversions, supraventricular and ventricular ectopy, atrial arrhythmias, and various forms of AV block, often the result of autonomic imbalance. ST-segment changes (both elevation and depression) and elevation of cardiac biomarkers may be seen as well. Predictors of increased mortality include atrial fibrillation, AV block, ST- and T-wave changes, and elevation of cardiac biomarkers. ■

A 59-year-old woman with dilated cardiomyopathy of unknown etiology is brought to the hospital emergency department by her sister after she spontaneously lost consciousness at home. On arrival, the woman is semi-conscious and moaning. A history is unobtainable. Telemetric monitoring is initiated and an ECG is obtained (17A) as vital

ECG 17A

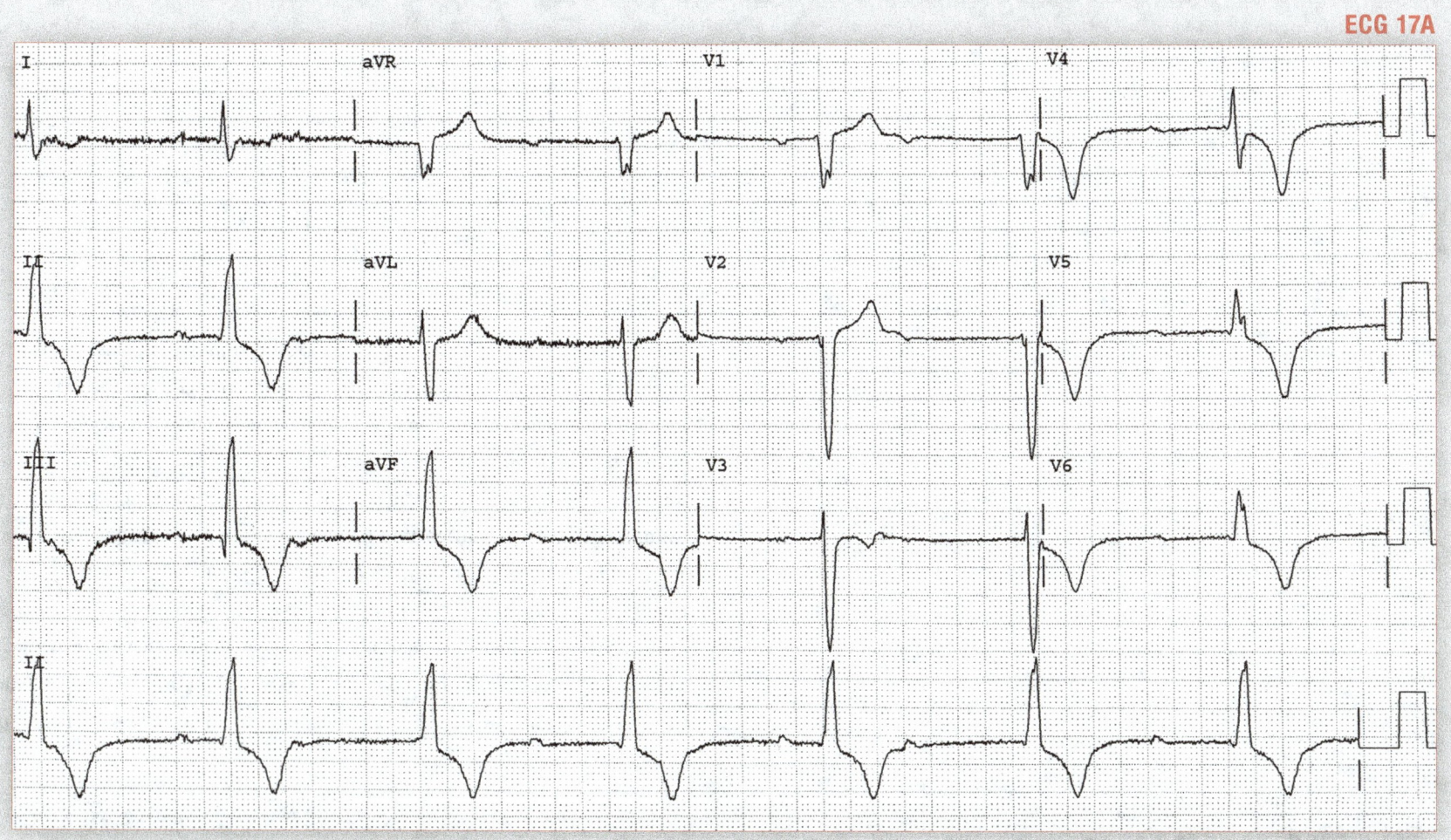

signs are gathered, a primary survey is completed, and preparations are made for intubation. Before any intervention can be performed, the woman's level of consciousness increases and she asks where she is and how she got there. You notice that her heart rate appears faster than on the ECG tracing you were provided. You request a second tracing (17B).

What do the tracings suggest regarding the location of the defect in her conduction system?

ECG 17B

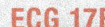

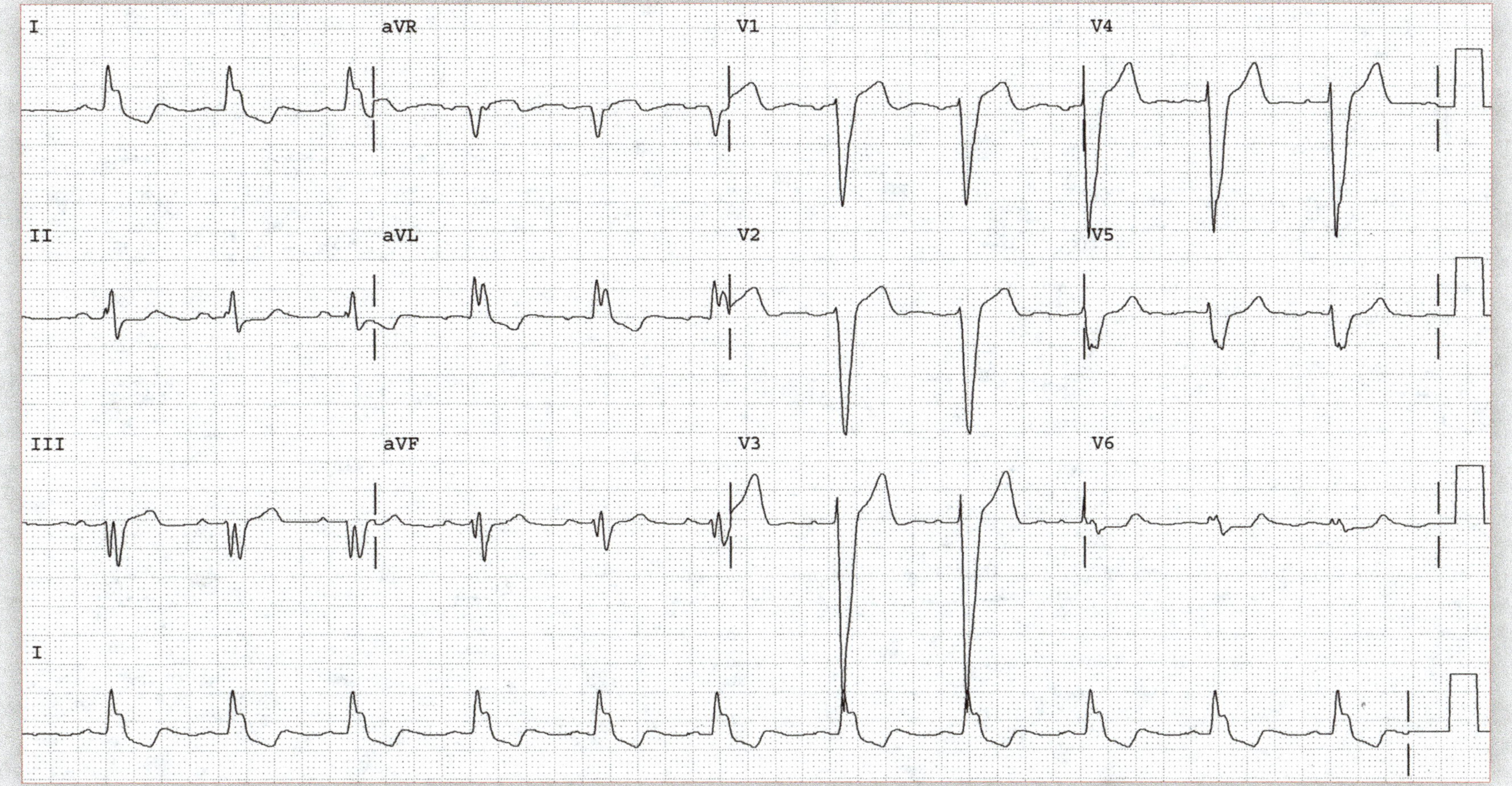

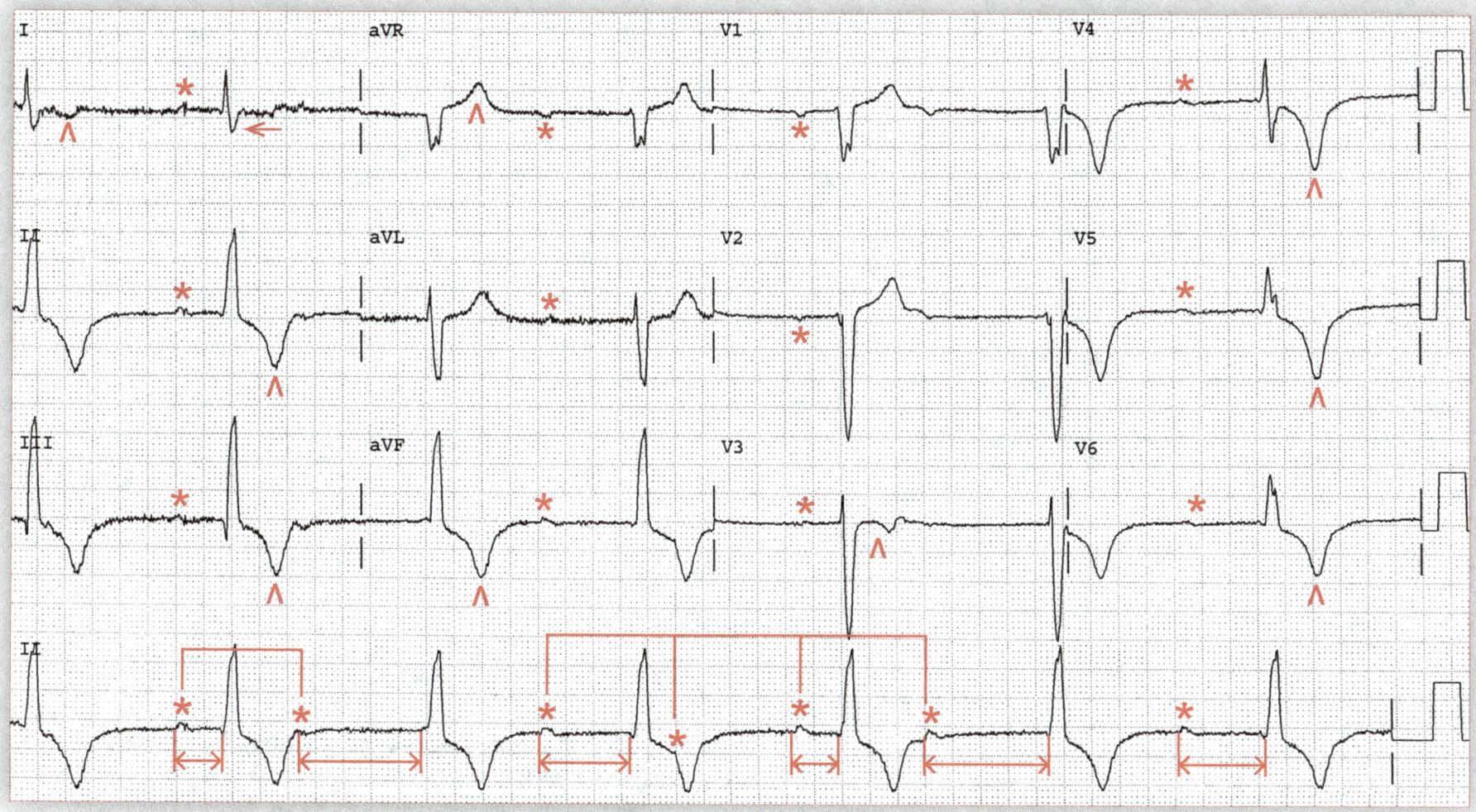

ECG 17A Analysis: Normal sinus rhythm, left atrial hypertrophy (abnormality), complete heart block, escape ventricular rhythm, diffuse T-wave inversions

In **ECG 17A**, there is a regular rhythm at a rate of 40 bpm. There are P waves (*) with a regular PP interval at a rate of 62 bpm (⊓). The P waves are positive in leads I, II, aVF, and V4-V6. The negative deflection of the P wave in lead V1 is prominent (> 1 mm wide and 1 mm deep), indicating left atrial hypertrophy. Hence this is a normal sinus rhythm. The PR intervals (↔) are not constant; hence there is AV dissociation. The atrial rate is faster than the ventricular rate, diagnostic for complete heart block. The QRS complexes are wide (0.14 sec) and have a left bundle branch block (LBBB)–like pattern, although it is a not typical LBBB as there is a terminal S wave (←) in lead I. There are no left-to-right forces seen with an LBBB. The axis is normal, between 0° and +90° (positive QRS complex in leads I and aVF). It is not certain whether the complexes are ventricular or junctional with an intraventricular conduction delay. Therefore, the location of the escape rhythm is not certain on this ECG. T-wave inversions can be seen in leads I, II, III, aVR (the positive T wave in this lead is actually inverted), aVF, and V3-V6 (^). The QT/QTc intervals are normal (500/410 msec).

continues

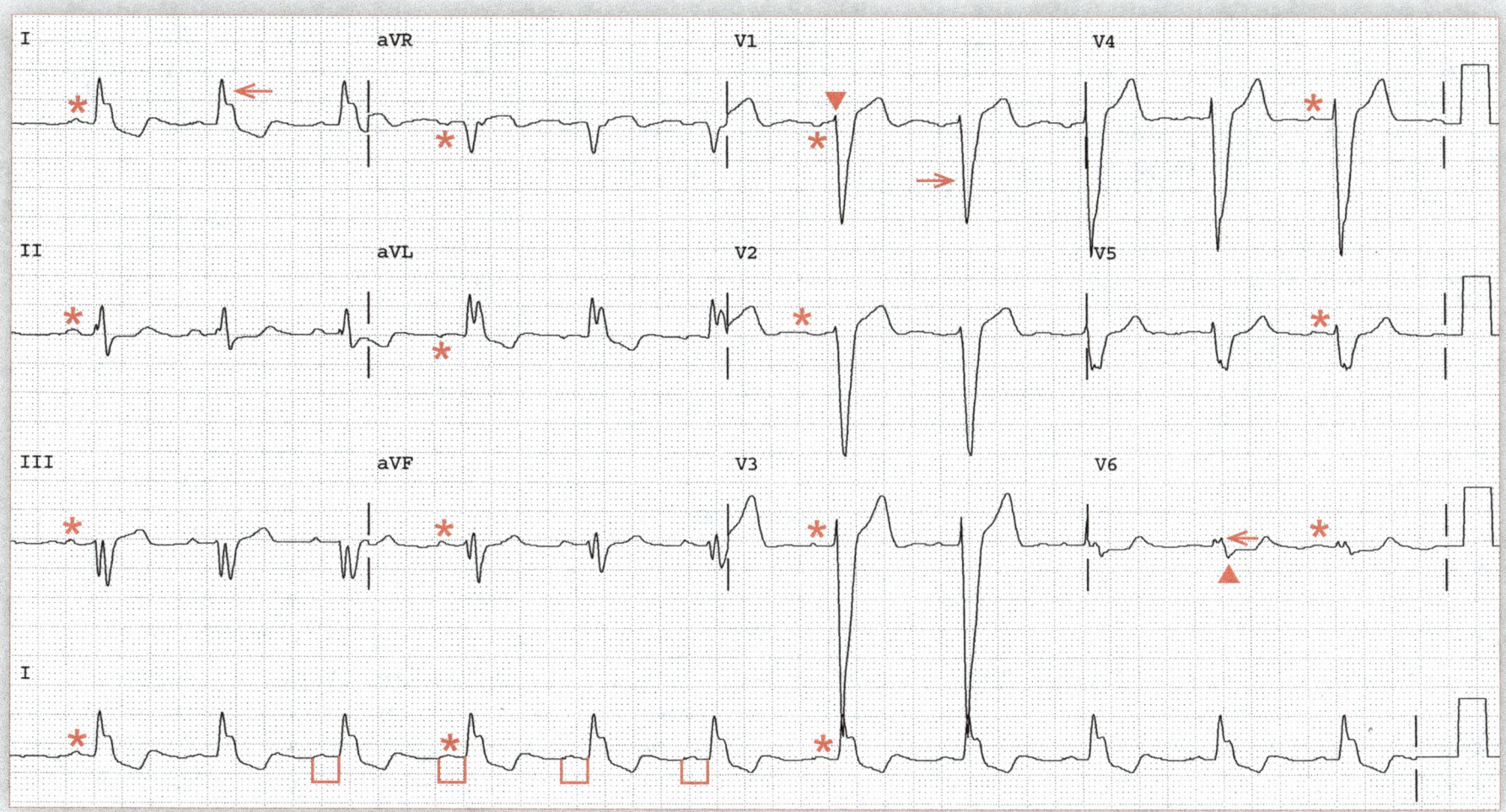

ECG 17B Analysis: Normal sinus rhythm, left atrial hypertrophy (abnormality), intraventricular conduction delay

ECG 17B shows a regular rhythm at a rate of 68 bpm. There is a P wave (*) before each QRS complex, and the PR interval (⊔) is stable at 0.20 second. The P wave is positive in leads I, II, aVF, and V4-V6. Therefore, this is a sinus rhythm. The QRS complexes are wide (0.16 sec) and have an LBBB-like pattern (broad R wave in leads I and V6 [←] and deep S wave in lead V1 [→]). However, there is a small initial R wave in lead V1 (▼), representing an initial septal force, which is not present in an LBBB. In addition there is a terminal S wave in lead V6 (▲), representing terminal left-to-right forces that are not seen with an LBBB. Therefore, this is an intraventricular conduction delay. The QT/QTc intervals are prolonged (440/470 msec) but are normal when the prolonged QRS complex duration is considered (360/385 msec). The QRS complexes seen in **ECG 17A** have a different morphology from these complexes, which are supraventricular in origin as this is a sinus rhythm. This confirms the fact that the escape rhythm in **ECG 17A** is ventricular in origin and that the location of the conduction block is infranodal. As this is complete heart block with an escape ventricular arrhythmia and it is associated with significant symptoms, a permanent pacemaker is indicated. If there is a delay in placing a permanent device, a temporary pacemaker would be indicated as an escape ventricular arrhythmia is not stable and is unpredictable with regard to rate. ■

Core Case 18

A 42-year-old man with a long history of drug abuse and known cocaine-associated dilated cardiomyopathy presents for routine follow-up. His review of systems is unremarkable, and his exam suggests that he is euvolemic. However, the physician notices that the patient's heart rate is

ECG 18A

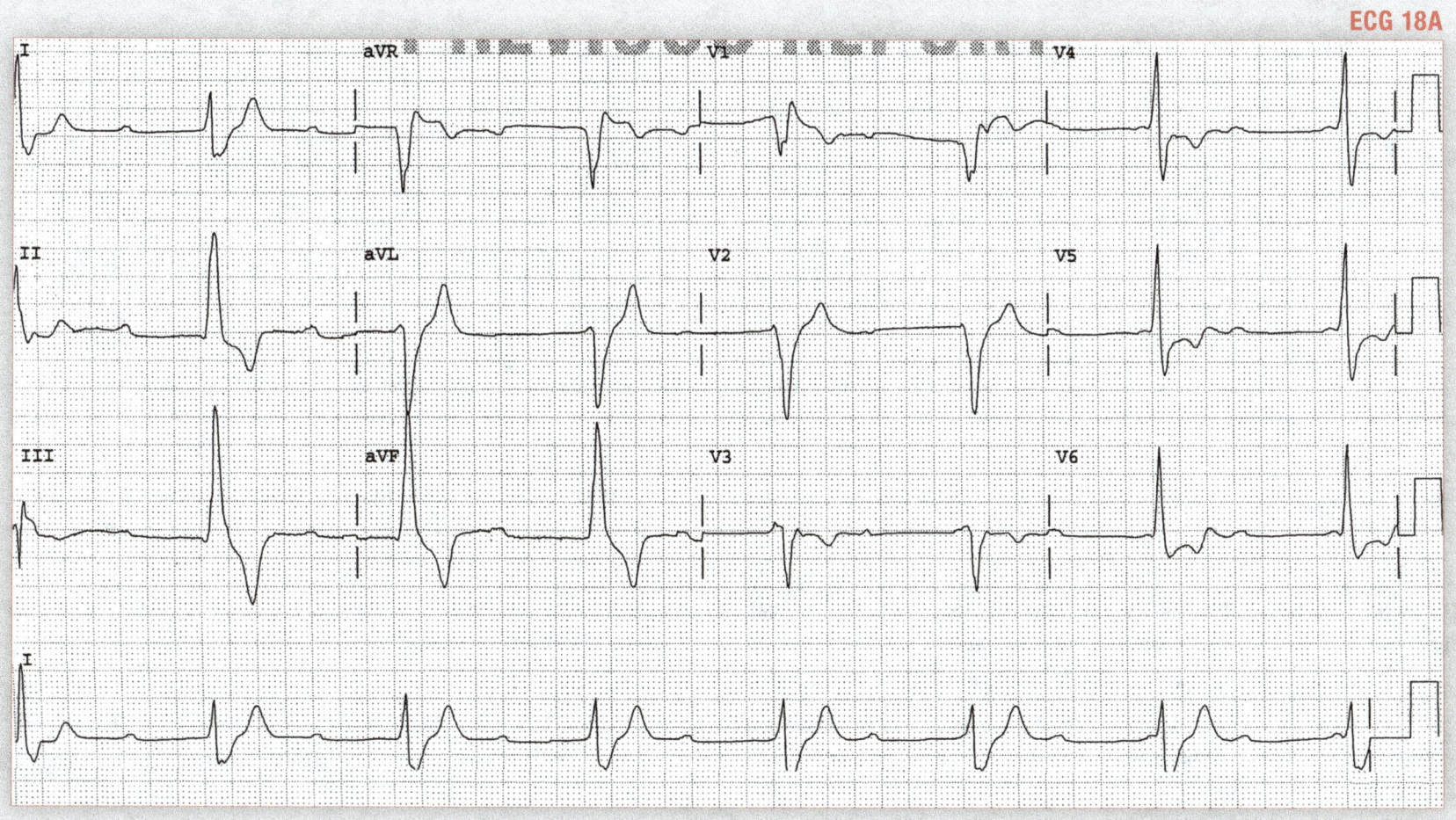

44 bpm and obtains an ECG (18A). The physician promptly admits the patient to the hospital and calls for an electrophysiology consult for pacemaker implantation. The following day, the physician obtains a follow-up ECG (18B) and is gratified to learn that his initial suspicion was correct.

What on the initial ECG was so concerning to the physician?

What on the follow-up tracing solidified the diagnosis?

ECG 18B

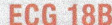

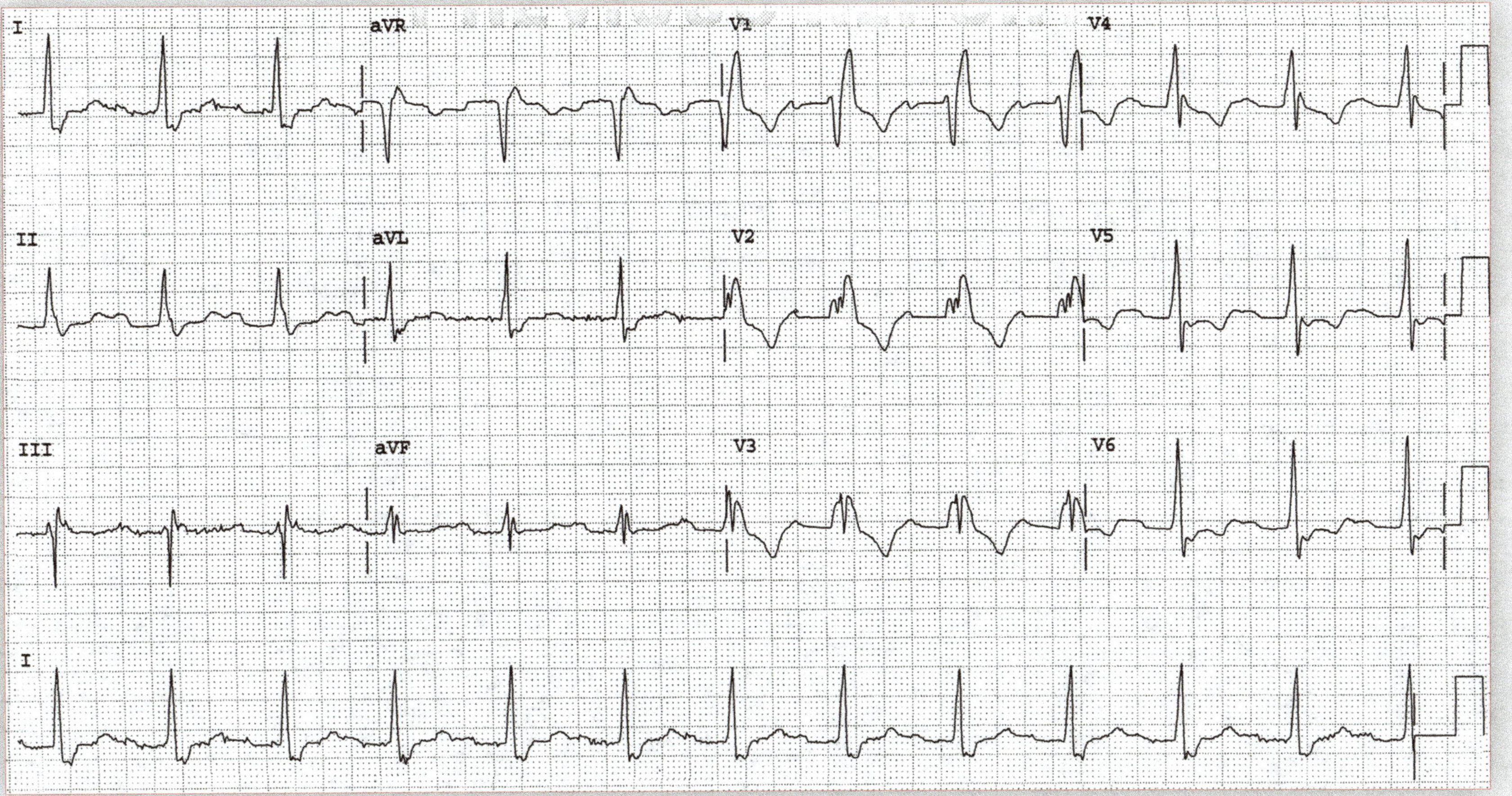

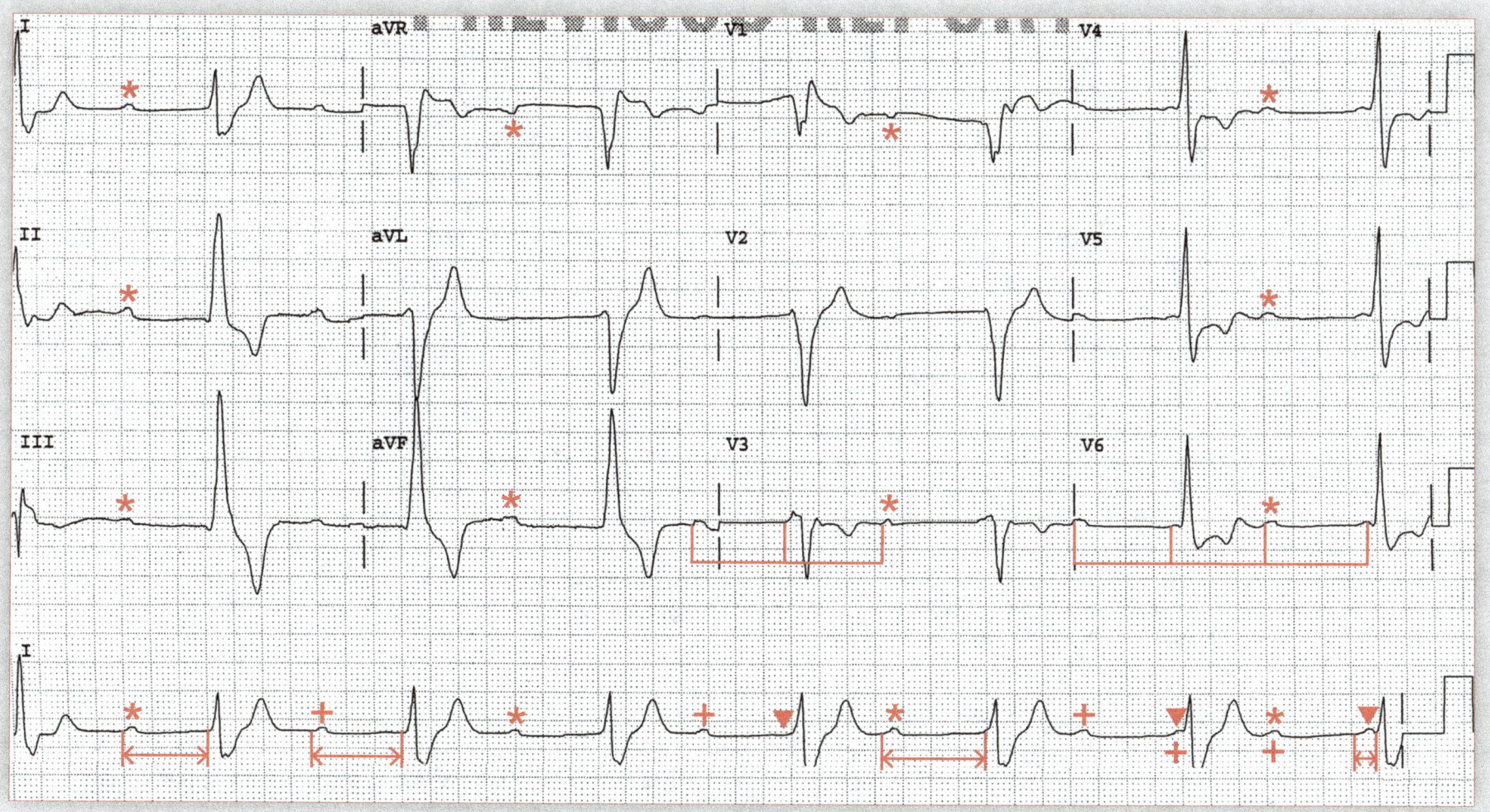

ECG 18A Analysis: Sinus rhythm, AV dissociation/complete heart block, ventricular escape rhythm

ECG **18A** shows a regular wide QRS complex rhythm at a rate of 44 bpm. The QRS complex duration is 0.20 second, and the morphology does not resemble either a left or right bundle branch block. It is likely a ventricular complex. The axis is normal, between 0° and +90° (positive QRS complex in leads I and aVF). The QT/QTc intervals are normal (440/380 msec). There are P waves (∗) that are positive in leads I, II, aVF, and V4-V6; hence they are sinus P waves. The P waves are not always visible as some are within or at the beginning of the QRS complex (▼). Two sequential P waves can be seen between the last two QRS complexes (+), and when this PP interval is used it can be seen that there is a regular PP interval (⊔) and the sinus rate is 90 bpm. Although some P waves are not seen, those that are obvious occur on time with a regular interval (⊔). There is variability of the PR interval (↔), indicating AV dissociation. Since the atrial rate exceeds the QRS complex rate, this is complete heart block with an escape ventricular rhythm.

continues

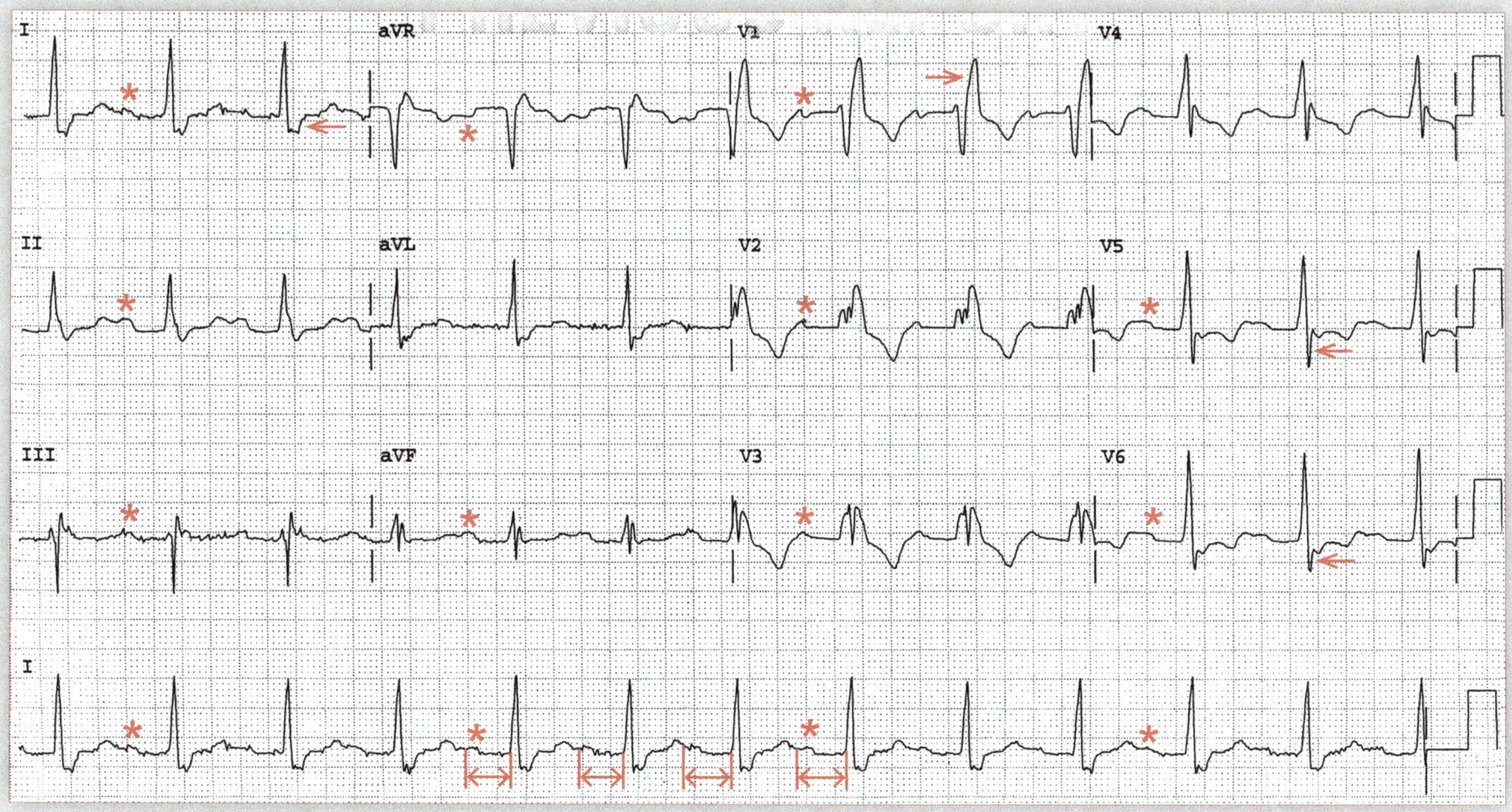

ECG 18B Analysis: Sinus rhythm, first-degree AV block (prolonged AV conduction), intraventricular conduction delay to the right ventricle

ECG **18B** shows a regular wide complex rhythm at a rate of 76 bpm. The QRS complex duration is very prolonged (0.20 sec). Although the morphology is that of a right bundle branch block (RSR′ morphology in lead V1 [→] with a very broad R′ wave and very broad S waves in leads I and V6 [←]), the QRS complex is much wider than what is seen with a bundle branch block. In general, the QRS complex width in a bundle branch block is 0.18 second or less. This suggests that this is an intraventricular conduction delay to the right ventricle (supported by the very broad R′ and S waves) caused by dilated cardiomyopathy with myocardial fibrosis. There is a P wave (*) before each QRS complex with a stable PR interval (↔), which is prolonged at 0.28 second (*ie*, this is sinus rhythm with first-degree AV block or prolonged AV conduction). The QRS complex is supraventricular and has a right bundle branch block pattern that is different from the QRS complex seen in ECG **18A**, establishing the fact that the escape rhythm in ECG **18B** is ventricular and hence the complete heart block is a result of His-Purkinje system disease. ◼

Notes

A 78-year-old woman with end-stage ischemic cardiomyopathy is admitted to the coronary care unit with decompensated heart failure. She is intubated on full inotropic support. The patient's heart rate has been stable. However, in watching the telemetry monitor, an astute medical student expresses concern about the patient's rhythm and obtains an ECG.

What conduction system abnormality is depicted on the ECG?

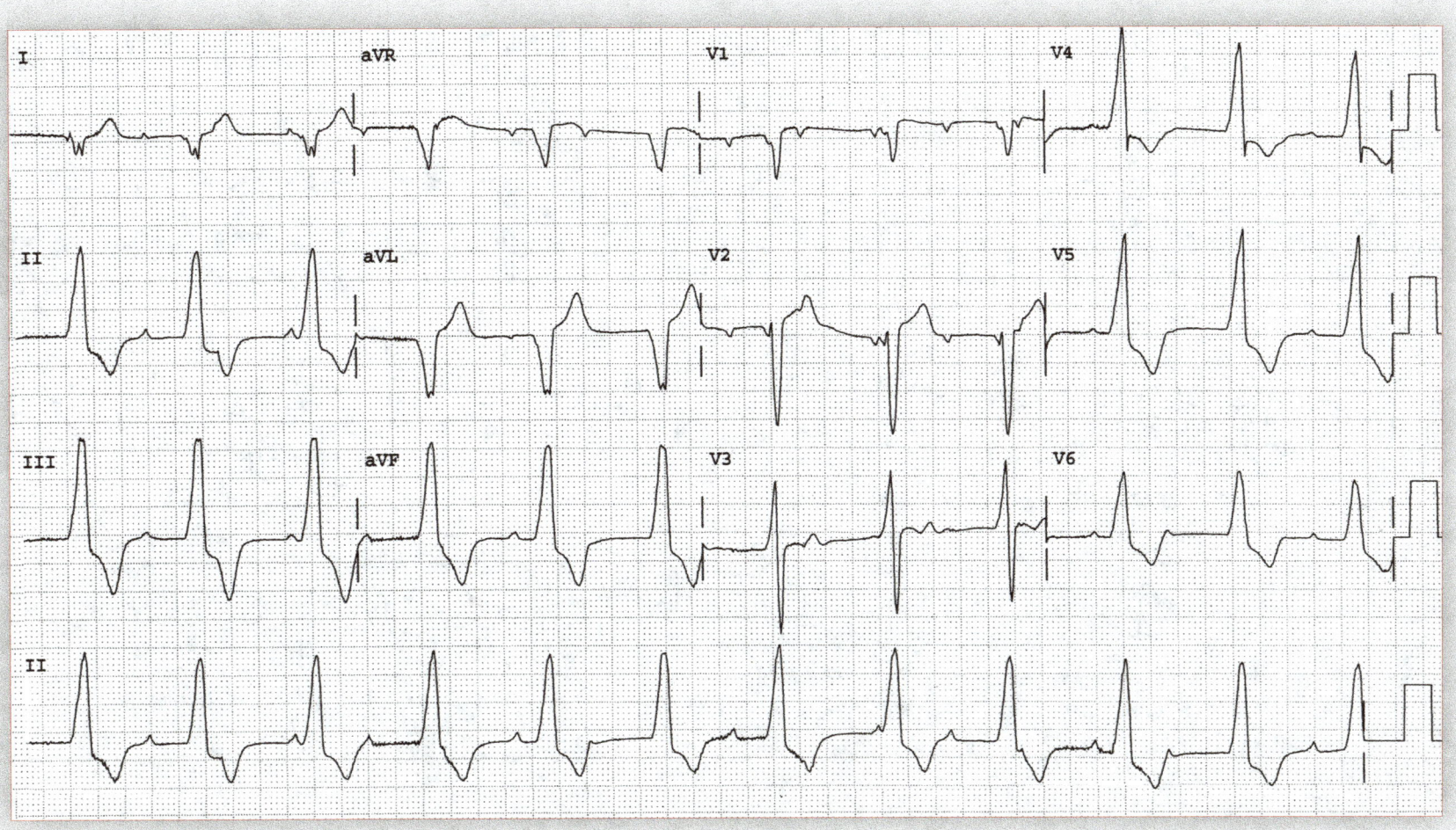

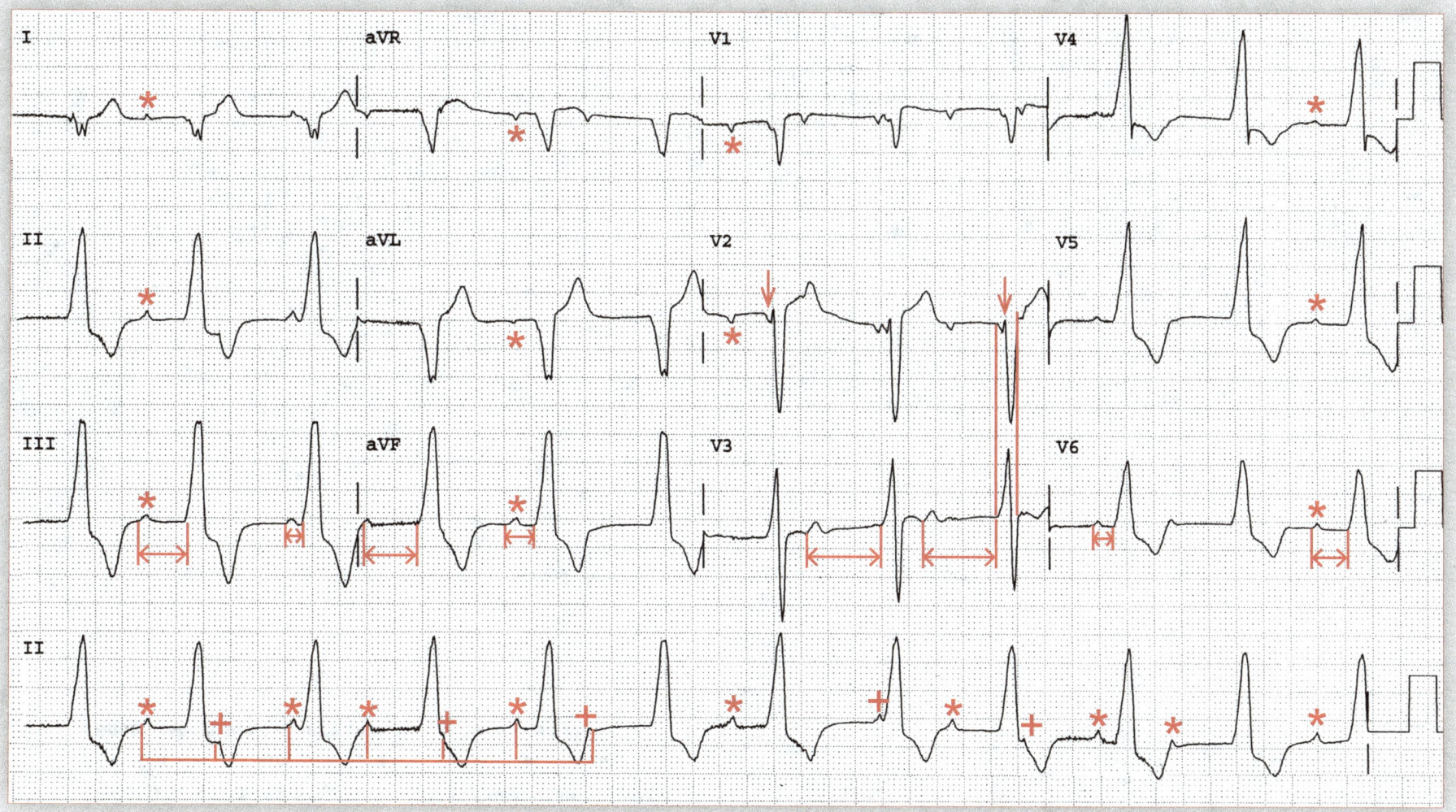

ECG 19 Analysis: Sinus tachycardia, AV dissociation/complete heart block, escape ventricular rhythm

There is a regular rhythm at a rate of 72 bpm. P waves can be seen (*), although occasionally the P wave is at the beginning or end of the QRS complex (+) and is not obvious. When seen, however, the P waves are occurring at a regular interval (⊔) at a rate of 110 bpm. The P waves are positive in leads I, II, aVF, and V4-V6. Hence there is sinus tachycardia. The PR intervals (↔) are not stable; therefore, the P waves are independent of the QRS complexes, thus defining AV dissociation. AV dissociation in this case is due to complete heart block since the atrial rate exceeds the rate of the QRS complex. The QRS complexes are widened, with a duration of 0.16 second and a right axis, between +90° and +180° (negative QRS complex in lead I and positive QRS complex in lead aVF). The QT/QTc intervals are prolonged (440/480 msec) but are normal when the prolonged QRS complex duration is considered (360/395 msec).

The QRS complexes do not have a pattern of either a right or left bundle branch block, but rather are wide with an unusual morphology. Hence there is an escape ventricular rhythm, even though the ventricular rate is 72 bpm. The fast ventricular rate is likely a result of an enhanced sympathetic state as the sinus rate is 110 bpm. As indicated, the location of the escape rhythm (junctional or ventricular) is based on the QRS morphology and not the rate. In this case the escape ventricular rhythm is 72 bpm, faster than is usually seen with an escape ventricular focus. However, this is in association with a sinus rate of 110 bpm, meaning that there is an increase in catecholamines or sympathetic tone that is driving both the sinus node and ventricular focus.

Noted in lead V2 are waveforms (↓) just before the QRS complex. These are not P waves, but rather are part of the QRS complex, established by measuring the maximum QRS complex width from simultaneously occurring complexes (in either lead V3 or the lead II rhythm strip) (‖). It can be seen that the waveform just before the QRS complex is part of the QRS complex and not a P wave. ■

Notes

A 74-year-old woman with a history of hypertension that has not been well controlled despite therapy with a β-blocker and an angiotensin-converting enzyme inhibitor presents to her physician with a complaint of fatigue that has been present for the past week. She denies chest discomfort, shortness of breath, and lightheadedness. The physical exam reveals a blood pressure of 170/90 mm Hg and a heart rate of 40 bpm, but is otherwise unremarkable. An ECG is obtained.

What abnormality is seen on the ECG?

Is this abnormality the result of the patient's medication?

What therapy is indicated?

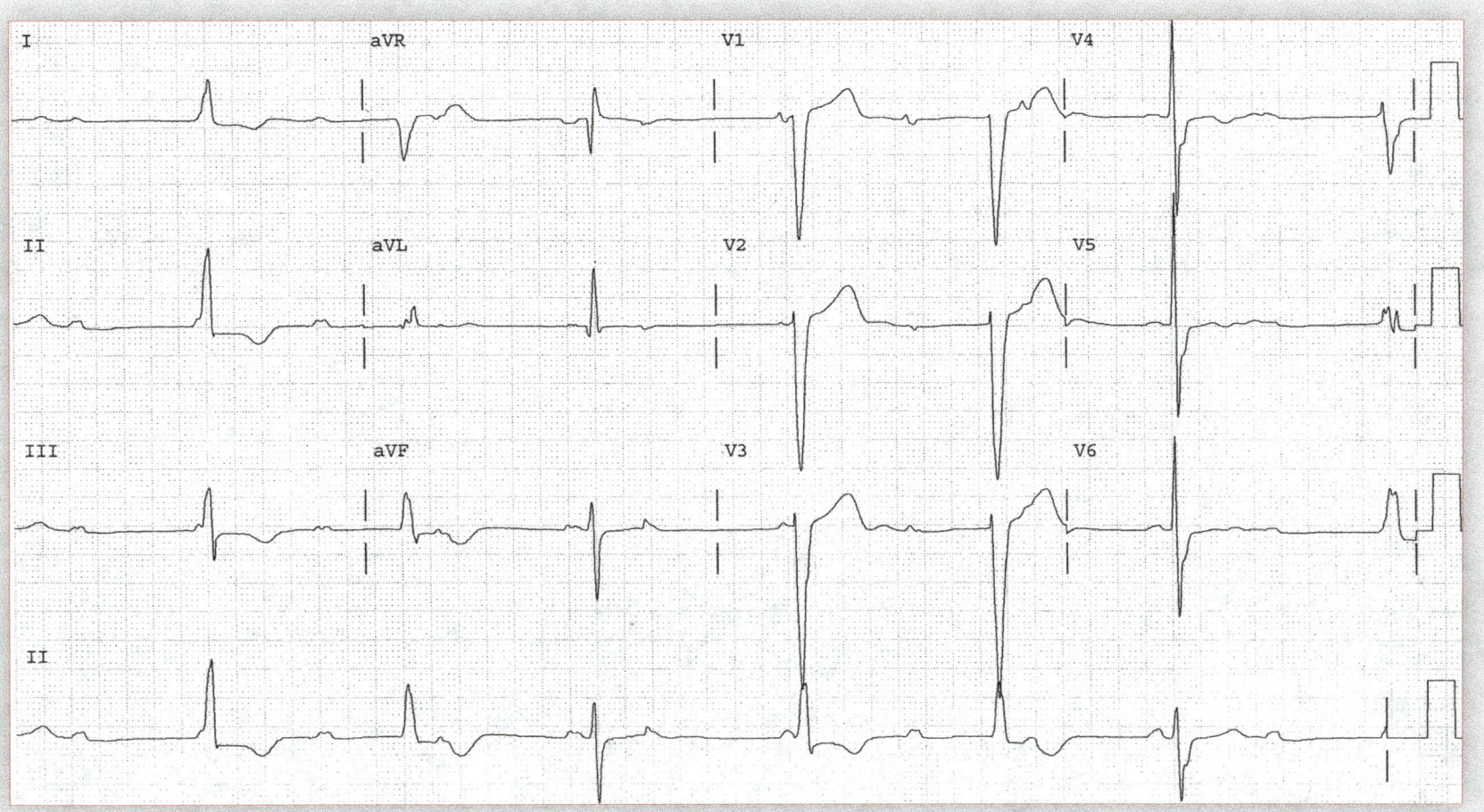

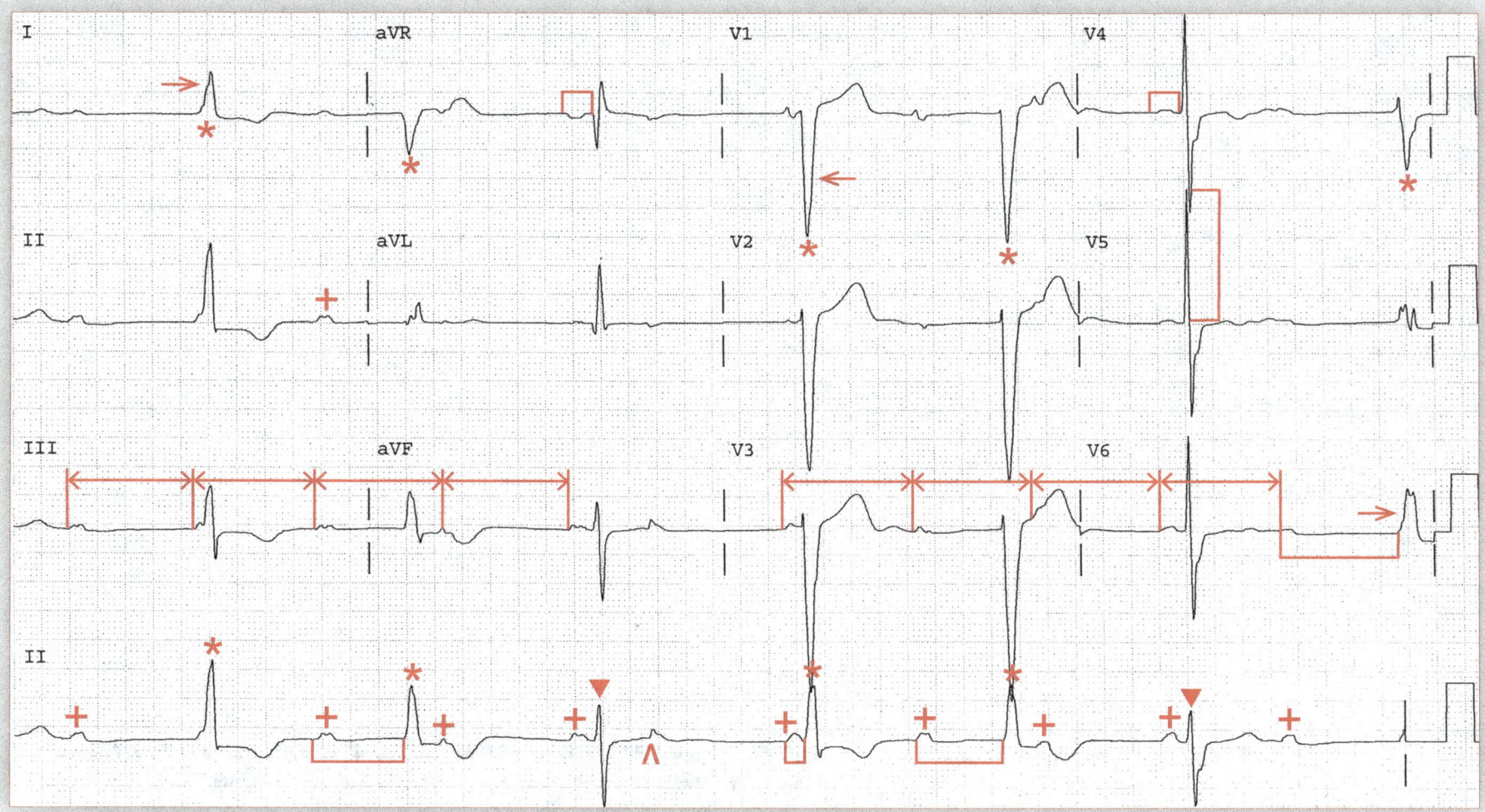

ECG 20 Analysis: Normal sinus rhythm, left atrial hypertrophy (abnormality), third-degree or complete heart block, escape ventricular rhythm, intermittent AV capture, premature atrial complex

There is a regular rhythm at a rate of 42 bpm. There is evidence of atrial activity (+), and the PP interval (↔) is generally regular at a rate of 64 bpm. The P waves are positive in leads I, II, aVF, and V4-V6. Hence there is a normal sinus rhythm. The P waves are broad and notched, particularly in leads II, III, and aVF, consistent with left atrial hypertrophy (or abnormality). There is no association between the P waves and the QRS complexes as the PR intervals are variable (⊔). Hence there is AV dissociation. As the atrial rate is faster than the ventricular rate, this is complete or third-degree AV block. There is a P wave that is premature (^), and it has a different morphology than the sinus P waves. This is a premature atrial complex, which resets the sinus P waves, accounting for the slight irregularity of the PP interval.

The QRS complexes have two different durations and morphologies. QRS complexes 1, 2, 4, 5, and 7 (*) have a wide duration (0.16 sec) and are associated with a variable PR interval (⊔). They have a left bundle branch block morphology with a broad R wave in leads I and V6 (→) and a QS complex in lead V1 (←). The narrow QRS complexes (complexes 3 and 6) (▼) have a normal duration (0.08 sec) and morphology. Although the narrow complex is not seen in lead I, the axis is likely very leftward, between –30° and –90°, as the QRS complex is negative in leads II and aVF. These are thus supraventricular complexes. The QRS amplitude is markedly increased in lead V5 (22 mm) ( ]).

Although it does not meet a criterion for left ventricular hypertrophy, a narrow QRS complex is not seen in leads V1-V3 and hence it is possible that left ventricular hypertrophy is present. The narrow QRS complexes are slightly early and both are preceded by a P wave with the same PR interval (0.18 sec) (⊓). Therefore, these two complexes are responding to the P wave that precedes them; hence they result from AV conduction. As the conducted QRS complexes have a normal duration and morphology that is different from the wide dissociated QRS complexes, the escape rhythm is ventricular and there is intermittent capture or AV conduction.

Although the patient does have a history of hypertension, her elevated blood pressure on presentation may be the result of the complete heart block. Elevated systolic pressure is often observed with complete heart block as a result of AV dyssynchrony and increased left ventricular stroke volume. With AV dissociation and the more rapid atrial rate there is an increase in ventricular filling with an increased left ventricular end-diastolic volume. Hence as a result of a Starling effect, left ventricular contractility and stroke volume are increased, resulting in systolic hypertension. Any decision about blood pressure and further medical therapy should wait until after a permanent pacemaker has been placed. ■

Notes

A 63-year-old man with end-stage renal disease is being evaluated by his nephrologist during a hemodialysis session. He complains of intermittent palpitations but is otherwise feeling well. On exam, the patient's heart rate is slow. On observation of the jugular venous pulse, intermittent brisk deflections to the angle of the jaw are noted (*ie*, cannon A waves). The cardiopulmonary exam is otherwise normal. These observations prompt recording of a surface 12-lead ECG.

What on the ECG explains the physical exam findings and the patient's symptoms?

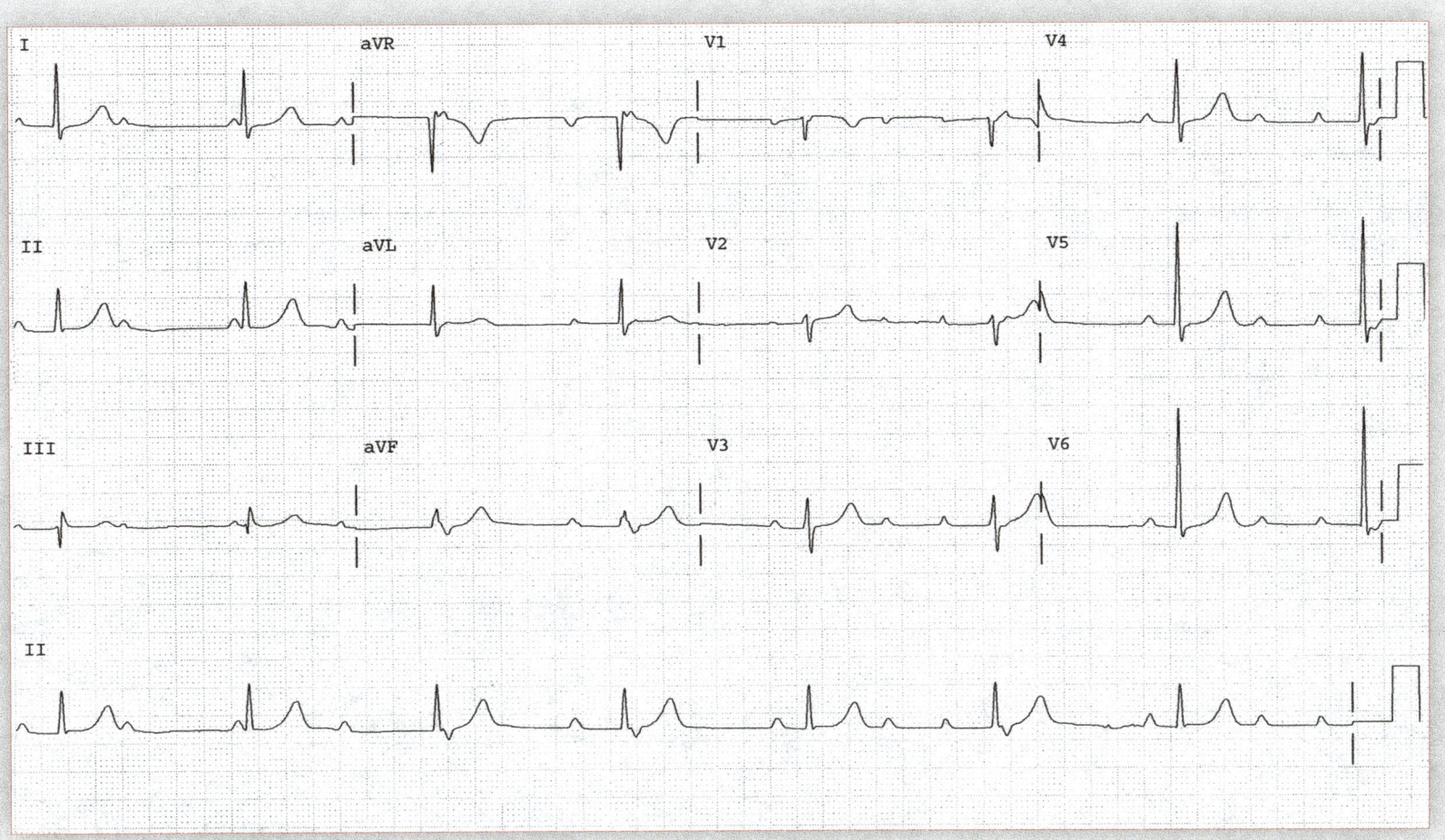

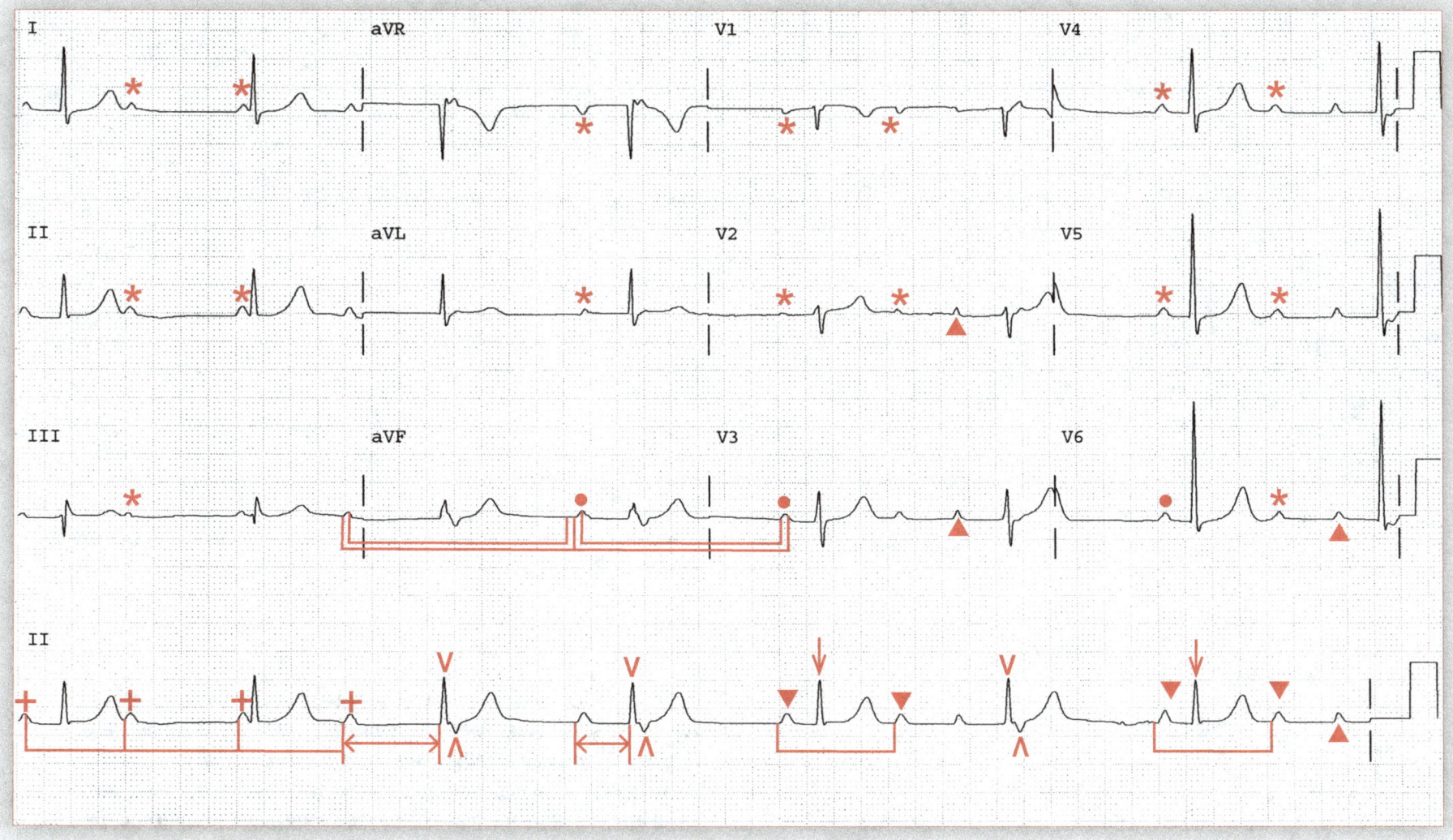

ECG 21 Analysis: Normal sinus rhythm, premature atrial complex, AV dissociation, third-degree or complete heart block, intermittent retrograde (ventriculoatrial) conduction

The RR intervals are regular at a rate of 44 bpm. The QRS complexes are narrow (0.08 sec), with a normal morphology and normal axis, between 0° and +90° (positive QRS complex in leads I and aVF). The QRS complexes are, therefore, supraventricular. The QT/QTc intervals are normal (480/410 msec). There are P waves (*), which are positive in leads I, II, aVF, and V4-V6. These are, therefore, sinus P waves. The PR intervals are variable (↔) and hence there is AV dissociation. The sinus rate is not constant. The first four P waves (+) occur with a regular interval (⊔) at a rate of 74 bpm. The P waves (▼) before and after the fifth and seventh QRS complexes (↓) have the same PP interval (⊔) (rate of 74 bpm). It is noted that the P waves after the third, fourth, and sixth QRS complexes (ie, the fifth, sixth, and ninth P waves) are late (●); that is, there is a longer PP interval (⊔⊔). The third, fourth, and sixth QRS complexes (ν) are different as there is a negative waveform (^) at the end of each complex. This is a retrograde P wave, with a fixed RP interval, indicating intermittent ventriculoatrial (VA) conduction from the junctional beat back to the atrium. As a result the sinus node is reset and hence the PP interval is altered and the P waves are late (⊔⊔).

Therefore, this is complete heart block with an escape junctional rhythm and occasional VA conduction. The VA conduction occurs whenever the atrium is able to be depolarized (ie, when the atrial activity is prior to the QRS complex with a long enough PR interval such that the AV node and atrium have had a chance to recover and are responsive to retrograde activation). It is important to note that even though there is complete antegrade AV block, there is still retrograde VA conduction, which is seen in about 20% to 30% of cases of complete AV block. As the antegrade and retrograde nodal properties are different, there may be intact retrograde or VA conduction even though there is no antegrade conduction. Alternatively, retrograde or VA conduction may be due to a concealed bypass tract, which usually conducts only retrogradely.

Also noted are additional P waves that are early (▲) (ie, after the fifth QRS complex and before the last [eighth] QRS complex). These are atrial premature beats that are not conducted.

The physical exam is consistent with complete heart block, particularly the presence of cannon A waves, which are due to atrial contraction against a closed tricuspid valve. This occurs whenever P waves superimpose on the QRS complexes, as in complete (third-degree) AV block.

Although there is complete AV block, it is not certain whether this is transient or permanent. Moreover, it is not clear whether this is related to electrolyte abnormalities associated with renal failure. While complete AV block is an indication for a permanent pacemaker, even though the escape rhythm is junctional, the risk for this must be weighed against the fact that the patient is on long-term dialysis, a factor that is associated with an increased risk for infection. ■

Notes

A 59-year-old college professor presents to the health clinic with complaints of intermittent palpitations but no other symptoms. Although he has no cardiac history, he states that he was told years ago that he had hypertension but has not been on any therapy. He is fully active and jogs about 6 miles per day. He has no symptoms while running. His physical exam and blood pressure are normal, and his heart rate is 90 bpm. An ECG is obtained.

What abnormality is noted?

Is a pacemaker indicated?

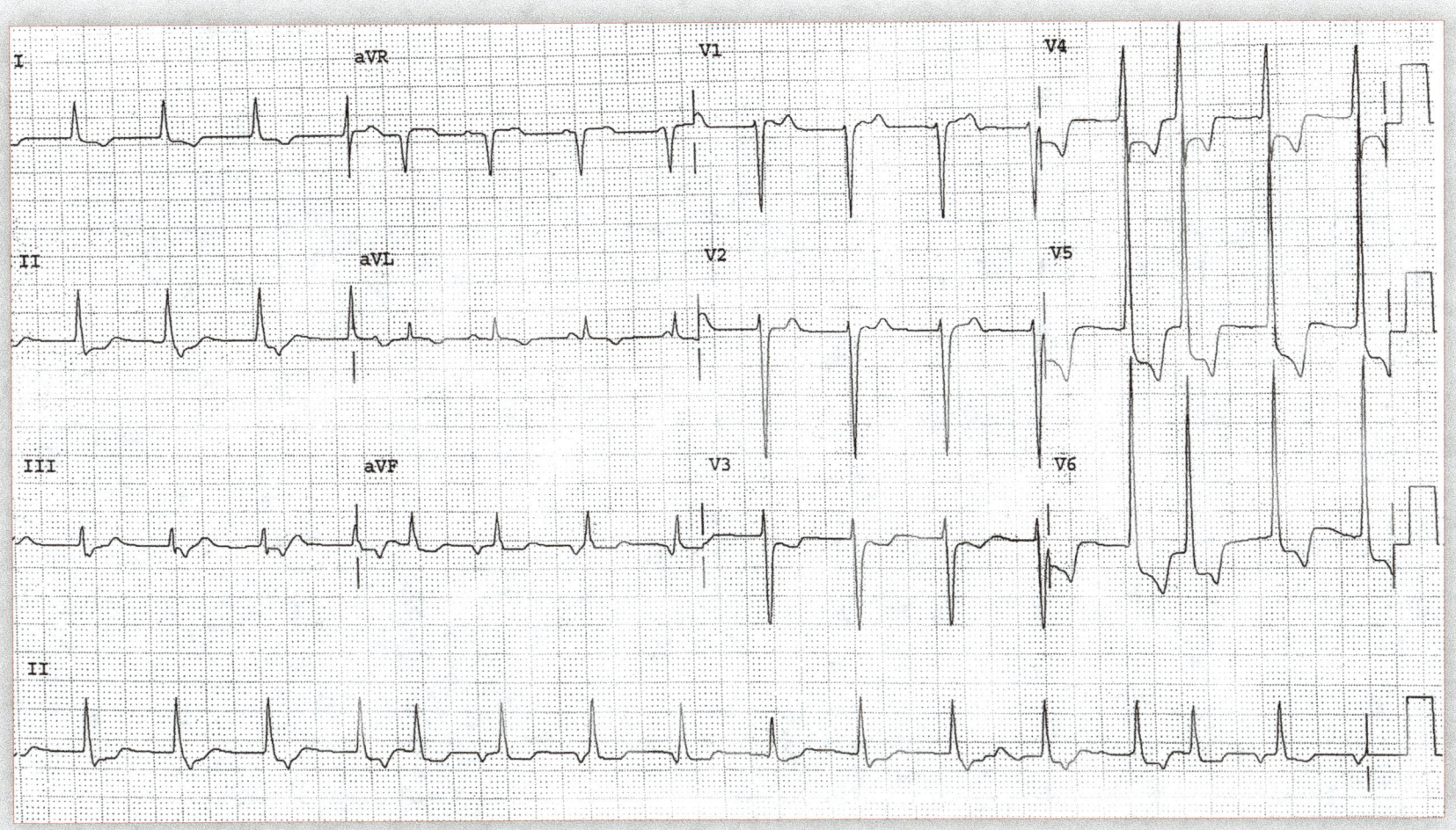

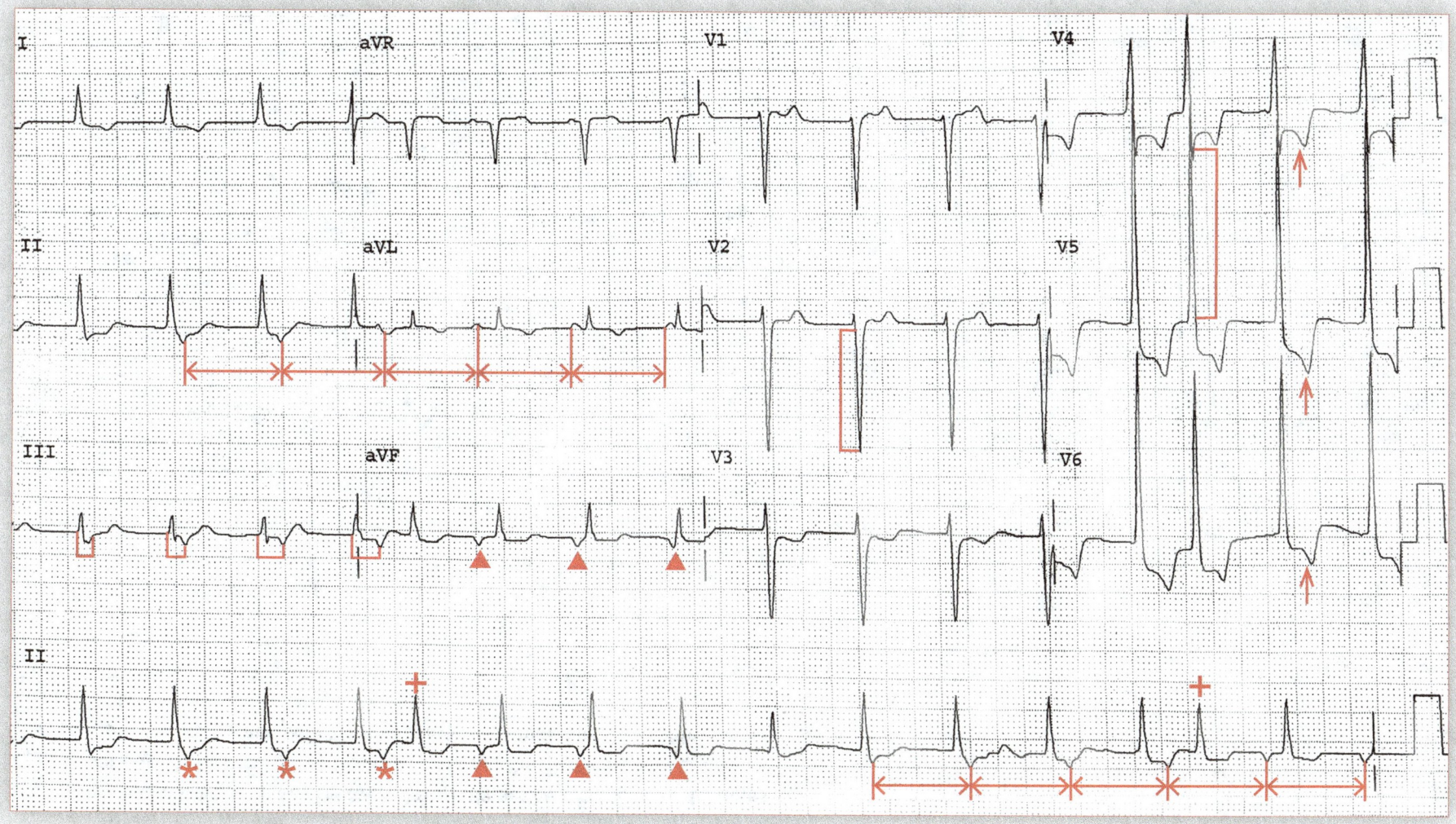

ECG 22 Analysis: Atrial rhythm, AV dissociation, accelerated junctional rhythm, occasional captured complex, left ventricular hypertrophy with associated ST-T wave changes

There is a regular rhythm at a rate of 94 bpm, although QRS complexes 5 and 14 (+) are early. The QRS complexes have a normal duration (0.08 sec) and a normal axis, between 0° and +90° (positive QRS complex in leads I and aVF). The QT/QTc intervals are normal (340/425 msec). The QRS complex has a tall R wave in lead V5 (32 mm) ( ]) and a deep S wave in lead V2 (22 mm) (S-wave depth in lead V2 + R-wave amplitude in lead V5 = 54 mm). This meets one of the criteria for left ventricular hypertrophy (ie, S-wave depth in lead V1 or V2 + R-wave amplitude in lead V5 or V6 ≥ 35 mm [or ≥ 45 mm if age under 45]). There are significant ST-T wave abnormalities seen in leads V4-V6 (↑), which are secondary to left ventricular hypertrophy and represent repolarization changes due to chronic subendocardial ischemia. Coronary blood flow goes from epicardium to endocardium and hence the last part of the myocardium to receive blood and oxygen supply is the subendocardial layer. When the myocardium is hypertrophied, the amount of blood or oxygen reaching the endocardial layer is limited, resulting in chronic subendocardial ischemia.

There are P waves seen (*,▲), and they are negative in leads II, III, and aVF. The P waves appear to be occurring after the QRS complex, suggesting that they are retrograde resulting from the junctional complexes. In addition, it appears that there is a progressively prolonging RP interval (⊔), suggesting retrograde or ventriculoatrial (VA) Wenckebach. If this were the case, the fifth and 14th QRS complexes, which are early and preceded by a negative P wave, would probably represent echo beats, resulting from retrograde or VA conduction stimulating the atria and then conducting antegradely through the AV node to reactivate the ventricles. However, the same negative P wave can be

seen before the sixth to eighth QRS complexes (▲), meaning that the P waves are in fact not retrograde but are antegrade. Indeed, there is a stable PP interval (↔) at an atrial rate of 86 bpm. The PR interval is not constant and hence there is AV dissociation. Since the atrial rate is slower than the ventricular rate, the AV dissociation is not the result of complete heart block (in which the atrial rate is faster than the ventricular rate). The AV dissociation is, therefore, the result of an accelerated junctional rhythm that is faster than the atrial rate. As the P waves are negative in leads II, III, and aVF, this is not a sinus rhythm but an atrial rhythm. The two early QRS complexes (fifth and 14th) (+), which have the same PR interval (0.24 sec), are thus captured complexes. The ability of the atrial impulse to conduct through the AV node and capture the ventricle depends on appropriate timing of the atrial impulse relative to the previous QRS complex. The AV dissociation is due to the fact that the junctional impulse retrogradely depolarizes the AV node, preventing antegrade impulse conduction from the atrium. If the AV node has recovered before the atrial impulse reaches it antegradely, the atrial impulse can be conducted through the node to capture the ventricle.

Since the AV dissociation is the result of an accelerated junctional rhythm and not complete heart block, there is no indication for the insertion of a pacemaker. An accelerated junctional rhythm can occur in many clinical scenarios but often is seen as a result of sinus or atrial bradycardia and an ectopic junctional focus that generates an impulse at a rate that is faster than the rate of the sinus node or atrial focus. ■

Notes

A 92-year-old woman is found unconscious by her family and brought to the local emergency department. Her daughter is not fully aware of her medical history, but states that her mother has been treated for hypertension, atrial fibrillation, and heart failure and is on medications for this. For the past several days, the patient had been complaining of abdominal pain and diarrhea but seemed to be doing fine otherwise. She has no other active medical conditions. On presentation, the patient's vital signs are notable for a heart rate of 36 bpm and a blood pressure of 84/58 mm Hg. She is quite somnolent and responds minimally to voice commands. She is anicteric, her lungs are clear on auscultation, and her heart has a nondisplaced point of maximal impulse and is regular without murmur, gallop, rub, or tap. Her extremities are cool, and skin turgor is decreased. No edema is evident. Her laboratory studies are notable for a serum sodium level of 156 mEq/L, potassium 3.2 mEq/L, blood urea nitrogen 92 mg/dL, and serum creatinine 4.6 mg/dL. Her cardiac biomarkers and complete blood count are normal. Intravenous fluid resuscitation is initiated and an ECG is obtained.

What abnormalities are depicted?

What medications are likely to cause these abnormalities?

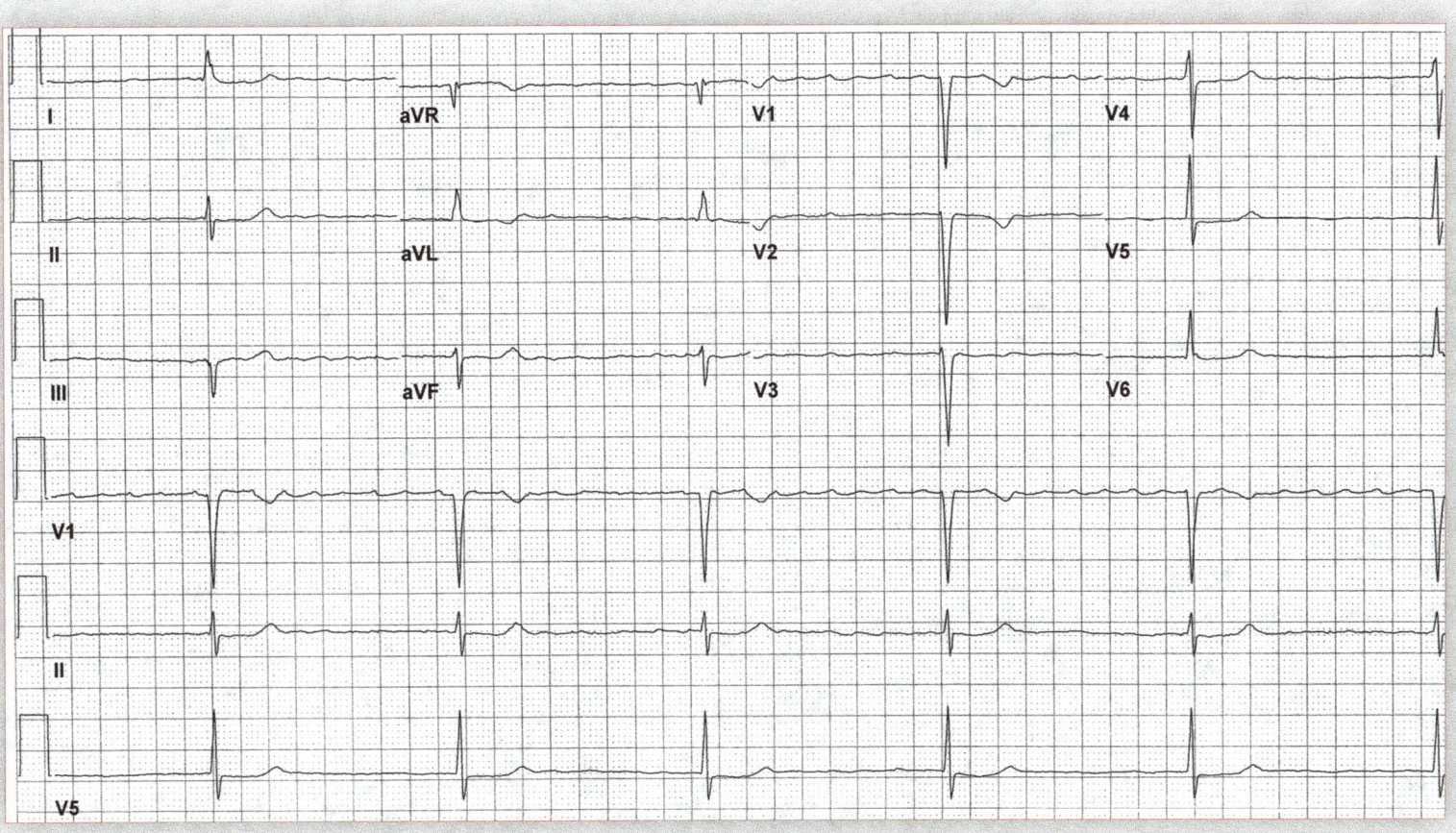

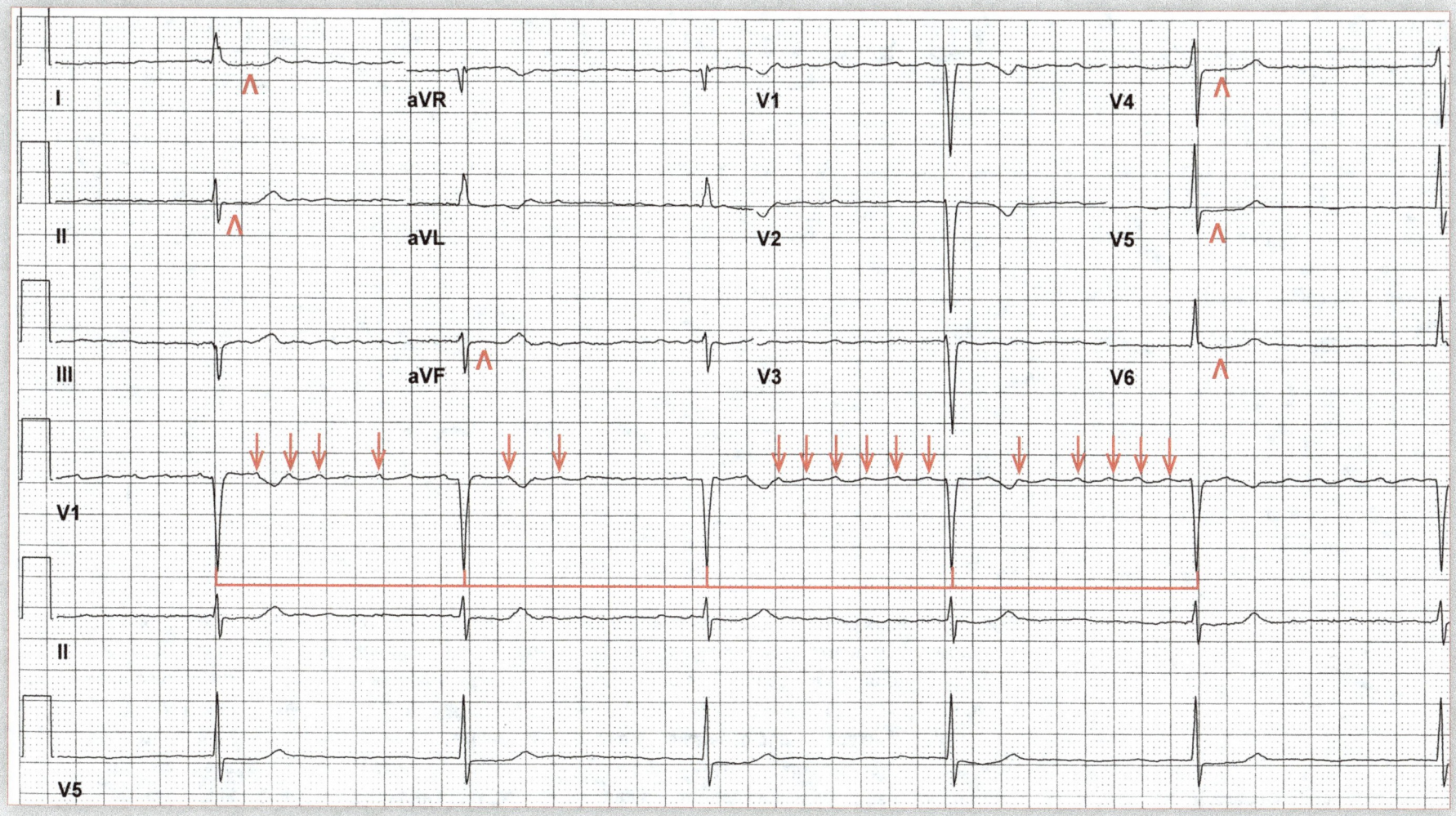

ECG 23 Analysis: Atrial fibrillation with complete heart block and escape junctional rhythm, clockwise rotation, nonspecific ST-segment abnormality

There are regular RR intervals (⊔) at a rate of 36 bpm. There are no organized P waves seen; however, there are rapid undulations (↓) of the baseline between each QRS complex; these undulations are irregular in morphology, amplitude, and interval. Hence the underlying rhythm is atrial fibrillation. The regularization of the QRS complex intervals indicates that there is complete heart block with an escape rhythm. The QRS complexes have a normal duration (0.08 sec) and morphology. Hence the escape rhythm is junctional. There is a left axis, between 0° and −30° (positive QRS complex in leads I and II and negative QRS complex in lead aVF). There is poor R-wave progression from lead V1 to lead V3 with late transition (ie, R/S > 1 in lead V5). This is consistent with a diagnosis of clockwise rotation in the horizontal plane. This is established by imagining the heart as viewed from under the diaphragm. With clockwise rotation, the left ventricular forces are directed more posteriorly and occur later in the precordial leads. In addition, there is flattening of the ST segments (^), as noted in leads I, II, aVF, and V4-V6. This is a nonspecific abnormality. The QT/QTc intervals are normal (520/400 msec).

The patient presents with signs, symptoms, and laboratory data suggesting significant dehydration, as a result of diarrhea, likely poor intake, and possibly the continued use of diuretics, although what drugs she is taking is unclear. She carries a diagnosis of heart failure, suggesting that she may be taking diuretics, and also atrial fibrillation for which digoxin, a β-blocker, or a calcium-channel blocker may be taken for rate control. Digoxin is cleared by the kidney, but in acute renal failure or prerenal azotemia, in this case due to dehydration in the context of an acute diarrheal illness, digoxin levels can increase acutely, leading to signs of digoxin toxicity that are manifest as significant conduction slowing through the AV node and the possibility of complete AV block, as seen in this ECG. Establishing digoxin toxicity in the presence of atrial fibrillation may be difficult. The earliest sign of excessive digoxin effect due to elevated digoxin levels (mediated by increased vagal tone) is the development of bradycardia, although the RR intervals remain irregularly irregular. With further elevation of digoxin levels there is the development of complete AV block, which is initially intermittent and presents with long RR intervals all of which have the same

continues

duration (intermittent regularization), indicating intermittent heart block with an escape focus. With further elevation of digoxin levels, the heart block becomes persistent, presenting as regularization of the RR intervals and the presence of an escape junctional rhythm, as is seen on this ECG. With further elevation of digoxin levels, the rate of the escape junctional rhythm increases (due to an increase in sympathetic output from the central nervous system), and nonparoxysmal junctional tachycardia occurs. Further elevation of digoxin levels results in His-Purkinje system abnormalities, with slowing of conduction through the bundles. This results in junctional tachycardia with alternating bundle branch block, called bidirectional tachycardia. Ultimately, there may be complete block within the bundles, resulting in an escape ventricular rhythm. The rate of the escape ventricular rhythm may be variable.

Another possible drug that she may be taking is a β-blocker (for hypertension and rate control of atrial fibrillation), which can also produce complete AV block. The two long-acting β-blockers, atenolol and nadolol, are cleared primarily by the kidneys. With reduced renal function, there may be an increase in the blood level and hence in the therapeutic effect of the β-blocker, leading to AV nodal blockade and the development of complete heart block.

In addition to rehydration, treatment is to withhold any agents that can affect AV nodal impulse transmission until there is resolution of the renal failure and the complete heart block. If the complete AV block is reversible, there is no indication for a pacemaker. ■

A 24-year-old man is admitted to the hospital with traumatic osteomyelitis. Because of marked bradycardia noted on exam, an ECG is performed. The patient's physical exam is notable for a soft, early diastolic murmur at the left upper sternal border. The ECG technician approaches you with the ECG, stating that he thinks the patient has Wolff-Parkinson-White syndrome.

Do you agree with the technician's diagnosis?

What further evaluation is warranted?

What therapy would help establish the diagnosis?

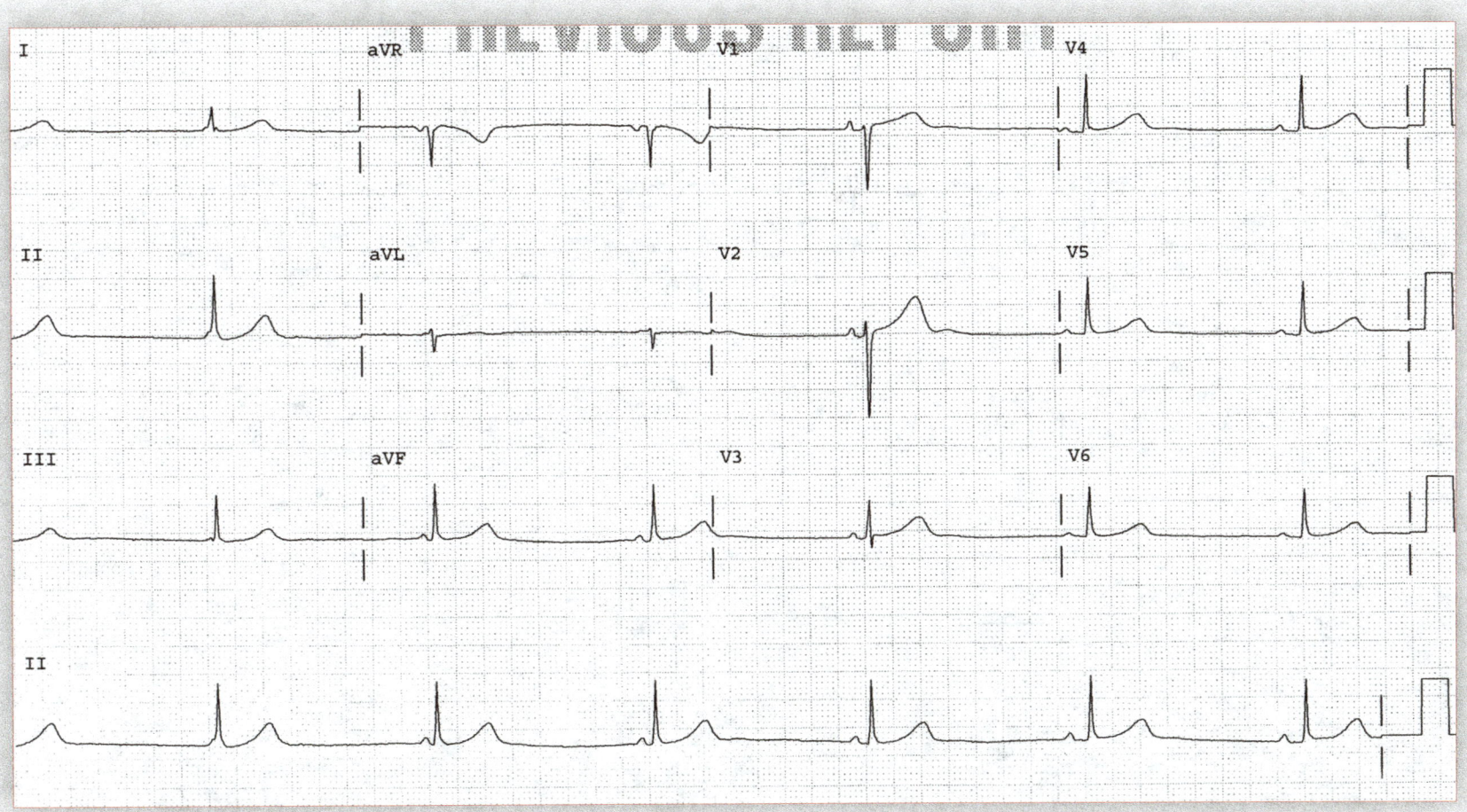

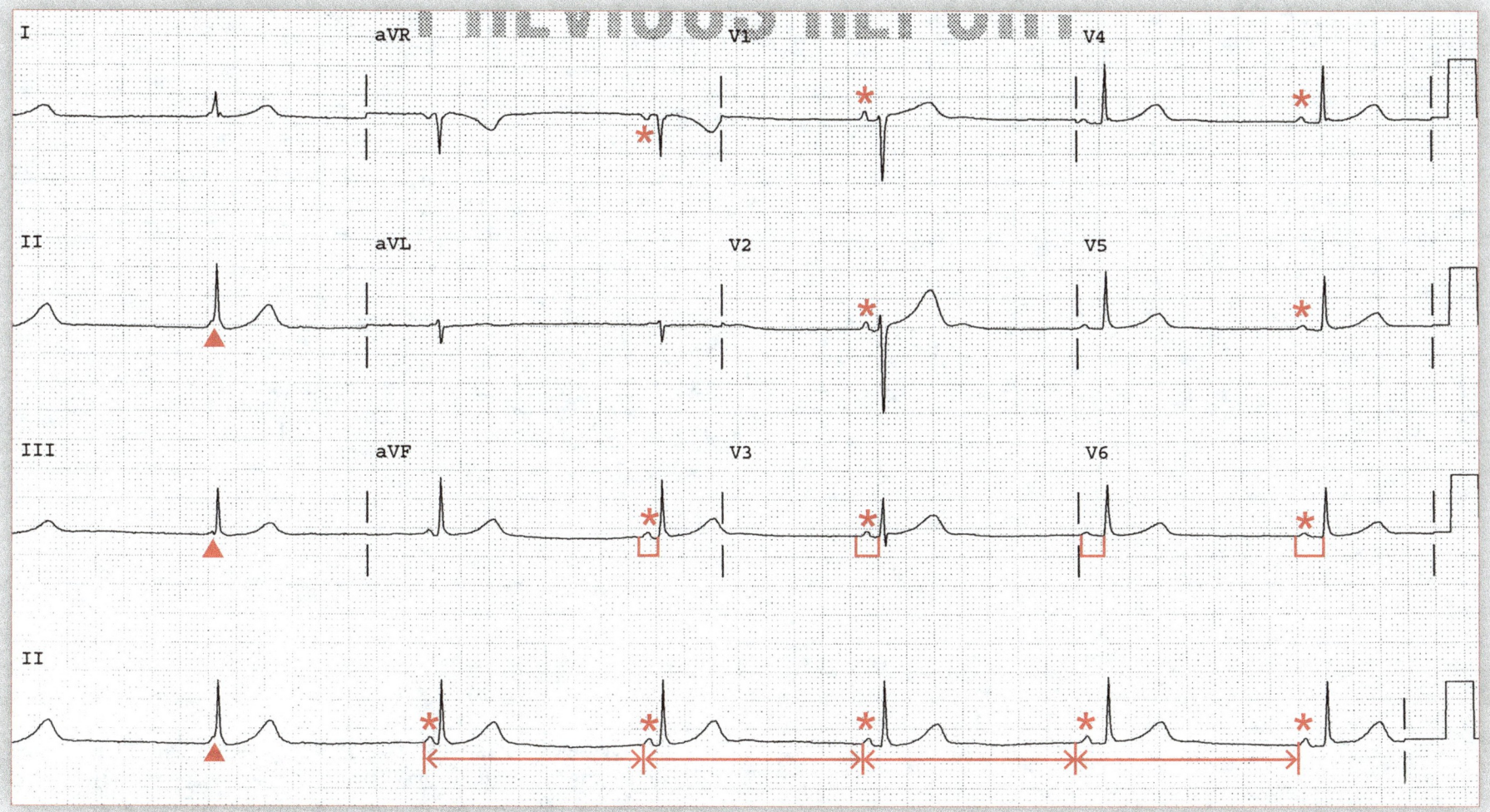

ECG 24 Analysis: Sinus bradycardia, isorhythmic AV dissociation, junctional rhythm

There is a regular narrow complex rhythm with a regular RR interval of 1.6 second and a rate of 38 bpm. The QRS complex duration is normal (0.08 sec) and there is a normal morphology and axis, between 0° and +90° (positive QRS complex in leads I and aVF). The QT/QTc intervals are normal (520/414 msec). Hence these are supraventricular complexes. P waves (*) are seen before each QRS complex, with a stable PP interval (1.6 sec) (↔) and an atrial rate of 38 bpm. The P waves are positive in leads II, aVF, and V4-V6. Hence this is a normal sinus rhythm. However, the PR intervals are not constant (⊔), becoming progressively longer. The P wave is actually superimposed on the first QRS complex (▲). As a result it looks like there is a delta wave; however, the apparent slurred upstroke is the P wave. Hence AV dissociation is present. As measured on the ECG when recorded at 25 mm/sec, the atrial and ventricular rates are identical. In this situation it cannot be established if there is complete AV block with an escape junctional rhythm (in which the atrial rate is faster than the junctional rate) or an accelerated junctional rhythm (in which case the atrial rate is slower than the junctional rate). Hence this is termed isorhythmic dissociation with a junctional rhythm.

The combination of possible heart block as well as a diastolic murmur suggestive of aortic regurgitation in a patient with osteomyelitis is concerning for aortic or mitral valve endocarditis. If endocarditis is present, complete (third-degree) AV block would be a more likely diagnosis. At this point no therapy is warranted as the junctional rhythm is stable. Even if the diagnosis were complete AV block, a temporary pacemaker would not be indicated, not only because of the absence of symptoms but also because of osteomyelitis and the possibility of endocarditis. Electrode catheters should not be inserted if there is an active infection because of the possibility of an infection occurring on the electrode catheter, which might result in a worsening of an underlying infection.

If clinically important, the etiology for the AV dissociation can be established with the use of atropine, which will increase the sinus rate but not affect the junctional rate. If there is capture with the increase in sinus rate, with consistent PR intervals, the mechanism for the isorhythmic dissociation would be established as an accelerated junctional rhythm. In contrast, if AV dissociation persisted with the increased sinus rate, the diagnosis would be complete heart block, as now the atrial rate would be faster than the junctional rate. ■

A 69-year-old man presents to the emergency department with complaints of substernal chest discomfort of 6 hours' duration. An ECG (25A) is obtained. His serum troponin level is elevated, and a diagnosis of non–ST-segment elevation myocardial infarction is made. The patient is

ECG 25A

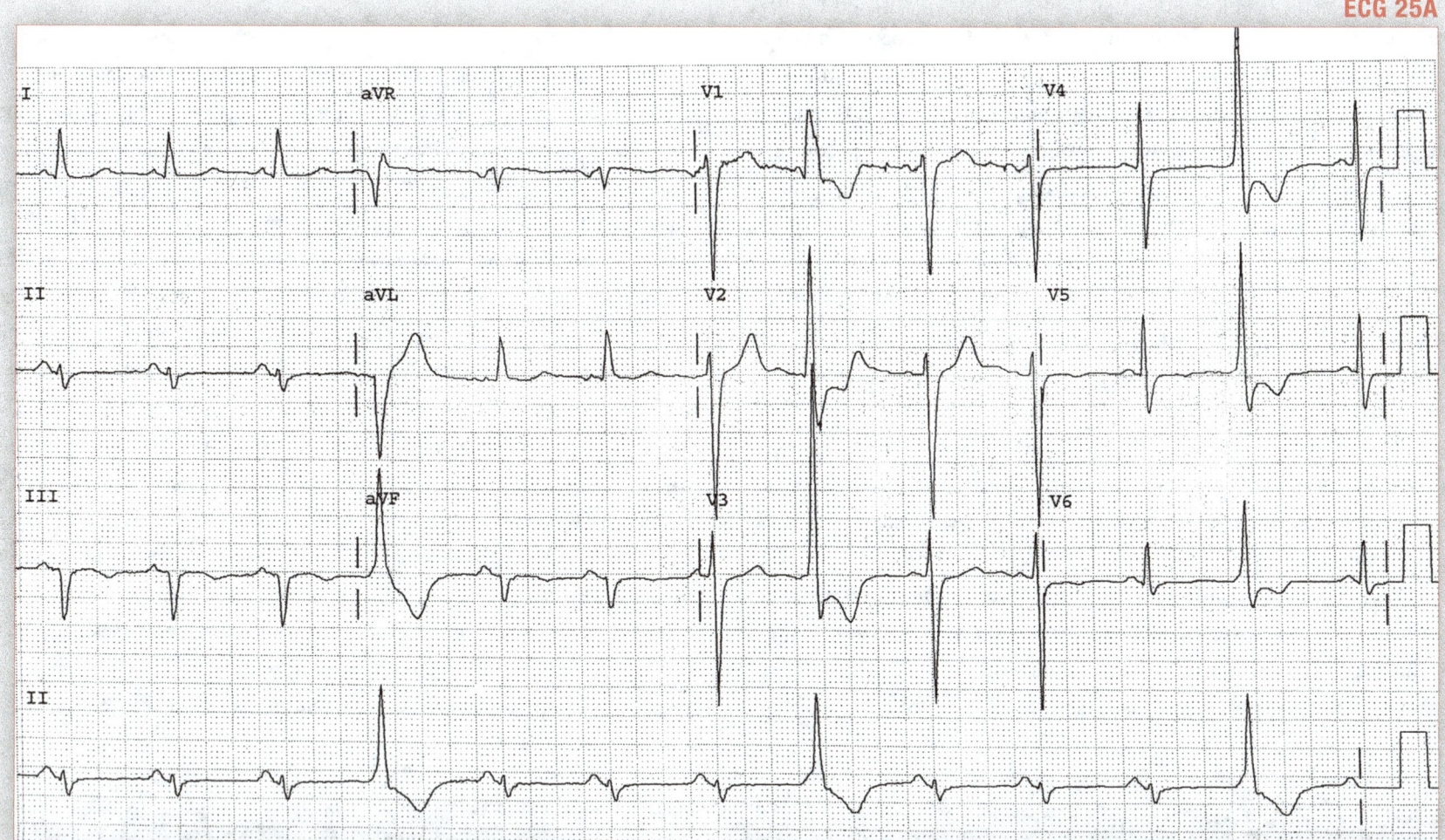

brought to the catheterization laboratory, where coronary angiography shows a thrombus in the first obtuse marginal artery. A drug-eluting stent is placed and the patient is brought to the coronary care unit. He is asymptomatic. A second ECG (25B) is obtained routinely.

What is noted on the ECGs?

What is the etiology of the rhythm on ECG 25B?

Is any therapy necessary?

ECG 25B

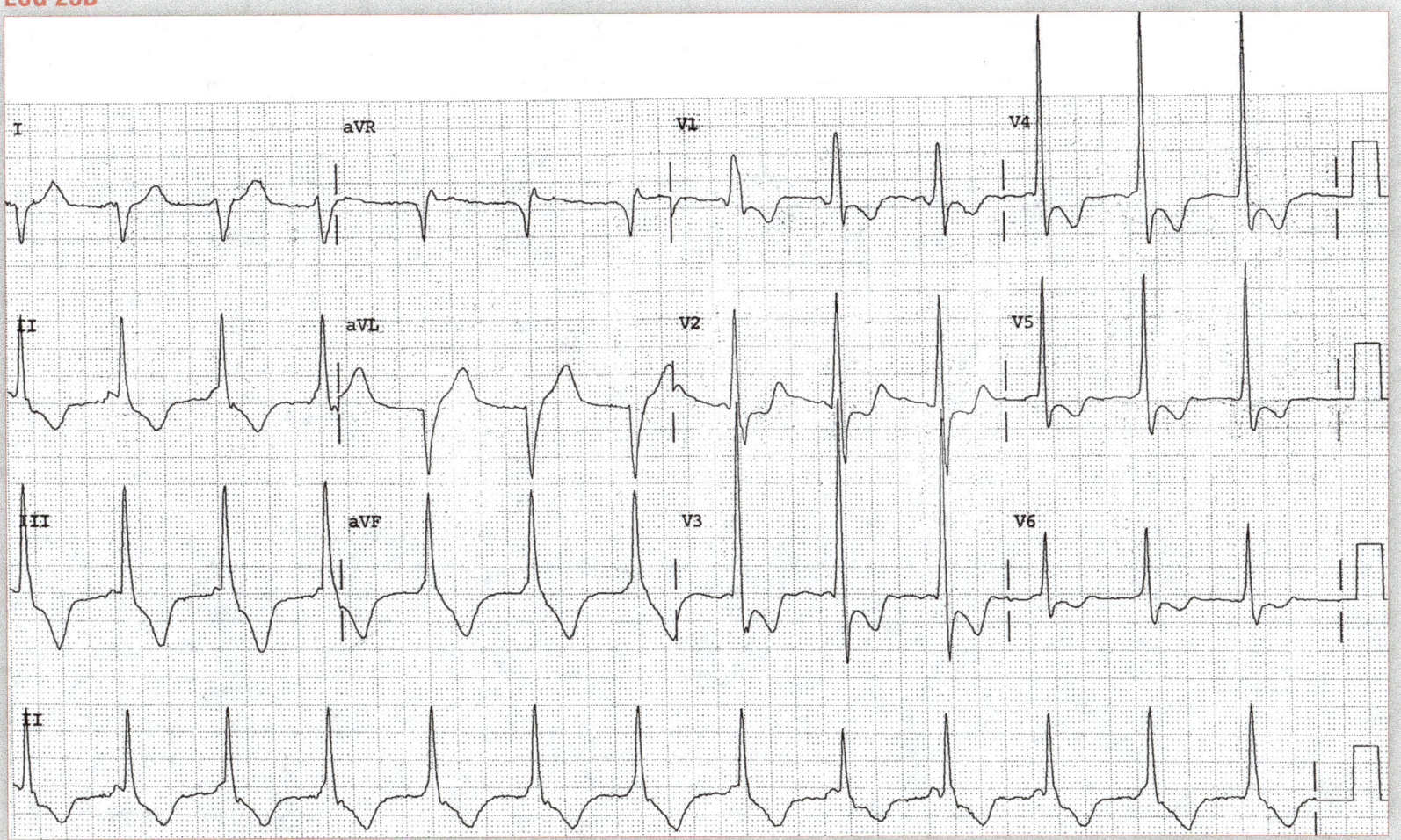

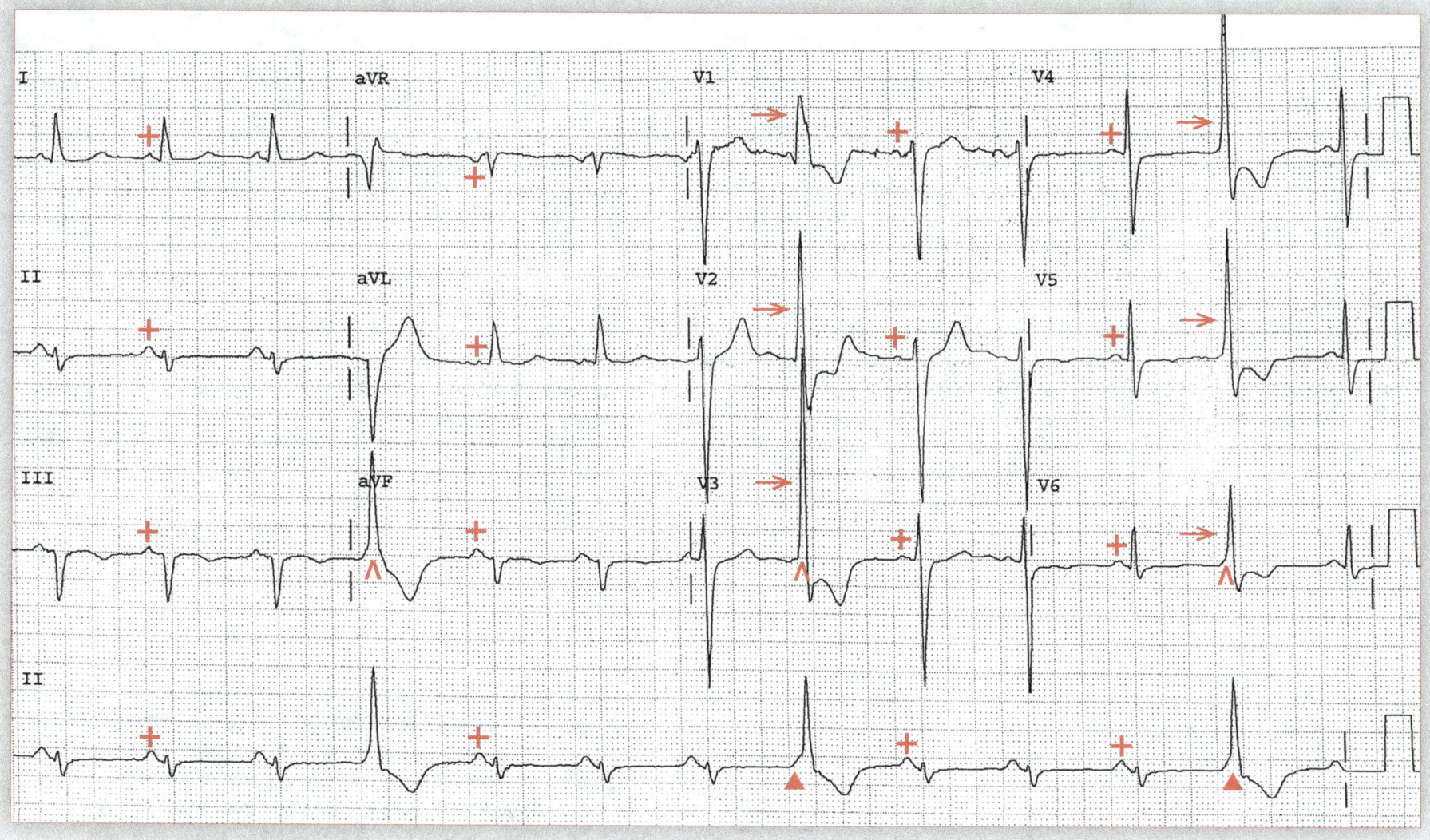

ECG 25A Analysis: Normal sinus rhythm, left anterior fascicular block, unifocal premature ventricular complexes, quadrigeminy

In **ECG 25A**, there is a regular rhythm at a rate of 72 bpm. There is a P wave (+) before each QRS complex with a stable PR interval (0.18 sec). The P waves are positive in leads I, II, aVF, and V4-V6. Hence this is a normal sinus rhythm. The QRS complex duration is normal (0.10 sec). The axis is extremely leftward, between −30° and −90° (positive QRS complex in lead I and negative QRS complex in leads II and aVF). As the QRS complexes have an rS morphology in leads II and aVF, this is a left anterior fascicular block. The QT/QTc intervals are normal (400/440 msec).

There are three premature QRS complexes (complexes 4, 8, and 12) (^), occurring every fourth beat; this is often termed quadrigeminy. They have an increased duration (0.16 sec) and an abnormal morphology, with positive concordance across the precordium (tall R waves in leads V1-V6 [→]). There is no distinct P wave before any of these QRS complexes, but there appears to be a P wave superimposed on the beginning of the eighth and 12th QRS complexes (▲). The P wave is not conducted as there is really no PR interval. Hence the wide and premature QRS complexes are premature ventricular complexes. Although there are no acute changes associated with a myocardial infarction, this is often the case with a lesion of the left circumflex artery or the obtuse marginal branch of the left circumflex artery. Infarction involving this vessel is not uncommonly electrically silent.

continues

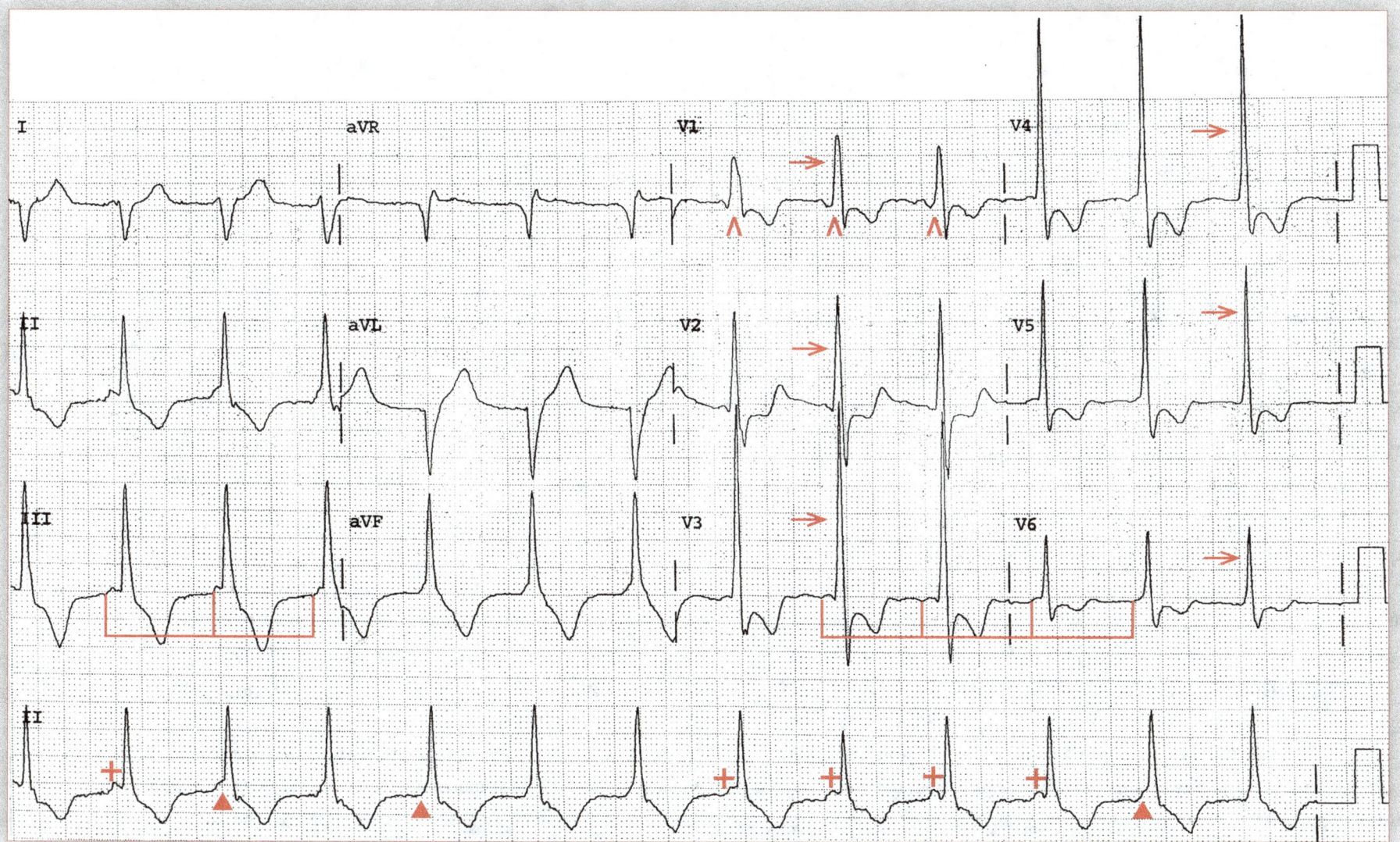

ECG 25B Analysis: Normal sinus rhythm, isorhythmic AV dissociation, ventricular rhythm

ECG 25B was obtained shortly after reperfusion of the first obtuse marginal artery. There is a regular rhythm at a rate of 75 bpm. The QRS complexes have the same duration and morphology as the premature ventricular complexes in ECG 25A. There is positive concordance across the precordium (tall R waves in leads V1-V6) (→), similar to the morphology of the premature ventricular complexes in ECG 25A. Also noted is a slight difference in the morphology of the QRS complexes in lead V1 (^). Lastly, there are P waves noted before some of the QRS complexes (+) but the PR interval is not constant. Some of the P waves are also superimposed at the beginning of the QRS complex (▲), which is evident by the slight widening of the initial portion of the QRS complex. Hence the P waves and QRS complexes are independent and there is AV dissociation. The axis is rightward, between +90° and +180° (negative QRS complex in lead I and positive QRS complex in lead aVF). The presence of AV dissociation, the positive concordance across the precordium, the slight variability of the QRS complex morphology noted in lead V1, and the fact that the QRS complex is identical to the premature ventricular complexes seen in ECG 25A establish the etiology as a ventricular rhythm. The PP intervals are regular (⊔) and the atrial rate is 75 bpm, which is identical to the ventricular rate. Hence this is isorhythmic AV dissociation and since the atrial and ventricular rates are identical it is not clear whether this is complete AV block with an escape ventricular rhythm or an accelerated idioventricular arrhythmia. However, based on the clinical scenario (*ie*, a non–ST-segment elevation myocardial infarction with reperfusion [stenting]), the most likely diagnosis is an accelerated idioventricular rhythm (AIVR), which is a reperfusion arrhythmia that often occurs after a percutaneous intervention or thrombolytic therapy for an acute myocardial infarction. An AIVR is usually benign and no therapy is typically required. However, if the ventricular rate were to accelerate and be associated with symptoms, then the ventricular arrhythmia should be suppressed with an antiarrhythmic, such as intravenous lidocaine, procainamide, or amiodarone. Therapy would likely be for a limited time as this arrhythmia is usually self-limited. ◼

Notes

An asymptomatic 58-year-old man presents for a routine physical. His review of symptoms, physical exam, and general laboratory evaluation are all normal. A routine ECG is obtained.

What abnormality is depicted?

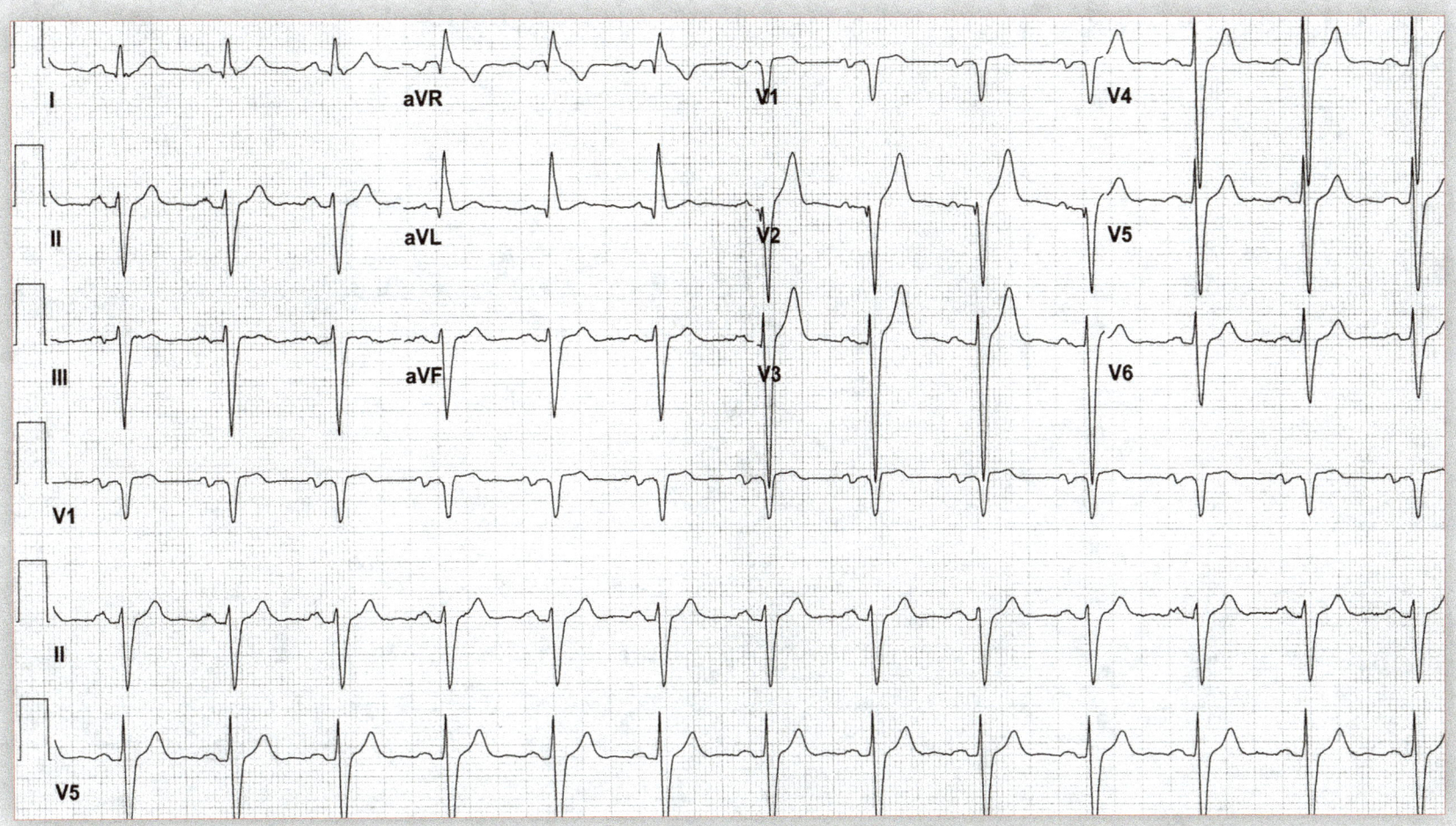

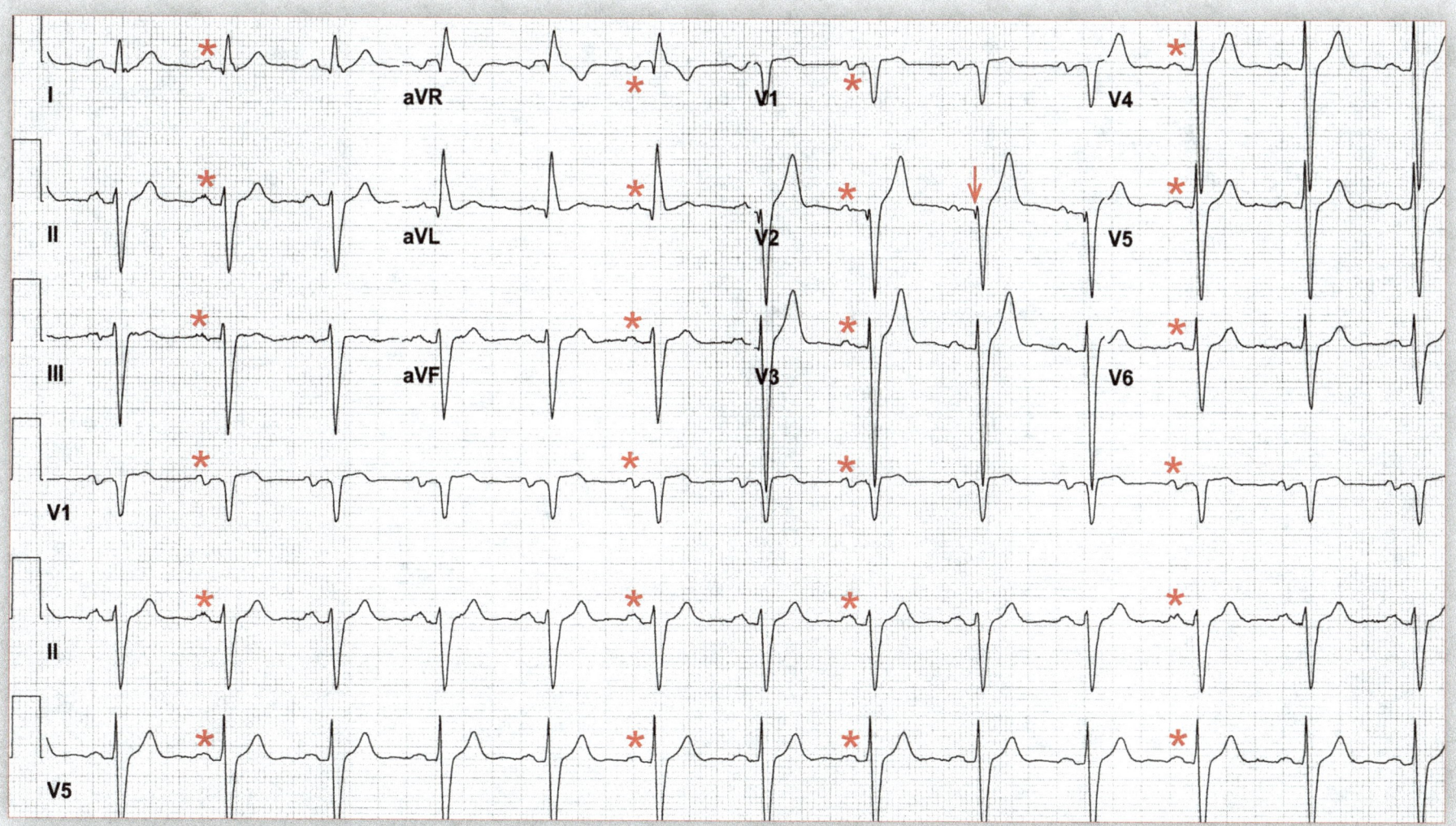

ECG 26 Analysis: Normal sinus rhythm, left anterior fascicular block (LAFB)

There is a regular rhythm at a rate of 78 bpm. There is a P wave (*) before each QRS complex with a stable PR interval of 0.18 second. The P waves are positive in leads I, II, aVF, and V4-V6. Hence this is a normal sinus rhythm. The QRS complexes are of a normal width (0.08 sec) and morphology. The axis is extremely leftward, between −30° and −90° (positive QRS complex in lead I and negative QRS complex in leads II and aVF). There are two reasons for an extreme left axis. The first is an inferior wall myocardial infarction (MI) (or a pseudo inferior wall MI, as seen in Wolff-Parkinson-White pattern), in which there are Q waves and a QS or Qr morphology in leads II and aVF. The second is a left anterior fascicular block (LAFB), also called a left anterior hemiblock, in which there are rS complexes in leads II and aVF. In this case, the left axis is due to an LAFB. The QT/QTc intervals are normal (380/430 msec).

The left bundle consists of two major fascicles (left anterior and left posterior) as well as a small septal branch. The concept of the hemi, or fascicular, block was put forth by Rosenbaum and colleagues in 1970. The definition of a fascicular block was based on the electrical axis of the heart in the frontal plane. An LAFB results in all of ventricular activation coming from the left posterior fascicle. The direction of the impulse is up and to the left. Hence the axis is extremely leftward (>−30°). Some authors consider an extreme left axis as >−45° or >−60°. A fascicular block results in an axis shift but does not cause any widening of the QRS complex. A widened QRS complex indicates the presence of an intraventricular conduction delay in addition to the fascicular block or might be an associated right bundle branch block.

Other causes for a left axis need to be excluded, primarily an inferior wall MI (which is also associated with a positive QRS complex in lead I and a negative QRS complex in leads II and aVF). The difference is related to the initial force. With an inferior wall MI the initial wave of the QRS complex is a Q wave (Qr or QS complex), while with an LAFB the initial wave is an R wave (rS complex). Another cause would be lead misplacement. However, in this situation the P wave would also be negative in leads II and aVF.

Also noted is a small Q wave in lead V2 (↓). Although this might be considered evidence of an anteroseptal MI, this pattern may be seen with conduction disease of the septal (median) branch that originates from the left bundle and is responsible for activation of the septum, which is the first part of the left ventricle to depolarize. The direction is from left to right, accounting for small initial R waves in leads V1-V2. The presence of Q waves suggest that in these leads the initial septal activation is from right to left, which is abnormal. This abnormality, along with the presence of an LAFB, may be predictive of the occurrence of a full left bundle branch block in the future.

The most common reason for an LAFB in the absence of heart disease is Lenègre's disease, which is a fibrotic sclerodegenerative disease. LAFB in the absence of apparent organic heart disease and not associated with block in the other fascicles is usually benign and infrequently progresses to bifascicular disease or complete heart block. There is no reason for any additional workup or therapy. ■

A 72-year-old man is brought to the emergency department after he suddenly lost consciousness while getting out of bed. The syncopal episode was observed by his wife, who called 911. The man states that the episode was preceded by a feeling of lightheadedness and weakness. He also reports that he has had abdominal cramps associated with diarrhea, nausea, vomiting, and anorexia for the past 2 days, during which time he has been unable to take in anything orally. When emergency medical services arrived, he was awake but diaphoretic and nauseated. In the emergency department he relates a history of a previous myocardial infarction (MI) but no other cardiac or medical problems. His current medications are aspirin, simvastatin, low-dose lisinopril, and low-dose metoprolol. The physical exam is unremarkable; his blood pressure is 110/60 mm Hg. Laboratory data are unremarkable, except for a blood urea nitrogen level of 45 mg/dL and a creatinine level of 1.3 mg/dL. An ECG is obtained.

What abnormality is seen?

Does the ECG suggest an etiology for the syncopal episode?

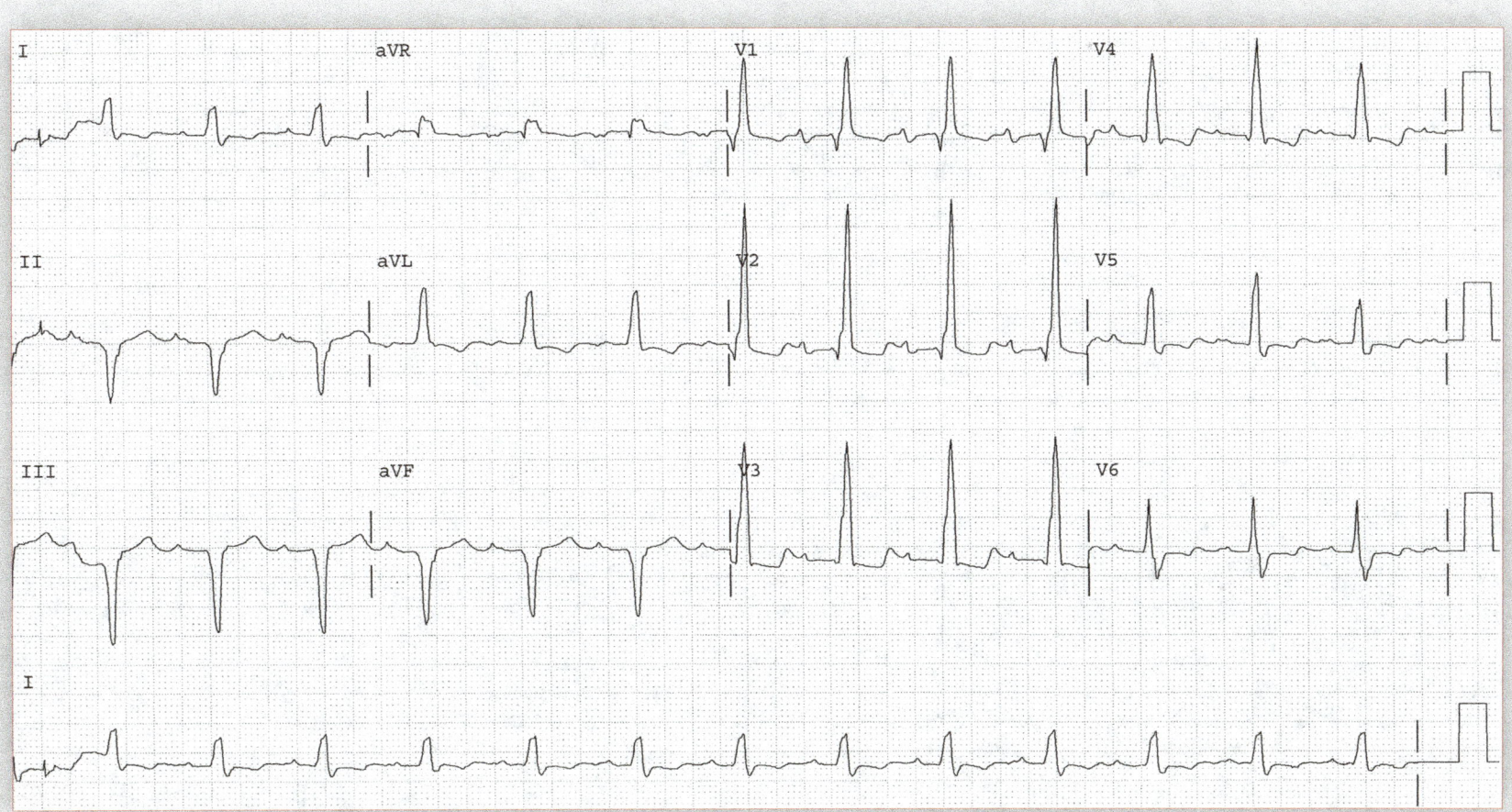

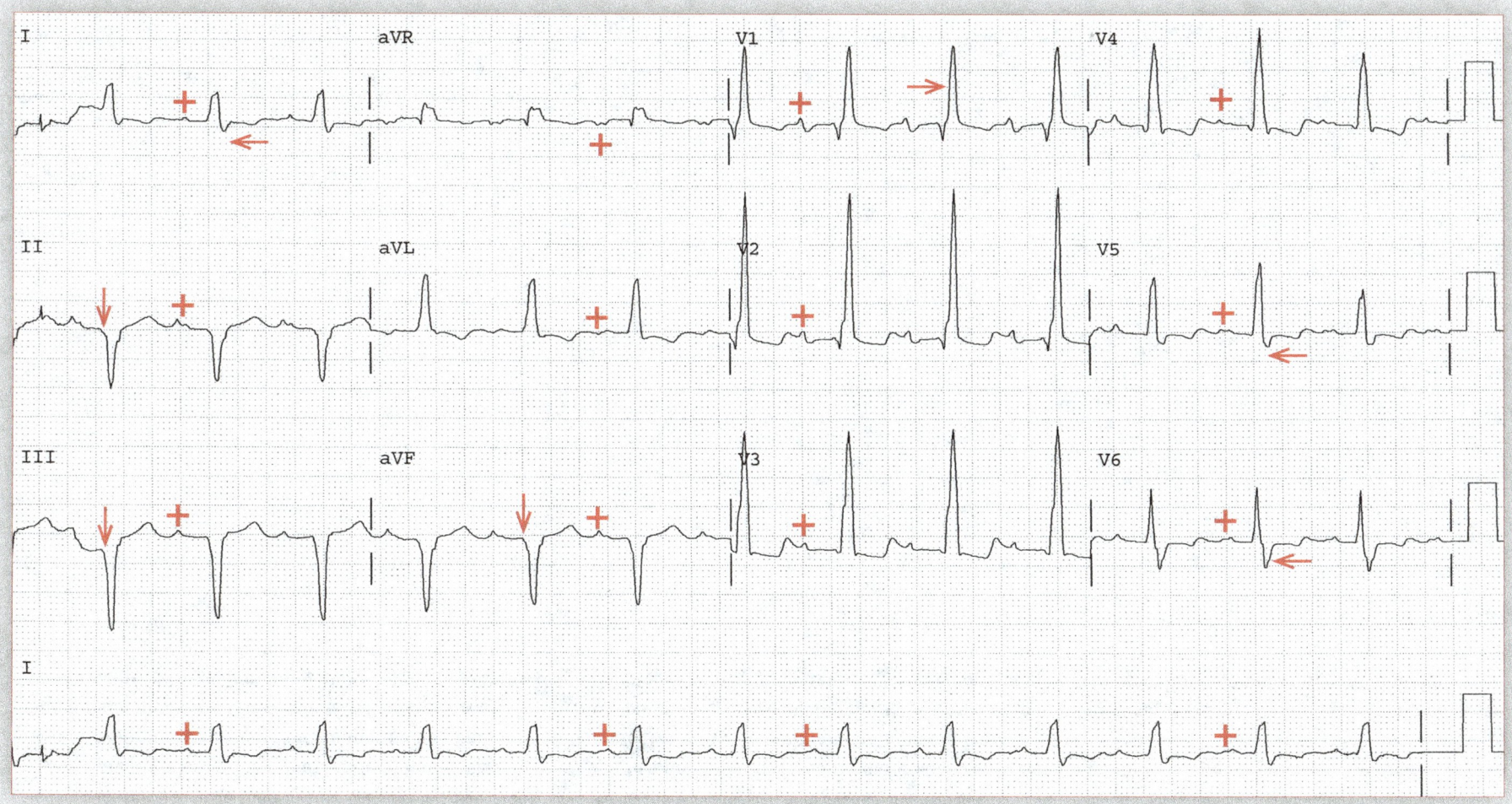

ECG 27 Analysis: Normal sinus rhythm, first-degree AV block (prolonged AV conduction), right bundle branch block, left axis, old inferior wall MI

There is a regular rhythm at a rate of 84 bpm. There is a P wave (+) before each QRS complex with a stable PR interval (0.28 sec). The P waves are positive in leads I, II, aVF, and V4-V6. Hence this is a normal sinus rhythm with first-degree AV block (prolonged AV conduction). The QRS complex duration is prolonged (0.14 sec), and it has a right bundle branch block (RBBB) morphology with an RSR′ complex in lead V1 (→) and a broad terminal S wave in leads I and V5-V6 (←). The QT/QTc intervals are prolonged (420/500 msec) but are normal when the prolonged QRS complex duration is considered (360/430 msec).

The axis is extremely leftward, between –30° and –90° (positive QRS complex in lead I and negative QRS complex in leads II and aVF). While the axis is consistent with a left anterior fascicular block (LAFB), the QRS complex has a QS morphology in leads II and aVF (↓), which is indicative of an old inferior wall myocardial infarction (MI). In contrast, a left anterior fascicular block has an rS morphology in leads II and aVF. Hence the left axis is not the result of a conduction abnormality but rather is due to an infarction.

The ECG suggests trifascicular conduction disease (ie, RBBB, left axis, and first-degree block). However, the left axis is due to an inferior wall MI and not a conduction abnormality; hence this is not trifascicular

disease. However, if trifascicular disease were present, the occurrence of syncope would suggest a more advanced conduction abnormality (ie, complete heart block with an escape ventricular rhythm). In this situation, further evaluation of the conduction system would be indicated. However, the presence of first-degree AV block in association with bifascicular disease (ie, RBBB and LAFB, if present) does not necessarily imply trifascicular disease as the prolonged PR interval might reflect an AV nodal conduction abnormality or slowing of conduction in the remaining fascicle (ie, the left posterior fascicle). In this case, since the left axis is not the result of an LAFB, the only definite conduction abnormality of the His-Purkinje system is an RBBB, while the first-degree AV block might be AV nodal or involve the remaining fascicles. This makes syncope from complete heart block far less likely. Indeed, the history strongly suggests that the patient was dehydrated as a result of 2 days of diarrhea, vomiting, and decreased oral intake. Further support for a diagnosis of volume depletion is the elevated blood urea nitrogen level, which is out of proportion to the serum creatinine level. The syncopal episode following a change in position is consistent with hypotension or perhaps a vasovagal episode as the etiology for the syncope. ■

An asymptomatic 58-year-old man presents for a routine checkup. His vital signs, physical exam, and general laboratory evaluation are all normal. An ECG is obtained.

What abnormality is depicted?

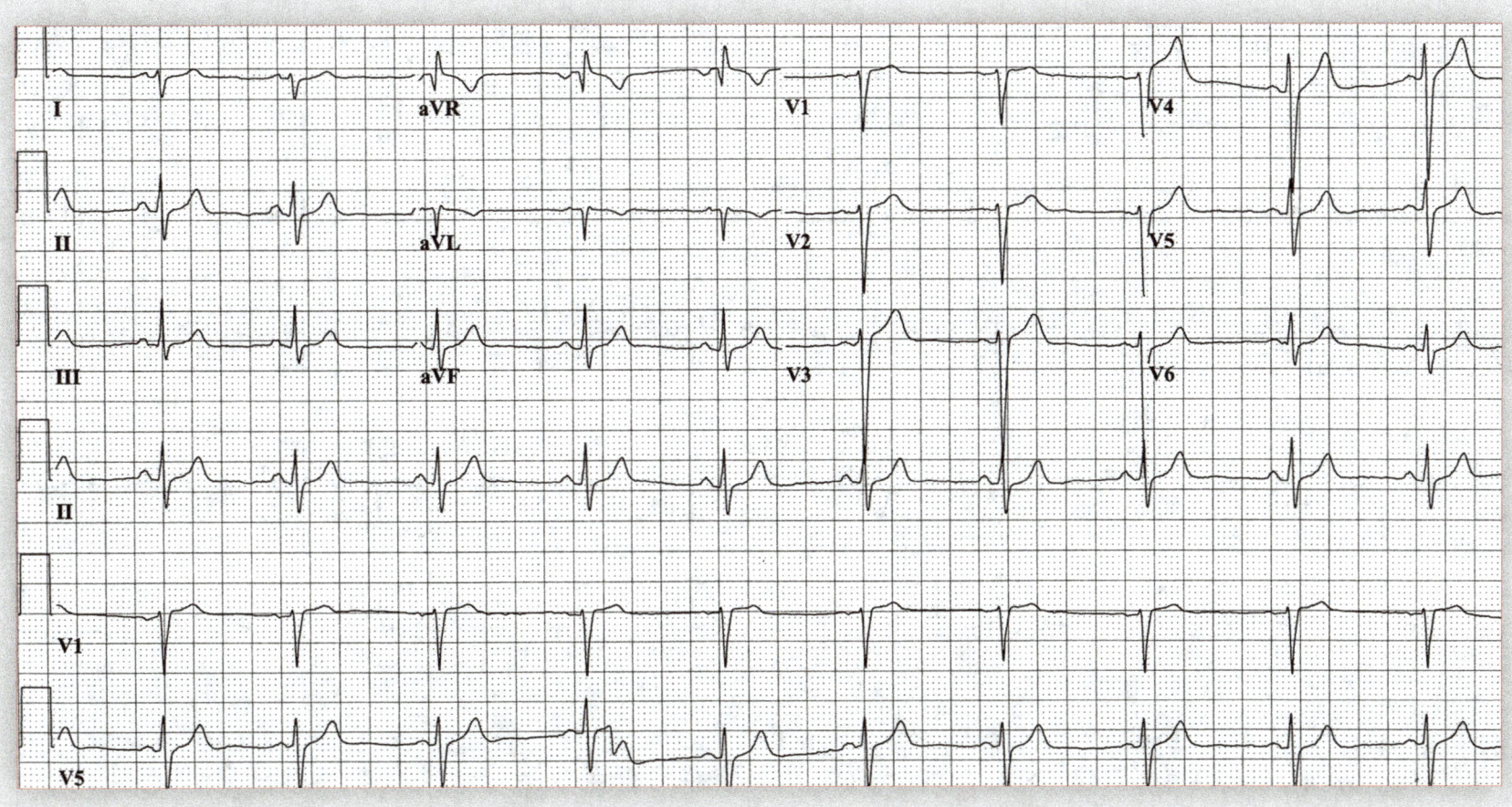

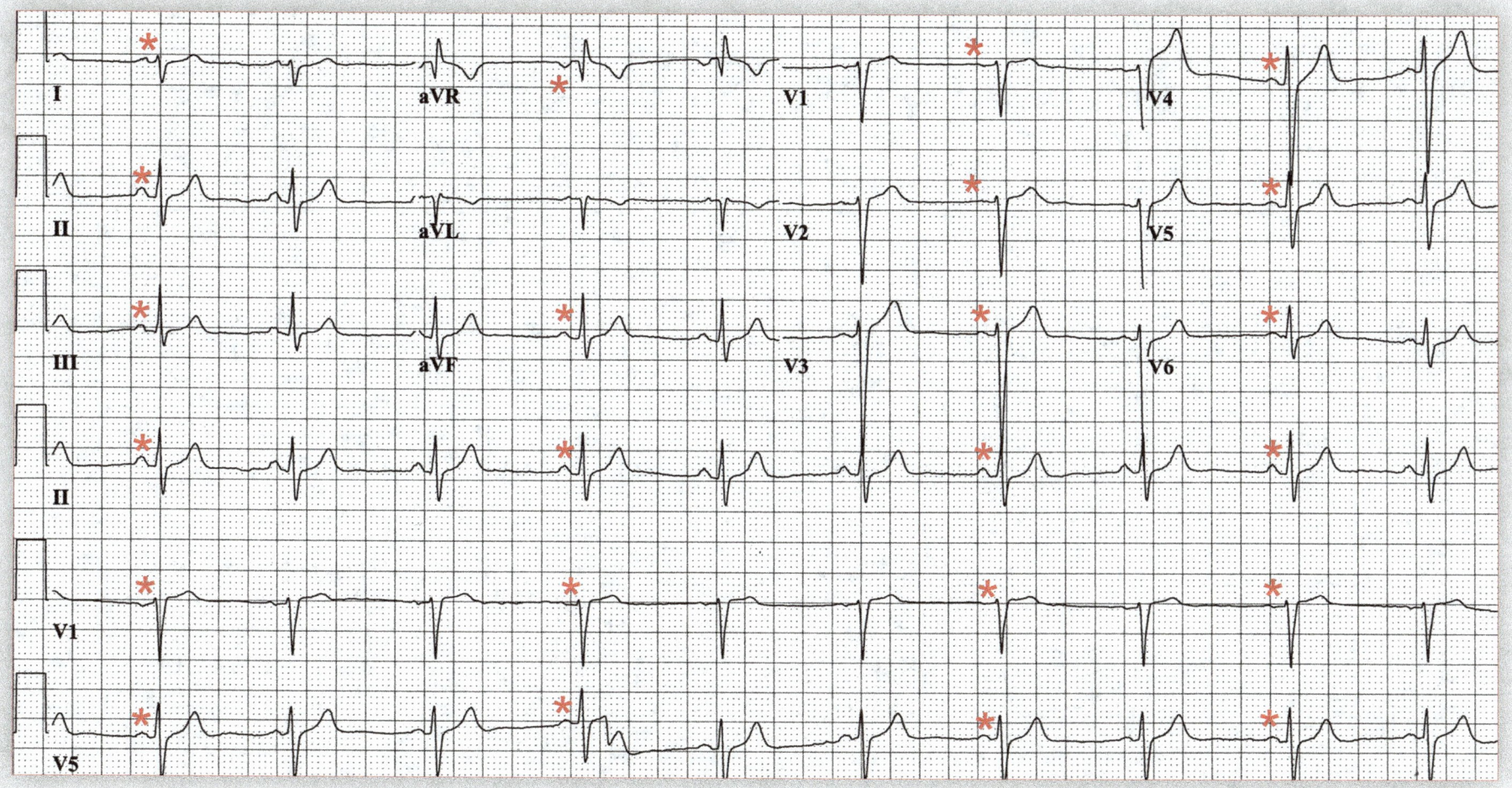

ECG 28 Analysis: Normal sinus rhythm, left posterior fascicular block

The rhythm is regular at a rate of 62 bpm. There is a P wave (*) before each QRS complex with a stable PR interval (0.16 sec). The P wave is positive in leads I, II, aVF, and V4-V6. Hence this is a normal sinus rhythm. The QRS complex is of normal duration (0.08 sec) and morphology. The QT/QTc intervals are normal (360/370 msec). The QRS complex is negative in lead I and positive in lead aVF. Hence the axis is rightward (between +90° and +180°). There are several etiologies for a right axis, including:

- Lateral wall infarct pattern, that is, an initial Q wave (Qr or QS) in leads I and aVL

- Right ventricular hypertrophy, which will be associated with a tall R wave in lead V1 and evidence of right atrial hypertrophy or abnormality (P pulmonale)

- Right–left arm lead switch, which is associated with negative P and T waves in leads I and aVL and positive P and T waves and positive QRS complexes in lead aVR

- Dextrocardia, in which there are inverted P and T waves in leads I and aVL and reverse R-wave progression across the precordium

- Right bundle branch block with a deep and broad S wave in lead I may be diagnosed as a right axis. In this situation the terminal S wave, which reflects delayed right ventricular activation, should be ignored as it is not reflective of left ventricular activation and hence not considered as part of axis determination.

- Wolff-Parkinson-White (WPW) pattern, which will be associated with a short PR interval and widened QRS complex resulting from a delta wave

- Biventricular pacemaker, which will have a QS or deep Q wave in lead I. Most often an indeterminate axis will be seen. With a pacemaker, pacemaker stimuli will be seen.

- Left posterior fascicular block (LPFB), with all left ventricular forces originating from the left anterior fascicle and directed down and to the right. This diagnosis is made when all other causes for a right axis have been excluded.

In this tracing, the QRS complexes have an initial R wave in leads I and aVL (rS complex), and there is no evidence for right ventricular hypertrophy, arm lead switch, dextrocardia, lateral infarction, WPW pattern, right bundle branch block, or pacemaker. Hence the right axis is due to an LPFB.

The left bundle divides into two major fascicles that innervate the left ventricle. The left anterior fascicle crosses the left ventricular outflow tract and terminates in the Purkinje system of the anterolateral wall of the left ventricle. The left posterior fascicle appears as an extension of the main bundle and fans out extensively posteriorly toward the papillary muscle and inferoposteriorly toward the free wall of the left ventricle. There is often a third, smaller fascicle that is a septal branch (median fascicle) that innervates the interventricular septum, which

continues

is the first part of the left ventricle to be activated (in a left-to-right direction). The left posterior fascicle is exposed to lower pressures and less turbulence than the left anterior fascicle; it also has a dual blood supply. These characteristics probably explain why isolated LPFB is an uncommon finding. Isolated LPFB can, however, be seen in the setting of extensive arteriosclerotic cardiovascular disease, as an association with inferior wall myocardial infarction and extensive coronary disease with diffuse myocardial fibrosis. LPFB can also occur with cardiomyopathies, hypertension with hypertrophy, myocarditis, hyperkalemia, acute cor pulmonale and, perhaps most commonly, chronic degenerative and fibrotic processes of the conducting system. An LPFB does not cause widening of the QRS complex, only a shift in axis. Hence any QRS widening is due to an associated intraventricular conduction delay or a right bundle branch block.

Isolated LPFB does not require any additional evaluation or therapy. However, additional evaluation may be required if there is evidence of trifascicular disease. ◼

A 54-year-old man presents to his primary doctor as a new patient. He has never had any meaningful medical care in the past. He comes today with complaints of shortness of breath with everyday activities that has progressed to the point that he cannot ascend a flight of stairs or even a slight grade incline without taking frequent rests to catch his breath. His review of systems is notable for a 40-pound unintentional weight loss over the past year. He has no known past medical history and does not take any medications. His family and social histories are remarkable for 35-year employment as a coal miner. He smoked cigarettes regularly for 20 years but quit 10 years ago. On exam, he appears emaciated. His heart rate is 90 bpm, his blood pressure is 92/60 mm Hg, and his lips are faintly blue. His head, ears, eyes, nose, and throat exam is notable for temporal wasting. His lungs are hyperinflated with poor air movement. His jugular venous pressure is 10 cm H_2O with taller CV waves. His precordium demonstrates a right ventricular lift. His point of maximal impulse is nondisplaced. His rhythm is regular, with a normal S1 and prominent P2. A respirophasic holosystolic murmur is noted at the right lower sternal border.

His abdominal, extremity, and neurologic exams are normal. Arterial blood gases confirm hypoxemia and hypercapnia. An ECG is obtained as part of his evaluation.

What abnormalities are noted?

To what cardiopulmonary process do these abnormalities point, as suggested by his exam and history?

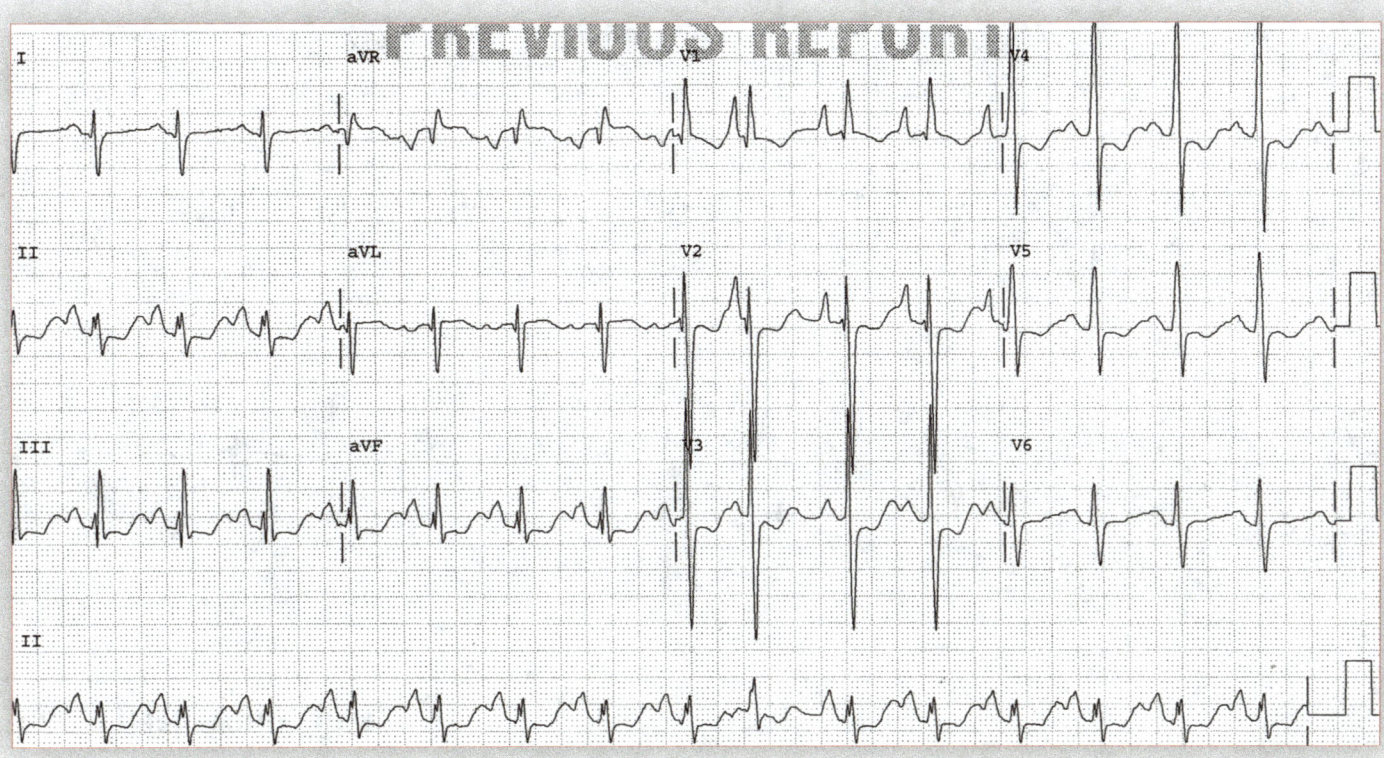

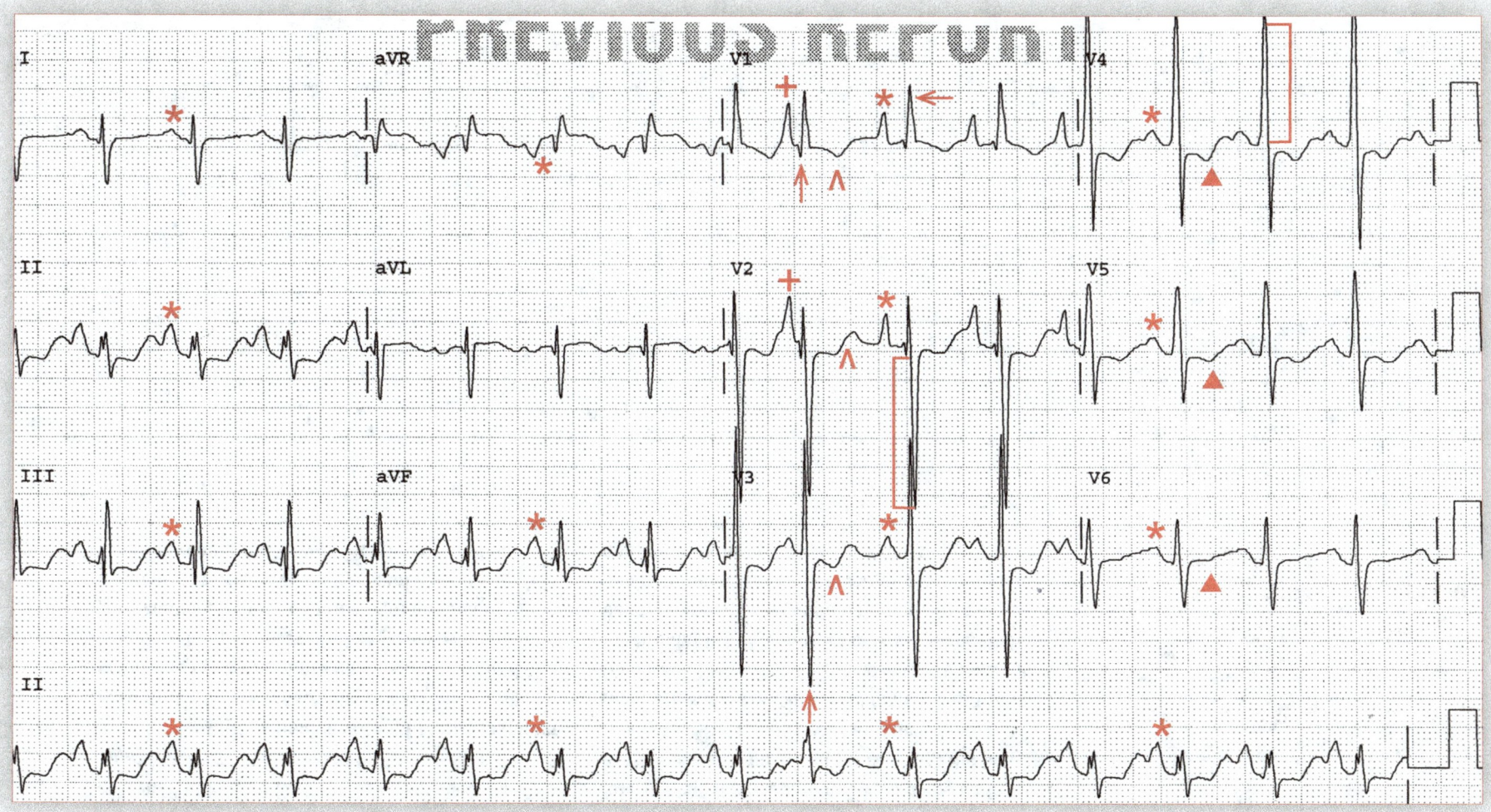

ECG 29 Analysis: Normal sinus rhythm, intraventricular conduction delay, right axis, right atrial hypertrophy (abnormality), P pulmonale, right ventricular hypertrophy (RVH) with ST-T wave changes, premature atrial complex, left ventricular hypertrophy (LVH) with ST-T wave changes, biventricular hypertrophy

The rhythm is regular at a rate of 90 bpm. There is a P wave (*) before each QRS complex with a stable PR interval (0.20 sec). The P waves are positive in leads I, II, aVF, and V4-V6. Hence this is a normal sinus rhythm. The P waves are very tall in leads II and aVF and also positive and tall in leads V1-V2; this is characteristic of right atrial hypertrophy or abnormality (P pulmonale). Given the height of the P waves in leads V1-V2, the term "Himalayan P waves" has been used. The QRS duration is slightly increased (0.12 sec), and there is an intraventricular conduction delay. The axis is rightward, between +90° and +180° (negative QRS complex in lead I and positive QRS complex in lead aVF). The QT/QTc intervals are prolonged (440/540 msec) even when the slightly prolonged QRS complex duration is considered (420/490 msec). There is a tall R wave (←) in lead V1. When associated with a right axis and P pulmonale, the tall R wave in lead V1 is indicative of right ventricular hypertrophy (RVH). Hence the right axis is the result of RVH and is not due to a left posterior fascicular block.

In addition, the S-wave depth in lead V2 is 26 mm [[ ], and the R-wave amplitude in lead V4 is 22 mm [ ]] (S-wave depth in lead V2 + R-wave amplitude in lead V4 = 48 mm), meeting the voltage criteria for left ventricular hypertrophy (LVH; S-wave depth + R-wave amplitude in any two precordial leads ≥ 35 mm). Therefore, there is evidence of biventricular hypertrophy. There are also ST-T wave abnormalities in leads V1-V3 (^), likely the result of RVH, while the ST-T wave abnormalities in leads V4-V6 (▲) are likely the result of LVH. The 10th QRS complex (↑) is early, is preceded by a premature P wave (+), and has the same QRS complex morphology as the sinus complexes. Hence it is a premature atrial complex.

This patient has signs, symptoms, and ECG evidence of RVH, the result of chronic obstructive lung disease from coal dust exposure as well as cigarette smoking. There is also evidence on the physical exam of tricuspid regurgitation (respirophasic holosystolic murmur and tall CV waves of the jugular pulsation). The patient should have an echocardiogram to evaluate pulmonary artery and right-sided pressures as well as left ventricular function. Initial therapy for pulmonary arterial hypertension as well as chronic obstructive lung disease consists of oxygen therapy. As there is no clinical evidence for fluid accumulation, diuretics are not needed. More advanced therapy includes treatment with prostanoids such as epoprostenol, endothelin receptor antagonists, phosphodiesterase 5 inhibitors such as sildenafil, or certain calcium-channel blockers (*eg*, a dihydropyridine or diltiazem). Patients with pulmonary hypertension who are selected for advanced therapy should undergo an invasive hemodynamic assessment prior to the initiation of advanced therapy. A vasoreactivity test with intravenous adenosine, intravenous epoprostenol, or inhaled nitric oxide is often performed at the time of hemodynamic assessment. The LVH may be the result of previous hypertension, although there is no clear history for this. ■

A 68-year-old diabetic woman presents to her primary care physician as a new patient. She states that "she had some heart trouble in the past" but is unaware of any specific diagnosis. She has stopped taking all medications that were previously prescribed. She declares, "No, I'm doing fine!" to all questions on a review of systems. Her vital signs and exam are unremarkable. As part of her evaluation, an ECG is performed.

What abnormalities are noted on the ECG, and to what pathology do they point?

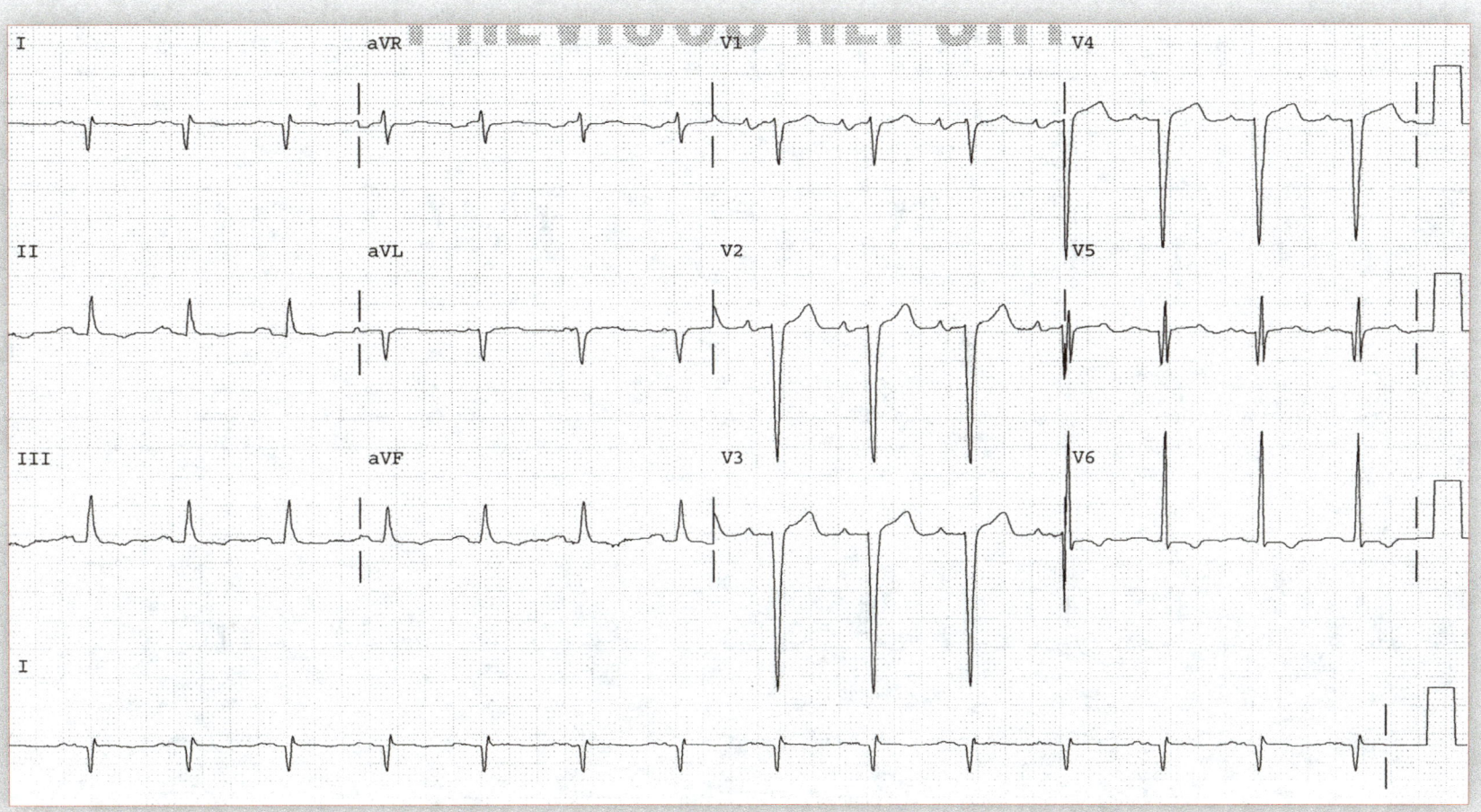

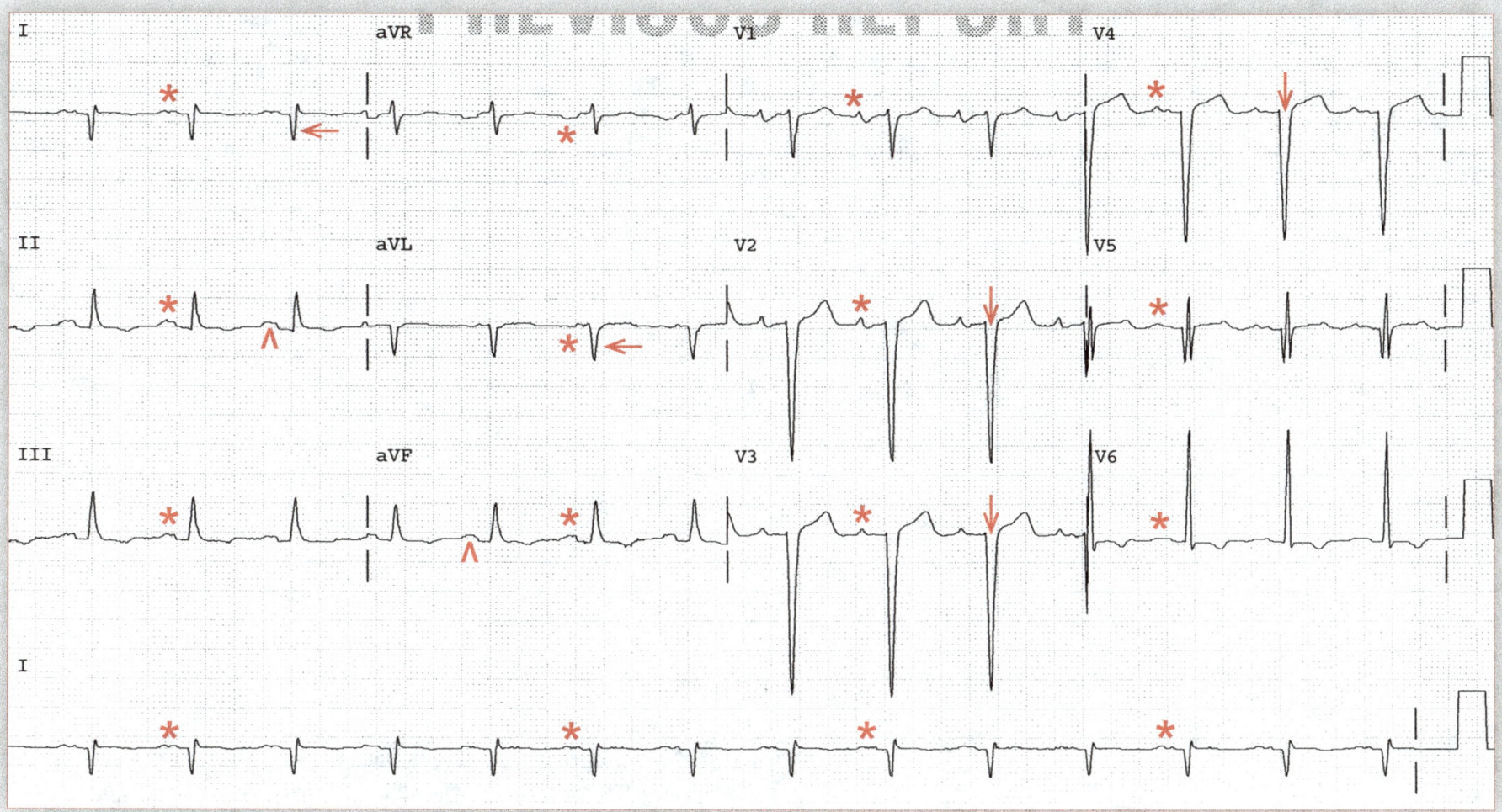

ECG 30 Analysis: Normal sinus rhythm, first-degree AV block (prolonged AV conduction), right axis, old lateral wall myocardial infarction (MI), old anterior wall MI, left atrial hypertrophy (abnormality)

There is a regular rhythm at a rate of 86 bpm. There is a P wave (*) before each QRS complex with a stable PR interval of 0.22 second. The P wave is positive in leads I, II, aVF, and V4-V6. Hence this is a normal sinus rhythm with first-degree AV block (prolonged AV conduction). However, the P waves are broad in leads II and aVF (^), suggesting left atrial hypertrophy or abnormality. The QRS complex duration is normal (0.10 sec). The axis is rightward, between +90° and +180° (negative QRS complex in lead I and positive QRS complex in lead aVF). However, the right axis is a result of a Q wave (←) in leads I and aVL (Qr morphology). This is, therefore, a lateral myocardial infarction (MI) and not a left posterior fascicular block. In addition, there are Q waves (↓) in leads V2-V5, indicating an anterior wall MI.

Although the patient does not provide any history to suggest a prior MI or its timing, the presence of Q waves indicates that the infarction is chronic or old. Although she claims a history of some heart problem in the past, she provides no specifics about this. Silent infarctions are not uncommon, especially in the diabetic patient. Her therapy should consist of aggressive risk factor modification, including aspirin; LDL-lowering therapy with statins; and good control of her diabetes. She is not having any symptoms, suggesting that there is no actual role for anti-ischemic medication, including β-blocker or nitrates. However, diabetic patients do have silent (discomfortless) ischemia, so exercise testing would be useful to document any ECG changes or symptoms that suggest underlying ischemia. ■

Core Case 31

A 42-year-old man without prior medical diagnoses but with a strong family history of myocardial infarction is seen by his nurse practitioner for a routine evaluation. He has no complaints on review of systems. His exam

ECG 31A

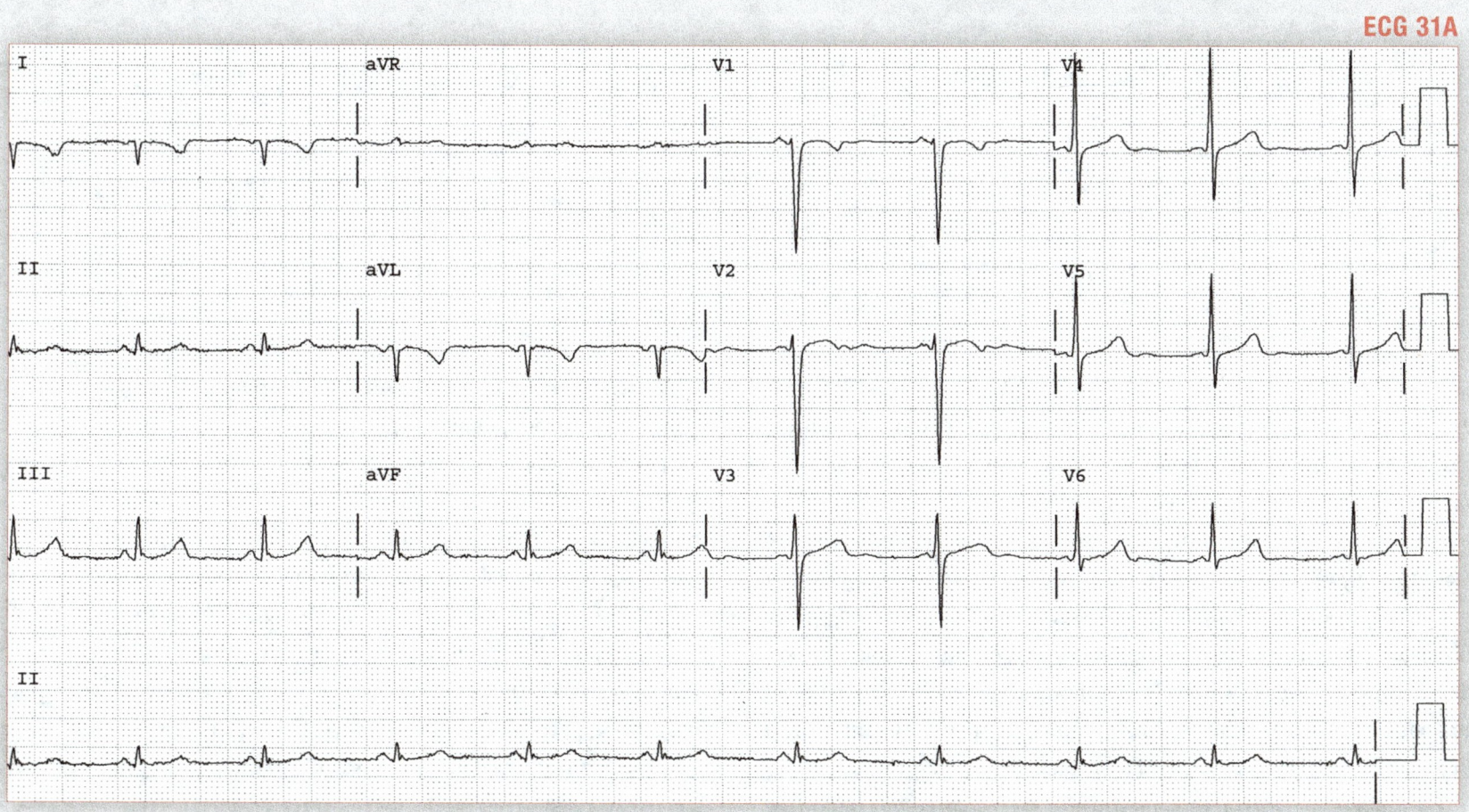

is normal. An ECG is obtained as part of his evaluation (31A). Upon viewing the tracing, the ECG technician becomes very concerned. The nurse practitioner then proceeds to repeat the ECG herself (31B).

What abnormality was noted on the initial ECG (31A)?

What is revealed by the subsequent ECG (31B)?

ECG 31B

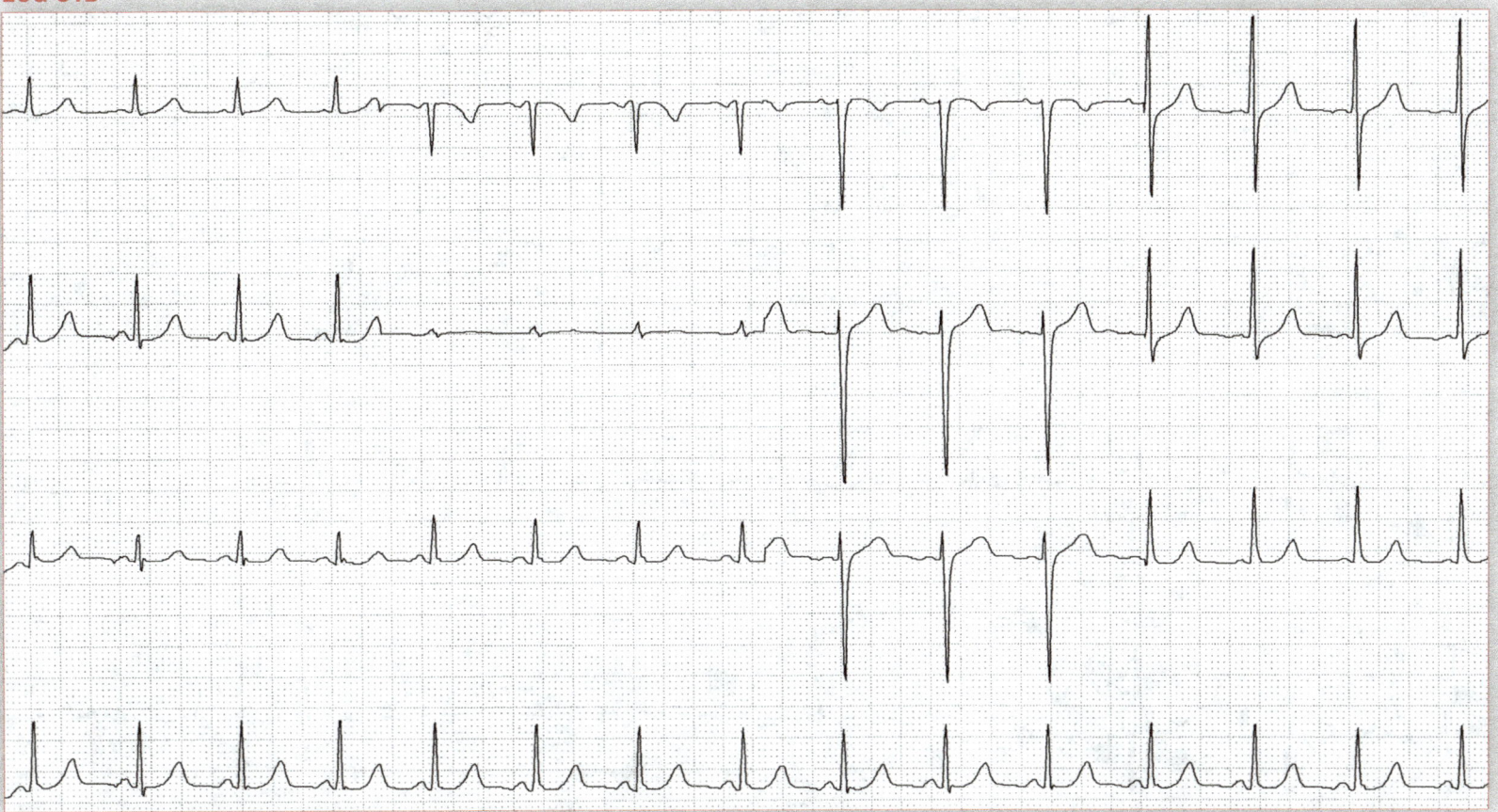

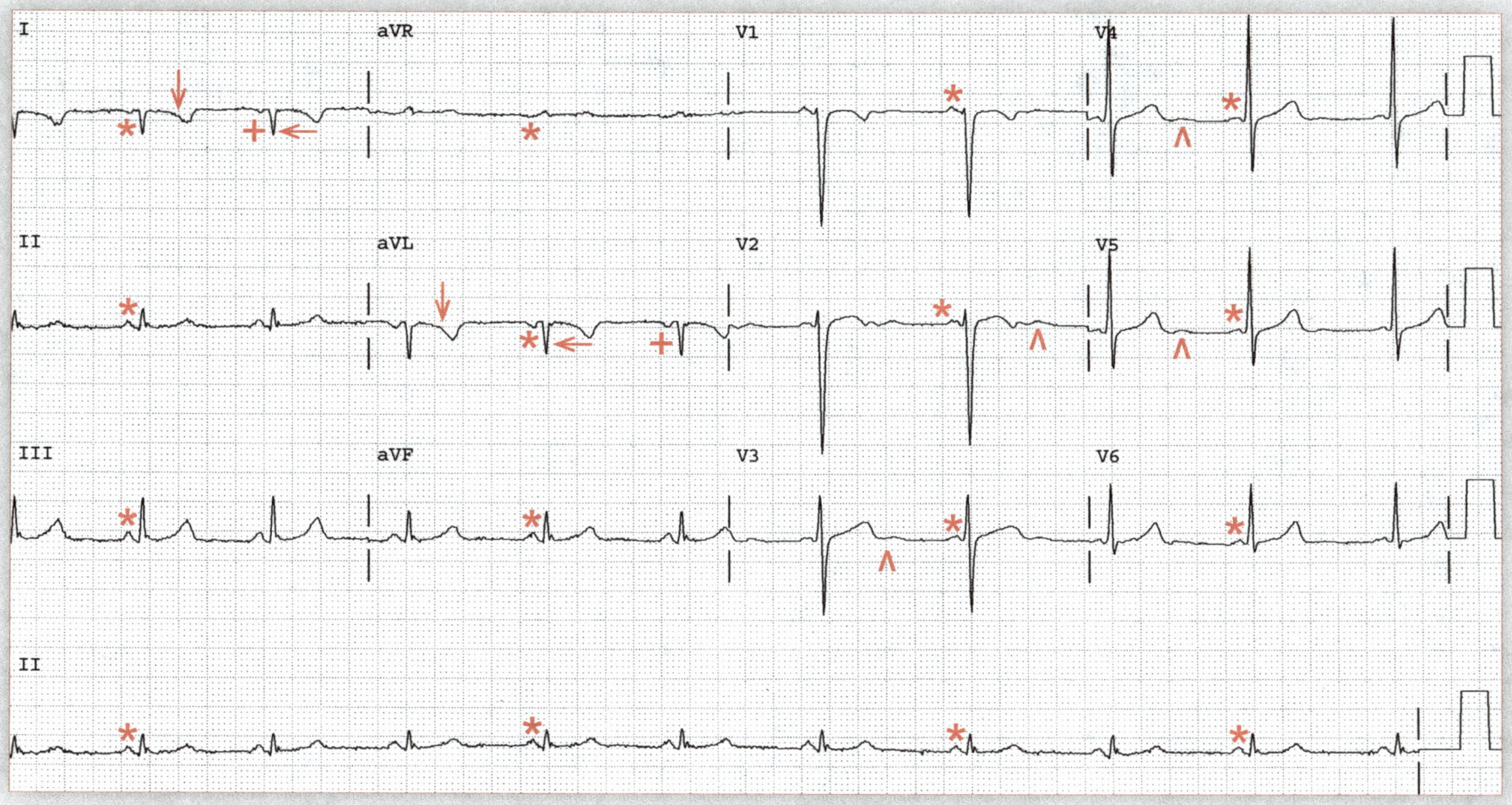

ECG 31A Analysis: Normal sinus rhythm, right axis, right–left arm lead switch, U waves

ECG **31A** shows a regular rhythm at a rate of 62 bpm. There is a P wave (*) before each QRS complex with a stable PR interval (0.14 sec). The QRS duration (0.08 sec) and morphology are normal. The axis is rightward, between +90° and +180° (negative QRS complex in lead I and positive QRS complex in lead aVF). However, the right axis is the result of a Q wave (←) in lead I and an rS complex in lead aVL. In addition, the P waves (+) and T waves (↓) are inverted in these leads. The P wave and QRS complex are positive in lead aVR, which is abnormal. Although the ECG suggests that the right axis is a result of a lateral wall myocardial infarction (and not left posterior fascicular block), the presence of negative P waves in leads I and aVL means that neither of these conditions is present but that the right axis is a result of right–left arm lead switch. This is suggested by the fact that all of the waveforms in leads I and aVL are negative and the waveforms in lead aVR are positive; this is abnormal. The QT/QTc intervals are normal (420/426 msec). Also noted are low-amplitude U waves in leads V2-V5 (^).

continues

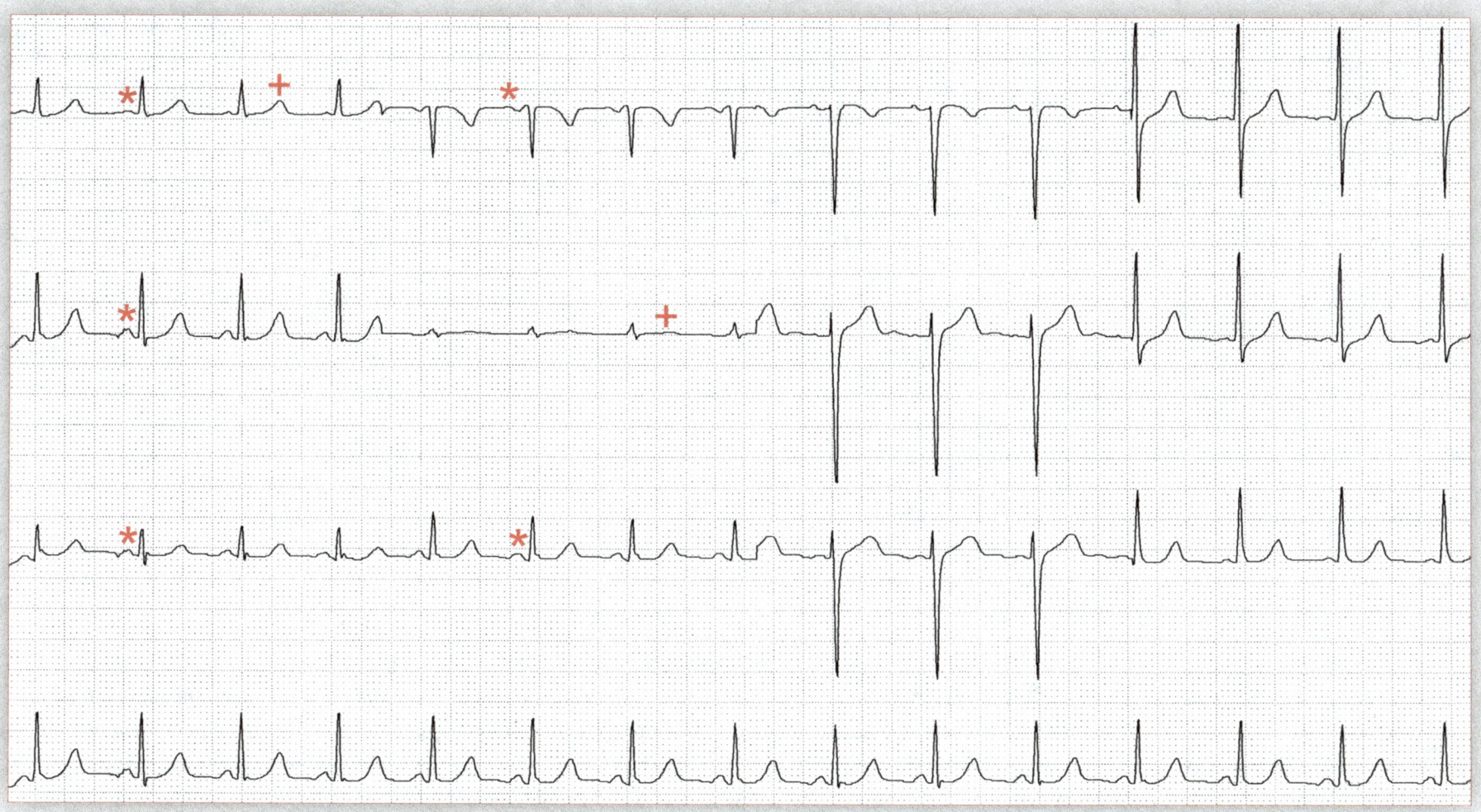

ECG 31B Analysis: Normal sinus rhythm, normal axis, normal PR interval, normal QRS complex, normal ECG

In **ECG 31B**, the leads are placed correctly and it can be seen that the axis is normal (positive QRS complex in leads I and aVF). The QRS complex has a normal morphology, and the P (*) and T (+) waves are normal in axis. The ECG is, therefore, normal.

Right–left arm lead switch is a common mistake made when recording the ECG. As the QRS complexes will be abnormal in leads I and aVL, a left posterior fascicular block or lateral wall myocardial infarction is often diagnosed in error. Hallmarks of lead switch, along with the abnormal QRS complex morphology, are negative P and T waves in leads I and aVF and a positive P and T waves and QRS complex in lead aVR, which are also abnormal. It should be remembered that dextrocardia will also present with the same P-wave, QRS complex, and T-wave abnormalities in leads I and aVL. However, there will also be abnormal QRS complexes in leads V1-V6, with reverse R-wave progression (R-wave amplitude progressively decreases). ∎

Core Case 32

A 70-year-old woman presents to the emergency department with complaints of fever, chills, burning with urination, and left-sided costovertebral tenderness. Her temperature is 103°F. A urinalysis shows

ECG 32A

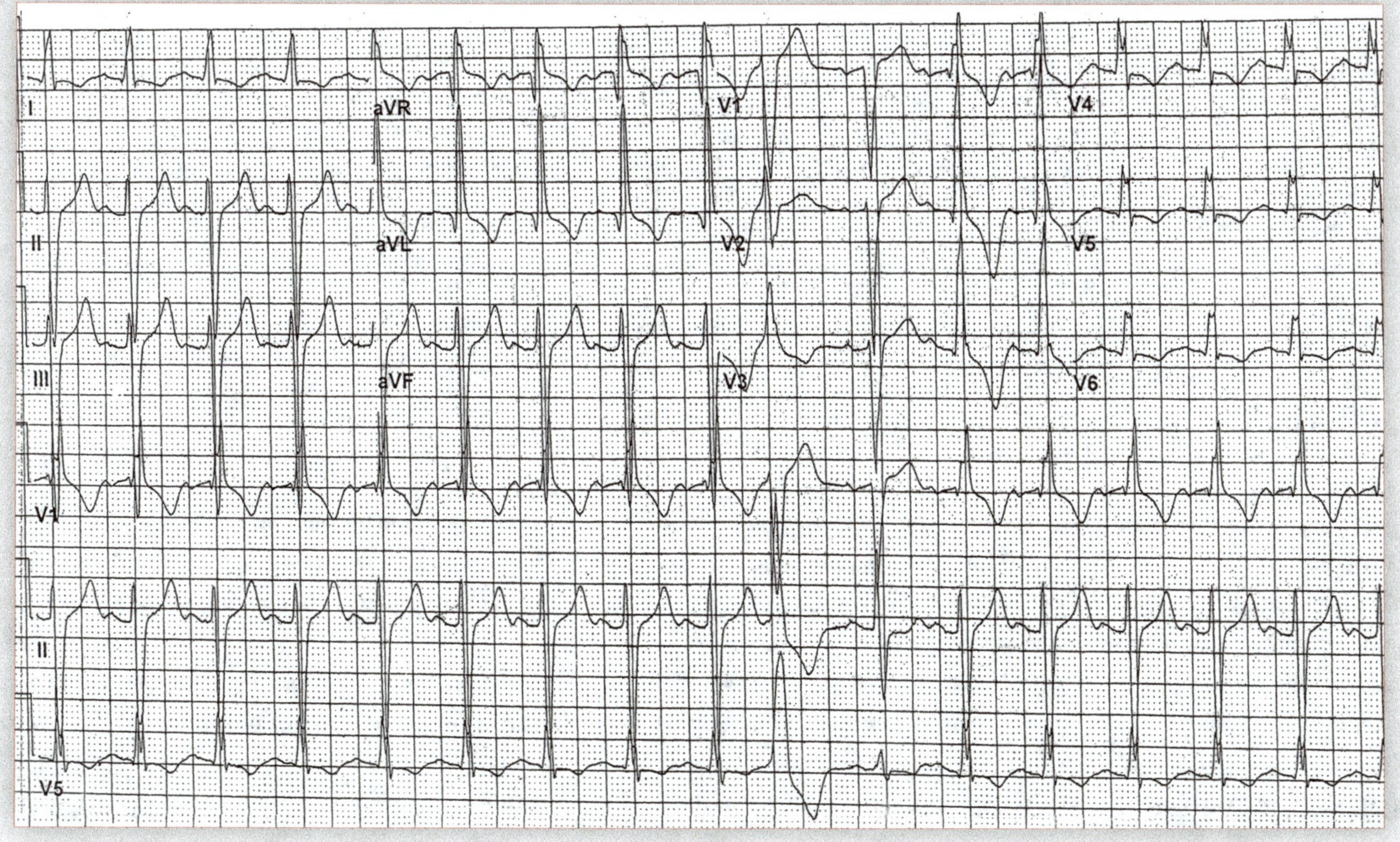

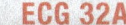

white blood cells and many bacteria. She is diagnosed with pyelonephritis, appropriate antibiotics are initiated, and an ECG is obtained (ECG 32A). She is afebrile on the following day, and another ECG is obtained (ECG 32B).

What is the difference between the two ECGs?

What is the etiology of the abnormalities?

ECG 32B

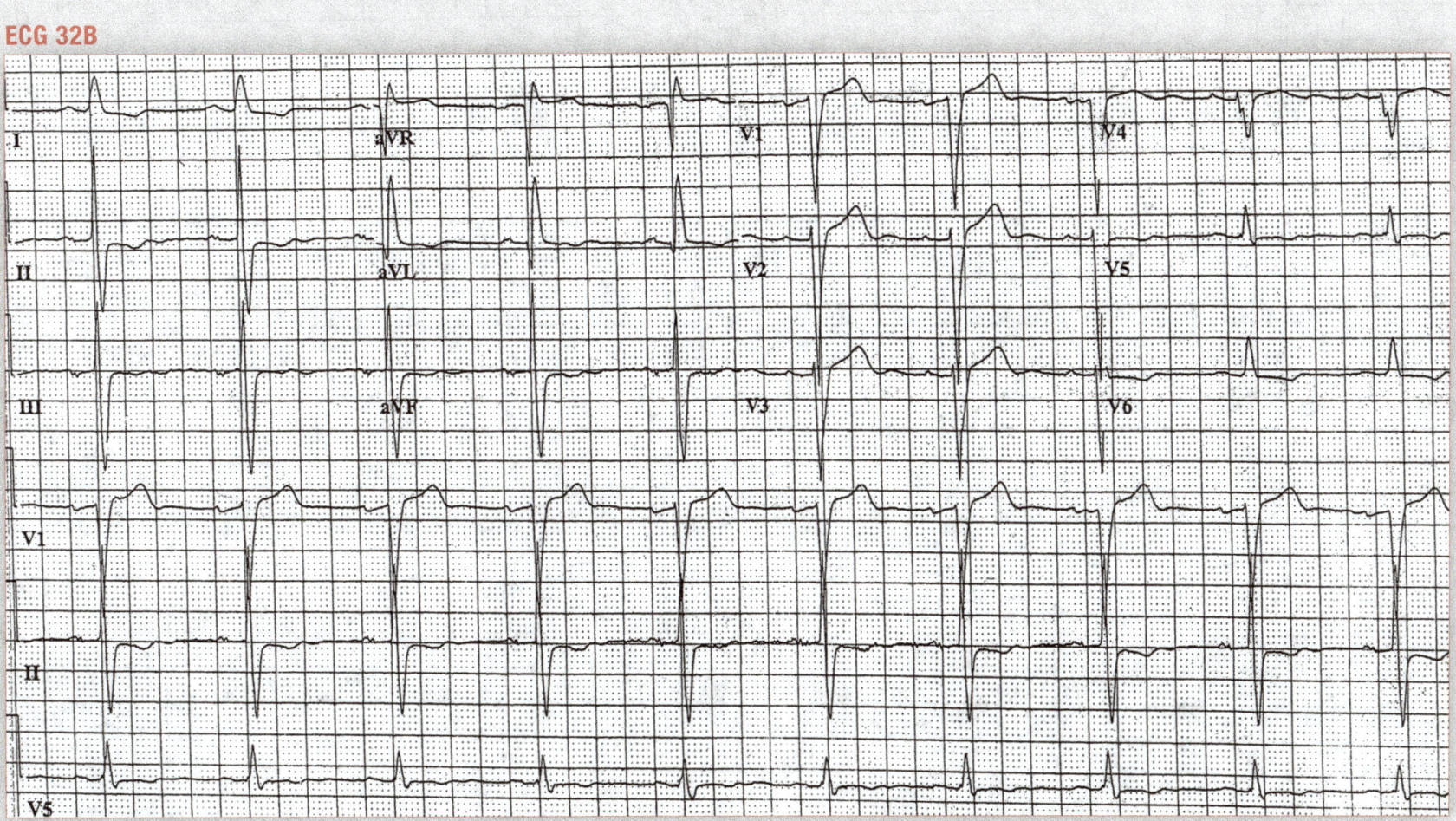

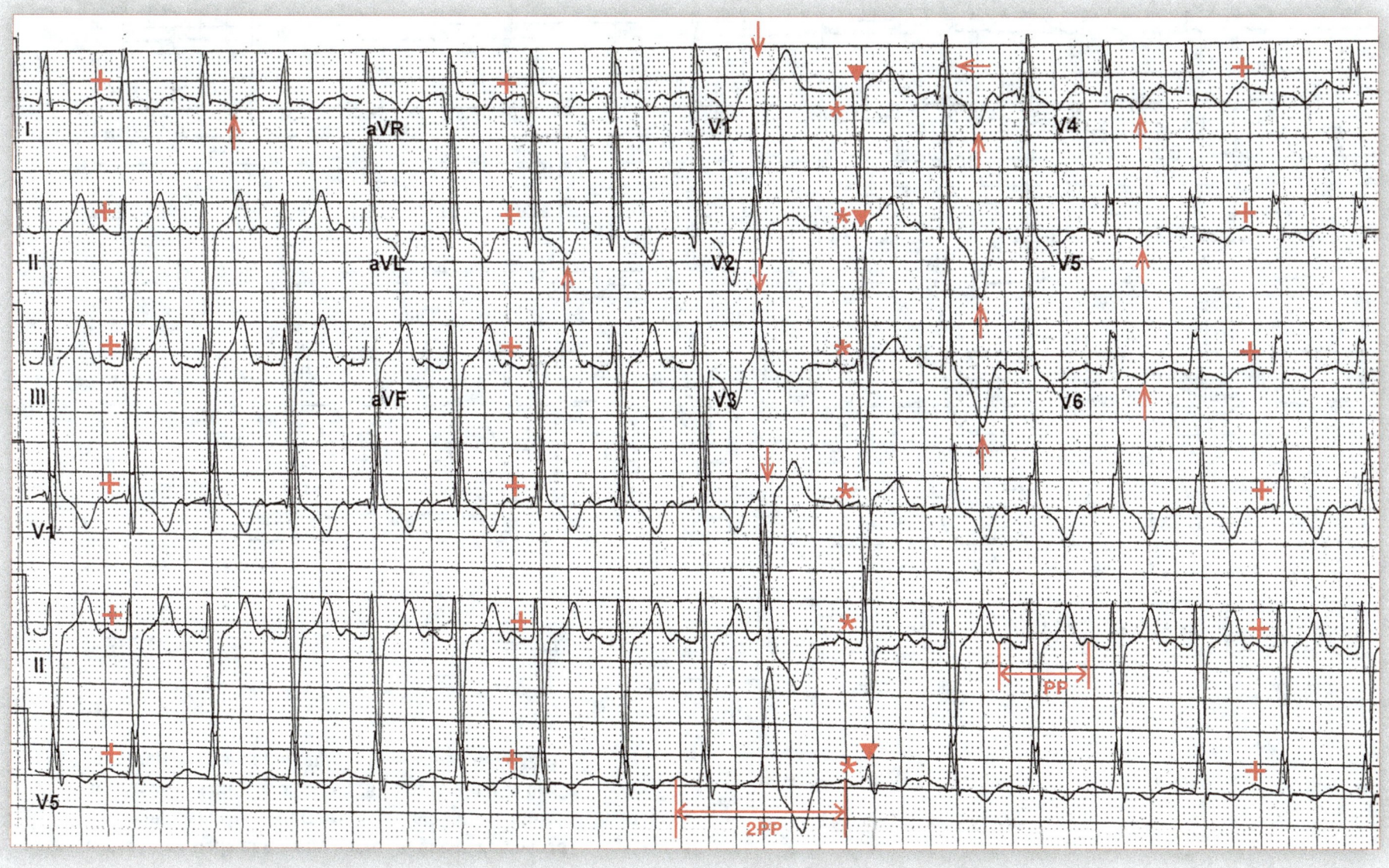

ECG 32A Analysis: Sinus tachycardia, premature ventricular complex, rate-related intraventricular conduction delay, rate-related left anterior fascicular block, long QT interval, diffuse T-wave abnormalities

In **ECG 32A**, there is a regular rhythm at a rate of 100 bpm. There are P waves (+) before each QRS complex with a stable PR interval (0.18 sec). The P waves are positive in leads I, II, aVF, and V4-V6. Hence this is sinus tachycardia. The QRS complex duration is prolonged (0.12 sec). There is an RSR' complex in lead V1 (←), but there are no terminal S waves in leads I or V5-V6. Thus while the morphology is suggestive of a right bundle branch block, it does not have a typical morphology. Therefore, it is an intraventricular conduction delay to the right ventricle. The axis is extremely leftward, between −30° and −90° (positive QRS complex in lead I and negative QRS complex in leads II and aVF). As the QRS complex does not have a QS or Qr morphology in leads II and aVF, the left axis is not due to an inferior wall myocardial infarction. This is a left anterior fascicular block. The QT/QTc intervals are prolonged (400/520 msec), even when the prolonged QRS complex duration is considered (380/490 msec). There are diffuse T-wave abnormalities (↑) seen in leads I, aVL, and V1-V6.

The 10th QRS complex is premature (↓). It is not preceded by a P wave, and it has a wider duration and an abnormal morphology. Hence this is a premature ventricular complex. Following this premature complex there is a full compensatory pause (↔) (*ie*, the PP interval around the premature complex is equal to two PP intervals). Following the premature ventricular complex is a narrow complex (▼) that is preceded by an on-time P wave (*). Unlike the other QRS complexes, it has a normal duration (0.10 sec) and does not have an intraventricular conduction delay. The axis is probably normal (*ie*, positive QRS complex in lead II). Hence it appears that there is a rate-related intraventricular conduction delay and a rate-related left anterior fascicular block, since after the pause and with a slower rate (longer RR interval) the conduction abnormalities are no longer present.

continues

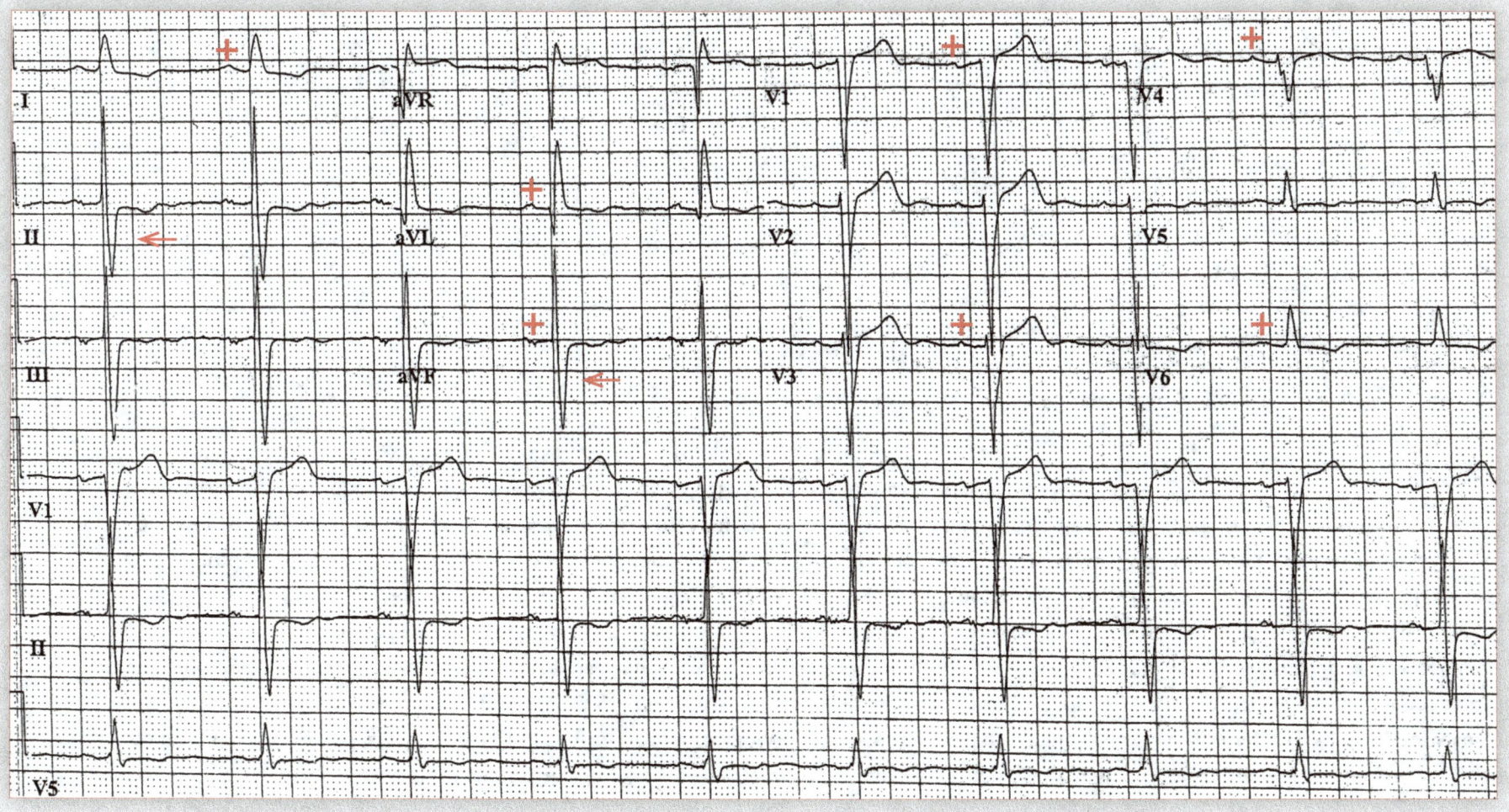

ECG 32B Analysis: **Normal sinus rhythm, diffuse T-wave abnormalities**

In **ECG 32B**, obtained on the day after admission when the patient was afebrile, there is a regular rhythm at a rate of 60 bpm. There is a P wave before each QRS complex (+) with a stable PR interval (0.18 sec), the same as the PR interval seen in **ECG 32A**. The P waves are positive in leads I, II, aVF, and V4-V6. Hence this is a normal sinus rhythm. The QRS complex duration is normal (0.10 sec). However, there are deep S waves seen in leads II and aVF (←), suggesting a slight conduction delay. Despite these S waves, the QRS axis is normal at about 0° (positive QRS complex in lead I and biphasic QRS complex in lead aVF). The QRS complex in **ECG 32B** has the same morphology as the QRS complex that follows the premature ventricular complex

in **ECG 32A**. The absence of an intraventricular conduction delay and left anterior fascicular block at the slower heart rate confirms the fact that they were rate related.

Although a rate-related right or left bundle branch block is more commonly seen, a rate-related intraventricular conduction delay and a rate-related left anterior fascicular block do occur, although the latter are not common. As with rate-related bundles, the presence of a rate-related fascicular block likely indicates underlying disease of this fascicle and the potential for a permanent left anterior fascicular block in the future. ▪

Notes

A 76-year-old man presents to his cardiologist with complaints of intermittent fatigue, during which time he notes that his pulse rate is slow. He denies any previous cardiac history except for hypertension, which is being treated with an angiotensin-converting enzyme inhibitor. His physical exam is unremarkable, but his pulse is noted to be slow and slightly irregular. His blood pressure is 180/100 mm Hg. An ECG is obtained.

What abnormality is noted?

Is any therapy needed?

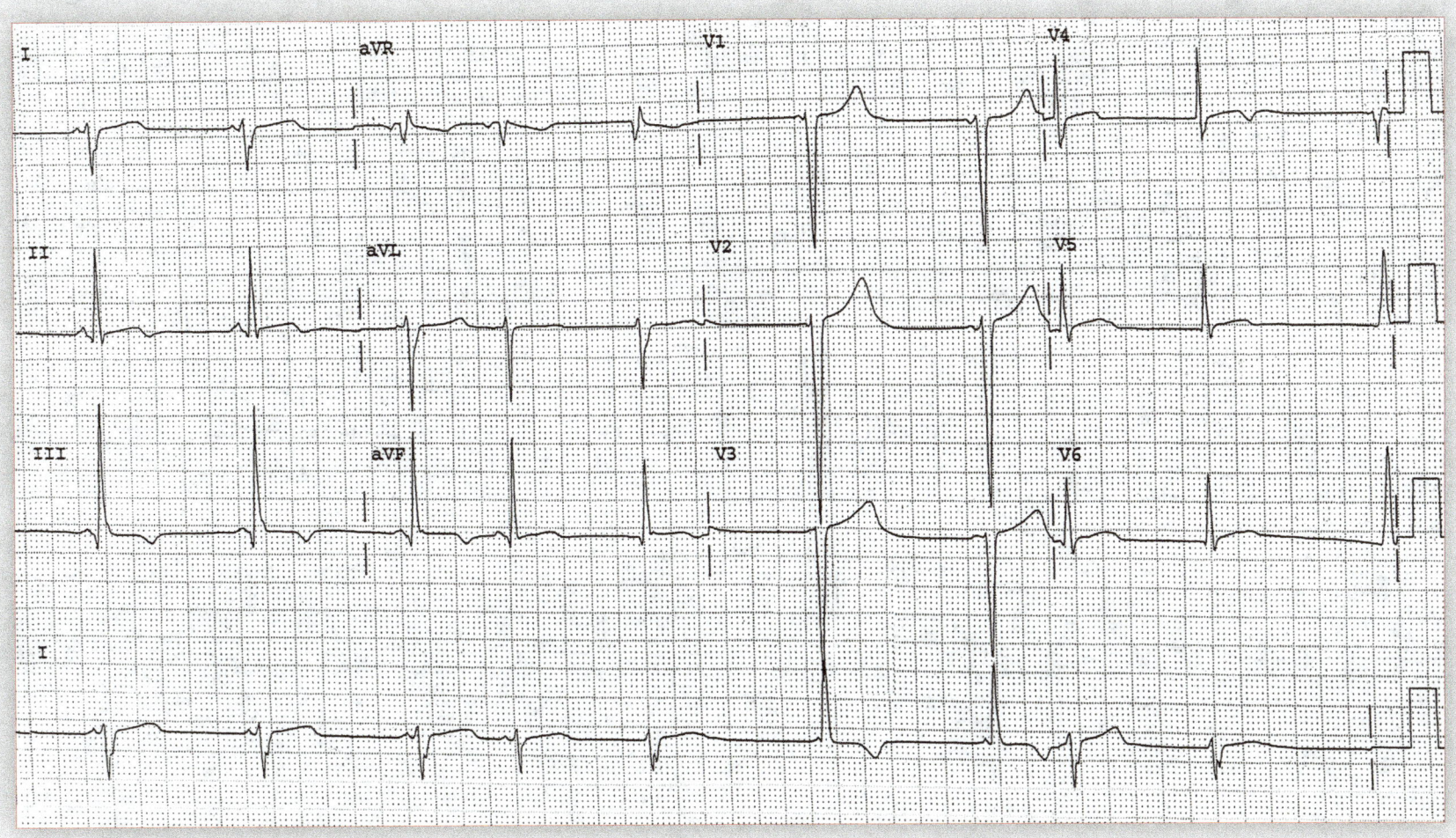

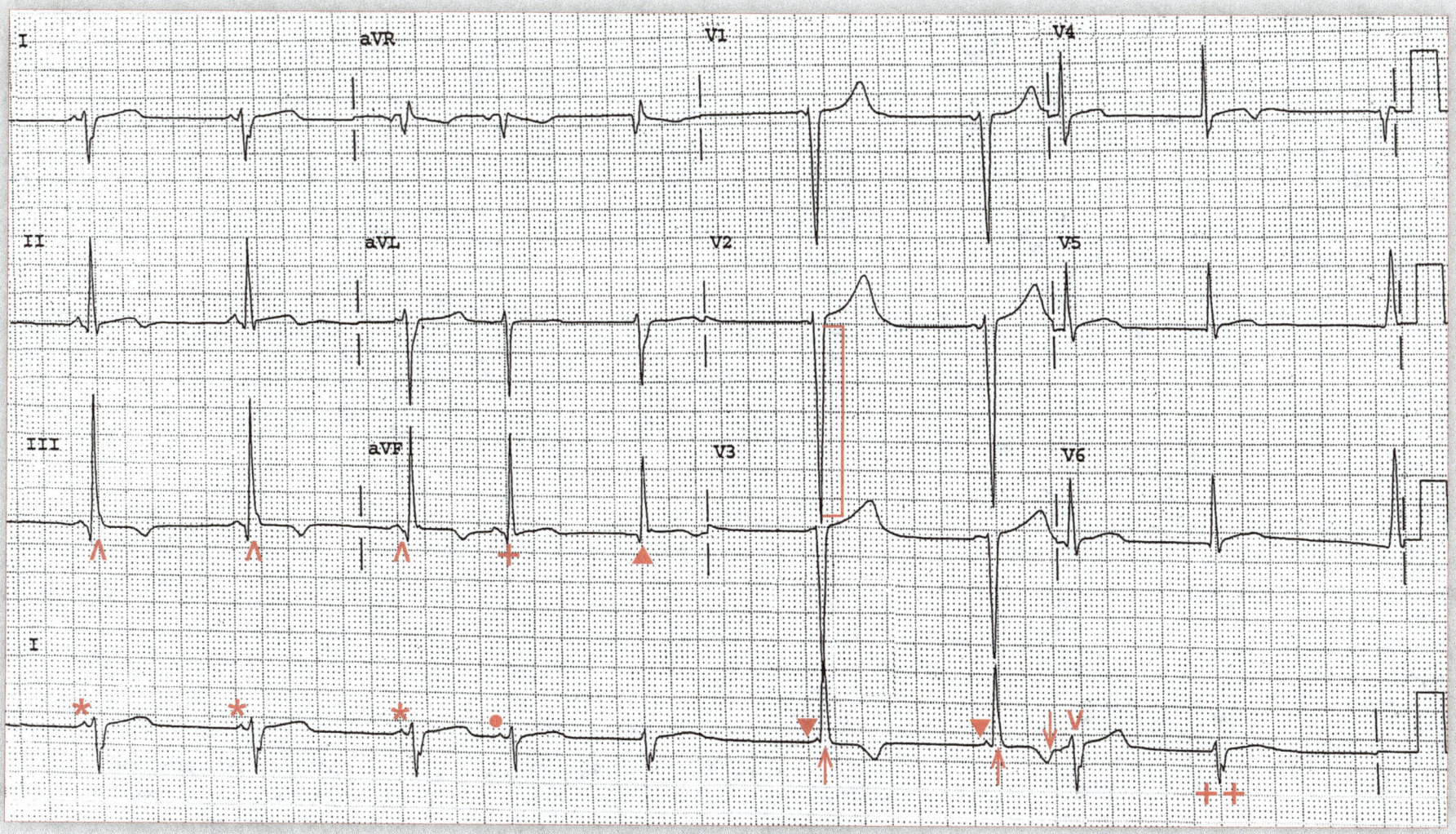

ECG 33 Analysis: Sinus bradycardia, accelerated AV conduction, premature atrial complexes, premature junctional complexes, escape junctional complexes, rate-related left posterior fascicular block, left ventricular hypertrophy

The rhythm is irregularly irregular. There are two different QRS complexes, but they both have a normal duration (0.10 sec). The first three QRS complexes (^) have P waves before them (*), and the PR interval is the same in each, but short (0.12 sec). These QRS complexes have a rate of 50 bpm. The P waves are positive in leads I, II, and aVF. This is, therefore, sinus bradycardia with accelerated AV conduction. The axis is rightward, between +90° and +180° (negative QRS complex in lead I and positive QRS complex in lead aVF). As the QRS complexes in leads I and aVL have an rS morphology, this is not a lateral infarction. The positive P waves in leads I and aVL eliminate lead switch as the cause. There is no evidence for right ventricular hypertrophy, pacemaker activity, or Wolff-Parkinson-White pattern. Hence, this is a left posterior fascicular block. The fourth QRS complex (+) is premature, and it is preceded by a P wave (●). Although the P wave looks similar to the sinus P waves, the PR interval is slightly longer (0.14 sec) and this is a premature atrial complex. The QRS complex that follows (complex 5) (▲) has the same morphology but is not preceded by a P wave. The RR interval of this complex is shorter than that of the sinus complexes; this is, therefore, a premature junctional complex. The next two complexes (complexes 6 and 7) (↑) occur after a pause of 1.32 seconds at a rate of 46 bpm. There is a P wave before both of these QRS complexes (▼), but the PR interval is very short, and shorter than the sinus complexes. In addition, the two PR intervals are different from each other. Hence these two complexes are not conducted. The QRS complex has the same duration as the sinus complexes; therefore, these are escape junctional complexes. The axis is different from what was seen with the conducted sinus complexes. The axis cannot be established as the junctional complexes are not seen in leads II and aVF. However, the axis is certainly not rightward, as the QRS complex is positive in lead I. It is likely to be a normal axis. The 8th QRS complex (∨) is premature and is preceded by a P wave. Hence this is a premature atrial complex with a QRS duration, morphology, and axis that are the same as the first sinus complexes. The last QRS complex (++) is identical in duration, morphology, and axis to the first three sinus complexes. There is no P wave before it and hence this is a premature junctional complex. The QRS complexes have an increased voltage, with an S-wave amplitude in lead V2 of 34 mm ( ]); this meets a criterion for left ventricular hypertrophy (*ie*, S-wave depth or R-wave amplitude in any precordial lead ≥ 25 mm). The QT/QTc intervals are normal (500/440 msec).

continues

It can be seen that the QRS complexes with a left posterior fascicular block always have a shorter RR interval (faster rate) compared with the two QRS complexes without a left posterior fascicular block (*ie*, complexes 6 and 7). Hence there is a rate-related left posterior fascicular block.

Although rate-related left and right bundle branch blocks are more common, a rate-related fascicular block may also occur as a result of conduction slowing present in only one of the fascicles from the left bundle. As with other rate-related conduction abnormalities of the bundles, the presence of a rate-related fascicular block may predict the development of a permanent fascicular block in the future.

In this patient it is not clear if the symptom of fatigue is related to the slow heart rate or the conduction abnormalities. One concern is the presence of significant hypertension, which may be associated with symptoms, including fatigue. Better blood pressure management is important. Although there is sinus bradycardia as well as evidence of junctional complexes, there is no definite indication for a pacemaker. ◼

The patient is a 14-year-old girl with a history of congenital heart disease, which she states required surgery when she was 8 years old. Review of her records confirms that she has an ostium primum atrial septal defect associated with an endocardial cushion defect and a cleft mitral valve.

What is the QRS complex axis on the ECG?

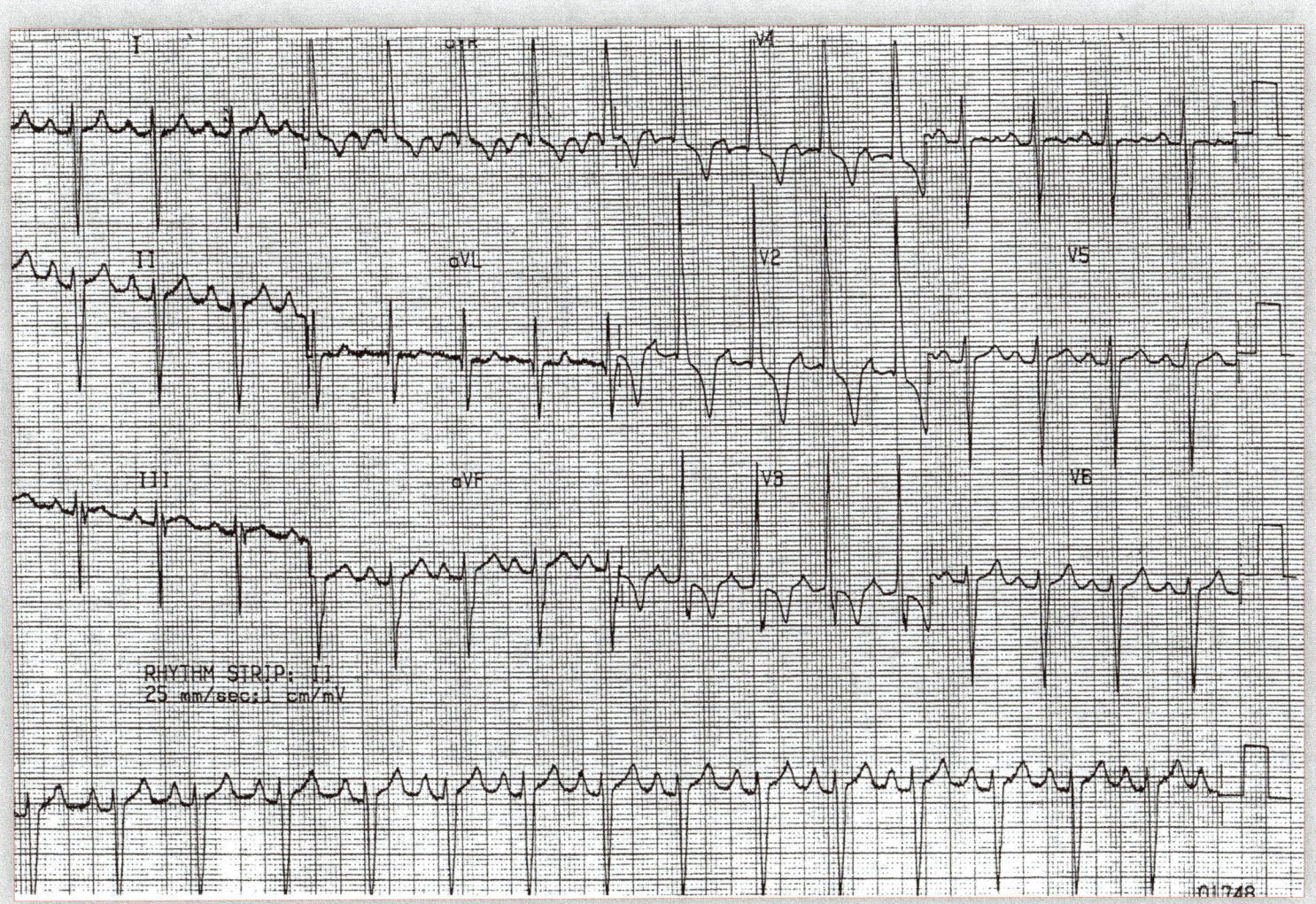

RHYTHM STRIP: II
25 mm/sec; 1 cm/mV

01748

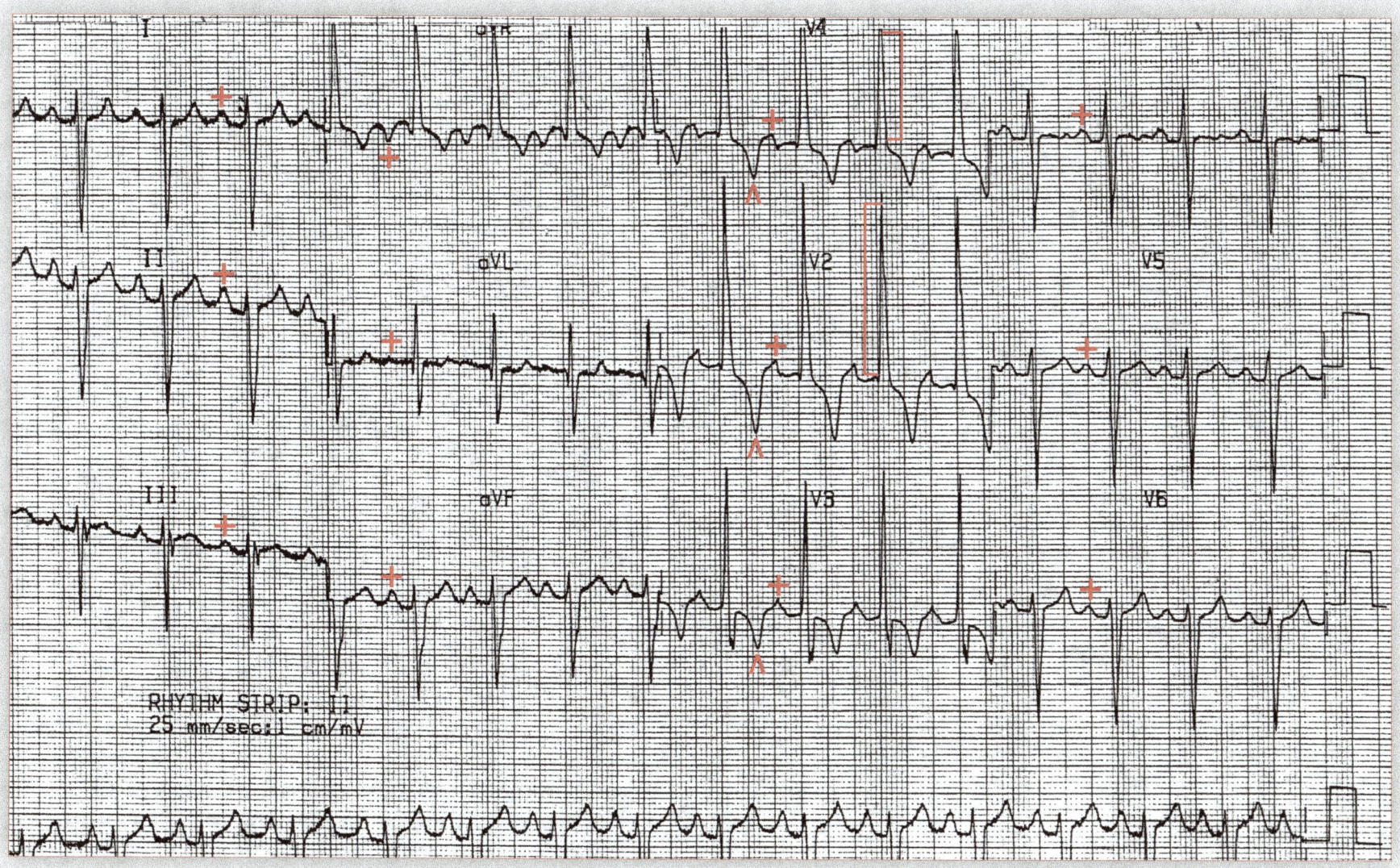

ECG 34 Analysis: Normal sinus rhythm, first-degree AV block (prolonged AV conduction), right atrial hypertrophy (P pulmonale), right ventricular hypertrophy (RVH) with associated ST-T wave changes, intraventricular conduction delay, indeterminate axis (due to left anterior fascicular block associated with a right axis due to RVH)

There is a regular rhythm at a rate of 94 bpm. (Note that the rhythm strip is not simultaneous with the 12-lead recording.) There is a P wave (+) before each QRS complex with a stable PR interval (0.22 sec). The P wave is positive in leads I, II, aVF, and V4-V6. Hence this is a normal sinus rhythm. The P wave is tall and peaked in lead II and primarily positive in lead V1; this is consistent with right atrial hypertrophy (or abnormality), termed P pulmonale. The QRS complex has a widened duration (0.12 sec), without any pattern of a right or left bundle branch block. Hence this is an intraventricular conduction delay. The R wave is tall in leads V1 (23 mm) ( ]) and V2 (33 mm) ([ ). In addition, the R/S ratio is less than 1 in leads V5-V6 (ie, the S-wave depth is greater than the R-wave amplitude). These features are consistent with a diagnosis of right ventricular hypertrophy (RVH, ie, R-wave amplitude in lead V1 > 7 mm or R/S ratio in lead V1 > 1 and R/S ratio in lead V6 < 1). Associated with the hypertrophy are ST-T wave abnormalities in leads V1-V3 (^). The RVH likely is the cause of the intraventricular conduction delay. The QT/QTc intervals are normal (320/410 msec). The axis is indeterminate, between −90° and +/-180° (negative QRS complex in leads I and aVF). This may be either an extreme right or extreme left axis.

An indeterminate axis is not uncommonly seen with a wide QRS complex, and in this situation typically reflects direct activation of the ventricular myocardium, as with a ventricular complex, a paced complex (particularly biventricular pacing), or Wolff-Parkinson-White pattern. However, an indeterminate axis is uncommon when there is a supraventricular and narrow QRS complex and typically results from an underlying conduction abnormality (ie, left anterior or left posterior fascicular block associated with another myocardial abnormality that causes an axis shift). For example, if there is an underlying left anterior fascicular block, the presence of RVH (which shifts the axis rightward) or a lateral wall myocardial infarction (with deep Q waves in leads I and aVL) can result in an indeterminate axis. The presence of a left posterior fascicular block associated with an old inferior wall myocardial infarction (with deep Q waves in leads II and aVF) is also associated with an indeterminate axis. Other combinations include an old inferior wall myocardial infarction with RVH and a right axis or both an inferior and lateral wall myocardial infarction.

Patients with an ostium primum atrial septal defect and endocardial cushion defect often have a congenital left anterior fascicular block and hence an extreme left axis. With left-to-right shunting and the development of RVH, the axis shifts rightward, resulting in an indeterminate axis. Therefore, the indeterminate axis in this patient is the result of a left anterior fascicular block with a right axis due to RVH. ■

A 76-year-old man with a long history of chronic obstructive pulmonary disease presents for a routine physical exam. He states that he had a previous myocardial infarction (MI) but is unable to provide any additional details.

His physical exam demonstrates decreased breath sounds and significant wheezes. His cardiac exam is normal. Arterial blood gases include an O_2 saturation of 86% on room air. He denies using supplemental oxygen at home. An ECG is obtained.

What does the ECG show?

What is the QRS complex axis?

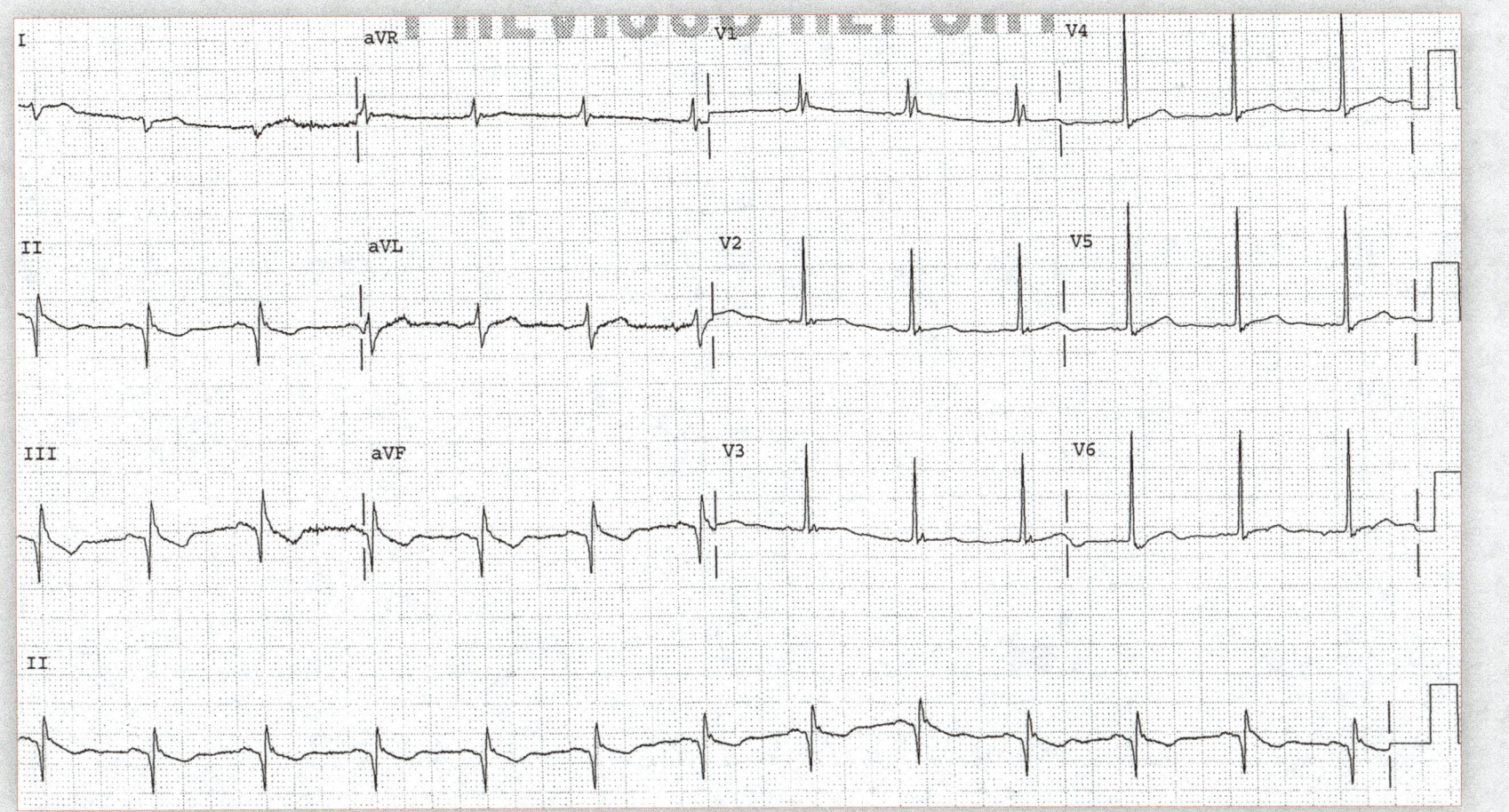

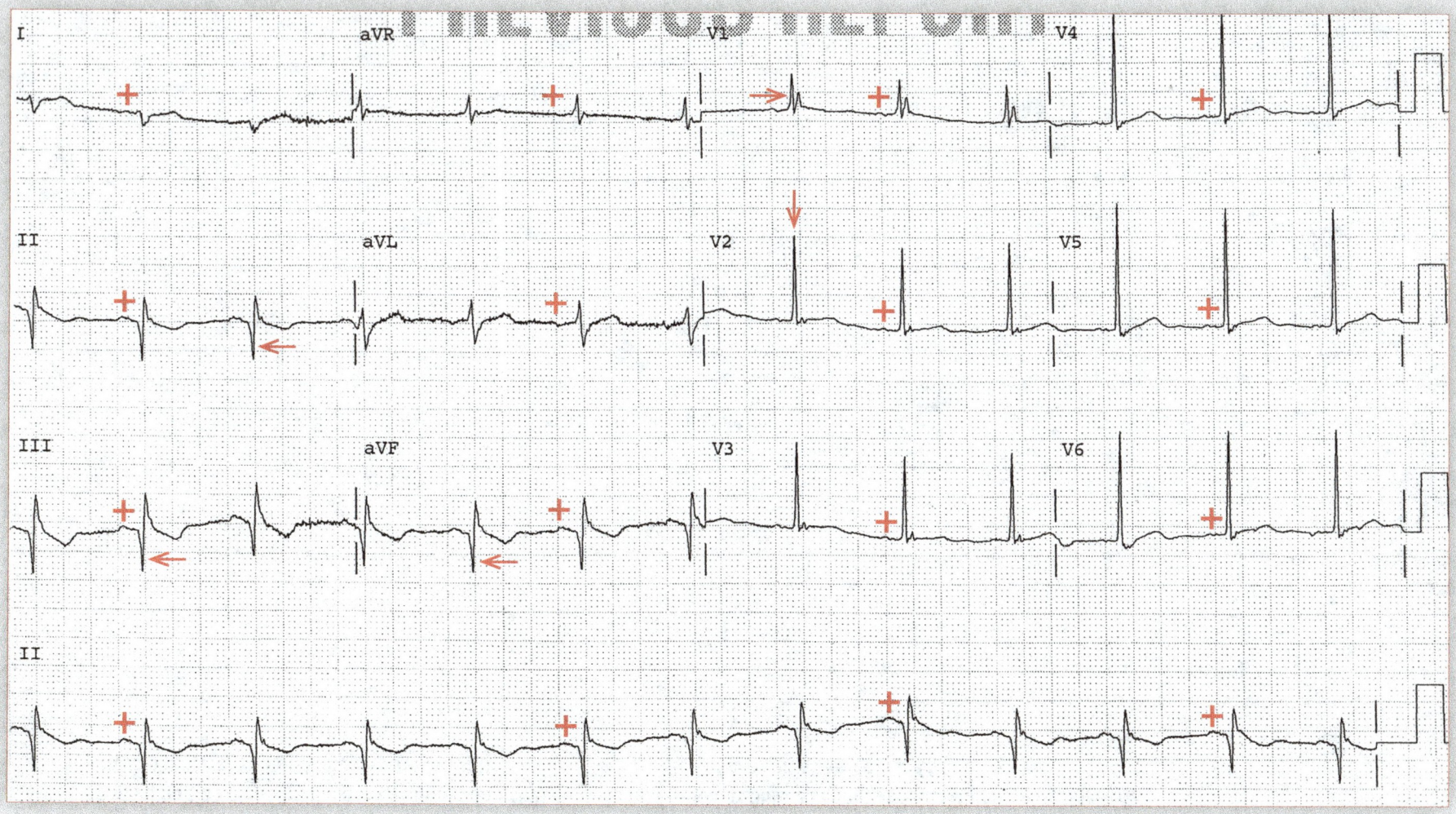

ECG 35 Analysis: Normal sinus rhythm, old inferoposterior wall MI, left posterior fascicular block, indeterminate axis, counterclockwise rotation (early transition)

There is a regular rhythm at a rate of 72 bpm. There is a P wave (+) before each QRS complex with a stable PR interval (0.18 sec). The P wave is positive in leads I, II, aVF, and V4-V6. Hence this is a normal sinus rhythm. The QRS complex duration is normal (0.10 sec). There are significant Q waves in leads II, III, and aVF (←), which are diagnostic for an old inferior wall myocardial infarction (MI). There is a tall R wave in lead V1 (→), which, in association with an inferior wall MI, is consistent with posterior wall involvement (or a posterior wall MI). There is also a tall R wave in lead V2, likely due to early transition or counterclockwise rotation of the electrical axis in the horizontal plane. This is established by imagining the heart as viewed from under the diaphragm. The right ventricle is anterior and the left ventricle is lateral. With counterclockwise rotation the left ventricular forces are shifted anteriorly and hence develop earlier in the right precordial leads, producing the tall R wave in lead V2. The QT/QTc intervals are normal (360/395 msec).

The axis in the frontal plane is indeterminate, between −90° and +/-180° (negative QRS complex in leads I and aVF). The QRS complex morphology in lead I is due to an rS complex, and this morphology is the result of a left posterior fascicular block. However, the negative QRS complex in leads II and aVF is the result of an old inferior wall MI (Qr complex). Therefore, the indeterminate axis is due to a left posterior fascicular block associated with a myocardial abnormality (a chronic inferior wall MI). ■

Notes

A 61-year-old man with longstanding multidrug-refractory essential hypertension is seen by a cardiologist. He states that he feels well and has been compliant with his medications, although on further questioning admits to some fatigue over the past few months. He denies dyspnea and angina. His exam is notable for a blood pressure of 152/88 mm Hg. As part of his evaluation, an ECG is obtained.

What abnormalities are noted?

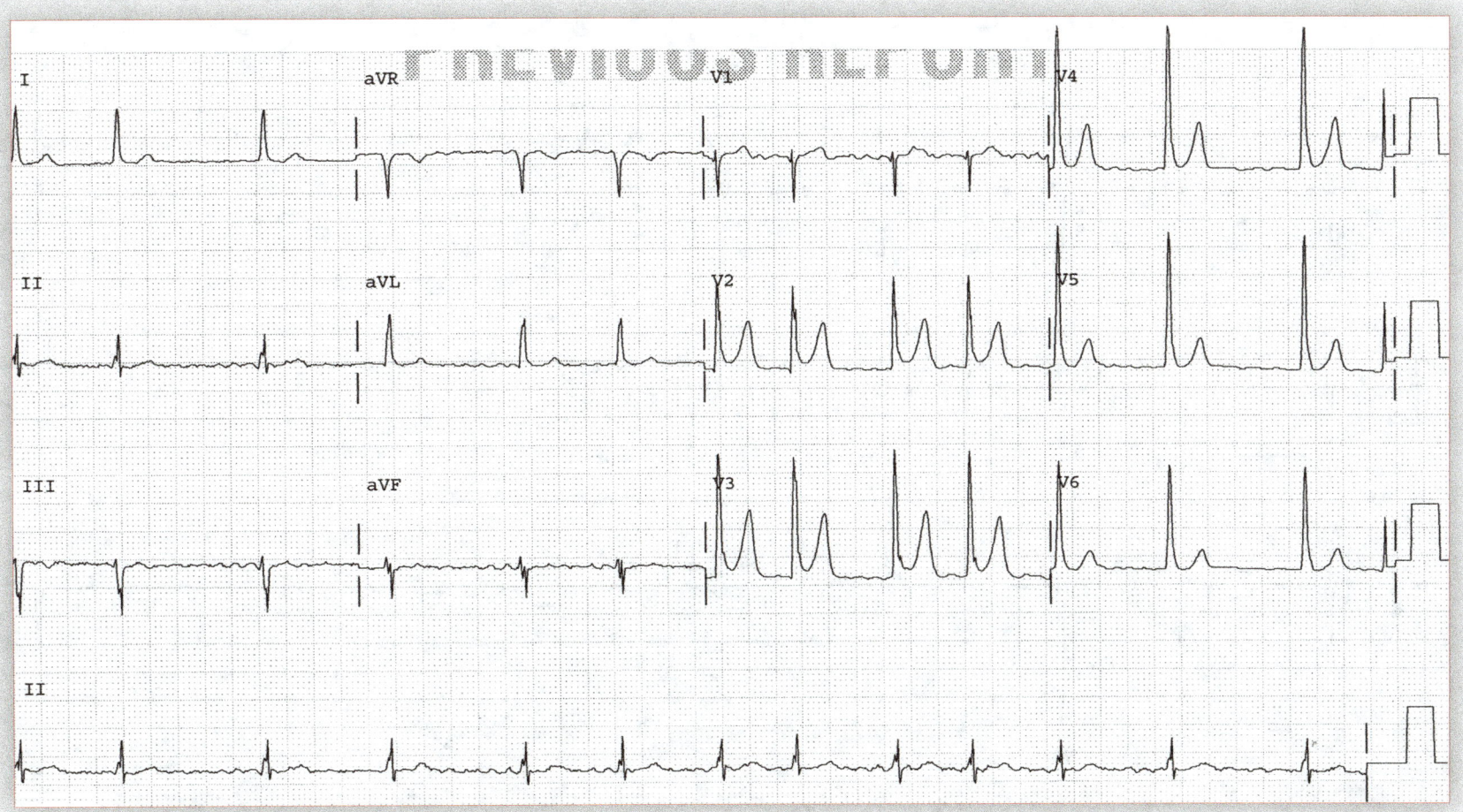

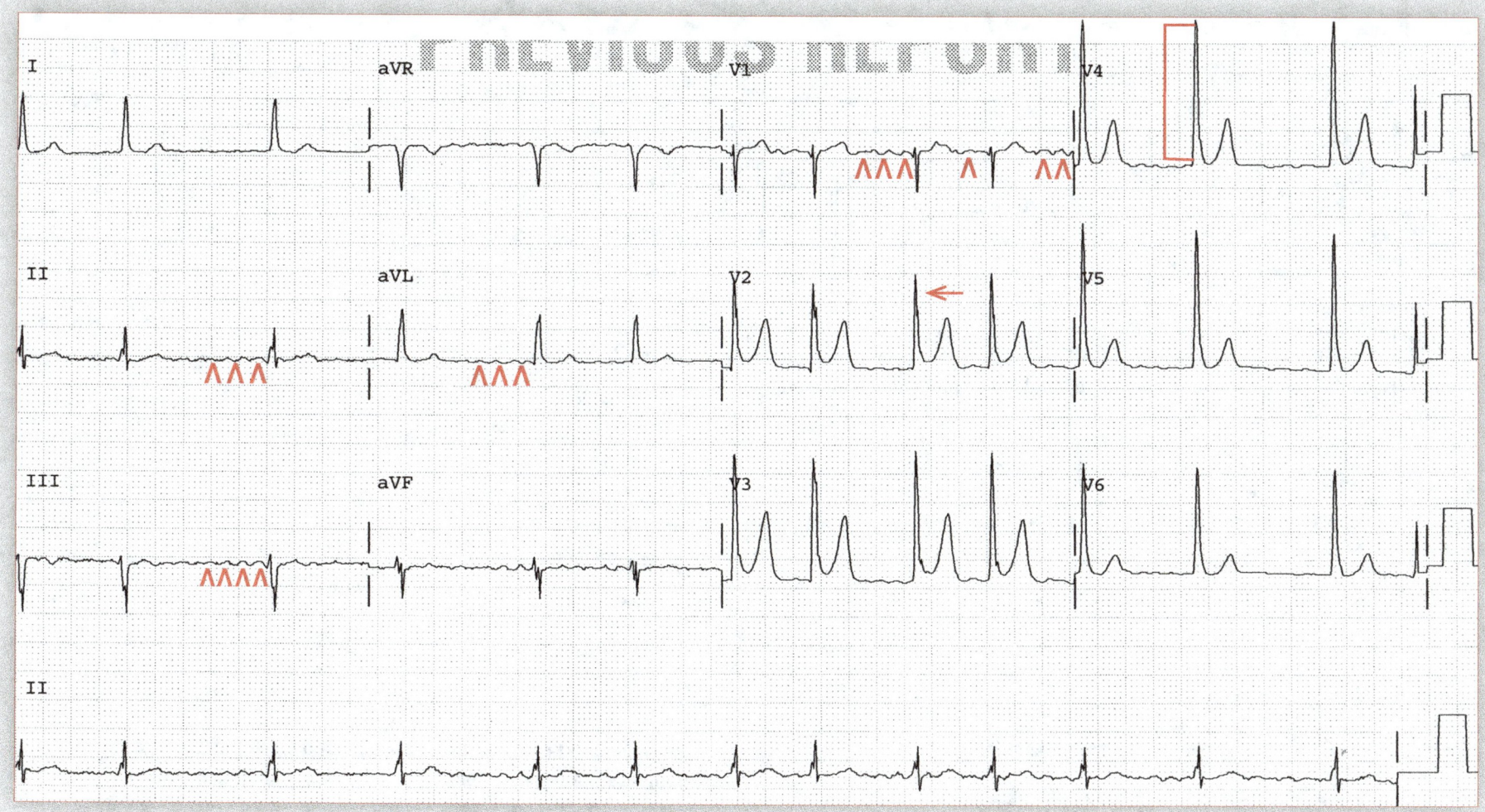

ECG 36 Analysis: Atrial fibrillation, counterclockwise rotation
(early transition), left ventricular hypertrophy

The rhythm is irregularly irregular (average rate of 78 bpm), and no organized atrial activity is seen. Rapid and irregular low-amplitude undulations of the baseline can be seen in leads II, III, aVF, and V1 (^). These are fibrillatory waves; therefore, the underlying rhythm is atrial fibrillation. The QRS complex duration is normal (0.08 sec). The axis is leftward, between 0° and −30° (positive QRS complex in leads I and II and negative QRS complex in lead aVF). Thus this is a physiologic left axis, which is a normal variant or may be seen with increased age or left ventricular hypertrophy (LVH). Borderline LVH is present based on an R-wave amplitude in lead V4 ([ ) of 26 mm (S-wave depth or R-wave amplitude in any precordial lead ≥ 25 mm is a criterion for LVH). Also noted is a tall R wave in lead V2 (←), which is termed early transition or counterclockwise rotation in the horizontal plane. The QT/QTc intervals are normal (340/390 msec).

In addition to the electrical axis of the heart in the frontal plane (normal, left, right, indeterminate), there is also an electrical axis in the horizontal plane, which is established by imagining the heart as viewed from under the diaphragm. From this direction, the right ventricle is in front and the left ventricle is to the left. When the heart is electrically rotated in a counterclockwise direction, the left ventricular forces appear earlier in the precordial leads, and hence there is early transition with the R wave being tall in lead V2. With clockwise rotation, the left ventricular forces are generated late, resulting in poor R-wave progression and late transition. It is important not to confuse the tall R wave in lead V2 as indicating right ventricular hypertrophy or a posterior wall myocardial infarction. In these situations, a tall R wave is also seen in lead V1 and not just in lead V2. The presence of counterclockwise rotation, which is only an electrical axis shift, has no clinical implications except for not confusing it with any other abnormality. ■

Notes

A 22-year-old woman presents to her primary care physician for a routine physical exam prior to joining a college basketball team. An ECG is obtained, raising questions about an abnormality that suggests there may have been a previous anterior wall myocardial infarction.

What is the abnormality?

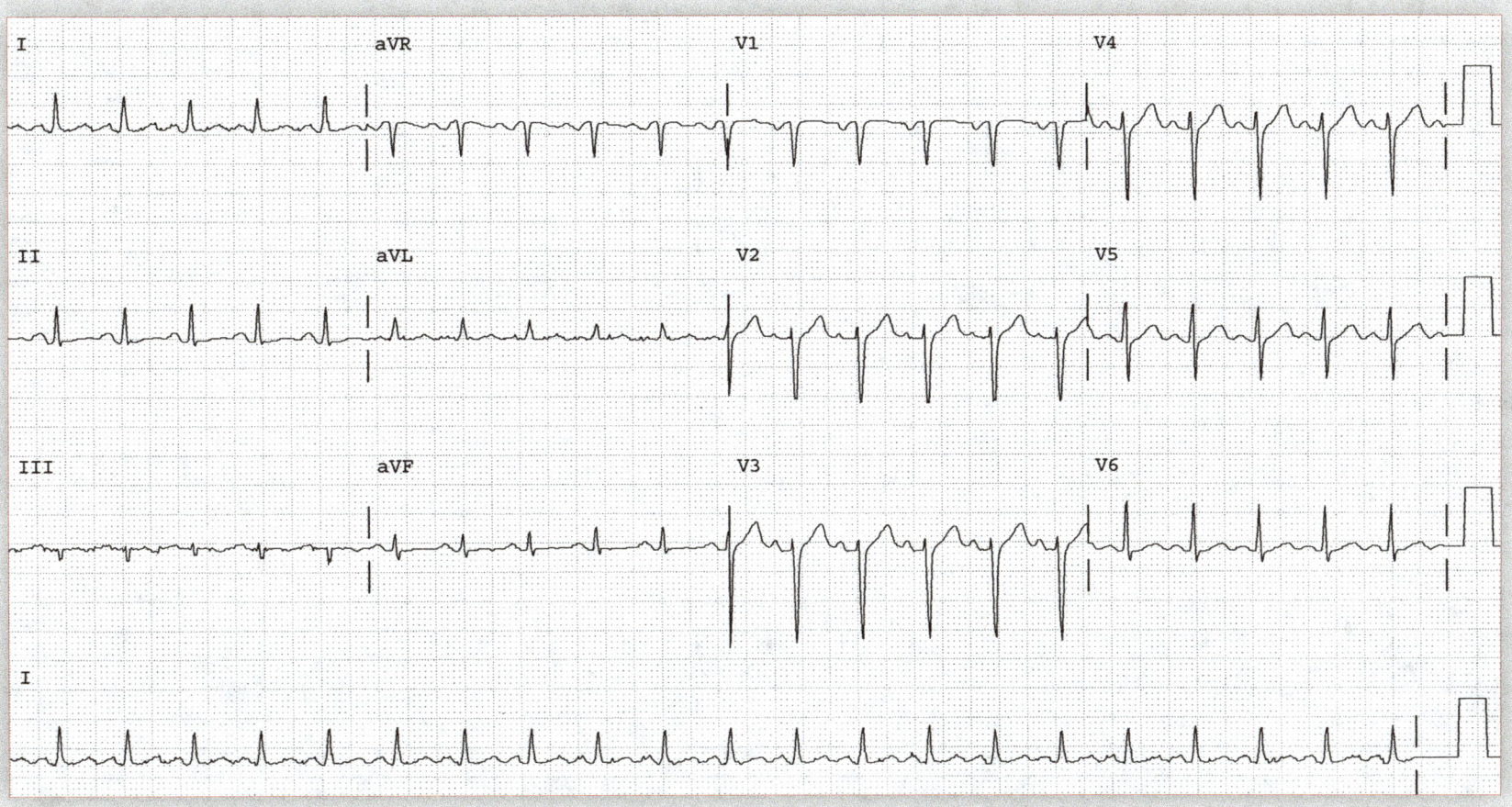

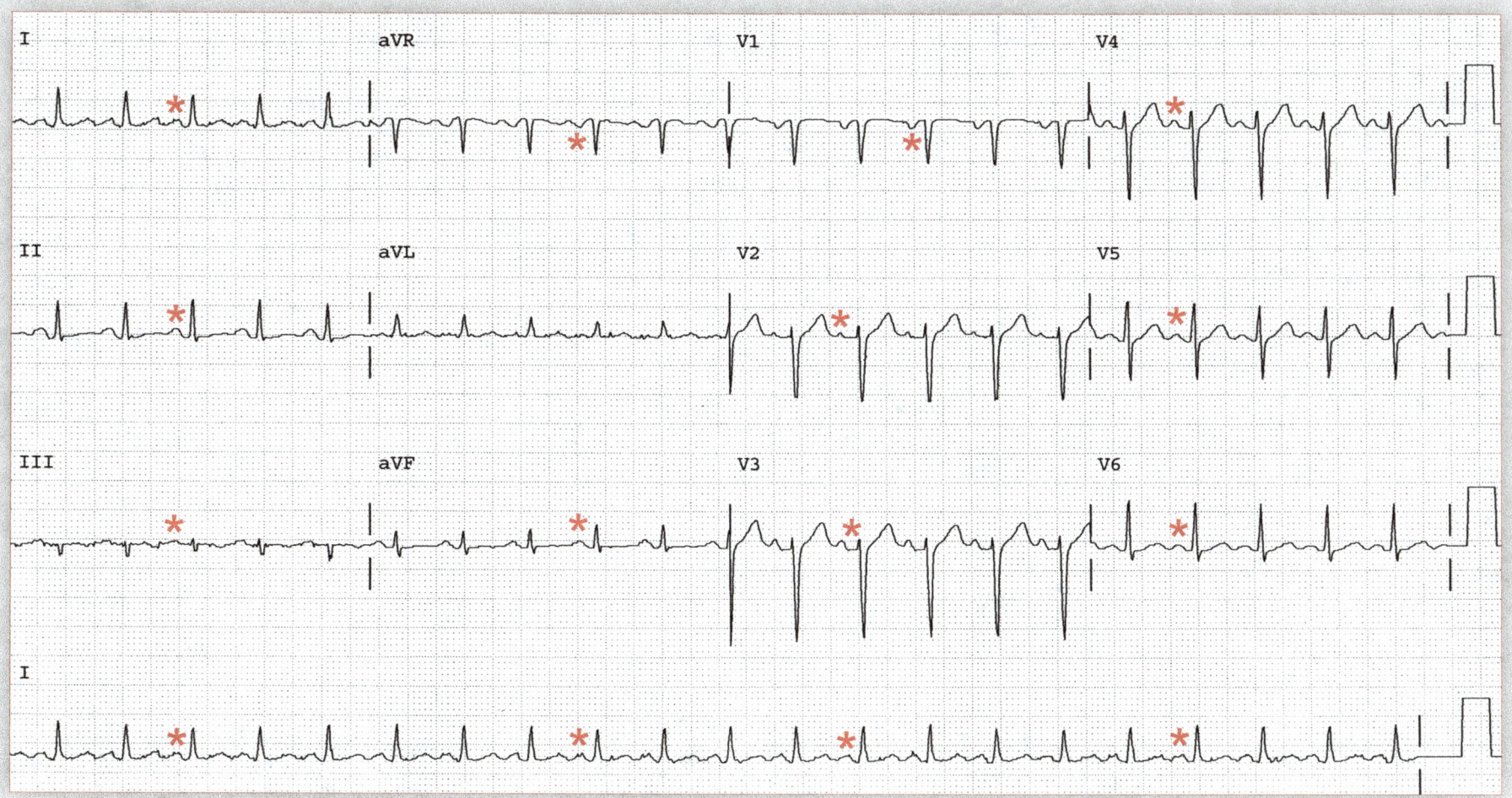

ECG 37 Analysis: Sinus tachycardia, clockwise rotation (late transition), poor R-wave progression

There is a regular rhythm at a rate of 130 bpm. There is a P wave (*) before each QRS complex with a stable PR interval of 0.16 second. The P wave is upright in leads I, II, aVF, and V4-V6. Therefore, this is sinus tachycardia. The axis is normal, between 0° and +90° (positive QRS complex in leads I and aVF). There is low voltage in the limb leads (QRS complex amplitude < 5 mm in each lead). The QT/QTc intervals are normal (300/440 msec). Poor R-wave progression is noted in leads V1-V3 (the R-wave amplitude does not become progressively taller), and there is also late transition (R/S > 1) in lead V6 rather than in leads V3-V4. This is also known as clockwise rotation in the horizontal plane.

In addition to the electrical axis of the heart in the frontal plane, there is an electrical axis in the horizontal plane, which is established by imagining the heart as viewed from under the diaphragm. From this direction the right ventricle is in front and the left ventricle is to the left. When the heart is electrically rotated in a clockwise direction in the horizontal plane, the left ventricular forces appear late and are seen in the lateral precordial leads. This results in poor R-wave progression and late transition. Poor R-wave progression is a normal variant and should not be confused with an anterior wall myocardial infarction, in which there are Q waves or QS complexes in the precordial leads and no initial R waves. With clockwise rotation there are normal anterior forces (ie, R waves), but their progression is delayed or slow. Clockwise rotation can be seen with a left anterior fascicular block or with significant lung disease. Women may have poor R-wave progression as a result of breast tissue attenuation of anterior forces. ■

Notes

A 38-year-old woman with metastatic breast cancer associated with a *BRCA* mutation is admitted for progressive shortness of breath and is found to have multiple, bilateral pulmonary emboli. She is hemodynamically stable, and her cardiopulmonary exam is normal. Her laboratory values show a mild elevation in brain natriuretic peptide of 400 pg/mL but undetectable troponin. An ECG is obtained.

What is the abnormality?

How is the abnormality related to the woman's current diagnosis?

What further evaluation is needed?

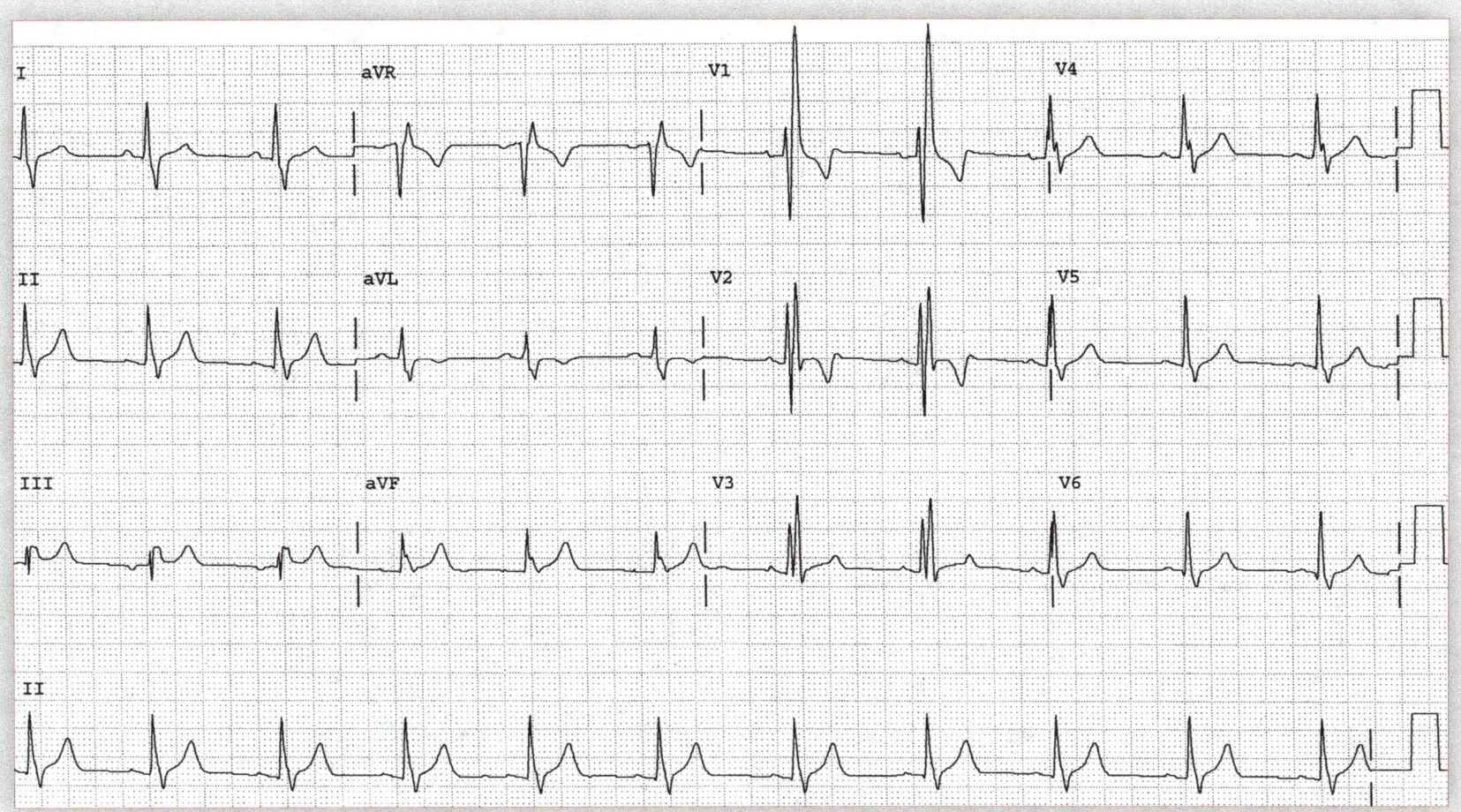

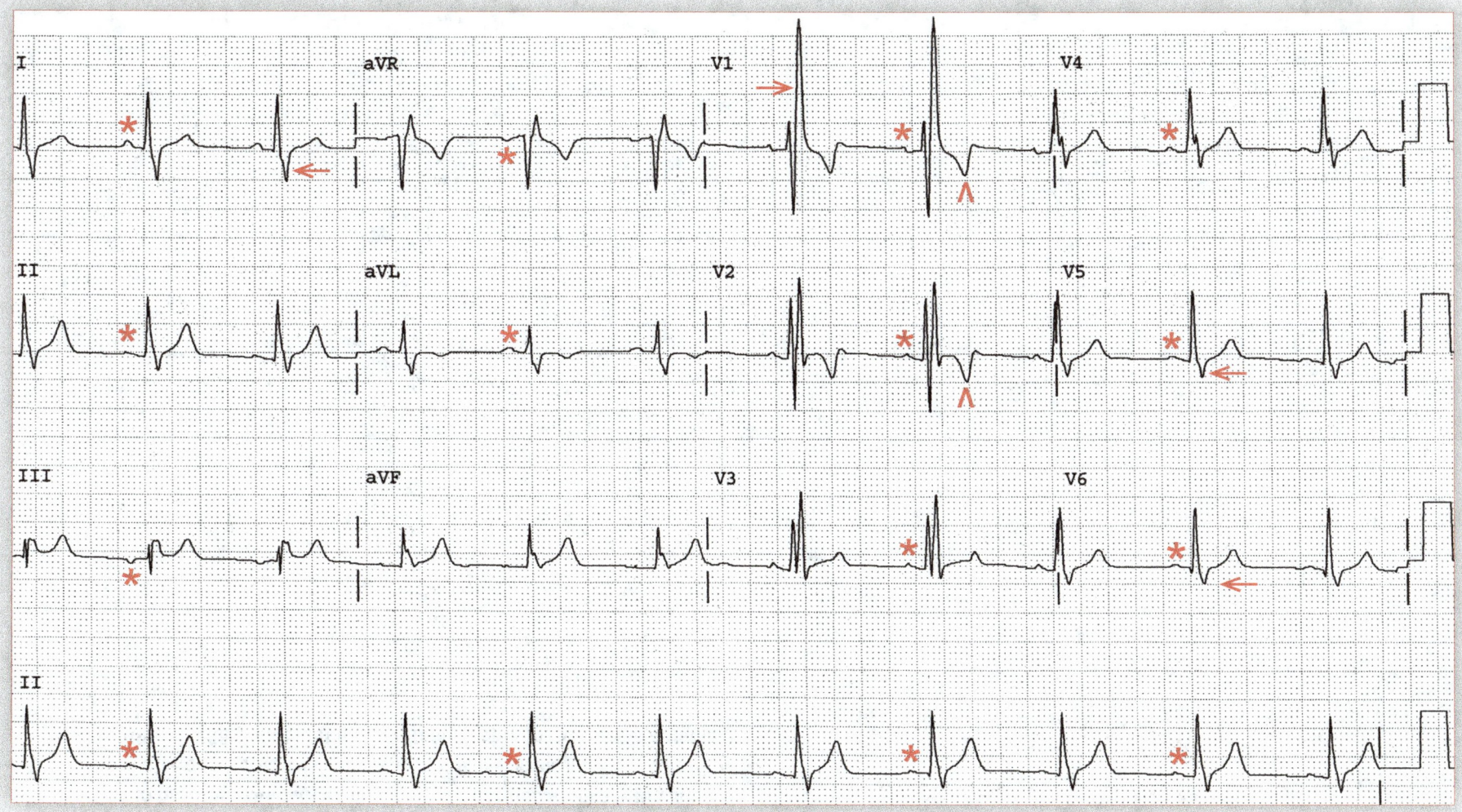

ECG 38 Analysis: Normal sinus rhythm, right bundle branch block with associated T-wave abnormalities

There is a regular rhythm at a rate of 64 bpm. There is a P wave (*) before each QRS complex with a constant PR interval (0.15 sec). The P waves are positive in leads I, II, aVF, and V4-V6. Hence this is a normal sinus rhythm. The axis is normal, between 0° and +90° (positive QRS complex in leads I and aVF). The QRS duration is increased (0.14 sec). The QT/QTc intervals are normal (410/420 msec and 350/360 msec when the increased QRS complex duration is considered). The QRS complex in lead V1 has an RSR′ morphology (→). The initial 0.08 second of the QRS complex is normal and the increased QRS duration is a result of the R′, which represents a delay in right ventricular activation, with the terminal forces being directed from left to right (toward lead V1). Leads I and V5-V6 have broad S waves (←) that also represent the terminal forces being directed from left to right (away from these leads), a result of delayed right ventricular activation. This is a pattern that indicates the presence of a right bundle branch block (RBBB). There are T-wave changes (^) in leads V1-V2 that are due to the RBBB. Although the R′ in lead V1 is very tall in amplitude, a diagnosis of right ventricular hypertrophy cannot be made on the ECG in the presence of an RBBB as right ventricular activation is abnormal, not occurring through the normal His-Purkinje system but rather directly through the right ventricular myocardium.

An RBBB is identified by the following characteristics:

- The QRS complex duration is 0.12 second or longer due to delayed activation of the right ventricle.

- Delayed right ventricular activation occurs directly through the right ventricular myocardium originating from the left bundle and left ventricle. Right ventricular activation, therefore, bypasses the normal His-Purkinje system. The terminal forces of the QRS complex are directed from left to right. Since conduction velocity is slow (due to direct myocardial conduction) the terminal forces are delayed, accounting for the widened QRS complex. Hence there is an RSR′ complex in leads V1-V2 (due to delayed right ventricular forces directed toward the right-sided leads V1-V2) and broad S waves in leads I and V5-V6 (due to delayed right ventricular forces directed away from the left).

- Right ventricular repolarization is also abnormal, and secondary ST-T wave changes are often seen in leads V1-V3.

- Since right ventricular activation is abnormal, right ventricular hypertrophy cannot be recognized.

- Since left ventricular activation is normal, the initial portion of the QRS complex (first 0.08 sec) is normal. Abnormalities affecting the left ventricle can be recognized (eg, left ventricular hypertrophy, infarction, ischemia, pericarditis).

continues

- An RBBB may also be associated with conduction abnormalities of the fascicles of the left bundle (*ie*, a left anterior or left posterior fascicular block). This is established by the presence of an extreme left or right axis in addition to the RBBB. The presence of an RBBB and fascicular block is termed bifascicular disease.

- An RBBB may be intermittent or related to increased heart rate (rate-related RBBB).

- A QRS complex duration of 0.10 to 0.12 second in conjunction with an RBBB-like morphology has been termed an incomplete RBBB. However, as conduction through the RBBB is all or none, it is more appropriate to term this an intraventricular conduction delay to the right ventricle.

There are multiple etiologies of isolated RBBB. Any entity that raises pulmonary pressures and induces geometric alteration of the right bundle may impair right bundle conduction. This is often in association with a rightward shift in the axis in the frontal plane. Cardiomyopathies, myocardial fibrosis from infarction, and myocarditis may also cause RBBB, generally with other ECG findings consistent with the underlying diagnosis. Idiopathic conduction system disease (Lev's or Lenègre's disease) may be isolated to the right bundle. In this case, chronic pulmonary emboli have likely raised pulmonary pressures to the point of right ventricular pressure overload (as evidenced by an elevated brain natriuretic peptide) but without physical findings of right ventricular hypertrophy or dilation (no parasternal lift on palpation, no murmur of tricuspid regurgitation). An echocardiogram would assist in evaluation of right ventricular morphology and pulmonary pressures. ■

A 48-year-old man with known obstructive sleep apnea presents to your clinic for routine evaluation. On review, the man admits that he is noncompliant with his continuous positive airway pressure (CPAP) machine as he is unable to sleep when wearing the mask. Due to severe dyspnea, his exercise capacity is severely diminished and he is limited to ambulating only within his home. He denies orthopnea or anginal symptoms. His heart rate is 100 bpm, and his blood pressure 162/110 mm Hg. His respiratory rate is 18 breaths/min, and his resting O_2 saturation is 94% on ambient air. His body mass index is 42. Cyanosis is absent. His lungs are clear. His jugular venous pressure is 14 cm H_2O with CV waves. His cardiovascular exam is notable for a precordial (right ventricular) lift, pulmonary artery tap, and a prominent P2 component of S2. A soft holosystolic murmur is noted at the left lower sternal border. Carvallo's sign (respiratory variation in the intensity and duration of the murmur) is noted. His abdomen is protuberant without gross hepatomegaly. His lower extremities display mild pitting edema bilaterally. An ECG is obtained.

What abnormalities are shown?

What is the underlying cause of these abnormalities?

What further diagnostic testing may be helpful?

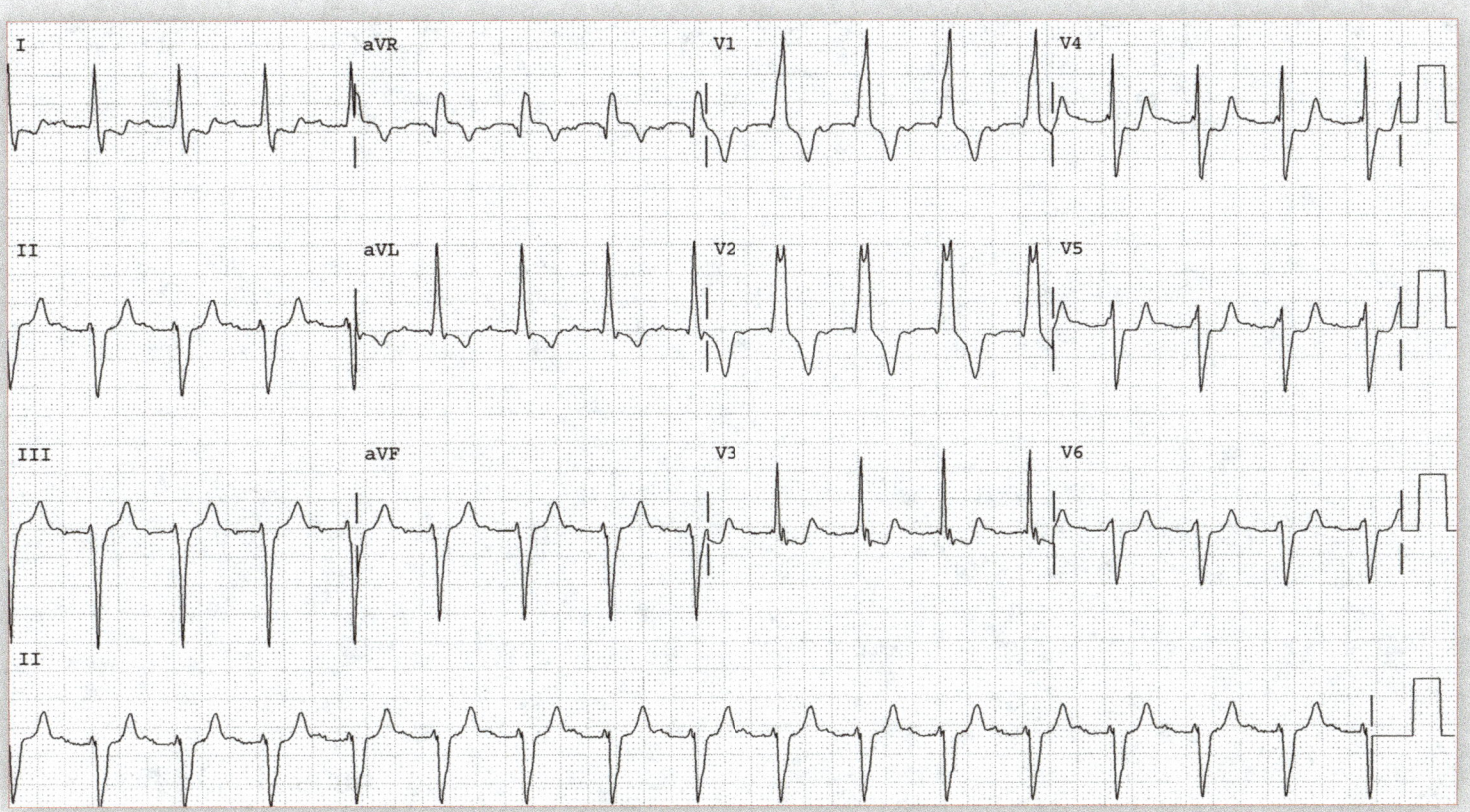

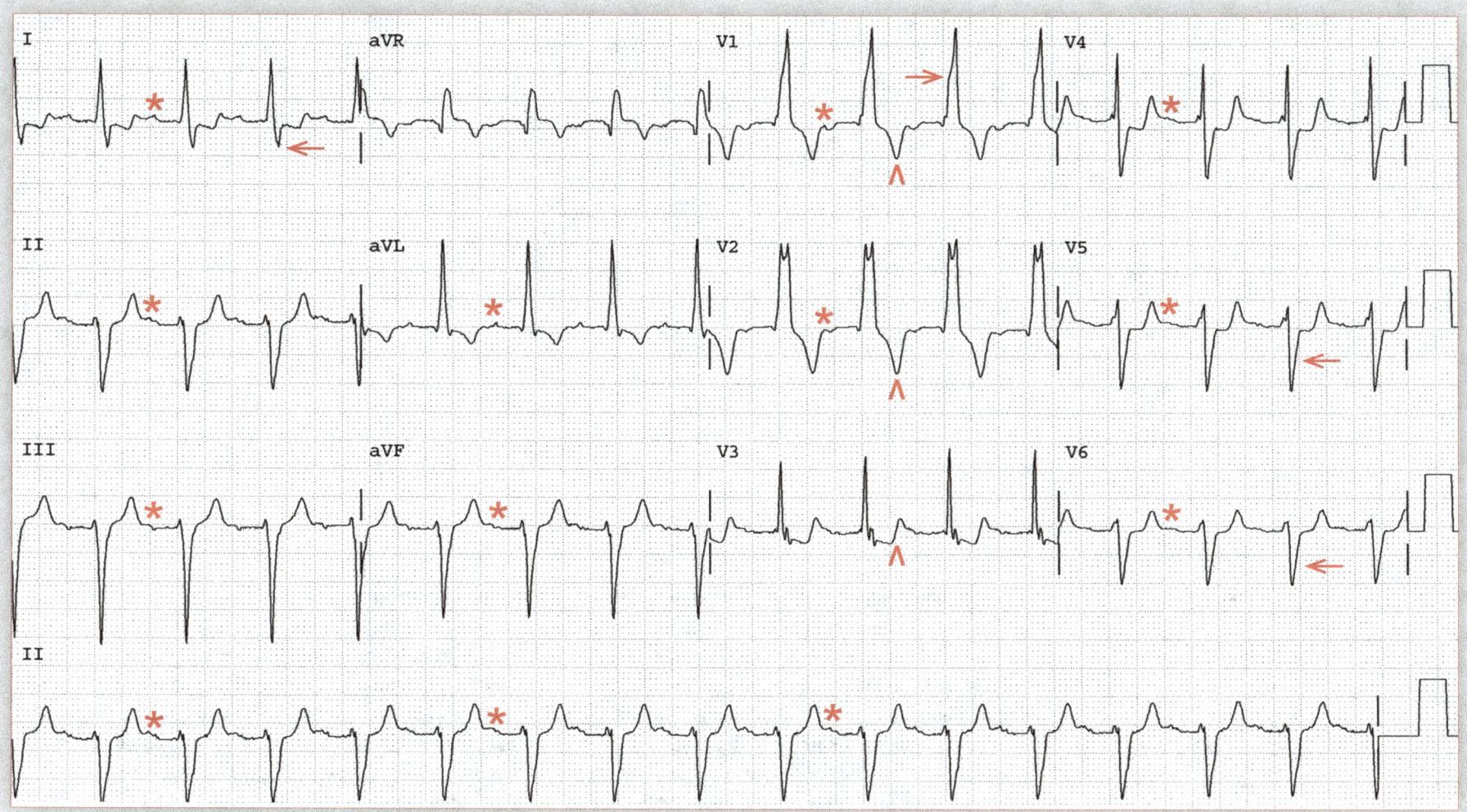

ECG 39 Analysis: Sinus tachycardia, first-degree AV block (prolonged AV conduction), right bundle branch block, left anterior fascicular block, bifascicular block

There is a regular rhythm at a rate of 100 bpm. There is a P wave (*) before each QRS complex with a stable PR interval of 0.24 second. The P wave is positive in leads I, II, aVF, and V4-V6 (although it is of very low amplitude in these leads). Hence this is sinus tachycardia with first-degree AV block (prolonged AV conduction). The complex duration is prolonged at 0.16 second, and the morphology is that of a right bundle branch block (RBBB; tall, broad R wave in lead V1 [→] and broad S waves in leads I and V5-V6 [←]). The QT/QTc intervals are prolonged (380/490 msec) but are normal when the prolonged QRS complex duration is considered (300/388 msec). There are associated ST-T wave changes (^) in leads V1-V3. The axis is extremely leftward, between −30° and −90° (positive QRS complex in lead I and negative QRS complex in leads II and aVF). The QRS complex has an rS morphology; hence this is a left anterior fascicular block and not an inferior wall myocardial infarction, in which the QRS complex would have a QS or Qr morphology. The presence of an RBBB and left anterior fascicular block is termed bifascicular block. In addition, there is first-degree AV block, which is often called "trifascicular block," implicating disease of all three fascicles. However, first-degree AV block may be the result of slow conduction through the AV node or the His-Purkinje system (ie, the remaining fascicle). Therefore, this should not be termed trifascicular disease. Trifascicular block can only be diagnosed on the ECG with either alternating RBBB and left bundle branch block (LBBB) or RBBB with alternating left anterior or left posterior fascicular block. Other situations in which trifascicular block can be diagnosed include (1) bifascicular block (ie, LBBB or RBBB with either left anterior or left posterior fascicular block) associated with Mobitz type II block or (2) bifascicular block with development of complete heart block with an escape ventricular rhythm.

Obstructive sleep apnea has been associated with advanced conduction system disease, and 70% of patients display a left anterior fascicular block. Other findings are persistent deep S waves in the lateral precordial leads and, less commonly, an RBBB (~5%). An RBBB may suggest pulmonary hypertension as a secondary phenomenon. In this patient, there is evidence on physical exam for significant pulmonary hypertension: a right ventricular lift (suggesting right ventricular enlargement), a pulmonary artery tap (suggesting enlargement of the pulmonary artery), a prominent P2, and a holosystolic murmur that demonstrates respirophasic changes in intensity (suggesting the presence of tricuspid regurgitation). Conduction system disease tends to progress in parallel with the severity of obstructive sleep apnea. An echocardiogram would be helpful in better delineating the extent of pulmonary hypertension and evaluating for right ventricular dysfunction suggested by the tricuspid regurgitation and peripheral edema. His tachycardia is quite concerning for incipient right ventricular failure. ■

Notes

An ECG of a 62-year-old man with known progressive, idiopathic conduction system disease is shown.

What portions of the conduction system are affected based on this tracing?

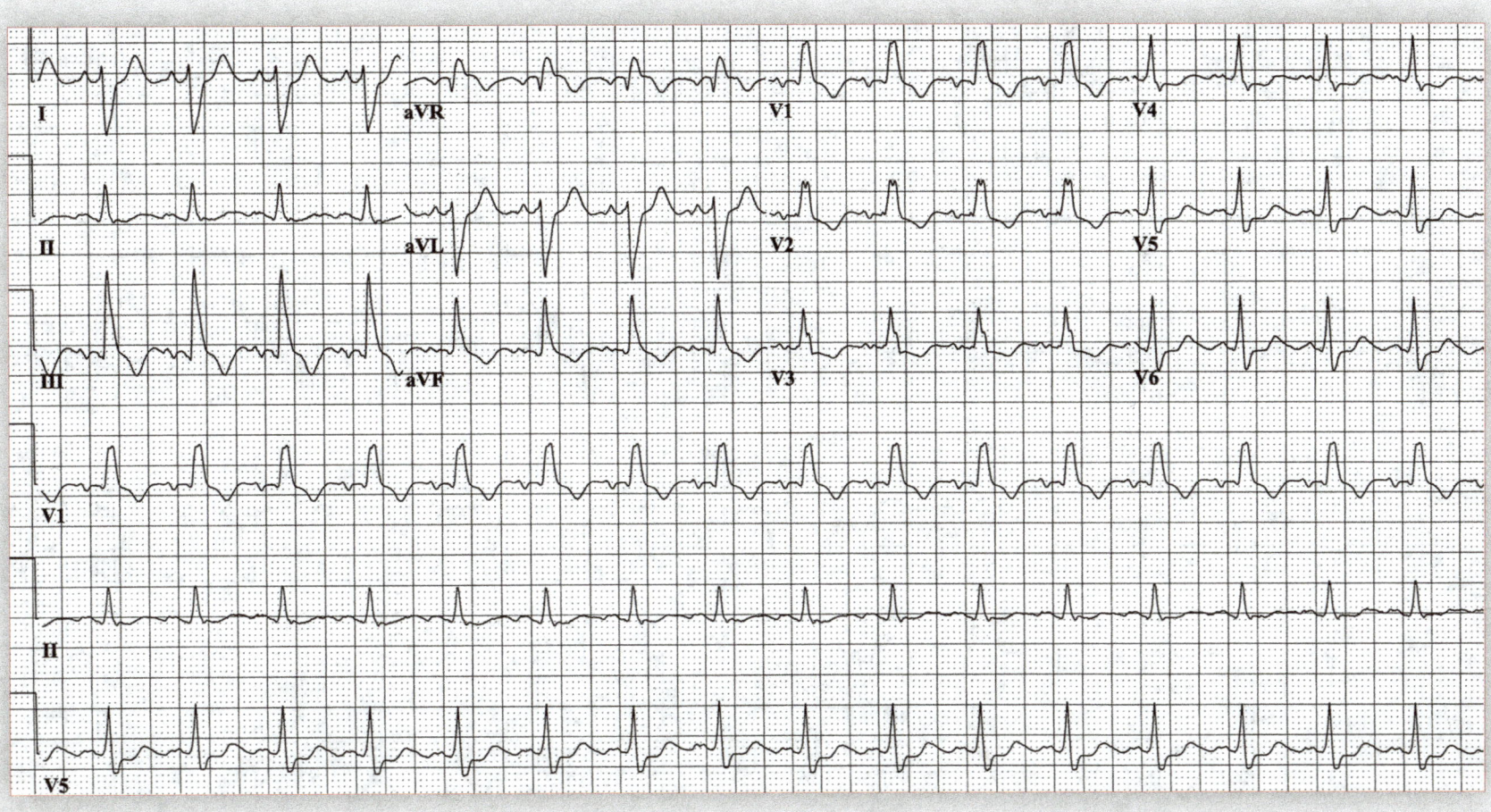

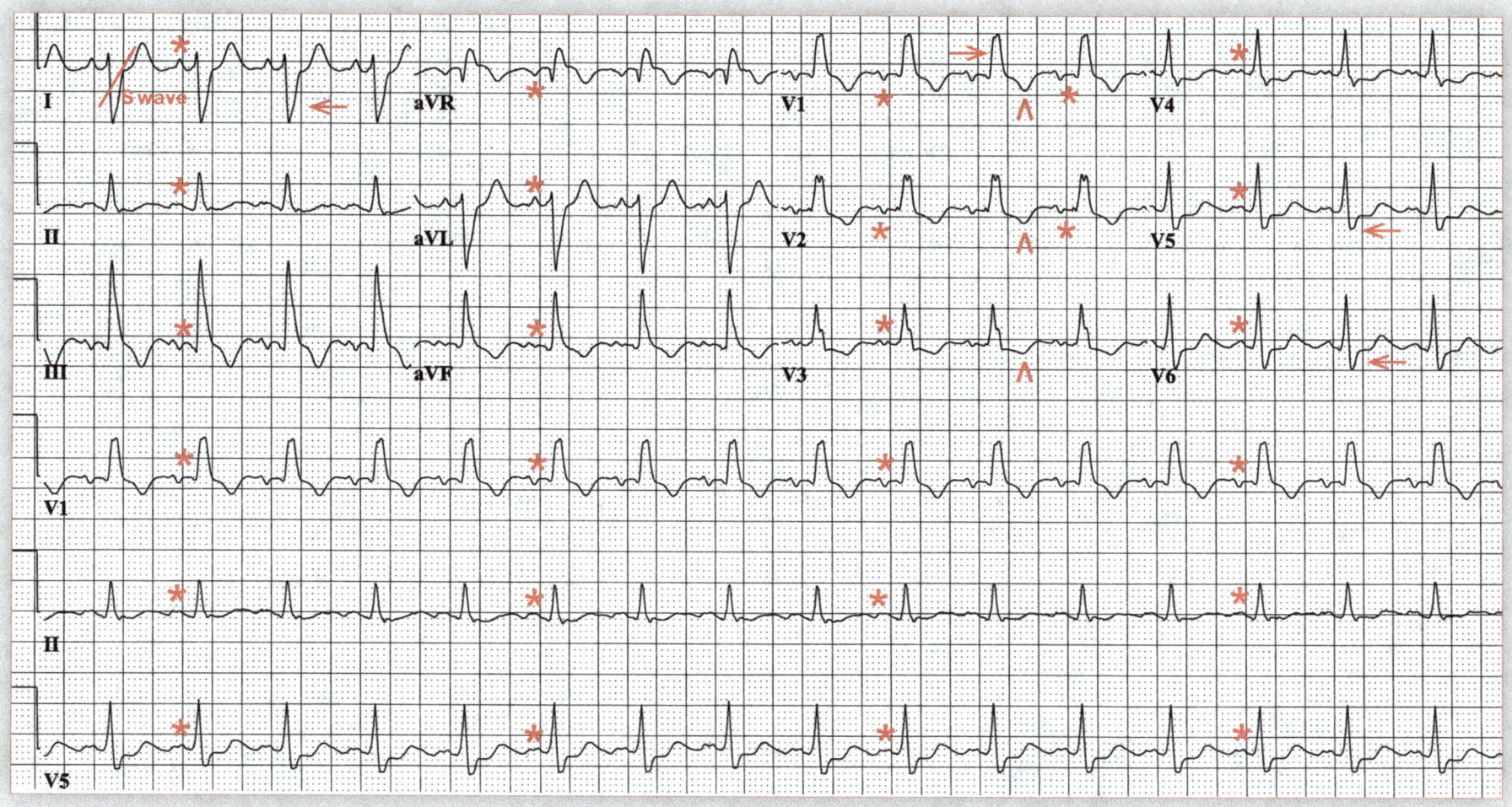

ECG 40 Analysis: Sinus tachycardia, left atrial hypertrophy (abnormality), left posterior fascicular block, right bundle branch block with associated ST-T wave changes, bifascicular block

There is a regular rhythm at a rate of 100 bpm. There is a P wave (*) before each QRS complex with a stable PR interval (0.16 sec). The P wave is positive in leads I, II, aVF, and V4-V6, consistent with a sinus rhythm. However, the P waves are broad in leads II and aVF and notched in leads V4-V6. There is also a prominent negative component to the P wave in leads V1-V2. Hence this indicates left atrial hypertrophy or abnormality. The QRS duration is prolonged (0.16 sec), and there is a pattern of a right bundle branch block (broad R wave in lead V1 [→] and broad S wave in leads I and V5-V6 [←]) with associated ST-T wave changes in leads V1-V3 (^). The QT/QTc intervals are prolonged (380/490 msec) but are normal when the prolonged QRS complex duration is considered (300/388 msec). The axis is rightward, between +90° and +180° (negative QRS complex in lead I and positive QRS complex in lead aVF). The QRS complex in lead I is negative even when the S wave in lead I (due to the right bundle branch block) is ignored. When there is a right bundle branch block, there is a broad terminal S wave in lead I that should not be considered as part of axis determination as it reflects a terminal delay in right ventricular activation. The axis in the frontal plane is based on the impulse direction in the left ventricle. Hence there is also a left posterior fascicular block associated with the right bundle branch block. This is termed bifascicular disease or block.

The presence of bifascicular block indicates more advanced conduction system disease. Bifascicular block due to a left posterior fascicular block is less commonly seen than a left anterior fascicular block, but it has the same implications for the future development of complete heart block. While such patients are at increased risk for complete heart block, the incidence is low. In several studies, the incidence of progression to complete AV block was about 1% to 1.5% per year. Indeed, mortality in these patients, often due to arrhythmia, was related to the underlying heart disease and not to the development of complete heart block. There is no specific therapy for bifascicular block except for discontinuation or avoidance of drugs that may further impair cardiac conduction. Pacemakers are not indicated for asymptomatic patients. However, insertion of a pacemaker should be considered (class II indication) for patients with a bifascicular block associated with syncope that can be attributed to transient complete heart block, based on the exclusion of other plausible causes of syncope. ■

Notes

A 48-year-old man with no previous cardiac history presents to the emergency department after 2 hours of severe substernal chest discomfort that radiates to his jaw and left arm and is associated with diaphoresis and nausea. An ECG shows evidence of an acute myocardial infarction (MI). He is taken urgently to the cardiac catheterization laboratory where angiography demonstrates a thrombotic occlusion of one of the coronary arteries. The vessel is stented in an uncomplicated procedure, and the patient is brought to the critical care unit. He remains stable, and an ECG is obtained the following day.

What was the location of the acute MI?

What other abnormalities are shown?

Is additional therapy necessary?

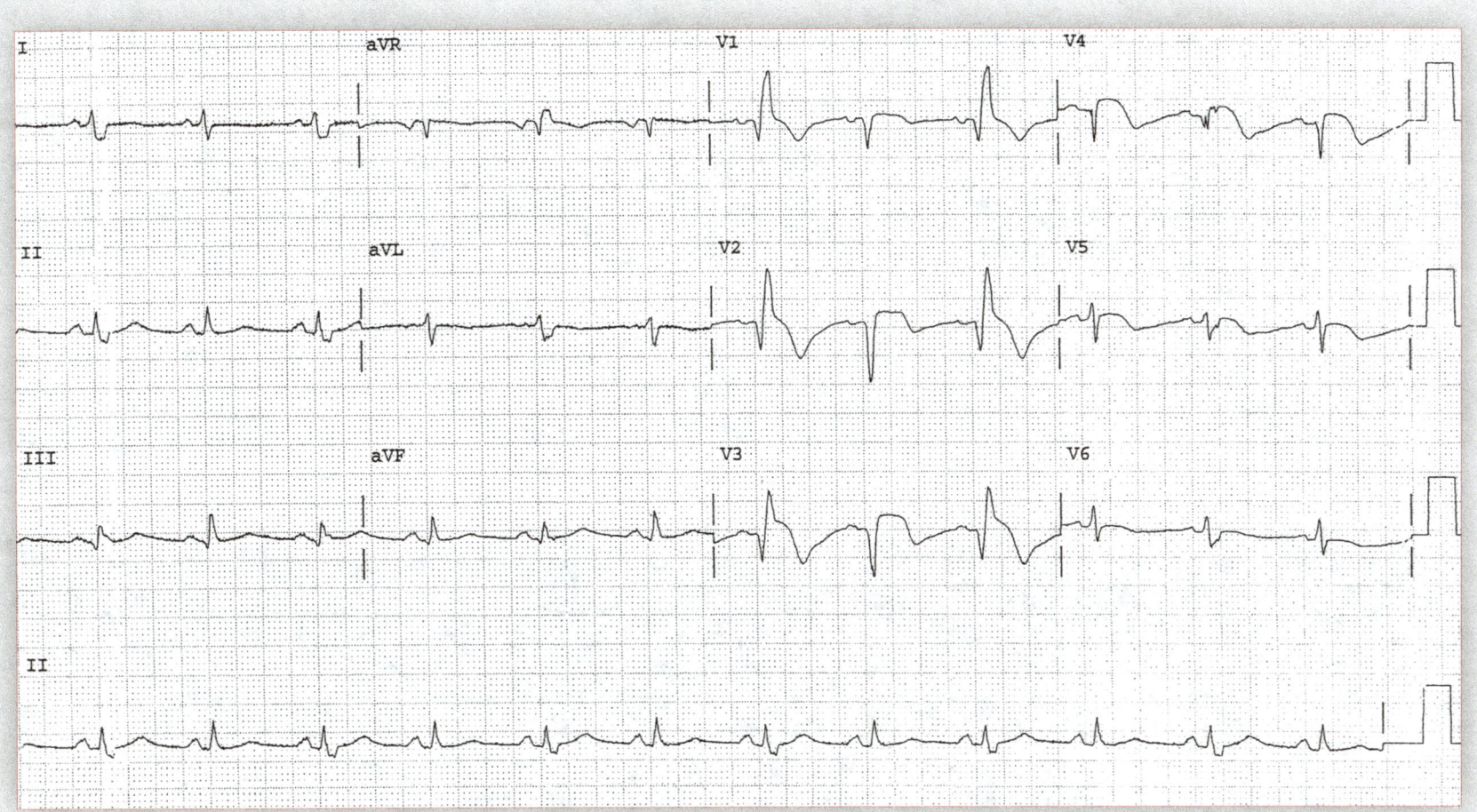

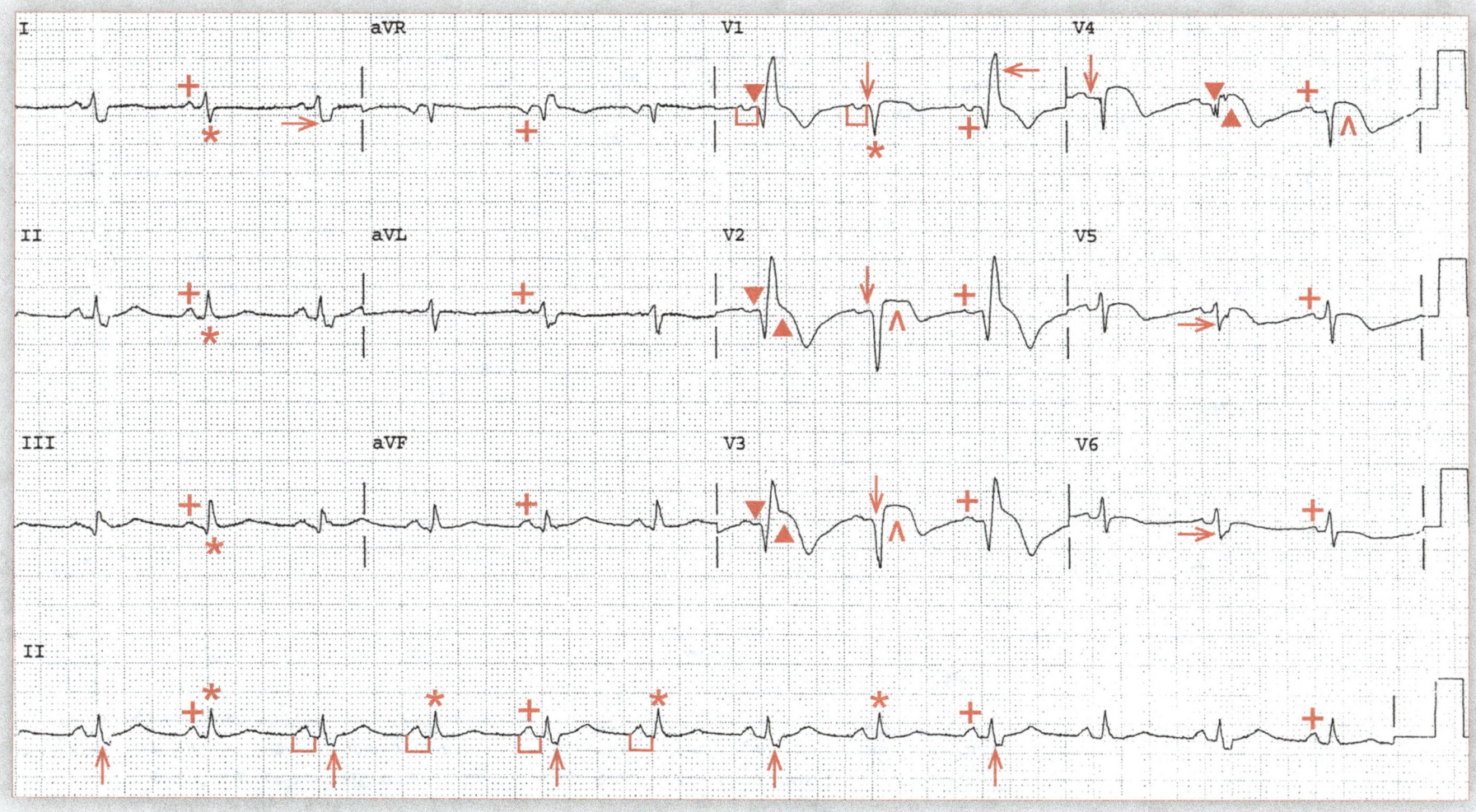

ECG 41 Analysis: Normal sinus rhythm, acute anterior wall
(septum and apex) MI, 2:1 right bundle branch block

There is a regular rhythm at a rate of 76 bpm. There are P waves (+) before each QRS complex with a stable PR interval (0.16 sec) (⊔). The P wave is positive in leads I, II, aVF, and V4-V6. Hence this is a normal sinus rhythm. The QRS complexes have two different morphologies that alternate in a repeating fashion. There are narrow complexes (duration, 0.08 sec) (*) that have a normal axis, between 0° and +90° (positive QRS complex in leads I and aVF). These QRS complexes have a QS morphology (*ie*, no initial R wave) in leads V1-V4 (↓), which indicates an anterior wall myocardial infarction (MI) (septum and apex). There is also ST-segment elevation in these leads (^), indicating that the anterior wall MI is recent.

The alternate QRS complexes have a wide duration (0.16 sec) (↑) with a qR morphology in lead V1 (←) and a broad terminal S wave in leads I and V5-V6 (→), typical for a right bundle branch block (RBBB). These QRS complexes also have a QS complex (▼) and ST-segment elevation (▲) in leads V1-V4, similar to what is seen with the narrow QRS complexes. Hence the alternating QRS complex (*ie*, normal conduction

and RBBB) is termed 2:1 RBBB. Importantly, left ventricular abnormalities can be recognized in the presence of an RBBB since the initial depolarization via the left bundle remains intact and normal, while the QRS complex widening is the result of a terminal delay in right ventricular activation. Hence both QRS complexes demonstrate the same changes that are consistent with a recent (acute) anterior wall MI. The QT/QTc intervals are normal (360/405 msec).

The presence of a new bundle branch block associated with an anterior wall MI indicates significant damage to the septum, which is where the bundle of His and proximal portion of the bundles are located. As the right bundle is located on the right side of the septum, the occurrence of an RBBB generally indicates more extensive infarction. It is possible that the 2:1 RBBB is in fact rate related and would become persistent at a faster heart rate. It is also possible that the RBBB will become permanent in the future. The occurrence of an RBBB, whether intermittent or permanent, is not an indication for permanent pacemaker implantation. No additional therapy is necessary. ■

Notes

A 56-year-old woman is admitted to the hospital for upper gastrointestinal bleeding. While on telemetry, the nurse notices an abrupt change in the patient's surface ECG tracing. He obtains a 12-lead ECG.

What abnormalities are noted?

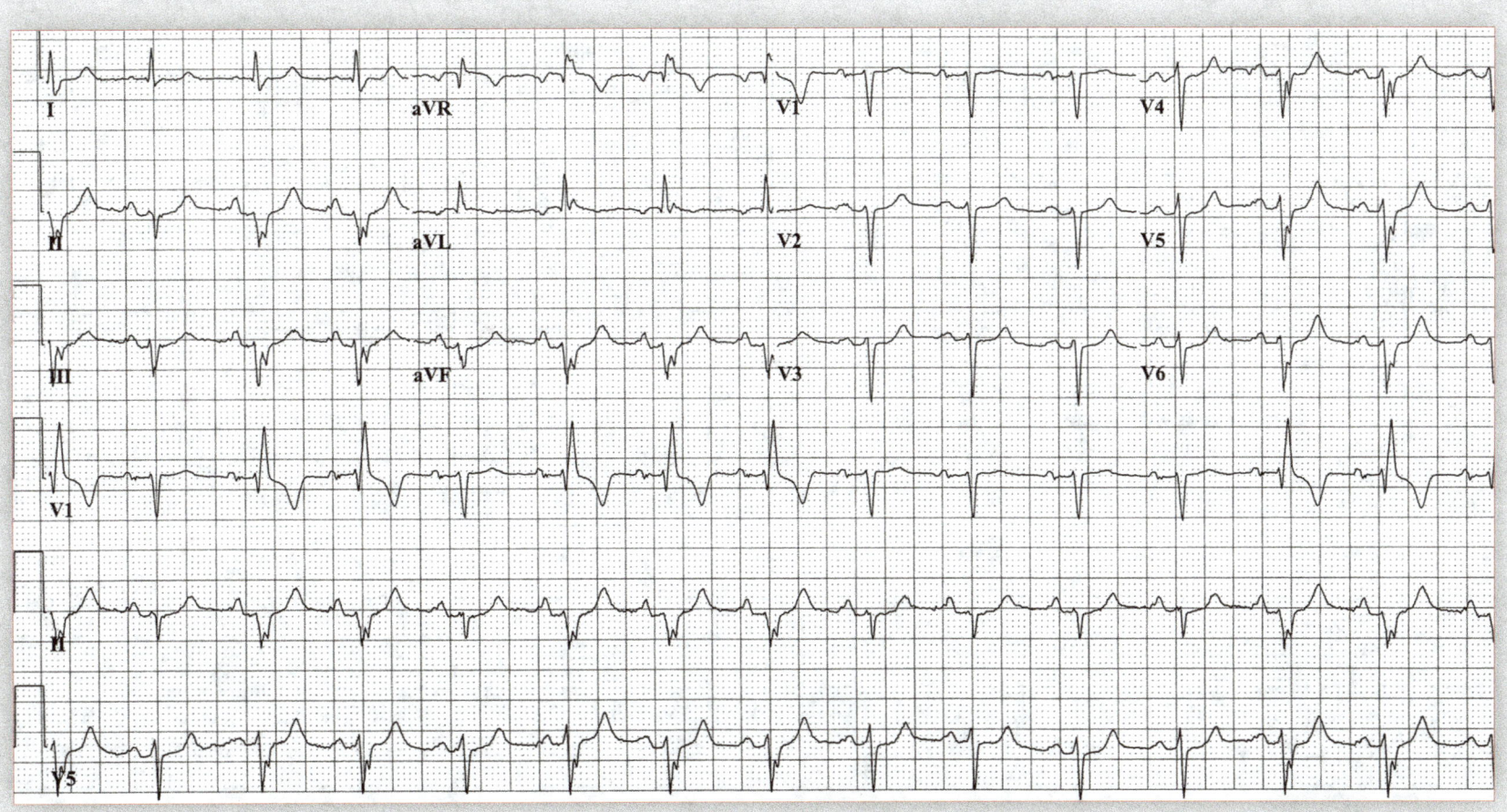

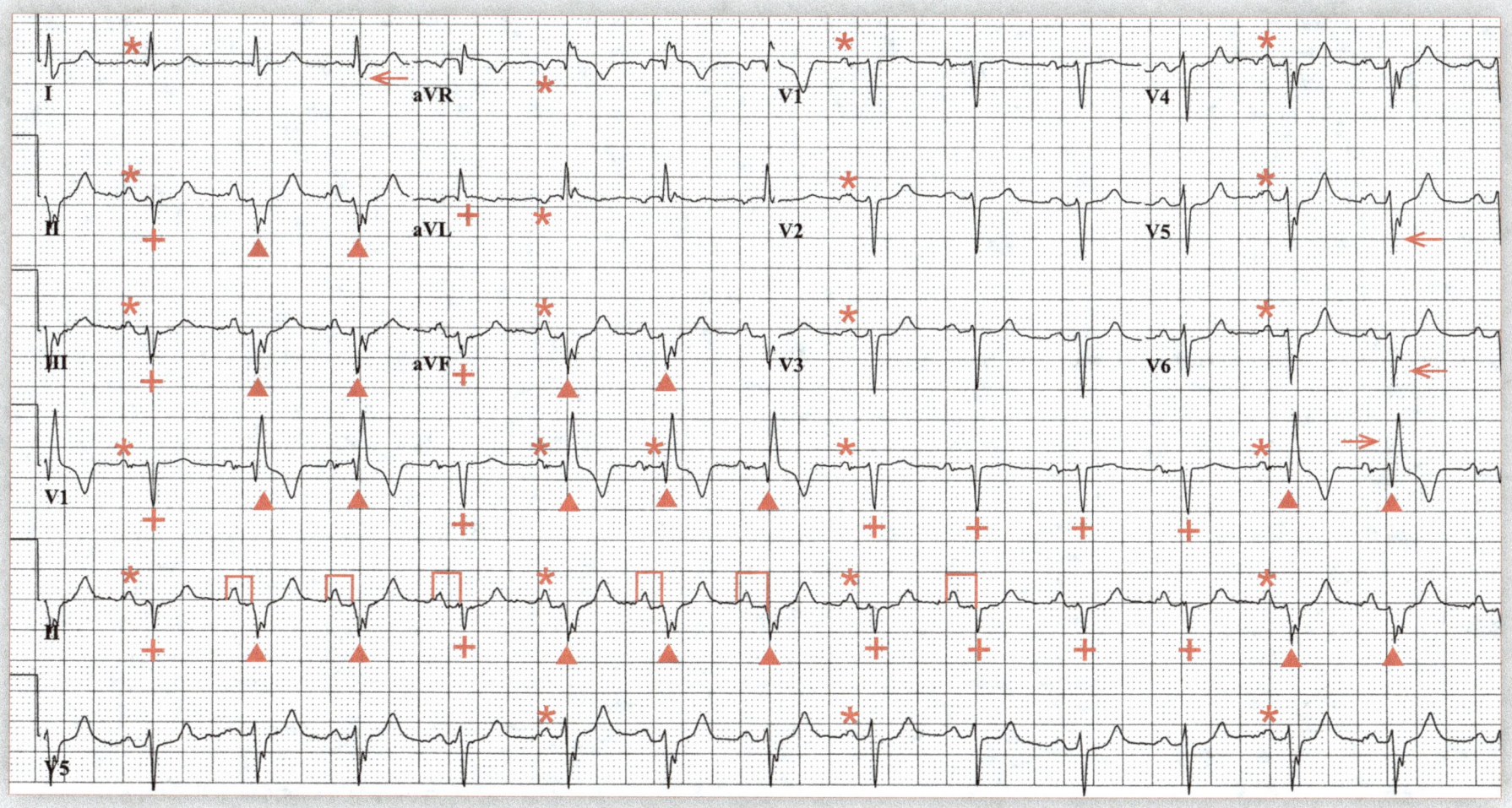

ECG 42 Analysis: Normal sinus rhythm, left anterior fascicular block, intermittent right bundle branch block, clockwise rotation (late transition)

The rhythm is regular at a rate of 86 bpm. There is a P wave (*) before each QRS complex with a stable PR interval (0.18 sec) (⊓). The P wave is positive in leads I, II, aVF, and V4-V6. Hence there is a stable normal sinus rhythm. There are two different QRS morphologies, both of which are preceded by a P wave that has the same morphology; the PR interval of both QRS complexes is the same. The narrow QRS complex (+) has a normal duration (0.08 sec) and morphology. The axis is extremely leftward, between −30° and −90° (positive QRS complex in lead I and negative QRS complex in leads II and aVF, with an rS complex). This is diagnostic for left anterior fascicular block.

Also noted are QRS complexes that are wide (▲) (0.14 sec) with a typical right bundle branch block (RBBB) morphology (RSR′ morphology in lead V1 [→] and broad S wave in leads I and V5-V6 [←]). This is an intermittent RBBB that does not appear to be rate related. However, subtle differences in rate may be present but not apparent when the ECG is recorded at slow speed (*ie*, 25 mm/sec). The P wave and PR interval before both the wide and narrow QRS complexes are the same. Of note is the fact that the intermittent RBBB, associated with a persistent left anterior fascicular block, indicates bifascicular disease. Both QRS complexes show poor R-wave progression across the precordium and late transition as a result of clockwise rotation in the horizontal plane. This is determined by imagining the heart as viewed from under the diaphragm. In this situation, the right ventricle is in front and the left ventricle is to the left. With clockwise rotation the left ventricular forces are delayed and develop later, occurring in the lateral precordial leads. Clockwise rotation can be seen with a left anterior fascicular block. The QT/QTc intervals for the narrow QRS complexes are normal (320/380 msec). The QT/QTc intervals for the QRS complexes with an RBBB are prolonged (380/455 msec) but are normal (320/380 msec) when correcting for the prolonged QRS complex duration.

Intermittent or rate-related RBBB is indicative of underlying conduction disease of the right bundle that becomes manifest most often when the heart rate is faster. Occasionally there is no change in heart rate. The onset of a widened QRS complex due rate-related bundle branch block is abrupt (*ie*, the widening of the QRS complex is not gradual). When an intermittent RBBB is present, the diseased bundle is unable to conduct at rapid rates and hence block develops within the bundle. This is often the precursor of a permanent RBBB. It has the same implications and prognosis as a persistent RBBB and a persistent bifascicular block. ■

A medical student is concerned about his patient's admission ECG. He notices an abnormality that prompts review by the patient's physician.

What abnormality is noted on the ECG?

What does it represent?

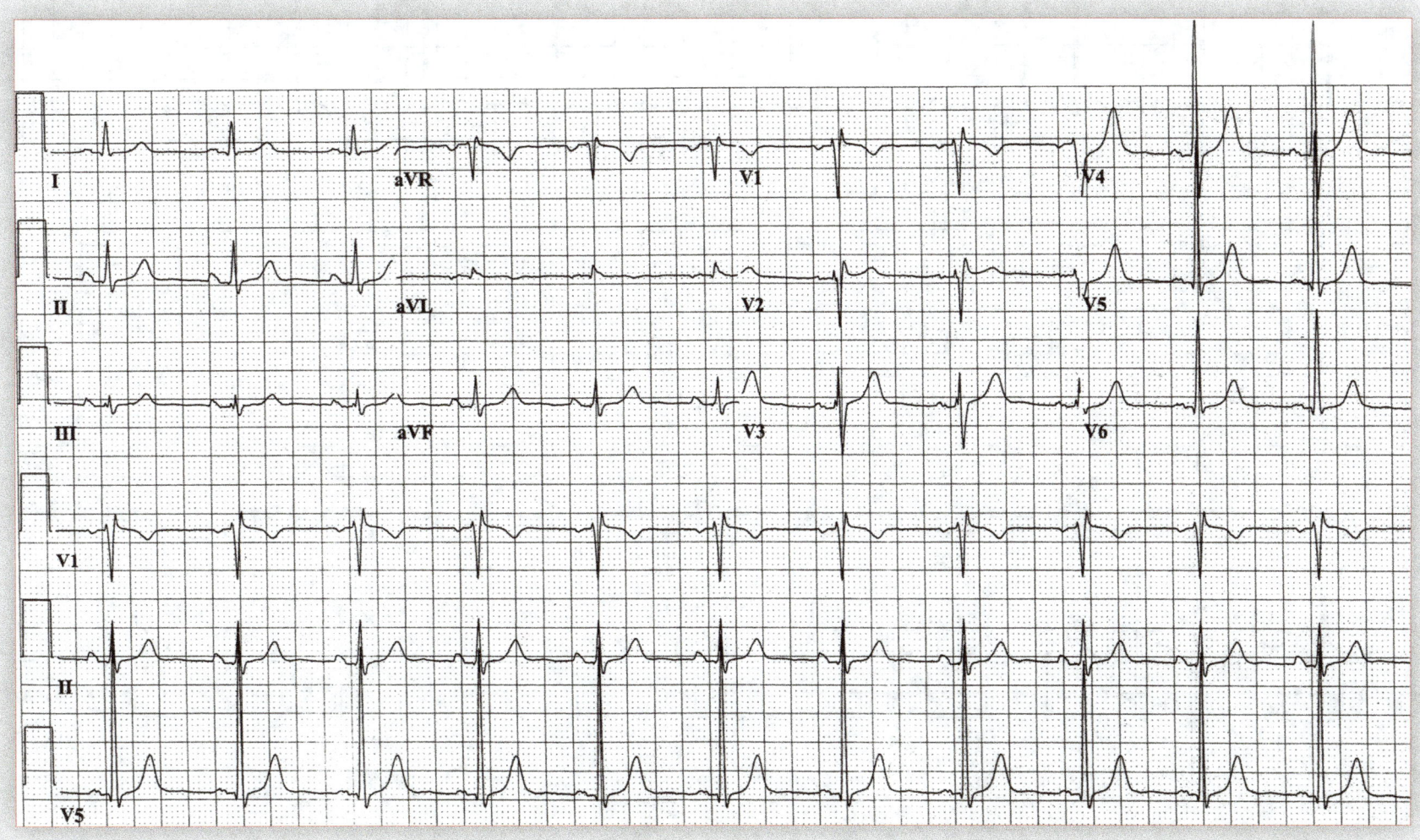

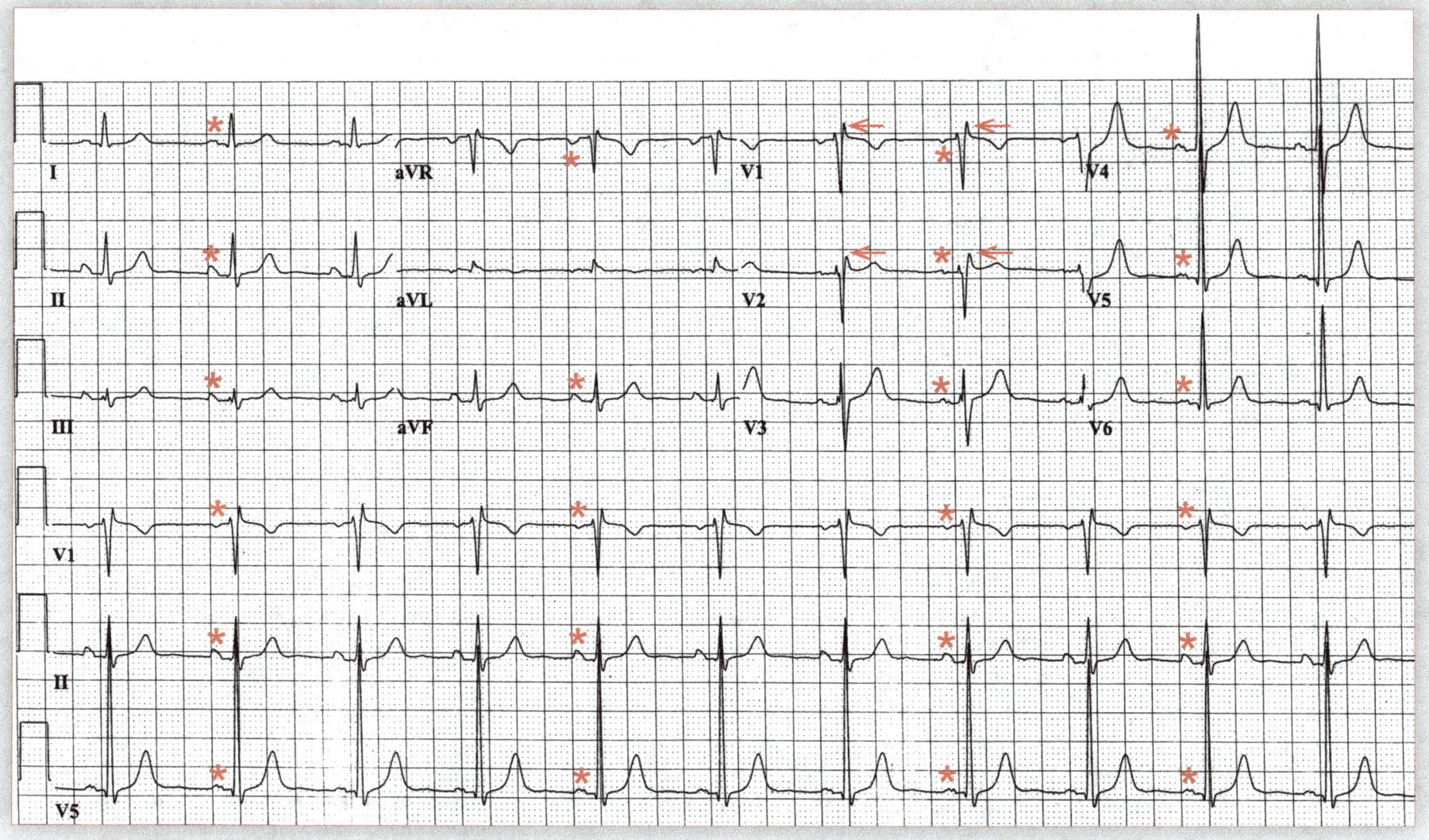

ECG 43 Analysis: Normal sinus rhythm, intraventricular conduction delay to right ventricle (crista pattern)

The rhythm is regular at a rate of 68 bpm. There is a P wave (*) before each QRS complex, and the PR interval is stable (0.16 sec). The P wave is positive in leads I, II, aVF, and V4-V6. Hence this is a normal sinus rhythm. The axis is normal, between 0° and +90°, and the QRS duration (0.10 sec) and morphology are normal. The QT/QTc intervals are normal (380/405 msec). However, the QRS complex in leads V1-V2 has an RSR′ morphology (←). This pattern represents a conduction delay to the right ventricle and has been called a "crista" pattern as the delay is in the last portion of the right ventricle to depolarize (*ie*, crista supraventricularis). It is a normal variant.

The RSR′ morphology seen in the early precordial leads (V1-V2) represents a spectrum of physiologic changes ranging from normal delayed depolarization of the crista supraventricularis of the right ventricle, to right intraventricular conduction delay, to pathologic right bundle branch block. The QRS complex duration defines the diagnosis. If the QRS complex duration is normal (< 0.10 sec), the morphology is deemed a normal variant and termed a crista pattern. If the QRS complex duration is slightly prolonged (between 0.10 and 0.12 sec), an intraventricular conduction delay (often referred to as an incomplete right bundle branch block) is present. The term incomplete right bundle branch block is not accurate, however, as the His-Purkinje system and bundles manifest all-or-none conduction characteristics; that is, the bundles either conduct (always at the same rate) or do not conduct. If the QRS complex duration is longer than 0.12 second, the diagnosis is a right bundle branch block. In this ECG there is a crista pattern present, which is a normal variant that does not have any clinical implications. ■

An 88-year-old woman who was diagnosed with hypertension in her 20s but has refrained from medical treatment is seen in your clinic. She has complaints of progressive dyspnea on exertion that has started to interfere with her daily 5-mile walks. She is otherwise asymptomatic, and a general review of systems is unremarkable. Her heart rate is 70 bpm, with a blood pressure of 154/90 mm Hg. Her cardiopulmonary exam is notable for normal jugular venous pressure, a slight lateral displacement of a prominent point of maximal impulse, an S4 gallop, and a soft holosystolic murmur at the apex. An ECG is obtained.

What abnormality is evident on the ECG?

What is the cause of this abnormality?

What further evaluation is warranted?

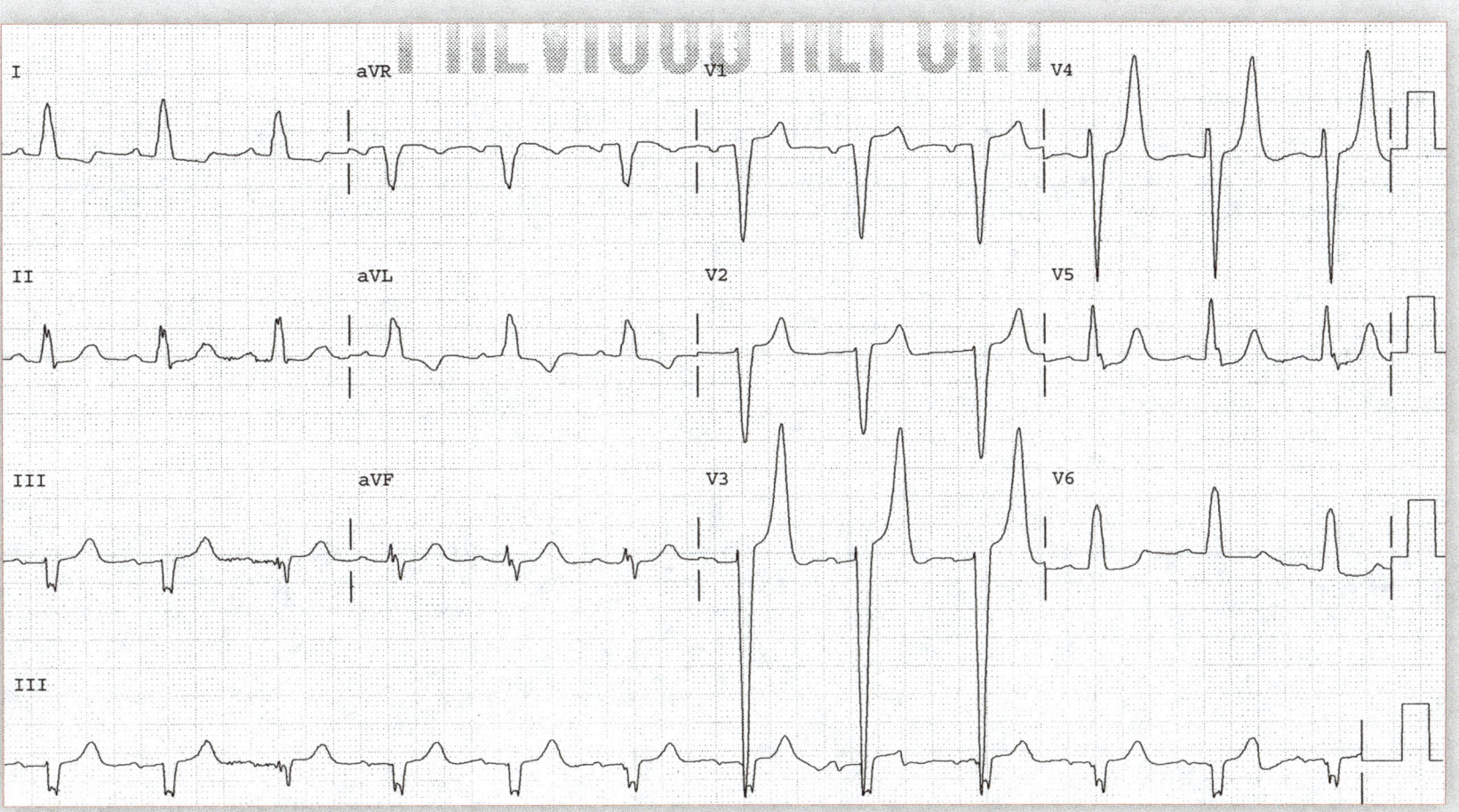

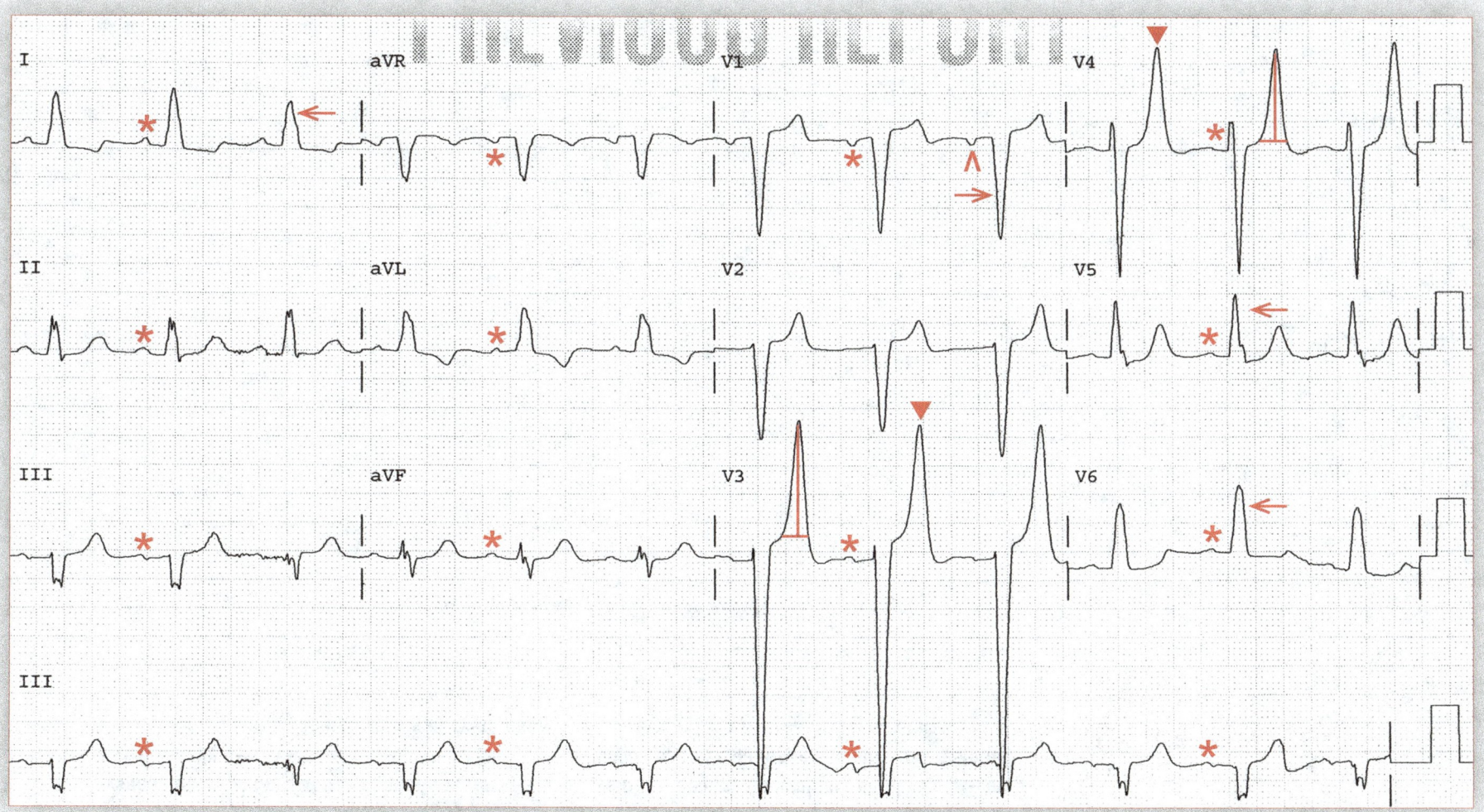

ECG 44 Analysis: Normal sinus rhythm, left atrial hypertrophy (abnormality), first-degree AV block (prolonged AV conduction), left bundle branch block

The rhythm is regular at a rate of 70 bpm. There is a P wave (*) before each QRS complex, and the PR interval is constant (0.24 sec). The P waves are positive in leads I, II, aVF, and V4-V6. Hence this is a normal sinus rhythm with first-degree AV block (prolonged AV conduction). The QRS duration is increased (0.16 sec). In leads I and V5-V6 there is a broad R wave (←), and in lead V1 there is a deep QS complex (→). This is the pattern of a left bundle branch block (LBBB). The QT/QTc intervals are prolonged (480/520 msec) but are normal when considering the prolonged QRS complex duration (400/430 msec). Noted are T waves that are tall and peaked in leads V3-V4 (▼); however, they are asymmetric and hence normal. The P wave in lead V1 is predominantly negative (^), suggesting left atrial hypertrophy.

An LBBB is identified by the following characteristics:

- The QRS complex duration is 0.12 second or longer due to delayed activation of the left ventricle. Left ventricular activation occurs after right ventricular activation.

- Left ventricular activation occurs from the right bundle and right ventricle directly through myocardium, bypassing the normal His-Purkinje system. Therefore, conduction is slow (causing the QRS complex to be widened) and all forces are directed from right to left (broad, tall R wave in leads I, aVL, and V5-V6; deep QS complex in leads V1 and possibly V2). No left-to-right forces should be seen (ie, there is no terminal S wave in lead I or V6).

- Since the interventricular septum is activated by a small septal branch (median fascicle) that comes from the left bundle and activates the septum in a left-to-right direction, no septal forces are seen (ie, no initial Q waves in lead I, aVL, or V5-V6 and no initial R wave in lead V1).

- Associated with the abnormal depolarization is abnormal repolarization. Hence diffuse ST-T wave abnormalities are seen.

- The axis may be normal or leftward. The left axis is not due to an isolated left anterior fascicular block as both fascicles are blocked as a result of the LBBB. Rather, the left axis is due to an abnormal direction of left ventricular activation from the right. A right axis is not seen with an LBBB as there should not be any left-to-right forces.

- Since left ventricular activation is abnormal and does not occur through the normal His-Purkinje system but rather through direct myocardial activation, left ventricular abnormalities (eg, left ventricular hypertrophy, infarction, ischemia, pericarditis) cannot be recognized.

continues

Longstanding hypertension may result in pathologic left ventricular hypertrophy, which is associated with diffuse fibrotic changes. This often produces chronic elevation of left ventricular filling pressure and diastolic dysfunction that result in secondary left atrial hypertrophy. These morphologic alterations of the left ventricle can result in disruption of the architecture of the conduction system and may lead to an LBBB as noted in this case. An echocardiogram may be helpful in corroborating the physical exam findings consistent with left ventricular hypertrophy (prominent point of maximal impulse, S4 gallop). Although left ventricular hypertrophy cannot be diagnosed on the surface ECG in the presence of an LBBB, left atrial hypertrophy is clearly seen and supports this diagnosis. ■

A 59-year-old man with premature coronary artery disease, a history of multiple myocardial infarctions, and ischemic cardiomyopathy is admitted with heart failure. His ECG is shown.

What abnormalities are evident?

What mechanism for the conduction abnormality does the ECG suggest?

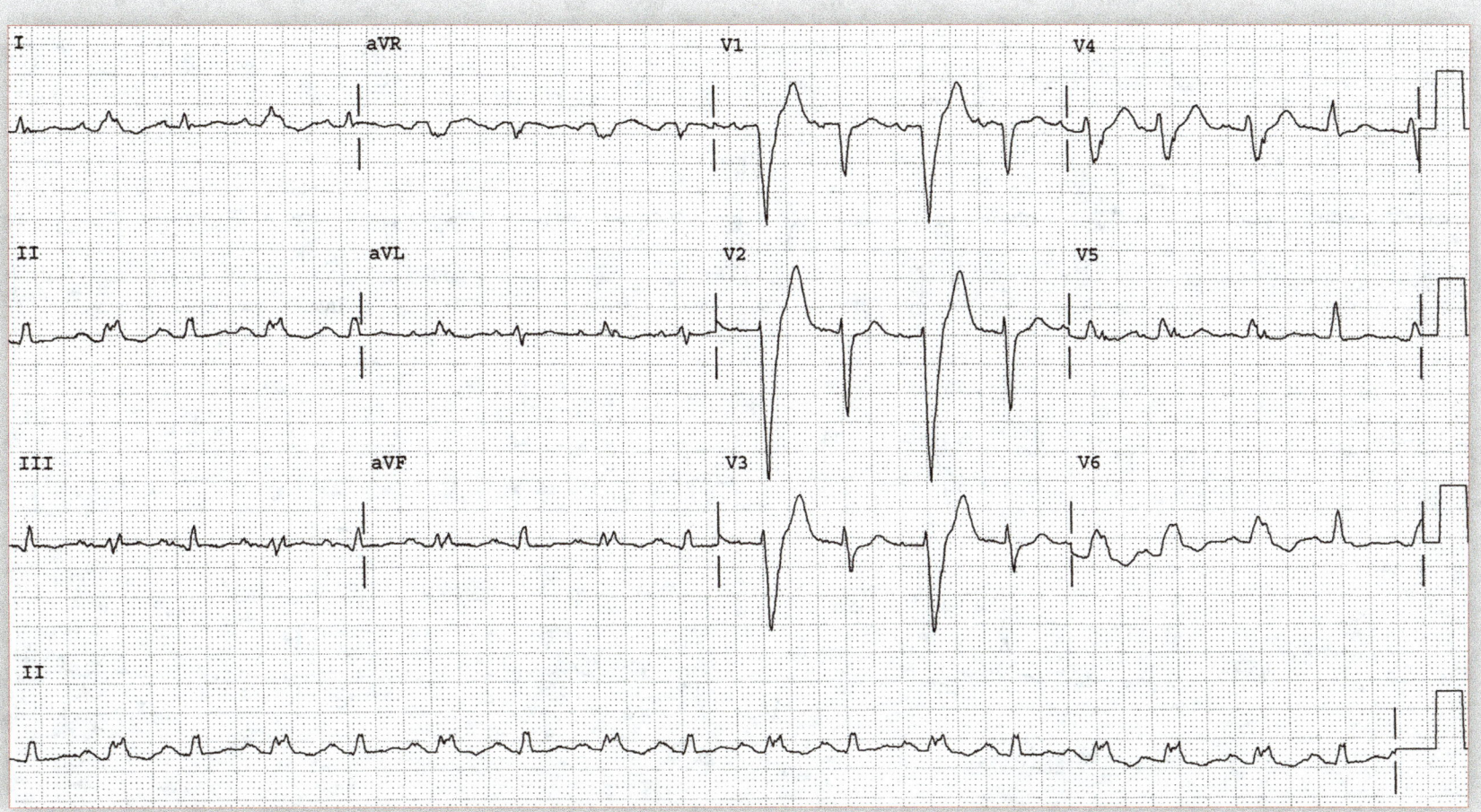

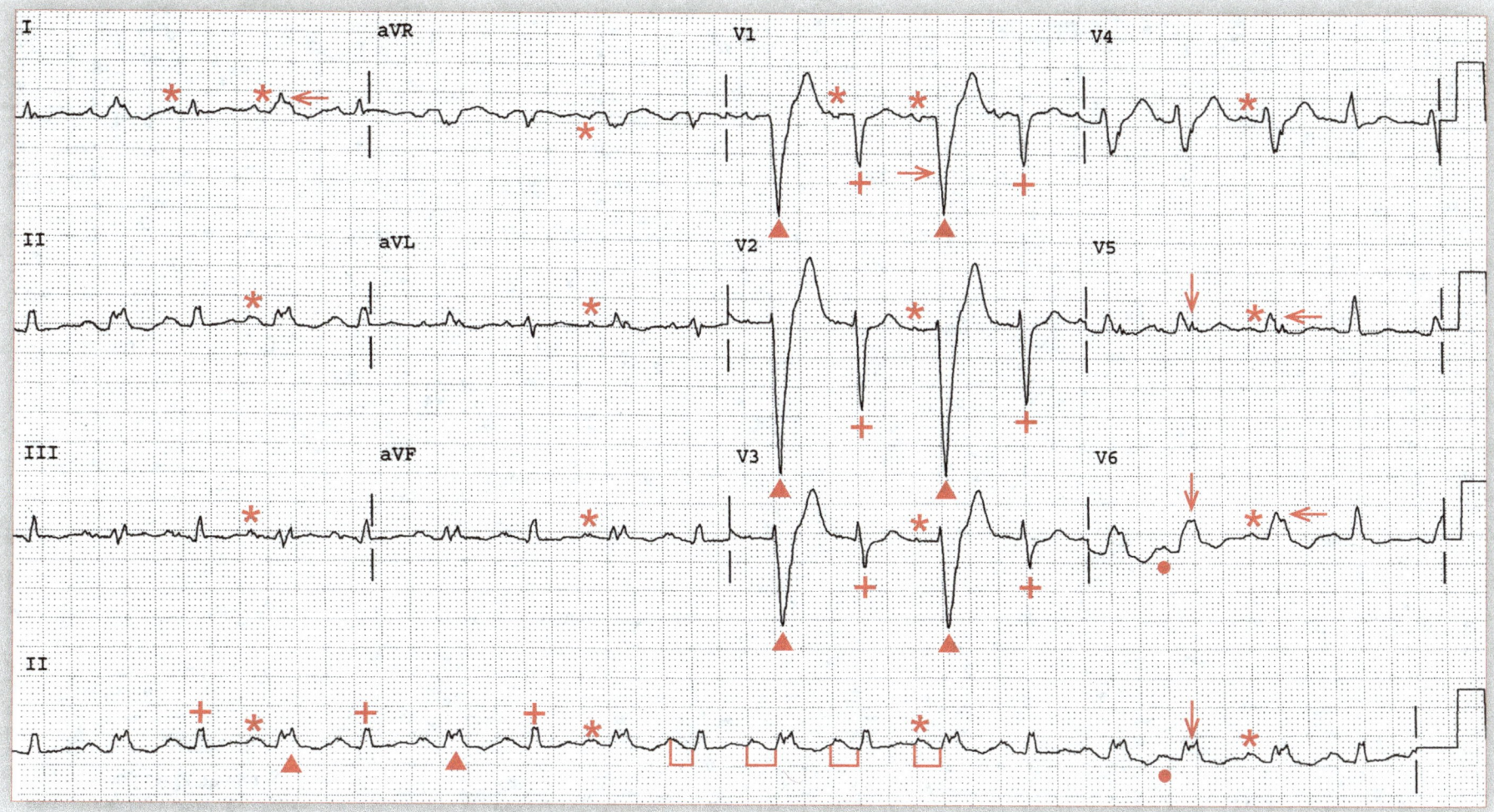

ECG 45 Analysis: Sinus tachycardia, intermittent (2:1)
left bundle branch block (possibly rate related), premature atrial complex

There is a regular rhythm at a rate of 100 bpm. There is a P wave (✱) before each QRS complex with a constant PR interval (⊔) (0.20 sec). The P waves are positive in leads I, II, aVF, and V4-V6. Hence this is sinus tachycardia. There are alternating changes in QRS complex width from beat to beat. The narrow QRS complexes (+) have a normal duration (0.10 sec) and morphology, while the wider QRS complexes (▲) (0.16 sec) have a left bundle branch block (LBBB) morphology (broad R wave in leads I and V5-V6 [←] and a deep QS complex in lead V1 [→]). The changes in QRS duration do not appear to be rate related. This is termed 2:1 LBBB. However, the 15th QRS complex (↓) is premature. A P wave with a different morphology than the sinus P waves (•) can be seen before this QRS complex; hence this is a premature atrial complex. This premature complex also has an LBBB morphology, suggesting that there is some relation to rate. The QT/QTc intervals of the wide QRS complexes are prolonged (400/516 msec) but are normal when corrected for the prolonged QRS complex duration (320/410 msec). The QT/QTc intervals of the narrow QRS complex are normal (320/410 msec).

The presence of 2:1 LBBB suggests that there is an underlying conduction abnormality in the left bundle such that it is not capable of conducting every QRS complex. Every other complex is blocked in the left bundle and hence not conducted through it. This is likely rate related, although it is difficult to establish this, except for the presence of a premature atrial complex that appears to have a rate-related LBBB. It is likely that in the future the patient will develop a permanent or persistent LBBB. There are no clinical implications to this finding, although it is important to recognize that the development of a persistent LBBB at a higher heart rate is not related to the presence of ischemia or another cause. ■

Notes

An ECG from a 67-year-old diabetic woman is shown.

What abnormalities are noted?

What pathology does the ECG suggest?

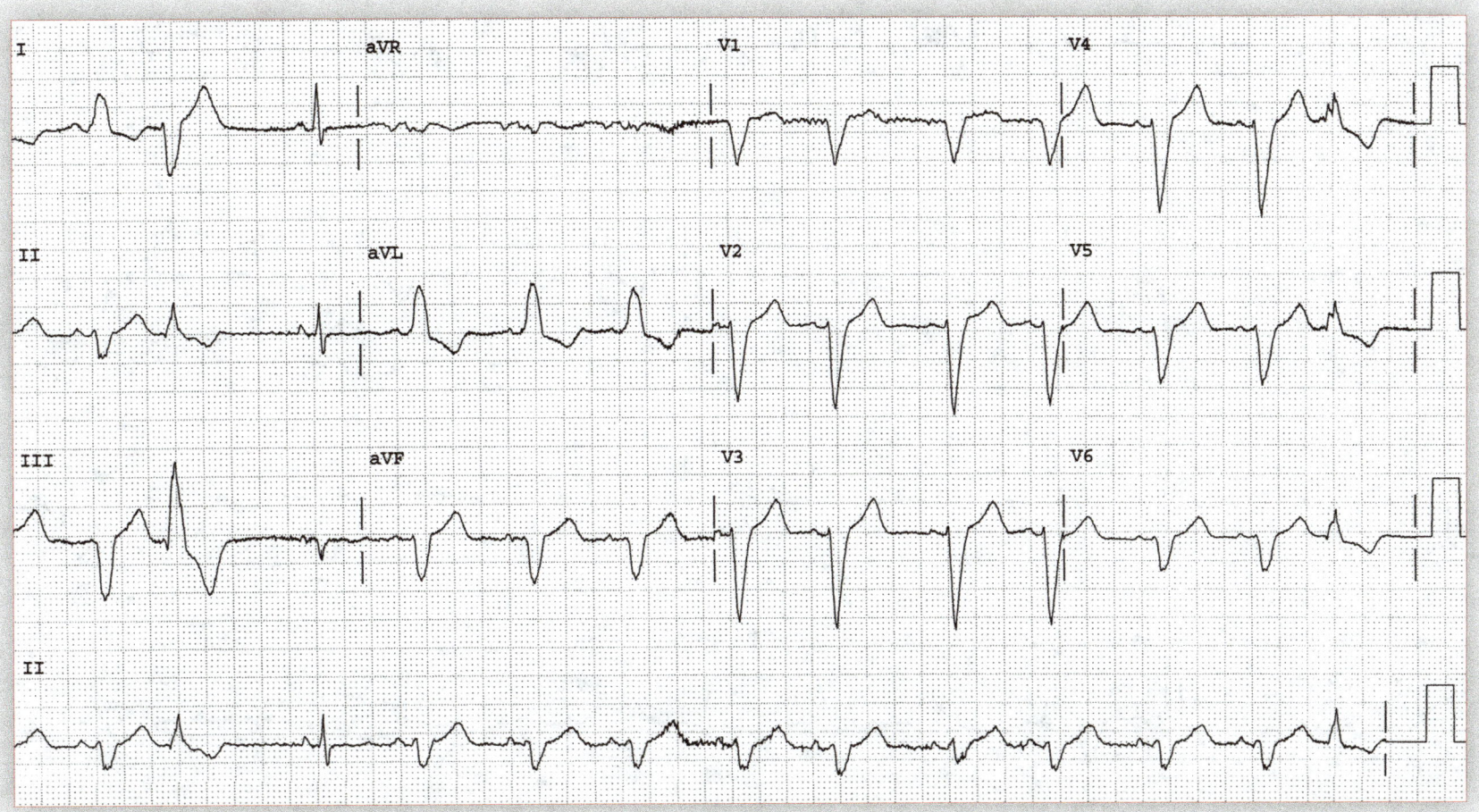

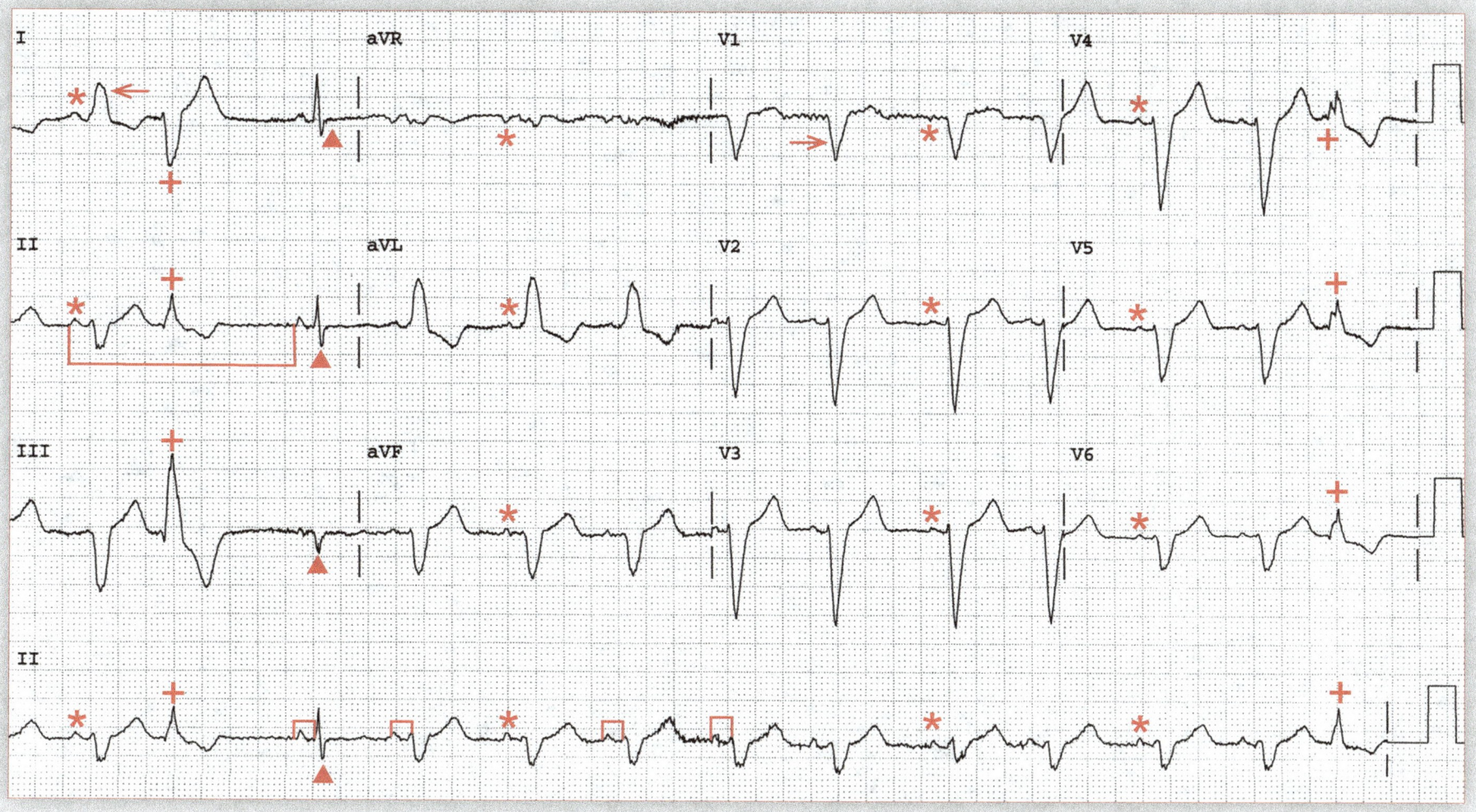

ECG 46 Analysis: Normal sinus rhythm, premature ventricular complex, rate-related left bundle branch block

There is a regular rhythm at a rate of 90 bpm. There is a P wave (*) before each QRS complex with a stable PR interval (0.16 sec) (⊓). The P waves are positive in leads I, II, aVF, and V4-V6. Hence this is a normal sinus rhythm. All of the QRS complexes, except for the third complex (▲), are wide (0.16 sec), and they have the morphology of a left bundle branch block (LBBB; broad R wave lead I [←] and QS complex in lead V1 [→]). Although there is an rS complex in leads V4-V6, this is still consistent with an LBBB.

An occasional premature complex (+) can be seen (complexes 2 and 13). There are no P waves before these complexes, and they are wider with a different morphology compared with the other QRS complexes. Hence these are premature ventricular complexes. Both of them have the same morphology, so they are unifocal. There is a compensatory pause (⊔) following the second QRS complex (ie, the PP intervals surrounding the pause are equal to two sinus PP intervals). A full compensatory pause is due to the fact that the on-time P wave that follows the premature ventricular complex does not conduct through the AV node, which is blocked as a result of retrograde conduction from the premature ventricular complex. As a result of the pause and a longer RR interval, the QRS complex following the ventricular premature complex (▲) is narrow, with the same PR interval (⊓) as the other complexes. This QRS complex is normal in both duration and morphology, as it does not have an LBBB. Therefore, the LBBB is rate related as it is not present when the rate is slower (ie, after the pause).

A diseased conduction system may manifest obvious abnormalities at faster rates. A rate-related conduction abnormality per se does not suggest a specific disease entity. Although this patient has no symptoms, underlying coronary artery disease with resultant myocardial fibrosis may be present. It is also possible that the underlying conduction system disease is due to idiopathic changes of the conduction system, as are seen with Lev's or Lenègre's disease. Lastly, the patient may have an underlying cardiomyopathy of any cause. Although the rate-related LBBB has no important clinical implications, a persistent or permanent LBBB may develop in the future. Importantly, an LBBB is not related to acute ischemia, although it may often be due to underlying ischemic heart disease and the presence of myocardial fibrosis or prior infarction.

No therapy is indicated. Generally, no further evaluation is necessary, although not uncommonly an echocardiogram will be obtained to assess for cardiac structural abnormalities. If an exercise test was indicated for diagnosing underlying coronary artery disease, nuclear or echocardiographic imaging would be essential as ST-segment changes could not be interpreted in the presence of a rate-related LBBB. ▪

Core Case 47

A 64-year-old man presents to the emergency room with complaints of substernal chest pressure and diaphoresis that began 1 hour earlier. He states that he has a history of hypertension and hyperlipidemia. He sees his primary care physician on a regular basis and remembers being told that he has some type of block on his ECG. His baseline ECG (47A) is

ECG 47A

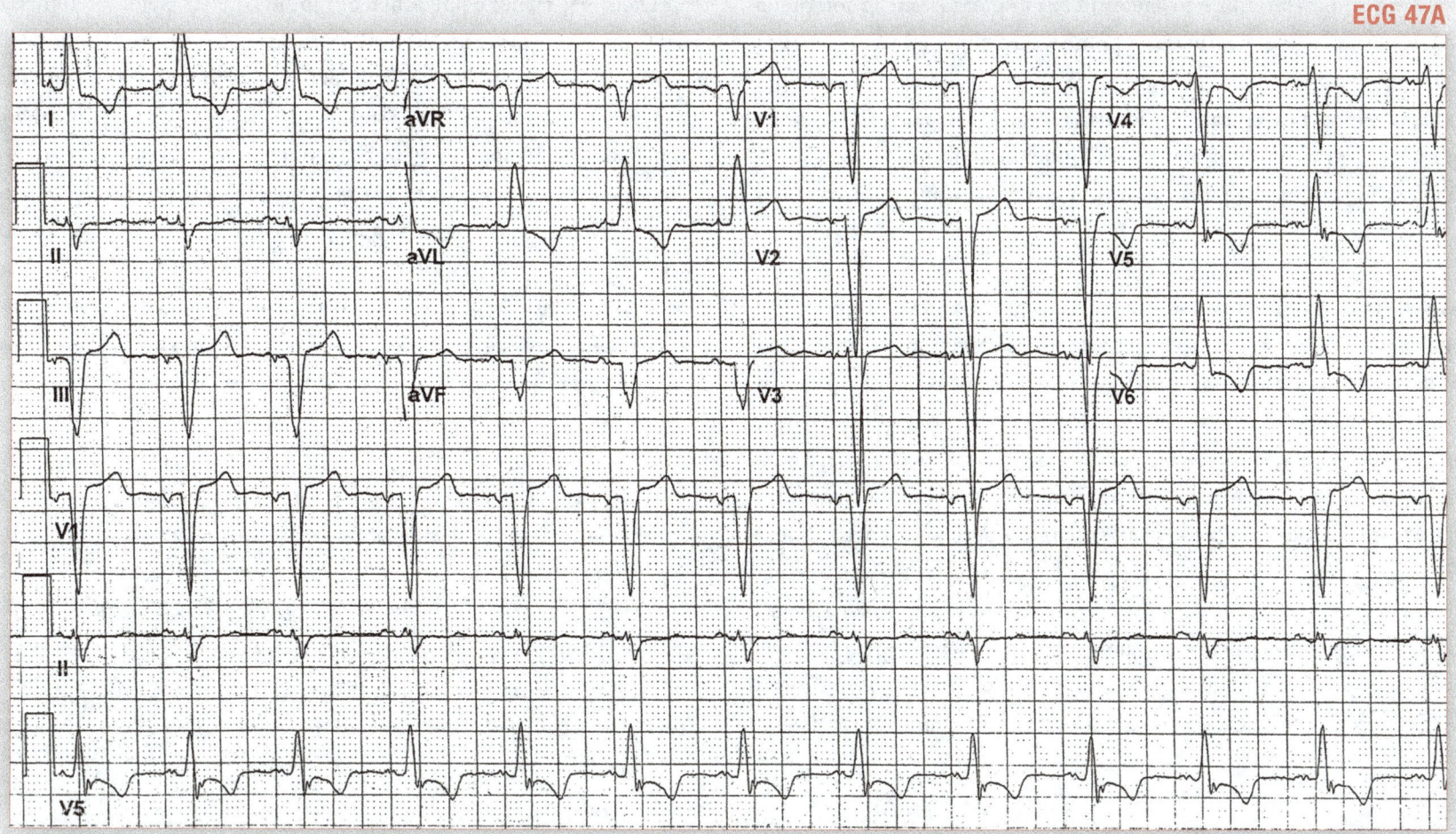

available for review. His initial vital signs are stable, with a blood pressure of 130/90 mm Hg and a pulse of 72 bpm. Physical examination is unremarkable, although he is noted to be very diaphoretic. Nitroglycerin is given for the chest discomfort, providing incomplete relief. Morphine is administered. A 12-lead ECG (47B) is obtained.

What type of "block" is shown on the baseline ECG (47A)?

What diagnosis can be made based on ECG 47B?

What therapy is indicated?

ECG 47B

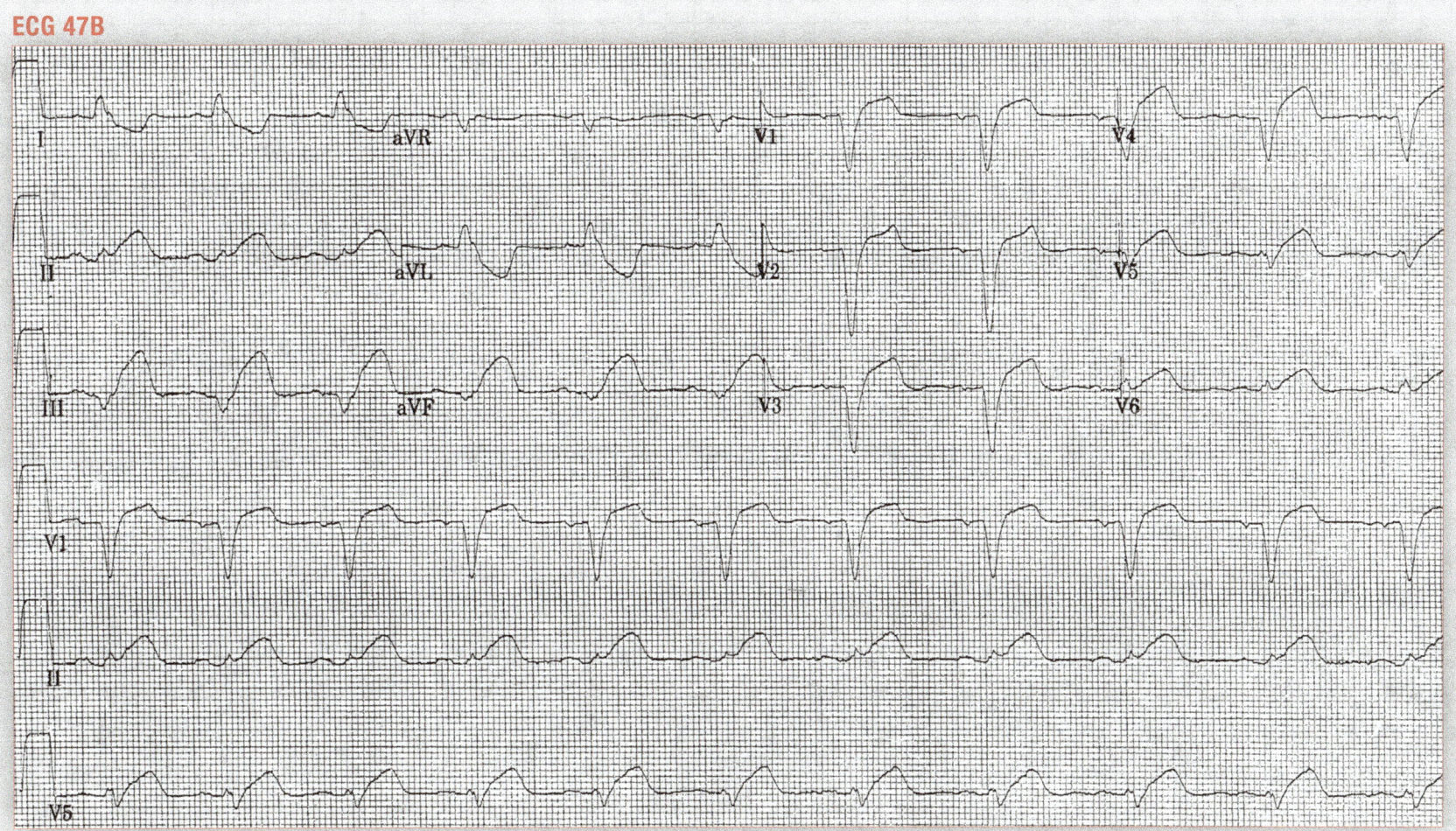

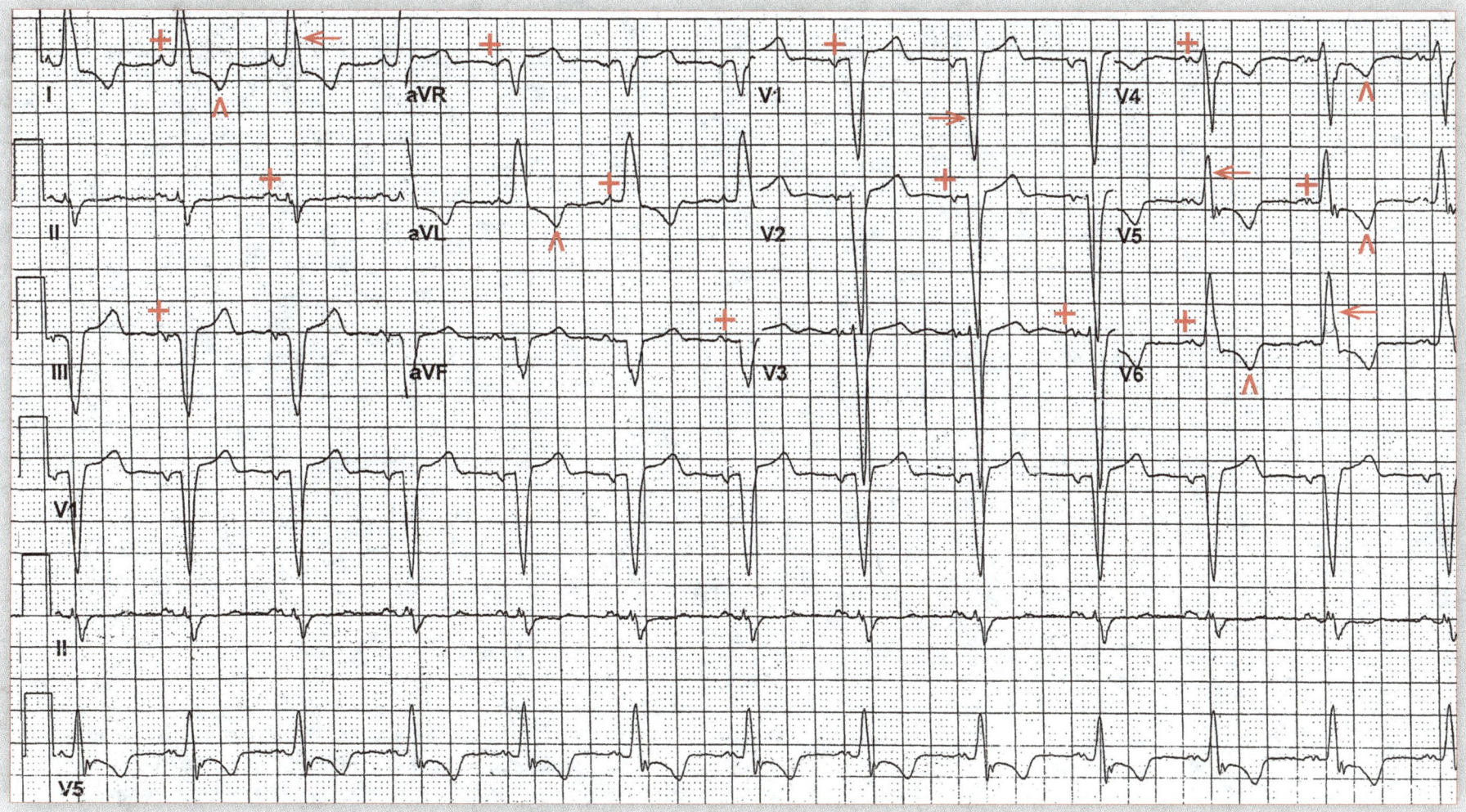

ECG 47A Analysis: Normal sinus rhythm, left atrial abnormality (hypertrophy), left bundle branch block with associated ST-T wave abnormalities

ECG **47A** shows a regular rhythm at a rate of 75 bpm. There is a P wave before each QRS complex (+), with a stable PR interval (0.18 sec). The P wave is positive in leads I, II, aVF, and V4-V6; therefore, this is a normal sinus rhythm. However, the P wave is broad and prominently notched in leads II and V3-V6 and is negative in leads V1-V2. This is consistent with left atrial hypertrophy (or abnormality). The QRS complex duration is increased (0.14 sec) and it has a typical left bundle branch block (LBBB) morphology, with a broad R wave in leads I and V5-V6 (←) and a deep QS complex in lead V1 (→). The axis is extremely leftward, between −30° and −90°. Although this axis is consistent with a left anterior fascicular block, this cannot be diagnosed in the presence of an LBBB as both fascicles (left anterior and left posterior) are blocked and not conducting an impulse to the ventricular myocardium. There are ST-T wave changes in leads I, aVL, and V3-V6 (^) that are secondary to the LBBB. The QT/QTc intervals are prolonged (420/470 msec) but are normal when the prolonged QRS complex duration is considered (380/425 msec).

continues

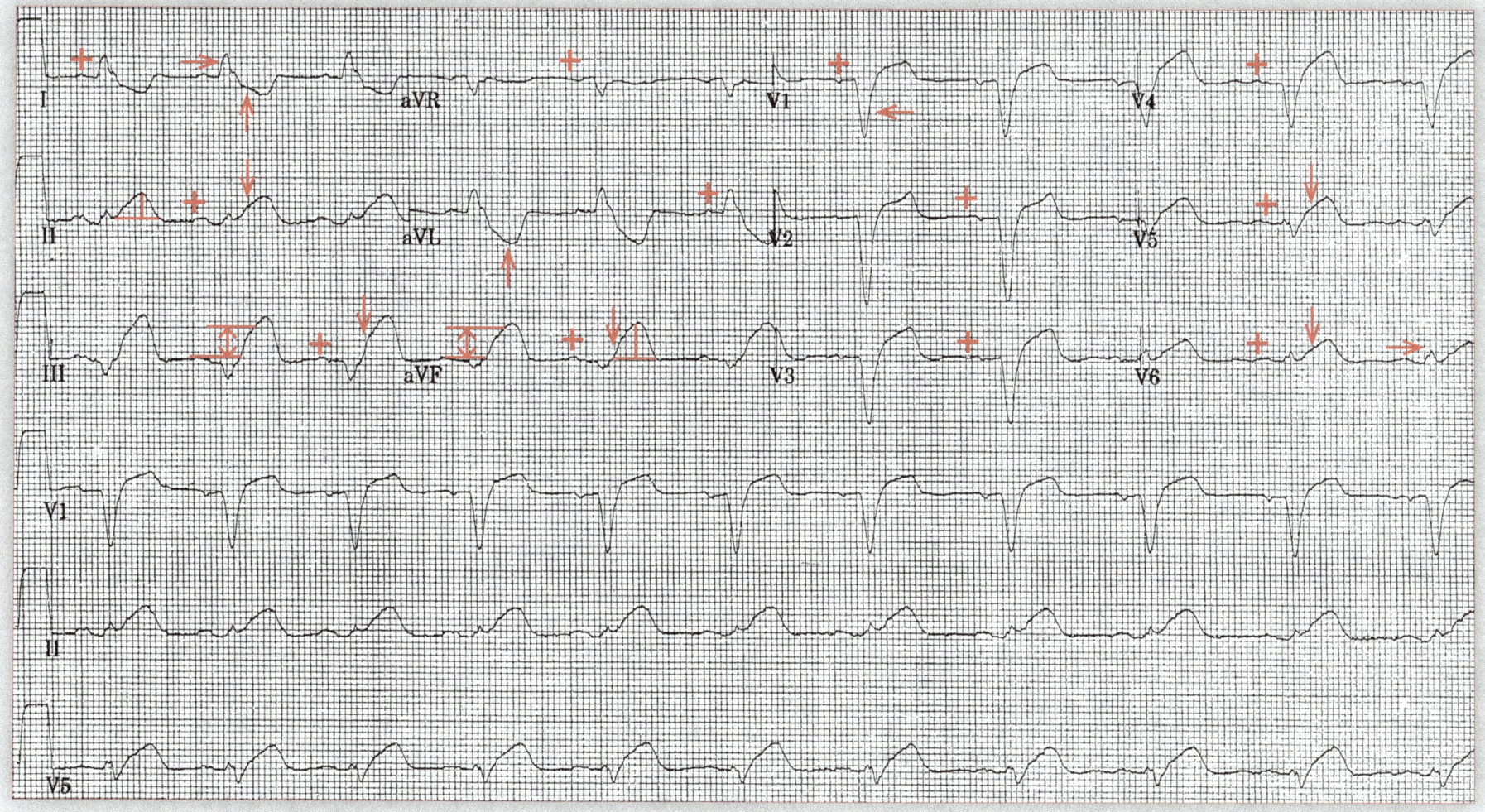

ECG 47B Analysis: Normal sinus rhythm, left bundle branch block, acute inferior wall and anterolateral wall myocardial infarction

In **ECG 47B** the rhythm is regular at a rate of 72 bpm. There is a P wave before each QRS complex (+) with a stable PR interval (0.18 sec). The P wave is positive in leads I, II, aVF, and V4-V6; hence this is a normal sinus rhythm. The QRS complex duration is increased (0.14 sec), and it has an LBBB morphology, with a broad R wave in leads I (→) and V6 and a deep QS complex in lead V1 (←). However, there is now significant ST-segment elevation (↓) in leads II, III, aVF, and V5-V6 that ranges from 2 to 5 mm (↕) as well as ST-segment depression in leads I and aVL (↑). These ST-segment depressions are more pronounced than those in the baseline ECG (**ECG 47A**) and are reciprocal changes seen with an inferior wall myocardial infarction (MI). In addition, the T waves in leads II, III, aVF, and V5-V6 are tall, domed, and symmetric. These changes are diagnostic for an acute inferior and anterolateral wall ST-segment elevation MI.

In the presence of an LBBB, left ventricular abnormalities (*eg*, left ventricular hypertrophy, pericarditis, ischemia, chronic MI, and axis) cannot be established reliably since left ventricular activation is no longer through the normal His-Purkinje system but instead is by direct myocardial activation from the right bundle and right ventricular myocardium. However, an acute ST-segment MI can be established based on the Sgarbossa criteria:

1. ST-segment elevation of ≥ 1 to 2 mm that is in the same direction (concordant) as the QRS complex in any lead.

2. ST-segment depression of ≥ 1 mm in any lead from V1 to V3

3. ST-segment elevation of ≥ 5 mm that is discordant with the QRS complex (*ie*, associated with a QS or rS complex)

Although the Sgarbossa criteria have been reported in patients with an LBBB, the same criteria have been found to be useful with a paced QRS complex and are likely also useful whenever there is direct myocardial activation, which would also include a ventricular complex and a Wolff-Parkinson-White pattern.

Even though this patient has an underlying LBBB, there are ECG changes that are diagnostic for an acute inferior wall ST-segment elevation MI, including the hyperacute T waves and the significant ST-segment elevation with reciprocal ST-segment depression. Important therapy would be prompt reperfusion either in the catheterization laboratory with percutaneous coronary intervention (stenting) or with a thrombolytic agent. ■

Notes

A 34-year-old man with a history of mild hypertension, well controlled on hydrochlorothiazide, presents to the emergency department with signs and symptoms of acute bronchitis. He has a productive cough and low-grade temperature and also notes pleuritic chest pain. A chest X-ray and white blood cell count are normal. An ECG is obtained, and the emergency department physician has some concerns about what it shows.

What is the abnormality?

Is it of any concern?

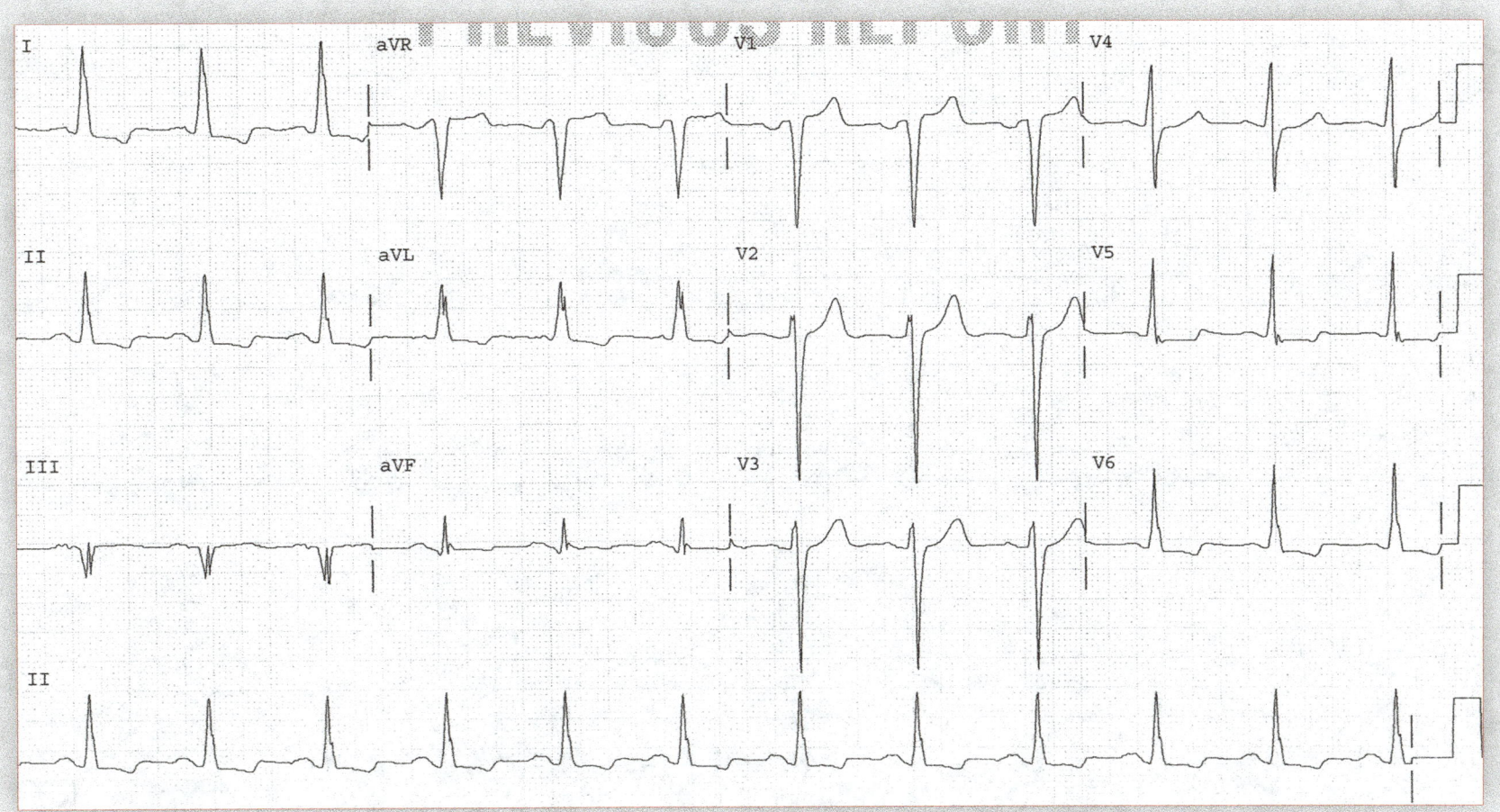

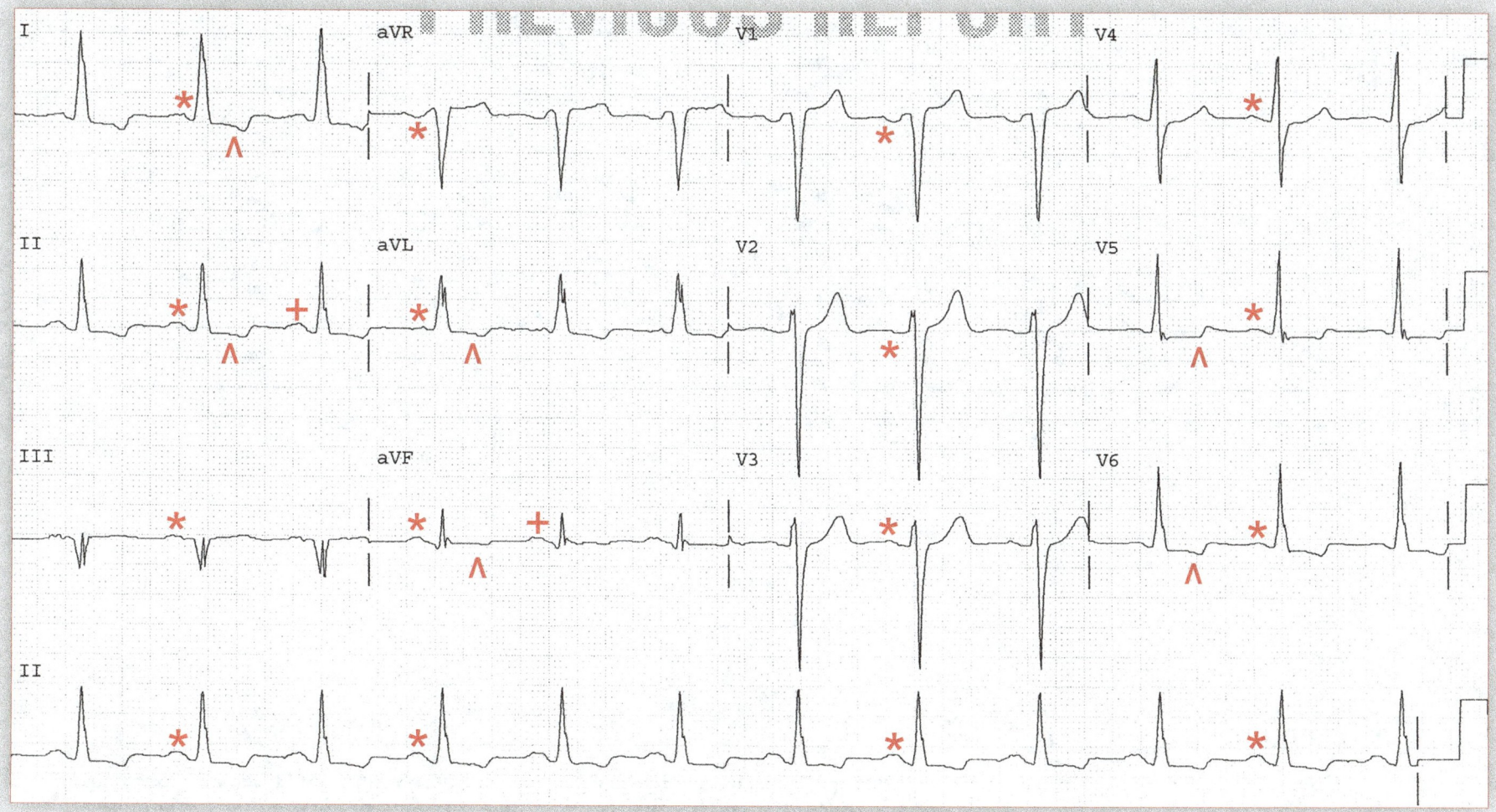

ECG 48 Analysis: **Normal sinus rhythm, left atrial hypertrophy (abnormality), nonspecific ST-T wave changes, intraventricular conduction delay (incomplete left bundle branch block)**

There is a regular rhythm at a rate of 72 bpm. There is a P wave (*) before each QRS complex with a stable PR interval (0.20 sec). The P wave is positive in leads I, II, aVF, and V4-V6. Hence this is a normal sinus rhythm. The P waves are broad (0.16 sec) in leads II and aVF (+) and negative in lead V1. These changes are consistent with left atrial hypertrophy (abnormality). The QRS complex duration is increased (0.11 sec) and there is a normal axis, between 0° and +90° (positive QRS complex in leads I and aVF). The QRS complex morphology is normal. There are nonspecific ST-T wave changes noted in leads I, II, aVL, and V5-V6 (^). The QT/QTc intervals are slightly prolonged (430/470 msec) but are normal when the prolonged QRS complex duration is considered (400/440 msec).

The major finding is the slightly prolonged QRS complex duration. Although it has a morphology resembling a left bundle branch block (LBBB; R wave in lead I and QS complex in lead V1), it is not wide enough for a true or complete LBBB. Therefore, this has been termed an incomplete LBBB. However, this is a misnomer since conduction through the bundles is all or none and not incomplete. The slight widening of the QRS complex is actually an intraventricular conduction delay to the left ventricle. Although this seems like only semantics, it is clinically important. An LBBB (complete or incomplete) means that the activation of the left ventricle bypasses (or partially bypasses) the normal His-Purkinje system. Thus activation of the left ventricle is not via the normal Purkinje system but directly through the ventricular myocardium. Therefore, abnormalities that affect the left ventricle (*eg*, ischemia, myocardial infarction, pericarditis, left ventricular hypertrophy) cannot be diagnosed. The presence of an intraventricular conduction delay means that impulse conduction still occurs through the normal conduction system, but there is diffuse slowing of conduction through the Purkinje network and ventricular myocardium. As the normal conduction system is used, abnormalities that affect the left ventricle can still be diagnosed.

As there is no major abnormality on the ECG, there is no reason for any concern and no need for any additional evaluation aside from making certain that blood pressure is well controlled. ■

Notes

A 40-year-old woman who recently emigrated from Brazil presents to a primary care physician as a new patient. On review, she states that she has become progressively limited in her activity over the past several months because of shortness of breath. She denies chest discomfort, orthopnea, or changes in weight. On exam, her heart rate is 62 bpm and blood pressure is 110/70 mm Hg. Her head, ears, eyes, nose, and throat exam is normal. Her jugular venous pressure is 12 cm H_2O with Kussmaul's sign. Her lungs are clear. Her precordium is notable for a diffuse point of maximal impulse. Heart sounds are regular, and an S3 gallop is evident. Her abdomen manifests a fluid wave. The remainder of her exam is normal. An ECG is obtained.

What abnormalities are evident?

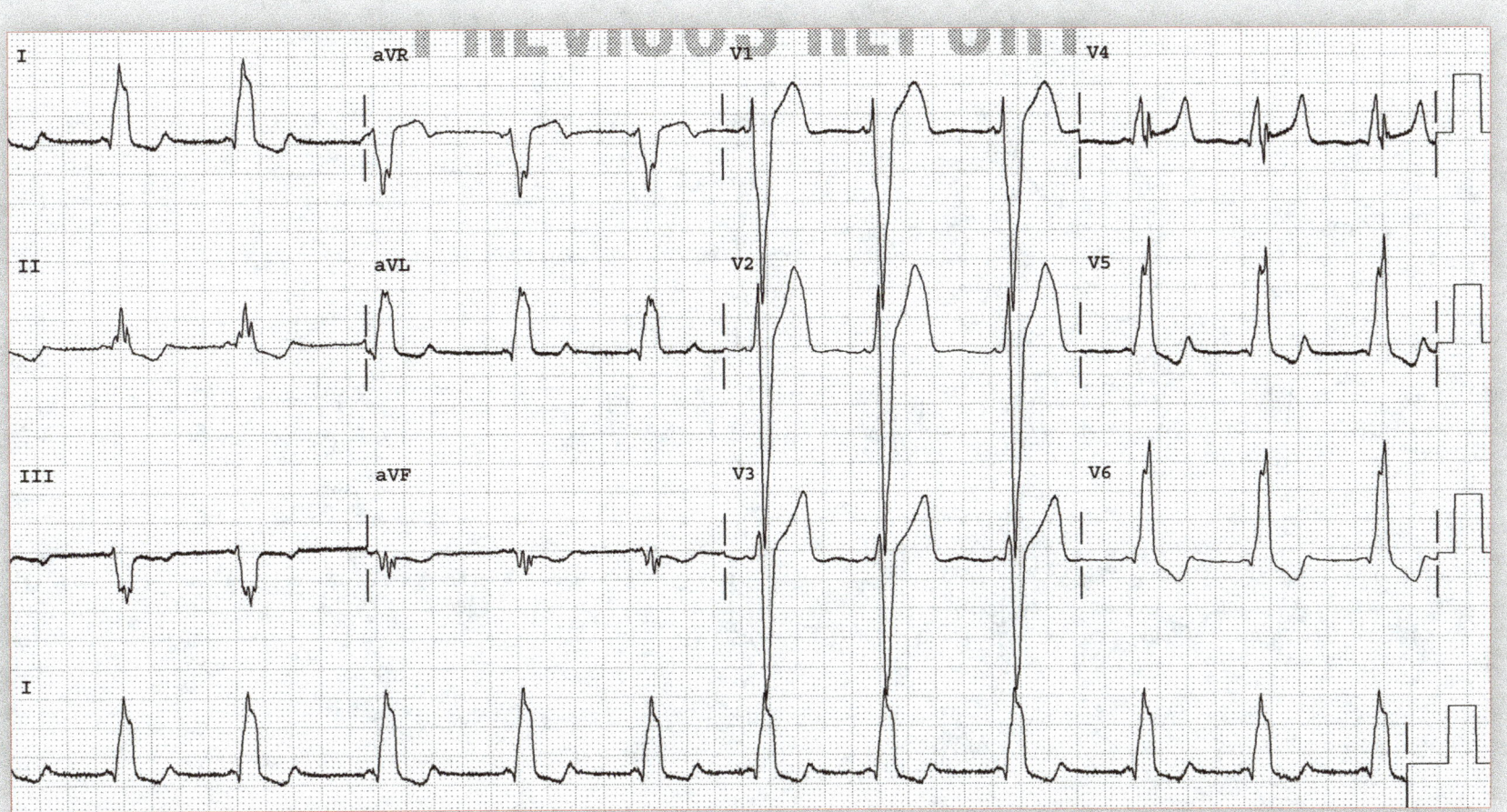

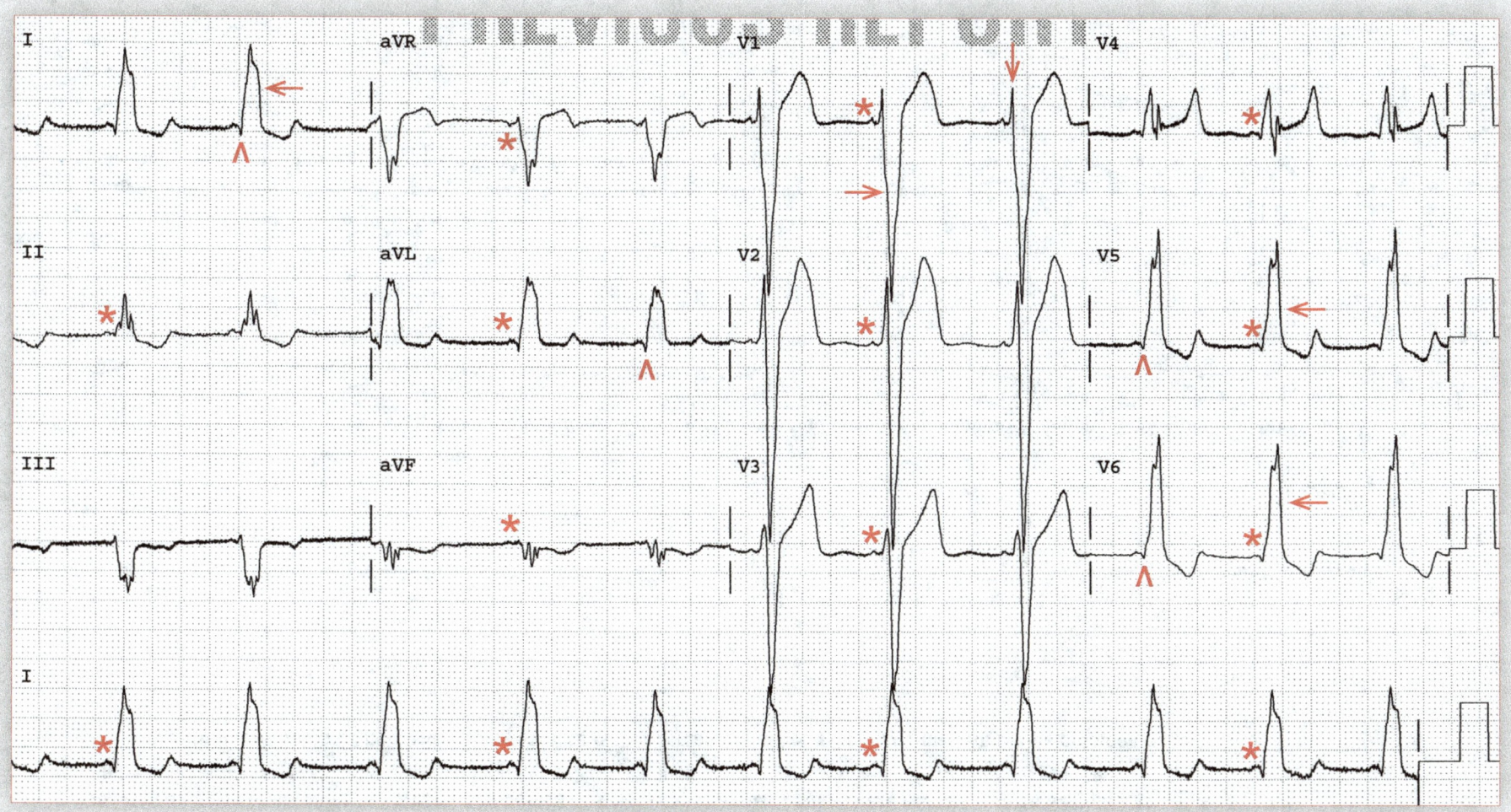

ECG 49 Analysis: Normal sinus rhythm, intraventricular conduction delay

There is a regular rhythm at a rate of 62 bpm. There is a P wave (*) before each QRS complex with a stable, short PR interval (0.12 sec). The QRS complex is wide (0.18 sec). Although the morphology looks like that of a left bundle branch block (broad R wave in leads I and V5-V6 [←] and deep S wave in lead V1 [→]), there are small septal Q waves (^) in leads I, aVL, and V5-V6 and a prominent septal R wave in lead V1 (↓). Septal Q waves cannot be present in a left bundle branch block, as septal activation is via the septal branch (median fascicle) from the left bundle. Hence the wide QRS complex is actually due to an intraventicular conduction delay. The QT/QTc intervals are prolonged (460/470 msec) but are normal when corrected for the wide QRS complex duration (360/370 msec).

With a left bundle branch block, activation of the left ventricle is not via the normal His-Purkinje system but rather is by direct myocardial activation. In contrast, the presence of an intraventricular conduction delay indicates that left ventricular activation is occurring via the normal conduction system but is diffusely slowed. Since the impulse travels along the normal His-Purkinje system, abnormalities that affect the left ventricle (*eg*, axis shift, acute and chronic myocardial infarction, ischemia, left ventricular hypertrophy, pericarditis) can be identified. Commonly a QRS complex that is this wide is the result of an underlying cardiomyopathy and is due to diffuse myocardial fibrosis and therefore marked slowing of impulse conduction. There is in fact a correlation between the left ventricular ejection fraction and the QRS complex duration with an intraventricular conduction delay. ■

Core Case 50

A 68-year-old woman presents to her physician with complaints of progressive shortness of breath. She is known to have nonischemic dilated cardiomyopathy with a left ventricular ejection fraction of 40%, but she has never had heart failure. Physical exam demonstrates an S3, a murmur of mitral regurgitation, and bibasilar rales. Her heart rate is 120 bpm, and an ECG demonstrates sinus

ECG 50A

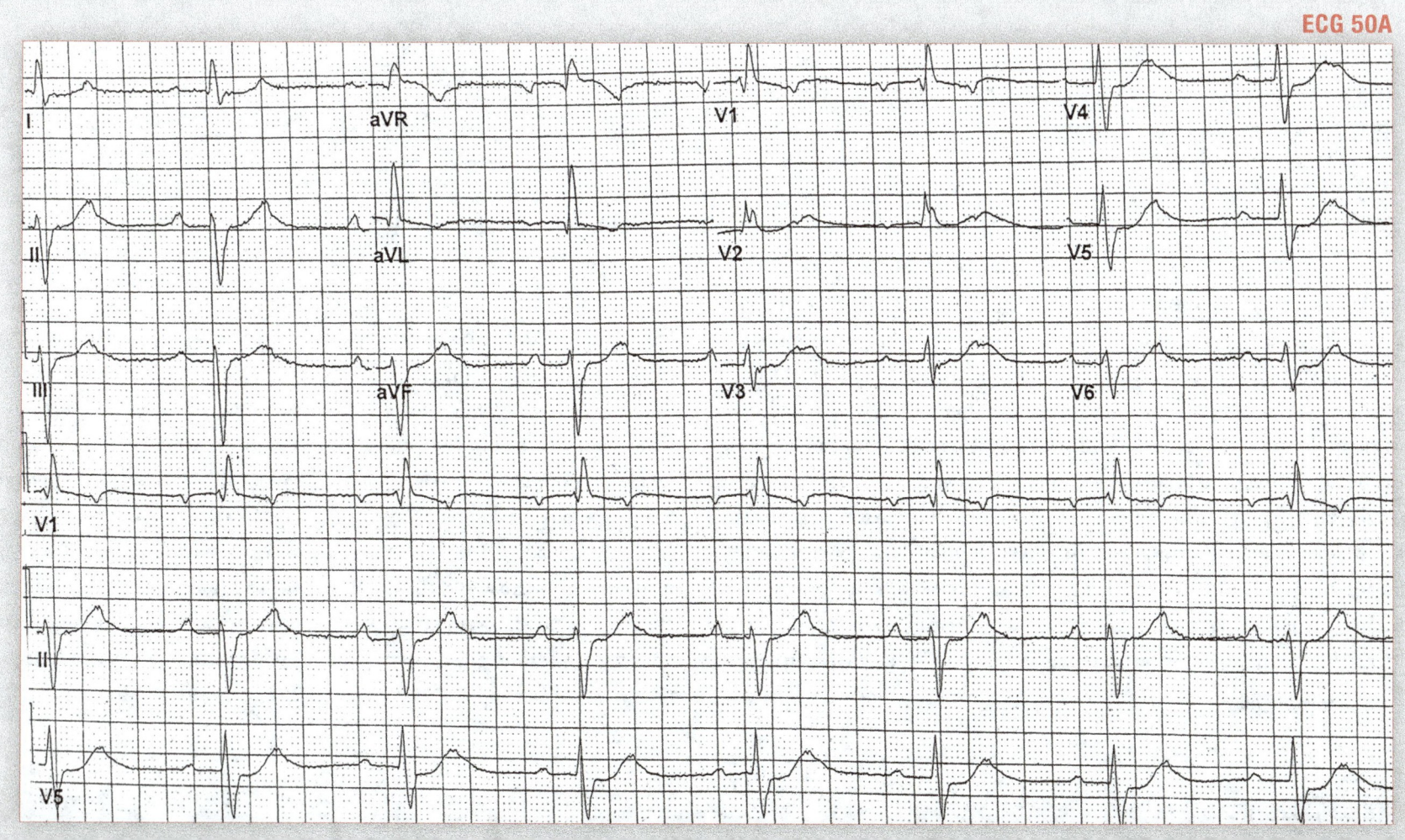

tachycardia. She is admitted to the hospital and treated with intravenous diuretics as well as an angiotensin-converting enzyme inhibitor. She responds well, and by the third hospital day she feels back to her baseline. A routine ECG is obtained (ECG 50A) prior to the institution of a β-blocker. Her physician is concerned about the ECG and later in the day orders another (ECG 50B).

Why is there a concern about the initial ECG?

What is the nature of the abnormality?

Could therapy with a β-blocker be safely instituted?

ECG 50B

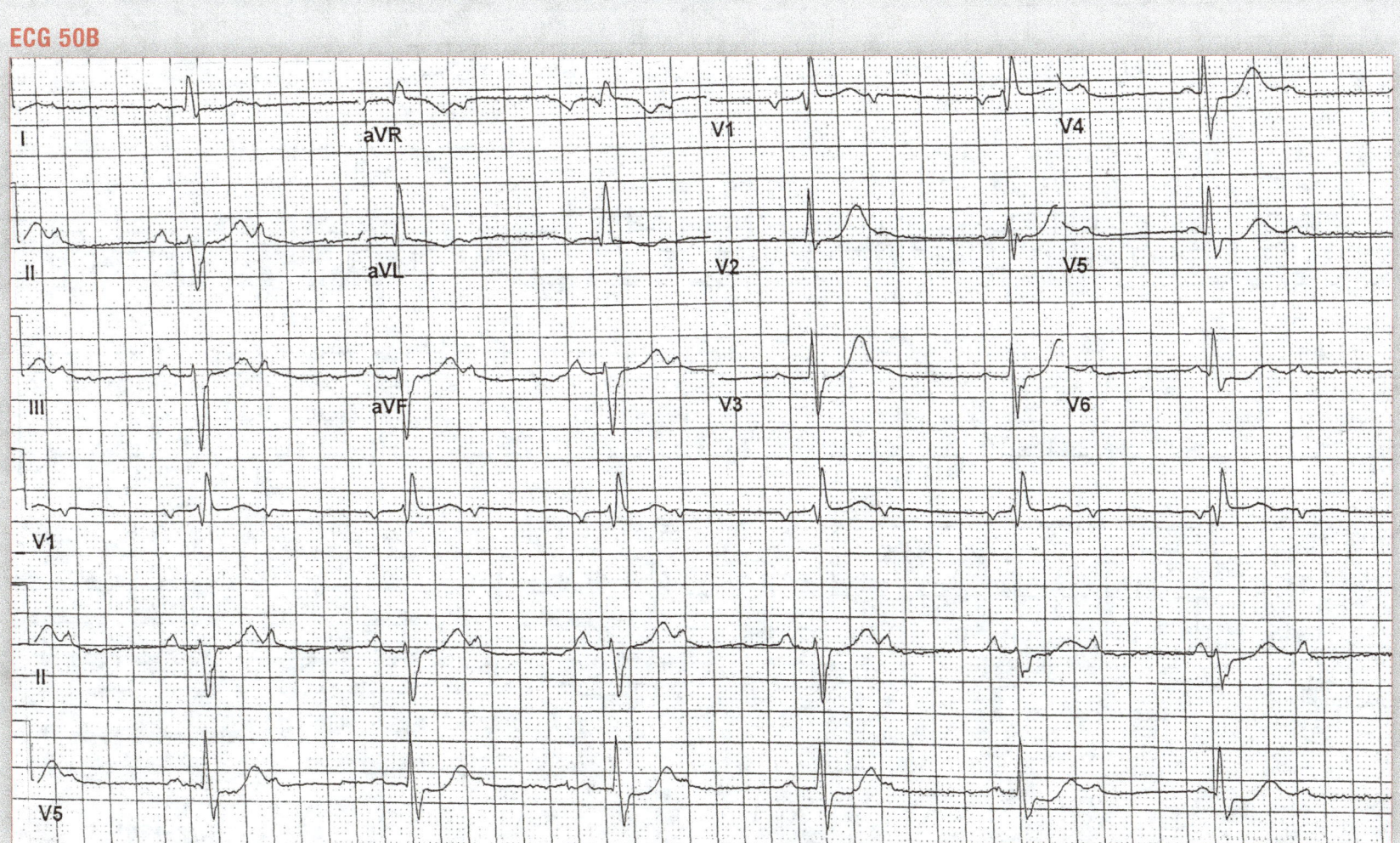

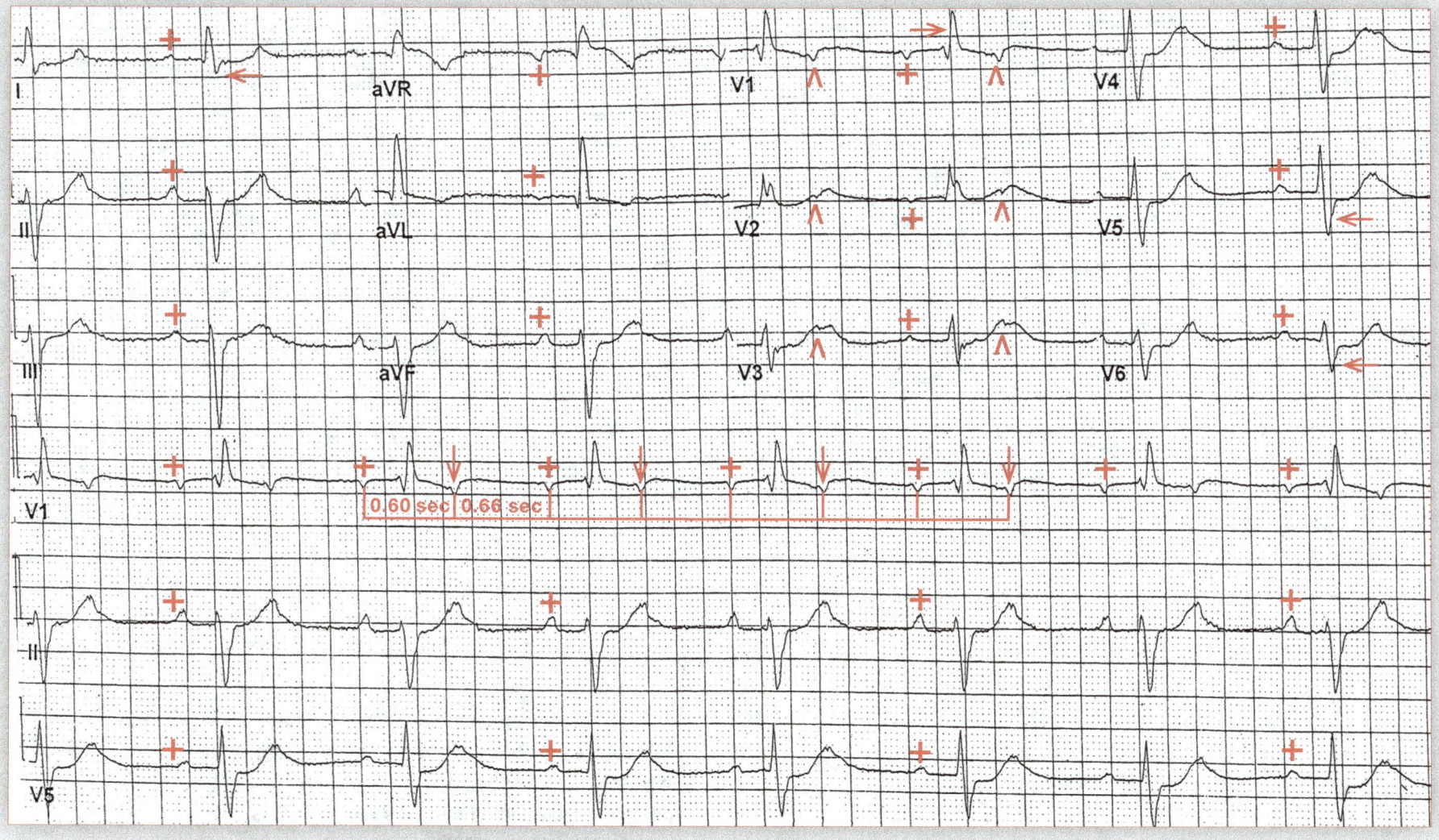

ECG 50A Analysis: Normal sinus rhythm, first-degree AV block (prolonged AV conduction), second-degree AV block with 2:1 AV conduction (2:1 AV block), right bundle branch block, left anterior fascicular block, bifascicular block, ventriculophasic arrhythmia

ECG 50A shows a regular rhythm at a rate of 46 bpm. There is a P wave (+) before each QRS complex with a stable PR interval (0.32 sec). A second P wave (↓) can be seen after each QRS complex. In some leads (V2-V3) the P wave is superimposed on the upstroke of the T wave (^), causing a notching of this waveform. The PP interval is slightly irregular (⊔), and the average atrial rate is 92 bpm. It can be seen that the PP interval surrounding the QRS complex is slightly shorter (0.60 sec) than the PP interval without a QRS complex (0.66 sec). This is termed ventriculophasic arrhythmia and is due to acute acceleration of sinus node activity with ventricular contraction. This may be seen with either 2:1 AV block or complete (third-degree) AV block. Proposed mechanisms include acceleration of sinus node automaticity due to augmentation of pulsatile blood flow through the sinus node artery, stretch of the right atrium resulting from ventricular contraction, or changes in autonomic tone due to changes in baroreceptor activity resulting from a stroke volume.

The P waves are positive in leads I, II, aVF, and V4-V6. Hence there is a normal sinus rhythm with first-degree AV block (prolonged AV conduction) and second-degree AV block with 2:1 conduction (2:1 AV block). The QRS complex duration is increased (0.16 sec), and it has a morphology of a typical right bundle branch block (RSR′ complex in lead V1 [→] and a broad terminal S wave in leads I and V5-V6 [←]). The axis is very leftward, between −30° and −90° (positive QRS complex in lead I and negative QRS complex in leads II and aVF, with an rS morphology). As the QRS complex has an rS morphology, this is a left anterior fascicular block. The QT/QTc intervals are slightly prolonged (520/455 msec) but are normal when the prolonged QRS complex duration is considered (440/385 msec).

Therefore, there is bifascicular disease (right bundle branch block and left anterior fascicular block) as well as first-degree AV block (prolonged AV conduction). Although this might be considered to represent trifascicular disease, this diagnosis cannot be established by this ECG as the first-degree AV block may be the result of either AV nodal disease (which would not be trifascicular disease) or disease of the remaining fascicle (which would represent trifascicular disease). Even though there is also second-degree AV block present with a pattern of 2:1 conduction, this may be either Mobitz type I or Mobitz type II. If the 2:1 AV block is Mobitz type II, then trifascicular disease can be diagnosed. If the 2:1 AV block is Mobitz type I, which is an AV nodal abnormality, then this would be bifascicular disease as well as AV nodal disease. The etiology of the 2:1 AV block can only be established if there was a change in the pattern of AV nodal conduction. Thus, if there were several sequential P waves that were conducted with a stable PR interval, then the diagnosis would be Mobitz type II. If the P waves were conducted with a progressive increase in the PR interval, the diagnosis would be Mobitz type I. If complete heart block were to develop, the etiology of the escape rhythm would also establish the etiology of the 2:1 AV block. That is, if there was a junctional escape rhythm the etiology would be Mobitz type I, while an escape ventricular rhythm would establish Mobitz type II as the etiology.

continues

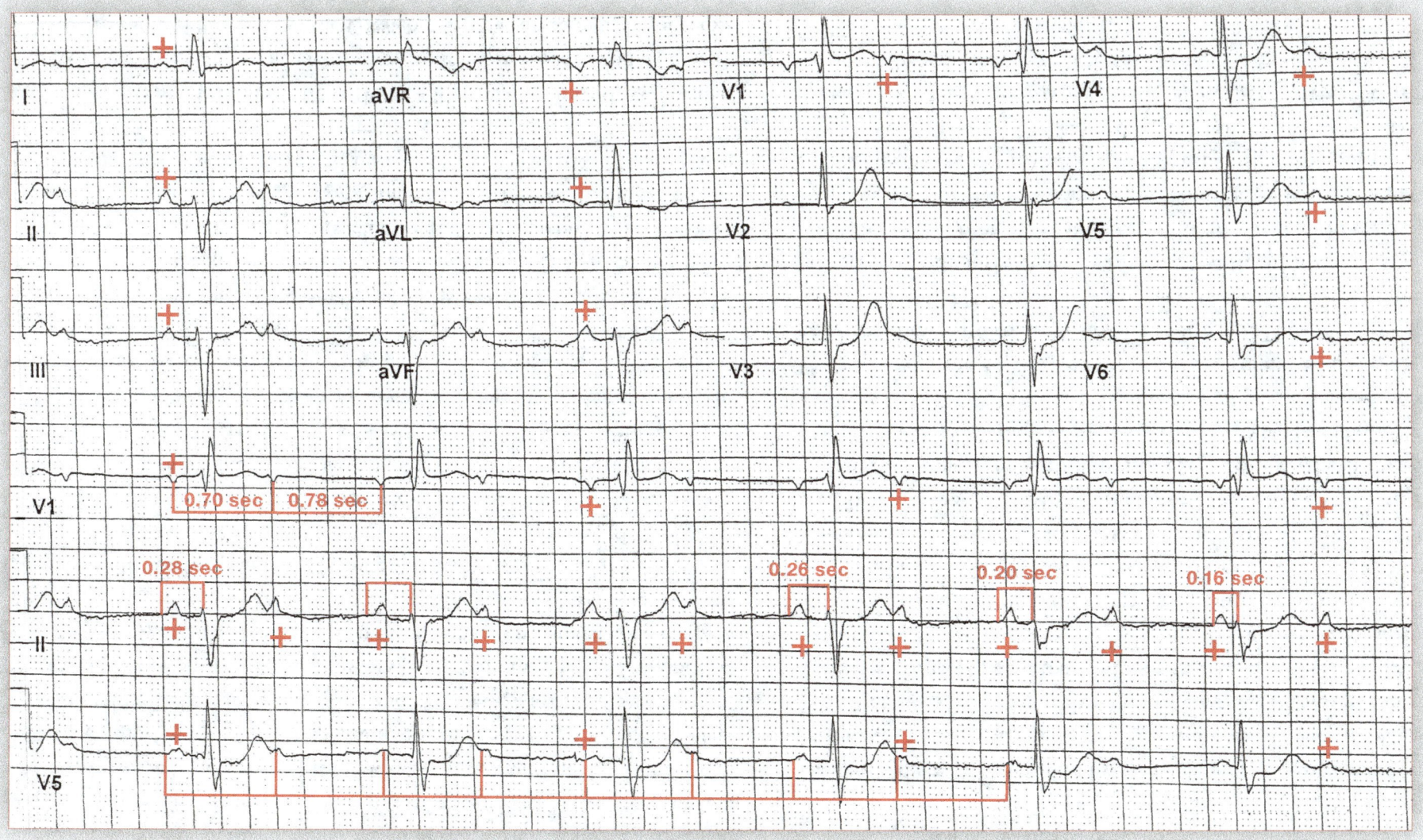

ECG 50B Analysis: Normal sinus rhythm, complete heart block, escape junctional rhythm, right bundle branch block, left anterior fascicular block, bifascicular block, ventriculophasic arrhythmia

In **ECG 50B**, there is a regular rhythm at a rate of 42 bpm. The QRS complex duration, morphology, and axis are identical to what was seen in **ECG 50A** (*ie*, right bundle branch block and left anterior fascicular block). The QT/QTc intervals are the same. P waves are seen (+), and the PP interval is fairly constant (⊔) with an average atrial rate of 84 bpm. As with **ECG 50A**, ventriculophasic arrhythmia is present and the PP interval surrounding the QRS complex (0.70 sec) is slightly shorter than the PP interval without an intervening QRS complex (0.78 sec) (⊔). However, the PR intervals are variable (⊓), particularly evident at the end of the ECG, indicating AV dissociation. As the atrial rate is faster than the ventricular rate, this is complete or third-degree AV block. The QRS complexes are identical to those seen in **ECG 50A**, so the escape rhythm is junctional. Therefore, the 2:1 AV block seen on **ECG 50A** is a result of Mobitz type I. The conduction abnormalities are not the result of trifascicular disease but rather are due to bifascicular disease with associated AV nodal abnormality. As the complete heart block is a result of failure of AV nodal conduction, a β-blocker should not be administered as this could exacerbate the presence of complete heart block and might depress an escape junctional focus, resulting in a slowing of the junctional rate. ◼

Core Case 51

A 36-year-old man with a family history of sudden death and dilated cardiomyopathy presents to the emergency department following 2 days of extreme fatigue and lightheadedness. On initial

ECG 51A

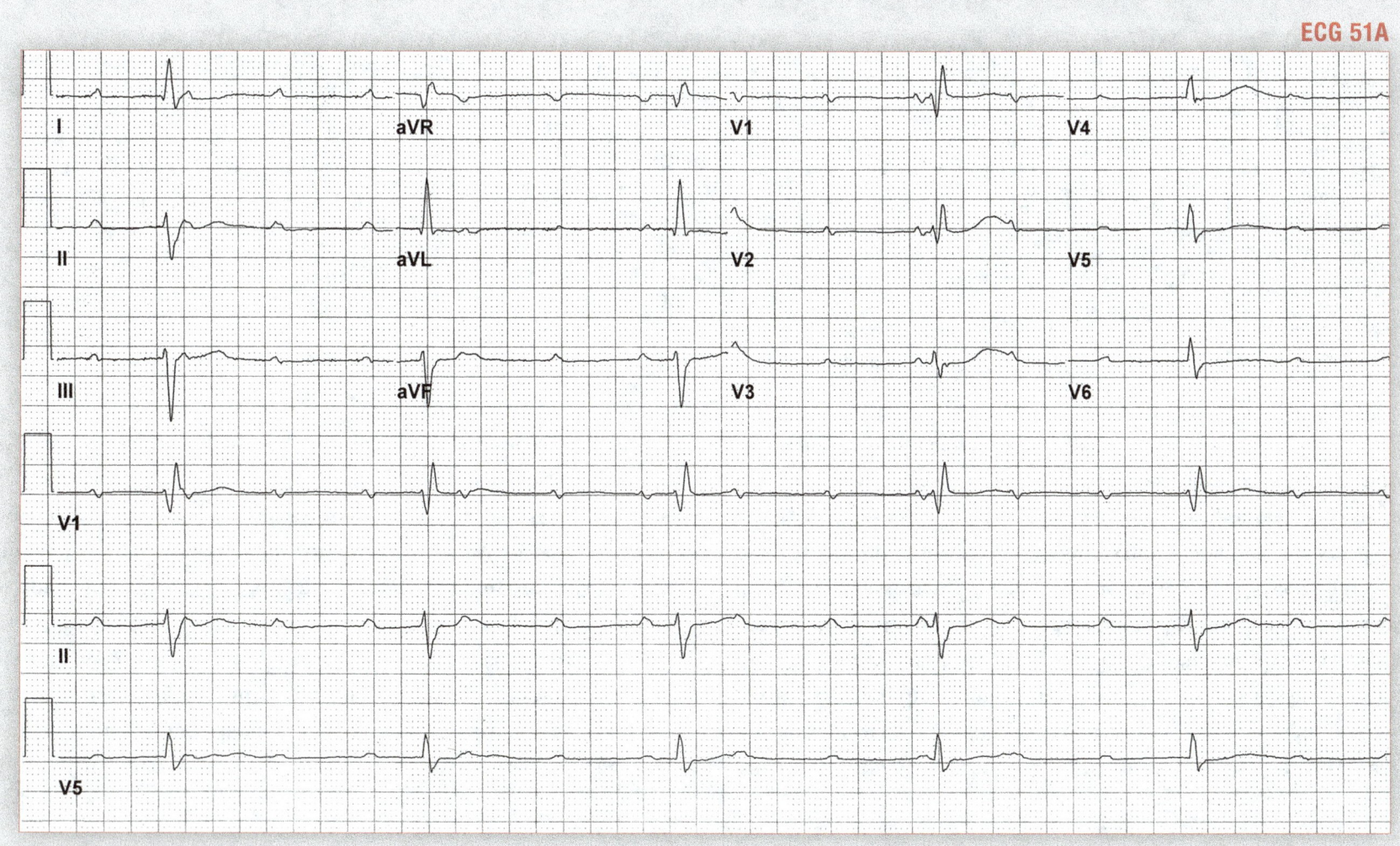

triage, his heart rate is 30 bpm with a blood
pressure of 90/60 mm Hg. An ECG (51A) is obtained.
The patient is admitted to the critical care unit
where a second ECG (51B) is obtained.

What abnormalities are shown?

What is the management?

ECG 51B

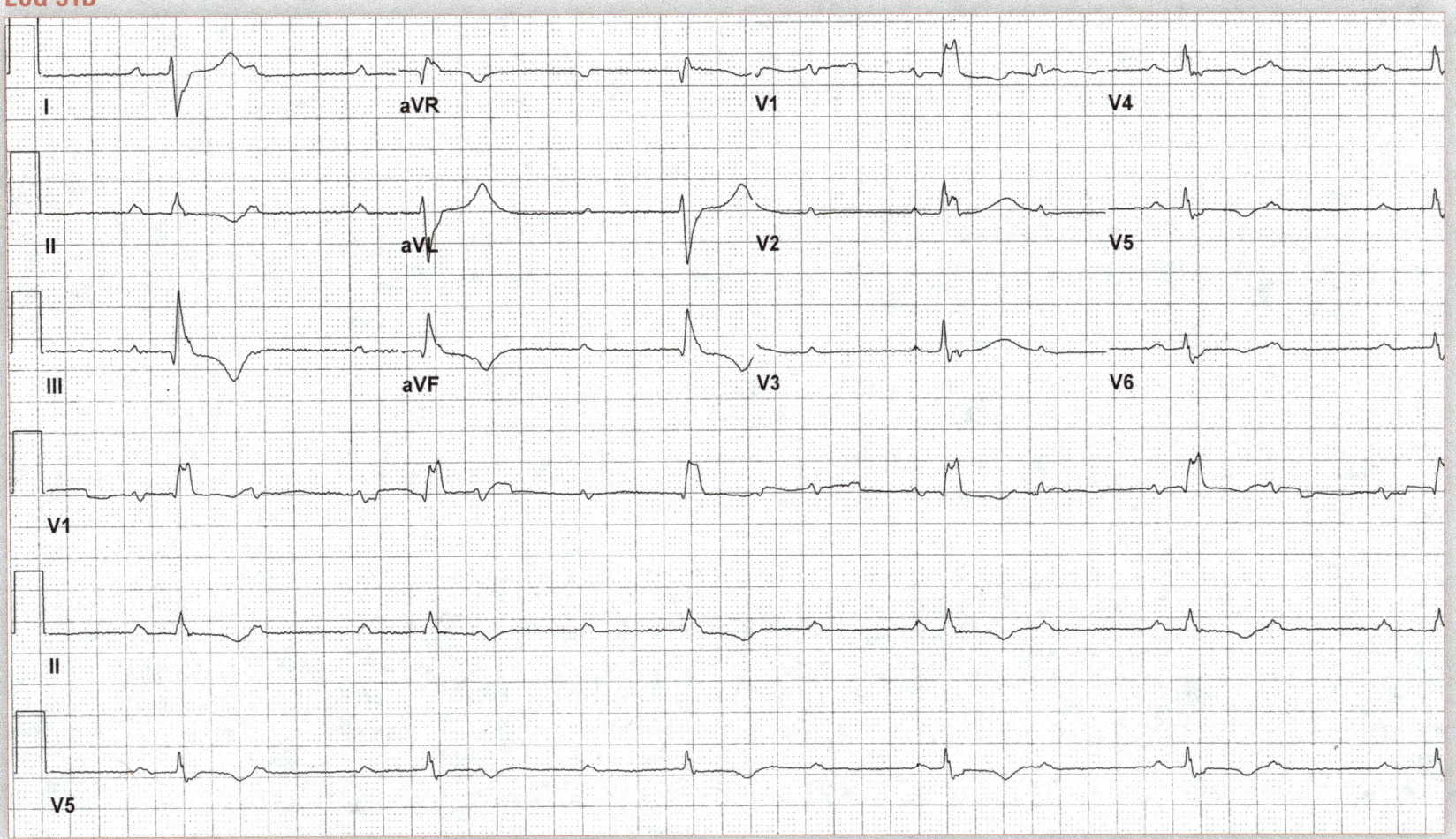

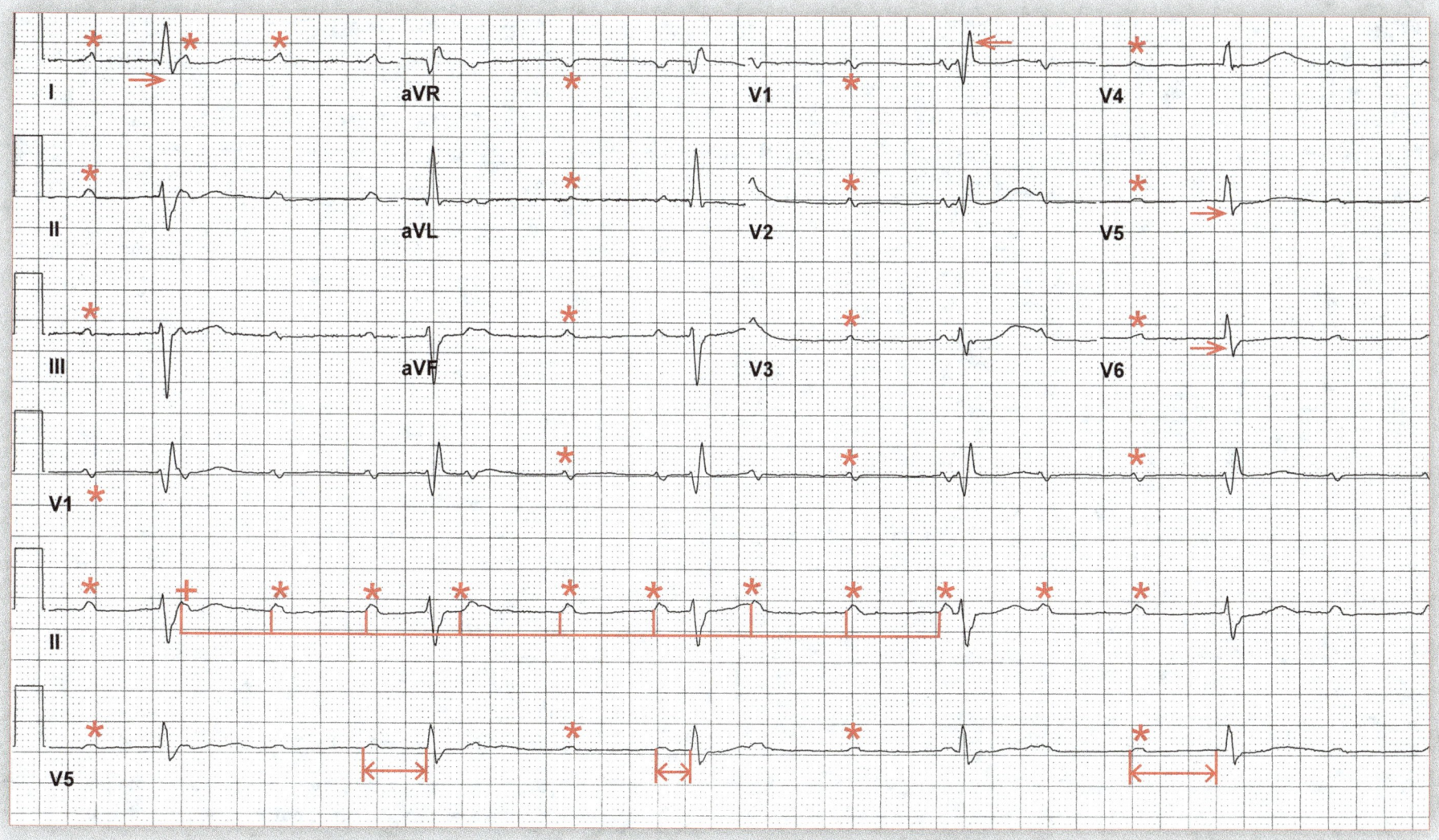

ECG 51A Analysis: Normal sinus rhythm, complete heart block, escape junctional rhythm with right bundle branch block (RBBB) and left anterior fascicular block (LAFB), bifascicular block

ECG 51A shows regular RR intervals at a rate of 30 bpm. There are P waves (*) seen, and they have a stable PP interval (⊔) at a rate of 90 bpm. Some of the P waves are not apparent (+) as they are either on T waves or superimposed on the QRS complexes. However, the PP intervals of the obvious P waves are regular (⊔). The P waves are positive in leads I, II, aVF, and V4-V6. Hence this is a normal sinus rhythm. The PR intervals (↔) are variable, indicating AV dissociation. The atrial rate is faster than the ventricular rate, and hence this is complete heart block. The QRS complexes are wide (0.16 sec) with a pattern of right bundle branch block (RBBB; RSR' morphology in lead V1 [←] and S wave in leads I and V5-V6 [→]). The axis is extremely leftward, between −30° and −90° (positive QRS complex in lead I and negative QRS complex in leads II and aVF, with an rS morphology), indicating a left anterior fascicular block (LAFB). Hence the escape rhythm is junctional with an RBBB and LAFB. The QT/QTc intervals are prolonged (560/400 msec) but are normal (480/340 msec) when adjusted for the increased QRS complex duration.

continues

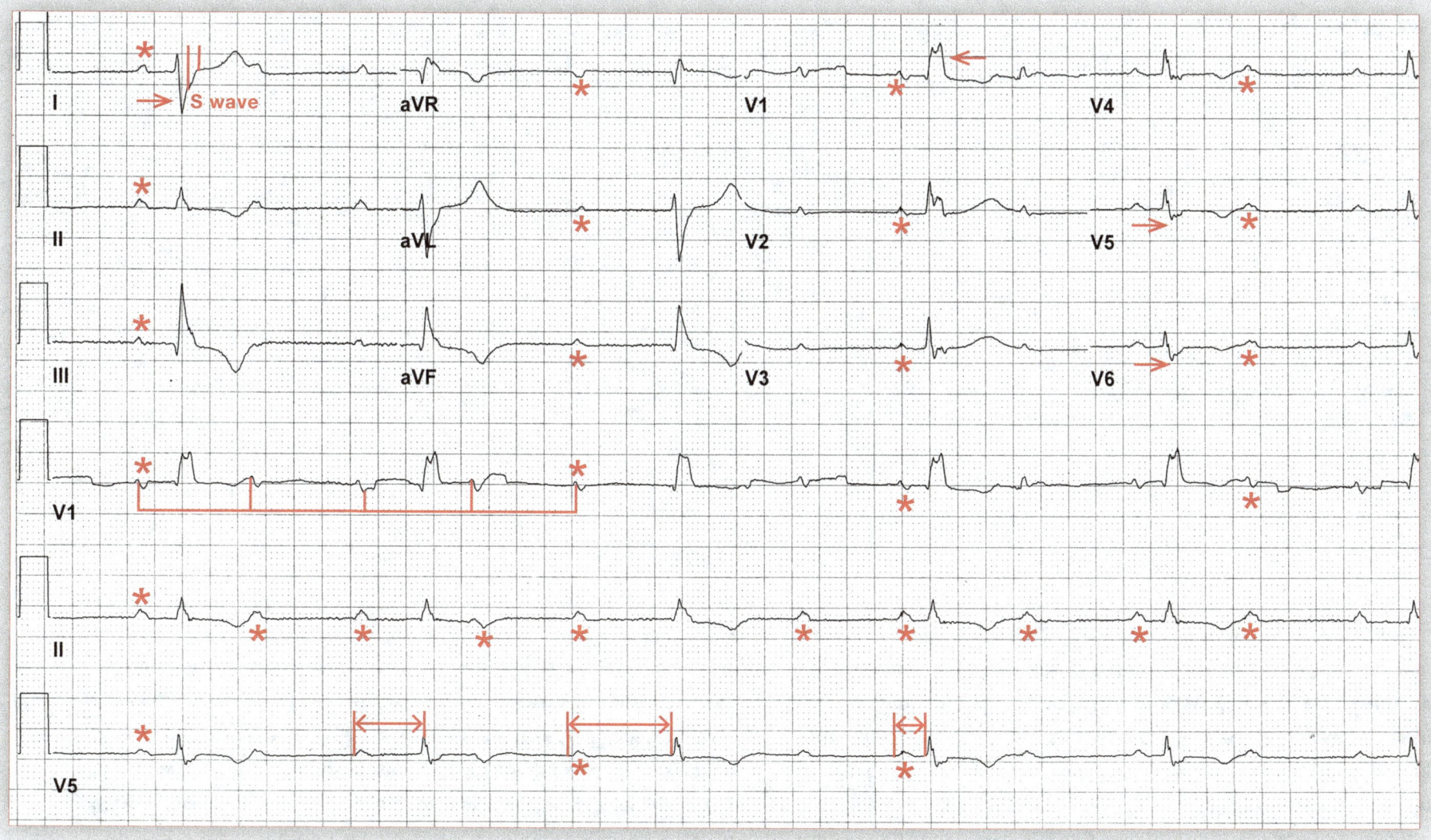

ECG 51B Analysis: Normal sinus rhythm, complete heart block, escape junctional rhythm with RBBB and left posterior fascicular block (LPFB), trifascicular block

In ECG 51B, there is a regular rhythm at a ventricular rate of 32 bpm. P waves (*) are seen, and they have a stable PP interval (⊔) at an atrial rate of 78 bpm. The PR interval (↔) is not constant, and hence there is AV dissociation as a result of complete heart block (the atrial rate is faster than the ventricular rate). The QRS complexes are wide (0.16 sec), similar to those in ECG 51A, with an RBBB pattern (RR′ morphology in lead V1 [←] and an S wave in leads I and V5-V6 [→]). The axis is rightward, between +90° and +180°. The QRS complex is negative in lead I (with an rS morphology), even when accounting for the terminal S wave caused by the RBBB, and positive in lead aVF. This is indicative of a left posterior fascicular block (LPFB). Hence the escape rhythm is junctional with an RBBB and LPFB. The QT/QTc intervals are the same as those seen in ECG 51A.

When compared with ECG 51A, the RBBB is still present in ECG 51B, with the same QRS complex duration and same QT/QTc intervals. However, there is also evidence of conduction disease involving both the left anterior and left posterior fascicles, as indicated by the axis change of the QRS complexes in the two ECGs (extreme left to right). Although the complete heart block is the result of block within the AV node (as the escape rhythm is junctional), there is also trifascicular disease present, as indicated by the RBBB associated with alternating LAFB and LPFB.

The diagnosis of trifascicular disease is made when there is evidence of conduction abnormalities affecting all three fascicles. This might be alternating RBBB and left bundle branch block (LBBB), also known as bi-bundle branch block or, as in this patient, RBBB with alternating LAFB and LPFB.

In this case, the escape junctional rhythm indicates a conduction abnormality of the AV node. However, there is also evidence of severe infra-Hisian disease of the His-Purkinje conduction system (ie, trifascicular disease). Insertion of a permanent pacemaker is indicated. In this patient with familial cardiomyopathy, the decision to place an implantable cardioverter-defibrillator in conjunction with the pacemaker will depend on the left ventricular ejection fraction (LVEF) and New York Heart Association (NYHA) functional class (LVEF < 35% and class II–III heart failure for non-ischemic cardiomyopathy based on current guidelines). In general, a biventricular pacemaker is not indicated when the widened QRS complex is the result of an RBBB. It has been shown that a biventricular pacemaker is effective primarily for patients with an LBBB and not those with an RBBB or an intraventricular conduction delay. However, this patient has complete heart block and will likely be pacemaker dependent. It has been suggested that biventricular pacing should be used in such patients who will, therefore, have continuous right ventricular pacing with an LBBB pattern. ■

Core Case 52

A 55-year-old woman with advanced HIV and related cardiomyopathy is admitted to the hospital with *Pneumocystis* pneumonia. An ECG is obtained (52A) as

ECG 52A

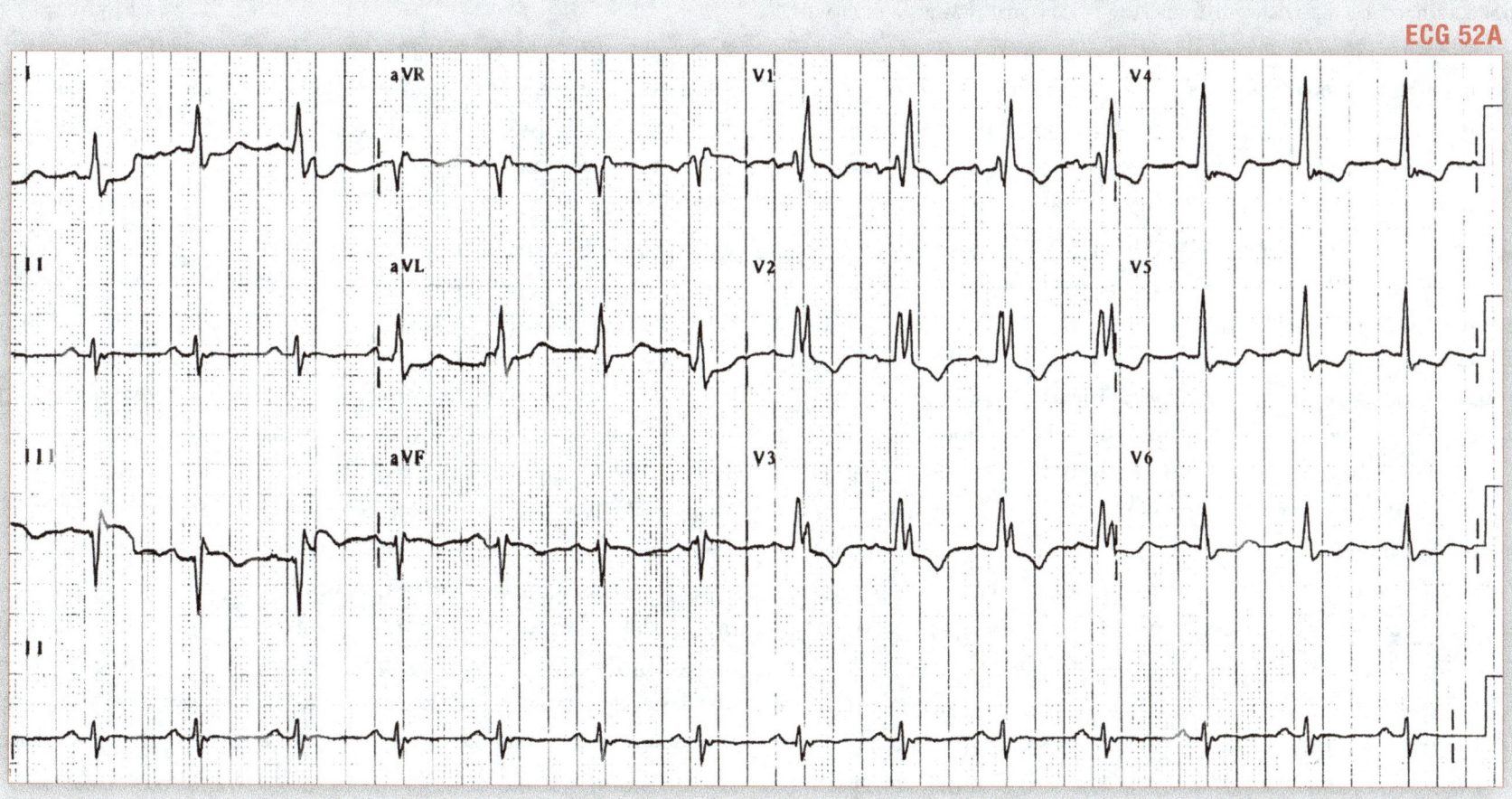

part of her initial evaluation. The following day, the attending physician notes a change in the appearance of her telemetry tracing and obtains a follow-up ECG (52B).

What abnormalities on the ECGs explain the physician's observations?

ECG 52B

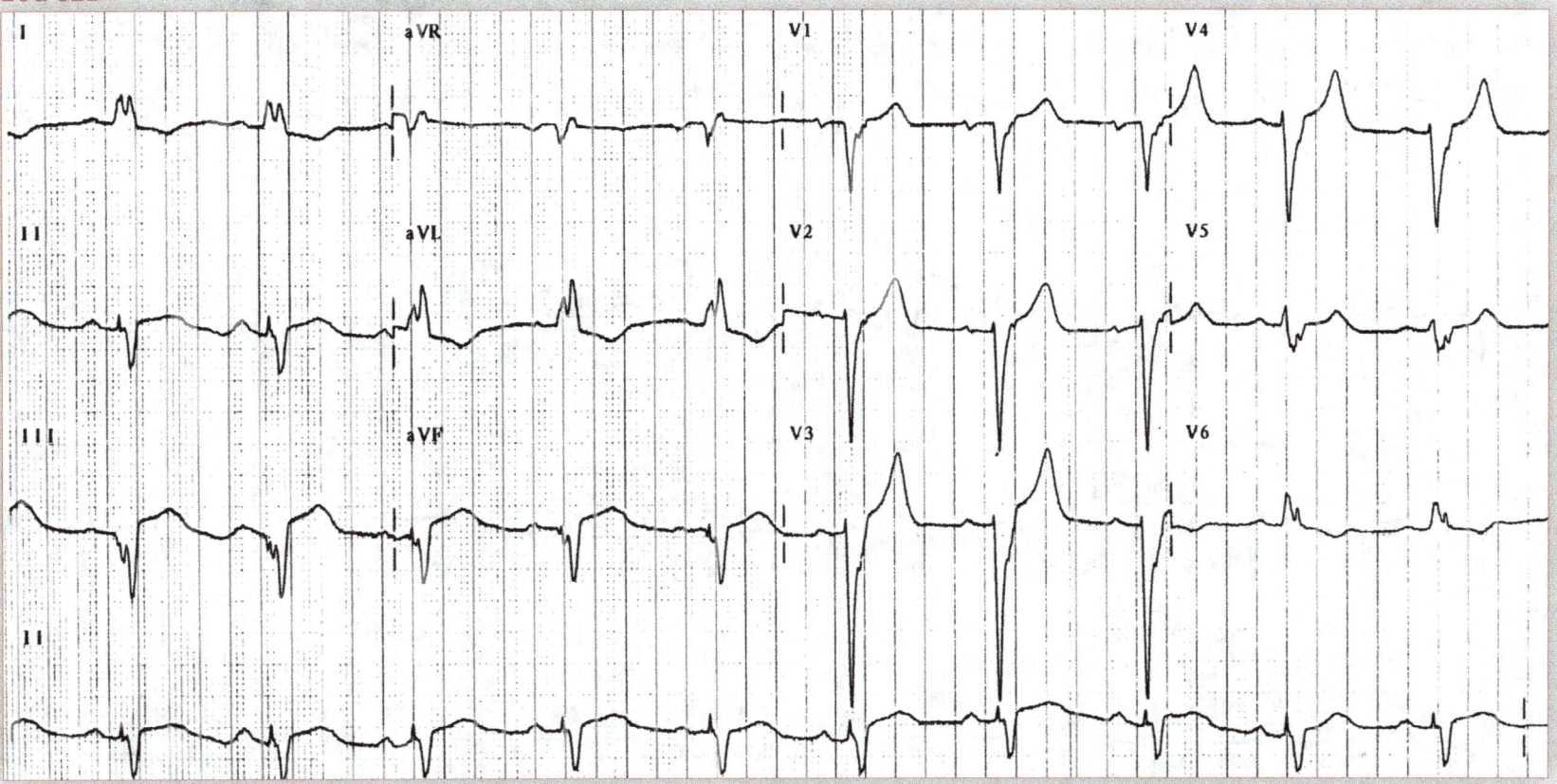

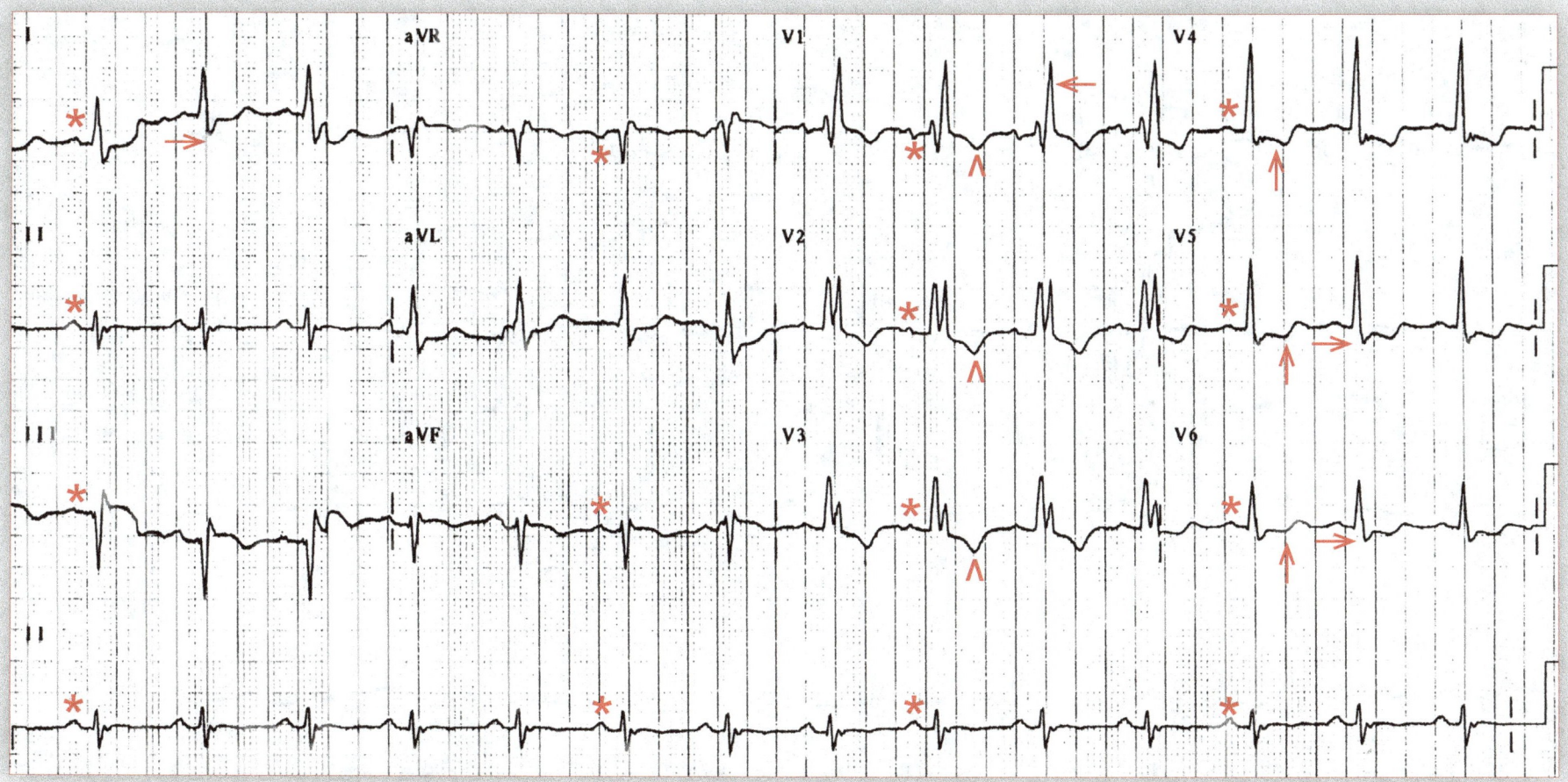

ECG 52A Analysis: Normal sinus rhythm, right bundle
branch block, nonspecific ST-T wave abnormalities

ECG 52A shows a regular rhythm at a rate of 86 bpm. There is a P wave (*) before each QRS complex, and the PR interval is constant (0.20 sec). The P waves are positive in leads I, II, aVF, and V4-V6. Hence this is a normal sinus rhythm. The QRS complex has a prolonged duration (0.16 sec) with a pattern that is typical for a right bundle branch block (RBBB; RSR′ morphology in lead V1 [←] and broad S wave in leads I and V5-V6 [→]). There is a physiologic left axis, between 0° and −30° (positive QRS complex in leads I and II and negative QRS complex in lead aVF). Nonspecific ST-T wave changes noted in leads V1-V3 (^) are associated with the RBBB. The ST-T wave changes seen in leads V4-V6 (↑) are, however, primary and not associated with the RBBB. The QT/QTc intervals are prolonged (420/500 msec) but are normal when the increased QRS complex duration is considered (340/410 msec).

continues

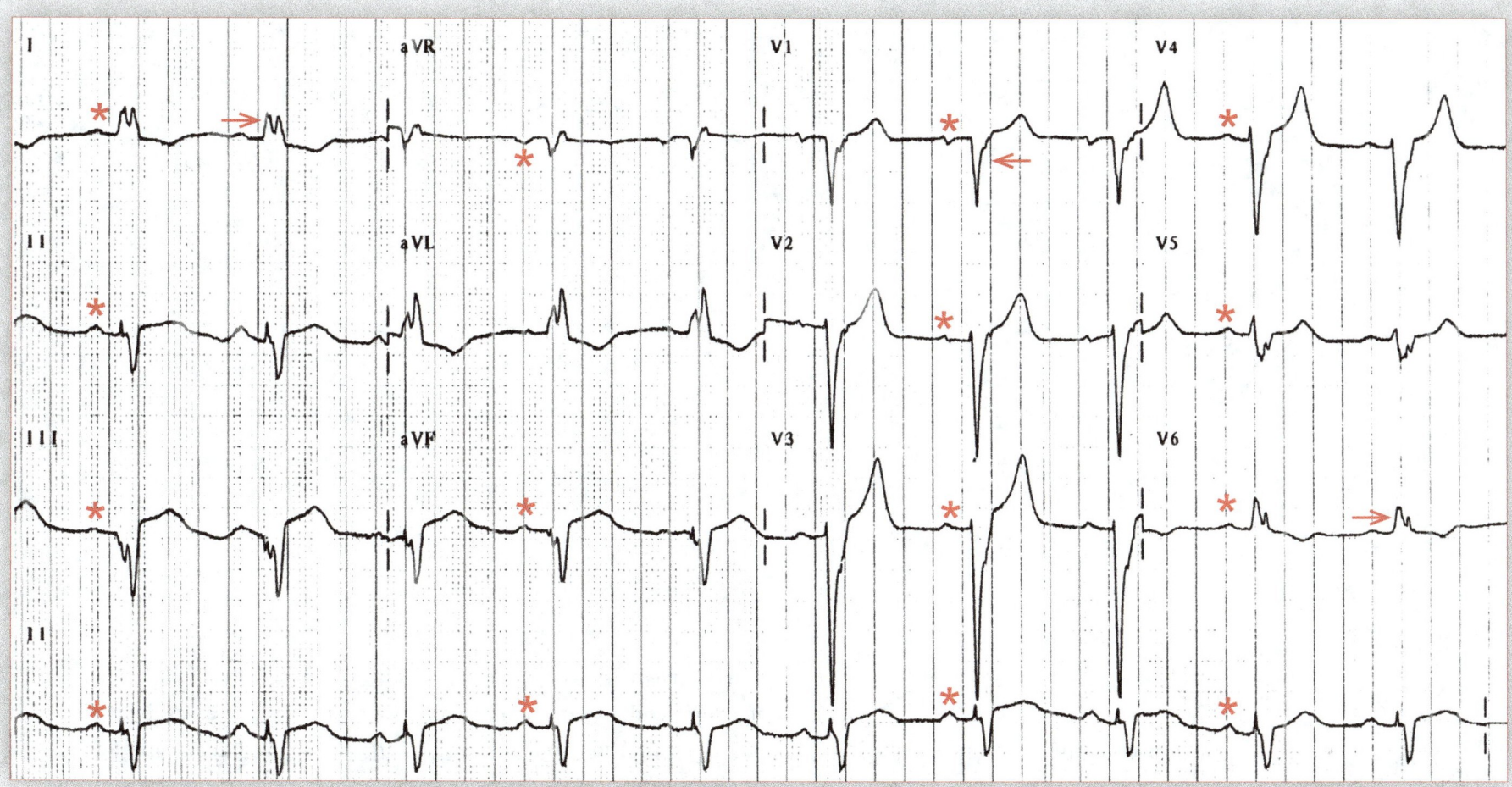

ECG 52B Analysis: Normal sinus rhythm, left bundle branch block, bi-bundle branch block (trifascicular disease)

ECG 52B, obtained the following day, shows a regular rhythm at a rate of 64 bpm. There is a P wave (*) before each QRS complex with a PR interval that is constant (0.20 sec). The P-wave morphology and PR interval are the same as in **ECG 52A.** The QRS complex duration is increased (0.16 sec), and the morphology is that of a left bundle branch block (LBBB; broad R wave in leads I and V6 [→] and QS complex in lead V1 [←]). The axis is now more leftward, between −30° and −90° (positive QRS complex in lead I and negative QRS complex in leads II and aVF). However, this is not a left anterior fascicular block as there is an LBBB present and hence both fascicles are not functional. The axis is due to the direction of left ventricular activation via direct myocardial activation. The QT/QTc intervals are the same as in **ECG 52A.** Hence the patient has evidence of both RBBB and LBBB, indicative of bi-bundle branch block or trifascicular disease.

The presence of both RBBB and LBBB represents high-grade conduction system disease of the His-Purkinje system, which is likely the result of the underlying cardiomyopathy. Although there is a high risk for complete heart block, which would be associated with an escape ventricular rhythm, a pacemaker is not indicated at this time. In the presence of bi-bundle branch block or trifascicular disease, a pacemaker is indicated for documented complete AV block, high-degree AV block (Mobitz type II) associated with symptoms, or a history of syncope that has no other definable etiology. ▪

Notes

A n ECG from a 24-year-old man with a history of palpitations associated with lightheadedness is presented.

What is your interpretation of this ECG?

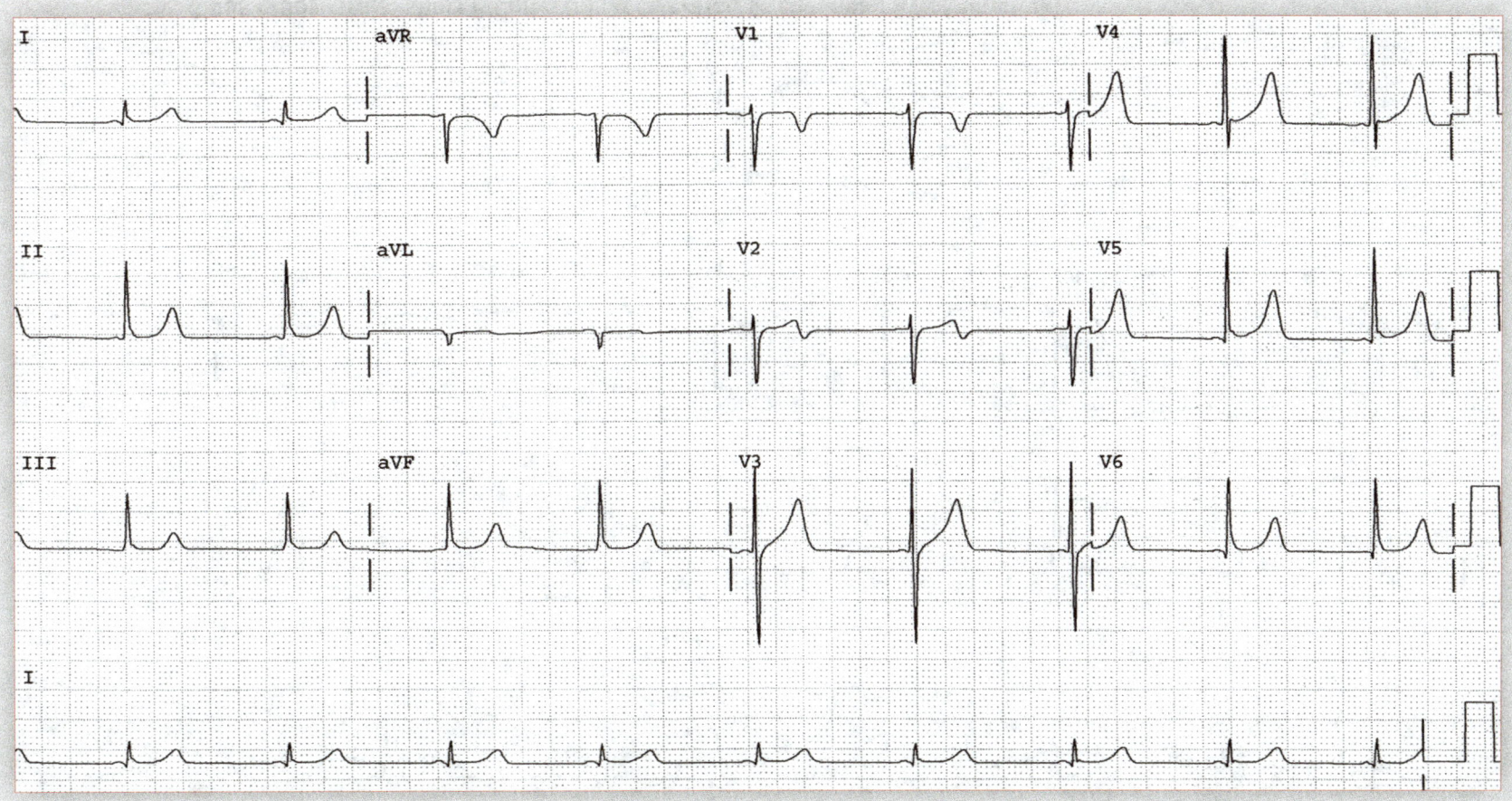

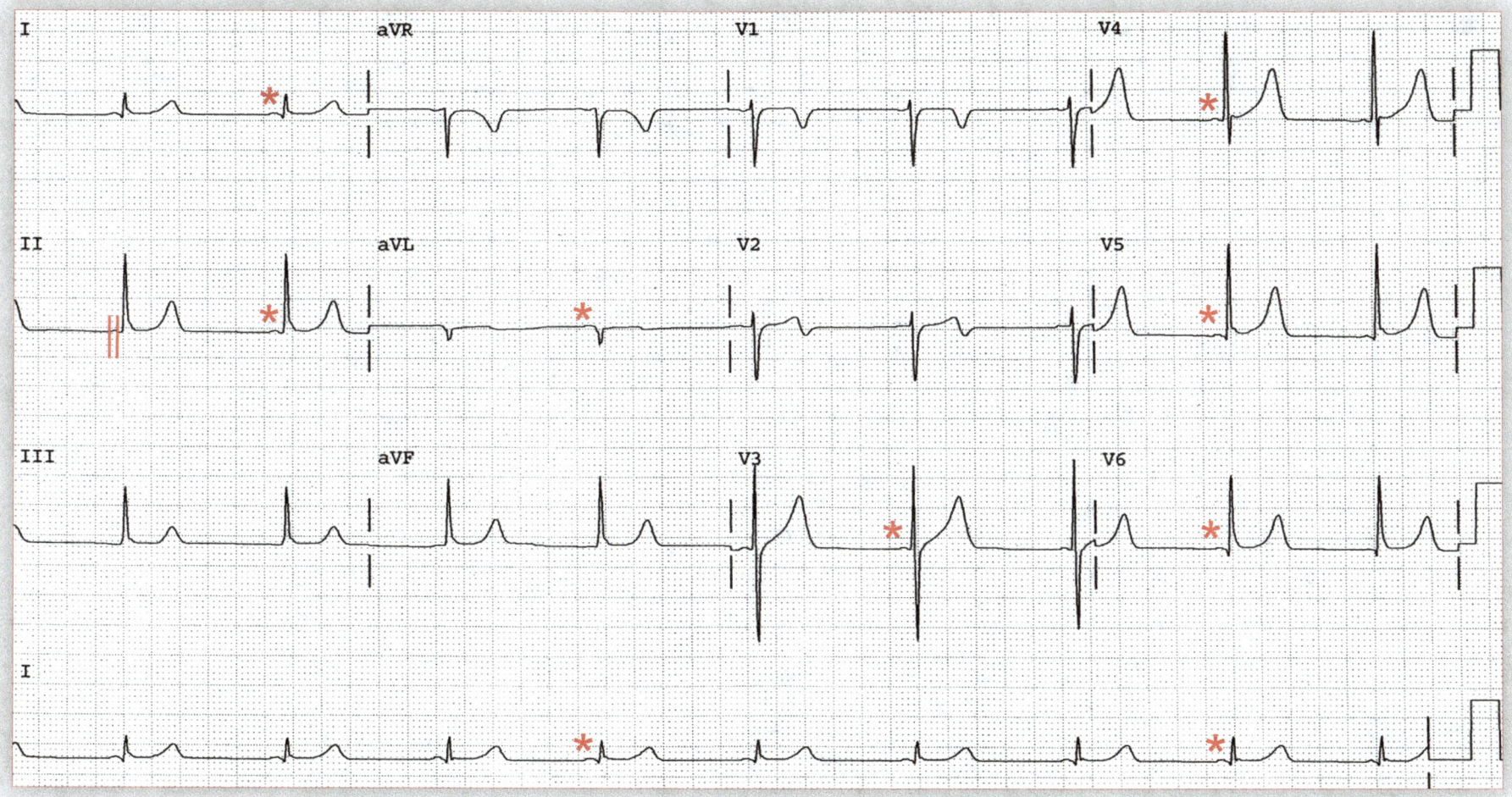

ECG 53 Analysis: Sinus bradycardia, short PR interval (accelerated or enhanced AV conduction)

There is a regular rhythm at a rate of 56 bpm. There is a P wave (*) before each QRS complex. The P wave is upright in leads I, II, and V4-V6 and is thus originating from the sinus node. The PR interval is constant but short (0.12 sec) (‖). Indeed, there is no PR segment seen. The QRS complex is narrow (0.08 sec) and has a normal morphology and normal axis, between 0° and +90° (positive QRS complex in leads I and aVF). The QT/QTc intervals are normal (420/406 msec). The short PR interval represents accelerated AV conduction, which is due to either enhanced AV nodal conduction or an accessory pathway that bypasses the AV node. Since the QRS complex is narrow, conduction to the ventricle is via the normal His-Purkinje system. When resulting from an accessory bypass tract, this pattern is known as Lown-Ganong-Levine (LGL) and is due to a bypass tract known as the bundle of James that links the atrium and the bundle of His. LGL pattern accounts for the short PR interval and normal QRS complex.

Since this patient has symptoms, it is important to perform ambulatory monitoring either with a Holter monitor if his symptoms are daily, or with an event recorder (or even an implantable loop recorder) if his symptoms are less frequent. LGL pattern is associated with a preexcitation syndrome, and the palpitations might be indicative of a reentrant arrhythmia involving a circuit that includes the accessory pathway and AV node. This arrhythmia is termed atrioventricular reentrant tachycardia. It is also possible that he could be experiencing another type of supraventricular arrhythmia in which the accessory pathway is being used as the conduction pathway to the ventricles. The documentation of an arrhythmia associated with an LGL pattern of the ECG is termed LGL syndrome. ■

Notes

A 24-year-old woman presents to your clinic with a history of episodic palpitations that occur several times per week. She has never felt lightheaded or experienced loss of consciousness. She is active, running 2 to 3 miles several times per week. She has no other medical problems and denies any family history of cardiac disease. Her vital signs and physical exam are normal. An ECG is obtained.

What abnormality is depicted?

What is the suggested cause of her symptoms?

What is the next step in her evaluation?

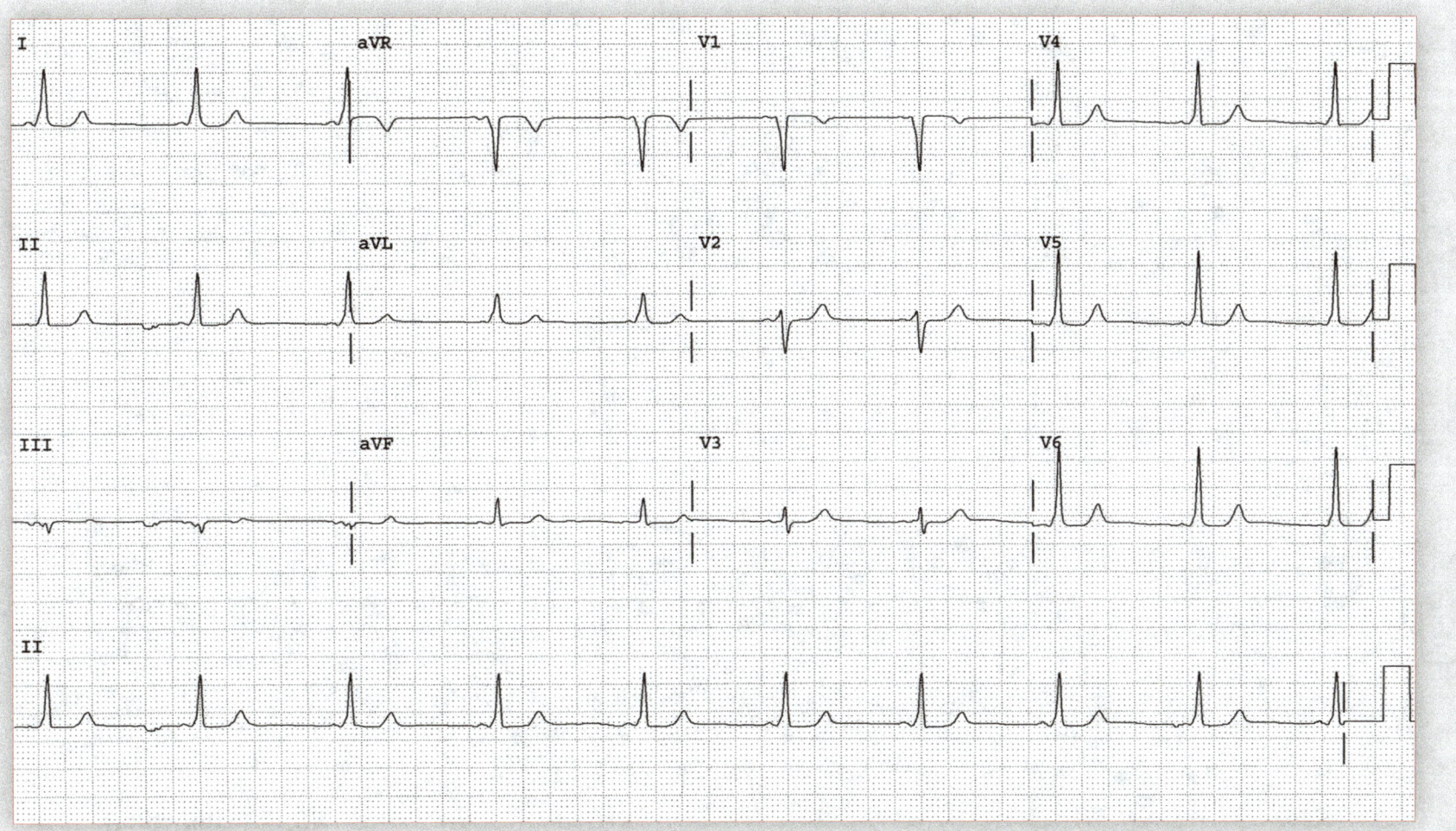

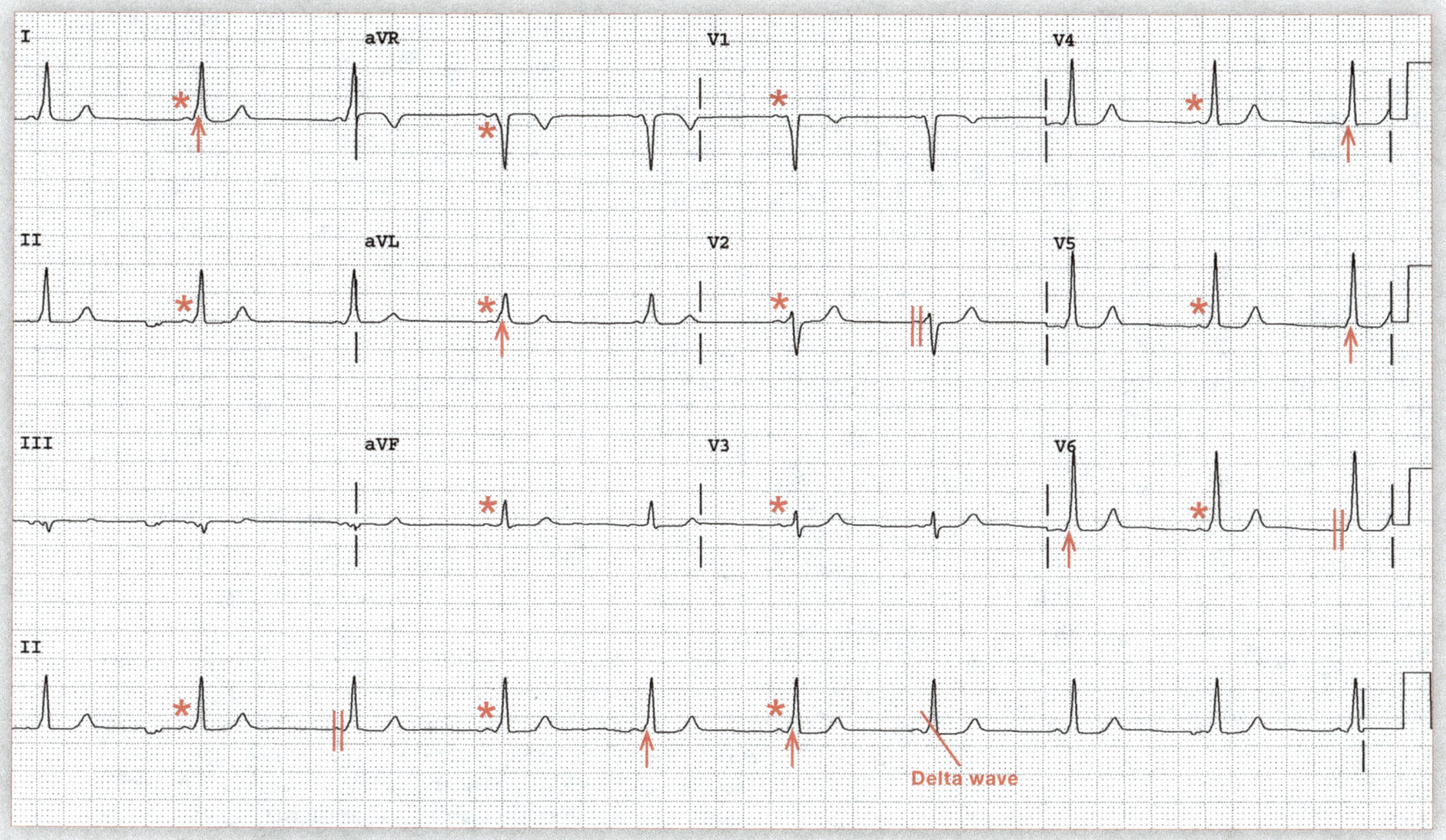

Delta wave

ECG 54 Analysis: Sinus bradycardia, Wolff-Parkinson-White pattern

There is a regular rhythm at a rate of 56 bpm. There is a P wave (*) before each QRS complex with a stable PR interval that is short (0.10 sec) (‖). The P waves are positive in leads I, II, aVF, and V4-V6. Hence this is sinus bradycardia. The QRS complex is widened (0.12 sec) as a result of a slurred upstroke (↑) of the initial portion of the QRS complex (producing a widening of the base of the QRS complex but not the peak). The axis is normal, between 0° and +90° (positive QRS complex in leads I and aVF). The QT/QTc intervals are normal (420/406 msec). This slurred upstroke, which can be seen in most but not all leads, is called a delta wave and indicates initial direct and slow myocardial activation via an accessory pathway. The presence of a short PR interval associated with the widened QRS complex and delta wave is known as Wolff-Parkinson-White (WPW) pattern. This is a form of preexcitation syndrome and may be associated with a specific reentrant arrhythmia that occurs as a result of the accessory pathway called atrioventricular reentrant tachycardia (AVRT). Other atrial arrhythmias may occur and use the accessory pathway to activate the ventricle; however, these arrhythmias do not require the accessory pathway for their occurrence. These arrhythmias may present with a wide QRS complex reflecting accessory pathway conduction.

WPW pattern is due to an AV nodal bypass tract called the bundle of Kent that serves as a direct connection between atrial and ventricular myocardium, bypassing the AV node and resulting in direct and early ventricular myocardial activation that precedes activation via the AV node (*ie*, preexcitation). The manifestation of this preexcitation is a short PR interval and an early and slurred upstroke of the QRS complex (reflecting initial direct myocardial activation) termed a delta wave. The QRS complex is widened as a result of this delta wave. The QRS complex is a fusion beat representing early ventricular activation initiated via the accessory pathway and slightly later activation via the normal AV node–His-Purkinje system. The QRS complex is thus widened and abnormal. The widening is more apparent at the base of the QRS complex, as a result of the delta wave, while the QRS complex is narrower at its peak. The width of the delta wave and the degree of aberration are related to balance between conduction through the AV node and accessory pathway. It is the AV nodal conduction properties that determine the extent of the delta wave and the QRS complex duration, as conduction through the accessory pathway is "all or none," similar to what is seen in His-Purkinje fibers. When AV nodal conduction is slow, more myocardium is activated via the accessory pathway; hence the PR interval is shorter, the delta wave is more prominent, and the QRS complex is wider. When AV nodal conduction is faster, less myocardium is activated via the accessory pathway; hence the PR interval is longer, the delta wave is less prominent, and the QRS complex is narrower.

continues

Palpitations have a broad differential diagnosis and may be related to an increase in sinus rate, isolated premature complexes, or a supraventricular tachyarrhythmia. Supraventricular arrhythmia (*ie*, atrial tachycardia, atrial flutter, atrial fibrillation) may conduct to the ventricles via the normal His-Purkinje system, by the accessory pathway, or via both conduction systems. AVRT is supraventricular tachycardia that is specific for a preexcitation syndrome and involves a macro-reentrant circuit (which includes the accessory pathway, AV node, normal His-Purkinje system, and the atrial and ventricular myocardium) that links these two pathways proximally and distally. The circuit must be complete for AVRT to exist.

The next step in this patient's evaluation is to correlate her symptoms with an arrhythmia via ambulatory monitoring, especially using an event or loop recorder that can record a patient's rhythm for up to 1 month. Documentation of an arrhythmia, particularly an AVRT, would be diagnostic for WPW syndrome and should prompt an electrophysiologic study with consideration of radiofrequency ablation of the bypass tract. Other supraventricular arrhythmias may also occur and may use the bypass tract to conduct to the ventricle. The treatment would depend on the type of supraventricular tachyarrhythmia documented and also whether the QRS complex during the arrhythmia was widened or preexcited. ■

An 18-year-old man has an ECG performed given his involvement in competitive athletics at the collegiate level and a family history of sudden death.

What abnormality is noted on the ECG?

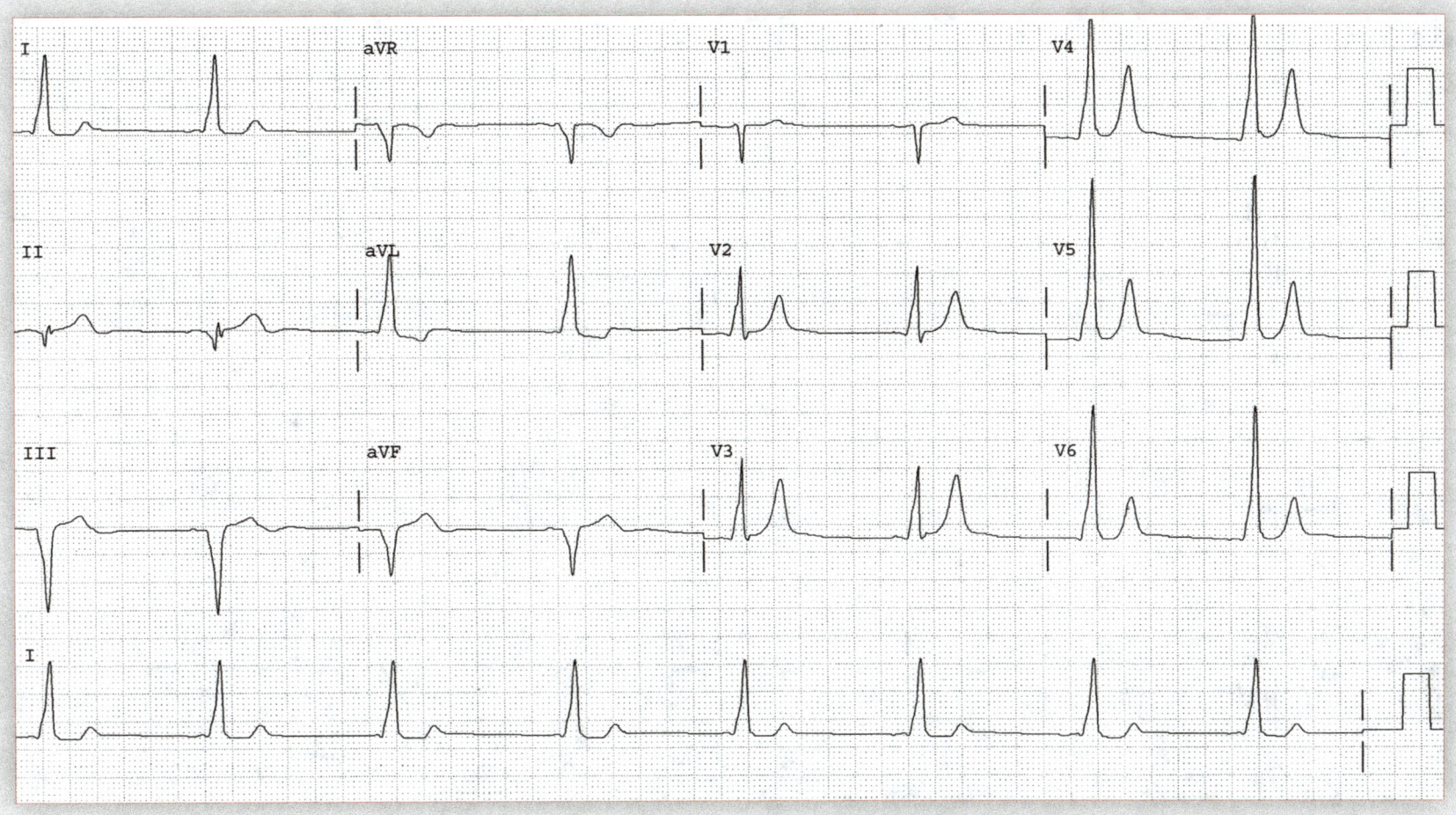

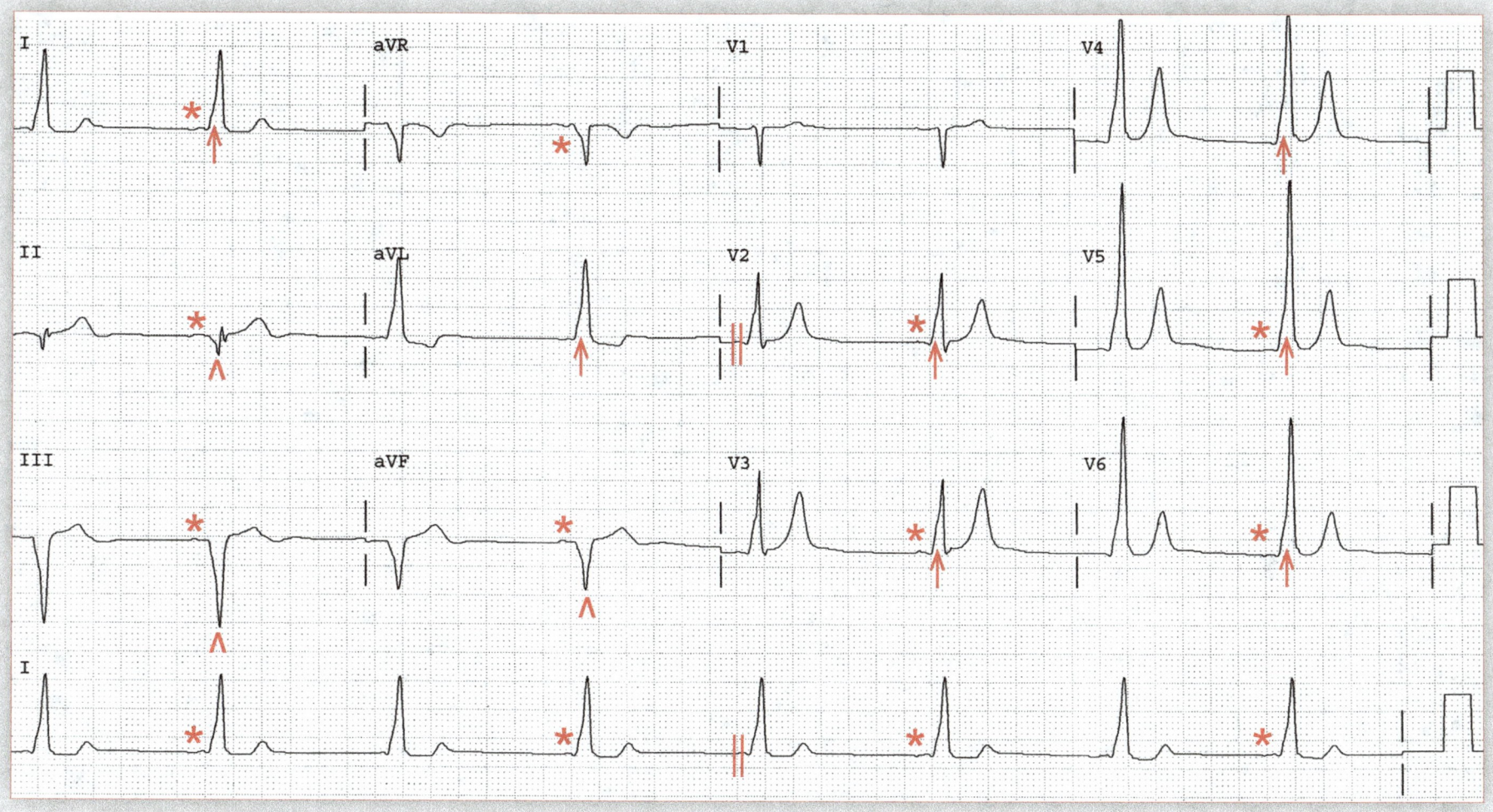

ECG 55 Analysis: Sinus bradycardia, Wolff-Parkinson-White pattern

There is a regular rhythm at a rate of 48 bpm. There is a P wave (*) before each QRS complex, and the PR interval is 0.10 second (‖). The P waves are positive in leads I, II, aVF, and V4-V6. Hence this is sinus bradycardia. The QRS complex is widened (0.18 sec) as a result of a slurred upstroke due to a very broad delta wave (↑). This is Wolff-Parkinson-White (WPW) pattern. The PR interval is very short, and the delta wave is wide. The delta wave presents as a negative waveform (Q wave) in leads II, III, and aVF (^). This is a pseudo inferior wall myocardial infarction pattern and is associated with a bypass tract located in the posterior septal wall. With WPW pattern initial ventricular activation is by direct myocardial activation, bypassing the His-Purkinje system. Therefore, a chronic infarction cannot be recognized or diagnosed; hence it is termed a pseudo infarction pattern. For the same reason, an extreme left axis due to a conduction abnormality of the His-Purkinje system (ie, a left anterior fascicular block) cannot be diagnosed in WPW pattern. Furthermore, other left ventricular abnormalities (eg, left ventricular hypertrophy, myocardial ischemia or infarction, pericarditis) cannot be diagnosed. As WPW pattern represents a fusion between conduction via two different pathways that connect the atria with the ventricles (accessory pathway and normal AV node–His-Purkinje system), the markedly short PR interval and wide delta wave indicate that the majority of ventricular activation is via the accessory pathway and less ventricular myocardium is being activated via the AV node–His-Purkinje system. This is due to the fact that conduction via the AV node is relatively slow, resulting in more ventricular myocardial activation through the rapidly conducting accessory pathway. The QT/QTc intervals are prolonged (560/500) but are normal (460/410 msec) when the increased QRS complex duration is considered.

Patients with WPW pattern are susceptible to a reentrant supraventricular arrhythmia known as atrioventricular reentrant tachycardia (AVRT). The reentrant circuit for this arrhythmia involves the accessory pathway and the normal AV node–His-Purkinje system, which are the two pathways (or limbs) that connect the atria and ventricles. These two limbs are connected via the atrial and ventricular myocardium, forming a macro-reentrant circuit. This entire circuit needs to be intact for an AVRT to exist. Other atrial arrhythmias may also occur, such as atrial fibrillation, atrial flutter, or atrial tachycardia.

continues

These arrhythmias originate in the atrium, and they use the normal His-Purkinje and accessory pathways to conduct impulses to the ventricles. Unlike AVRT, they do not depend on the conduction system or accessory pathway for their existence.

Any supraventricular arrhythmia may be associated with symptoms. However, the major concern is a risk for sudden cardiac death in patients with WPW syndrome. Sudden death occurs primarily in those patients who experience atrial fibrillation with an atrial rate in excess of 350 to 450 bpm. If the refractoriness of the accessory pathway is very short, it is capable of rapid conduction and may transmit the atrial fibrillatory impulses to the ventricle at very rapid rates. In this situation the ventricle, even if normal, may develop ventricular fibrillation, which is the mechanism for sudden death. Although the actual incidence of sudden death in patients with WPW pattern on their ECG is low, this patient has a family history of sudden death. In addition, he is involved in competitive sports. Radiofrequency ablation is often performed in this type of patient, even in the absence of symptoms. ◼

A 52-year-old woman is seen by her physician because of complaints of palpitations. However, the etiology for these symptoms has never been documented. Her physician recommends an exercise test. When she presents for this study, a resting ECG is obtained. The exercise technician thinks the ECG is abnormal, and he cancels the test.

What abnormality is noted?

What is the significance of this finding?

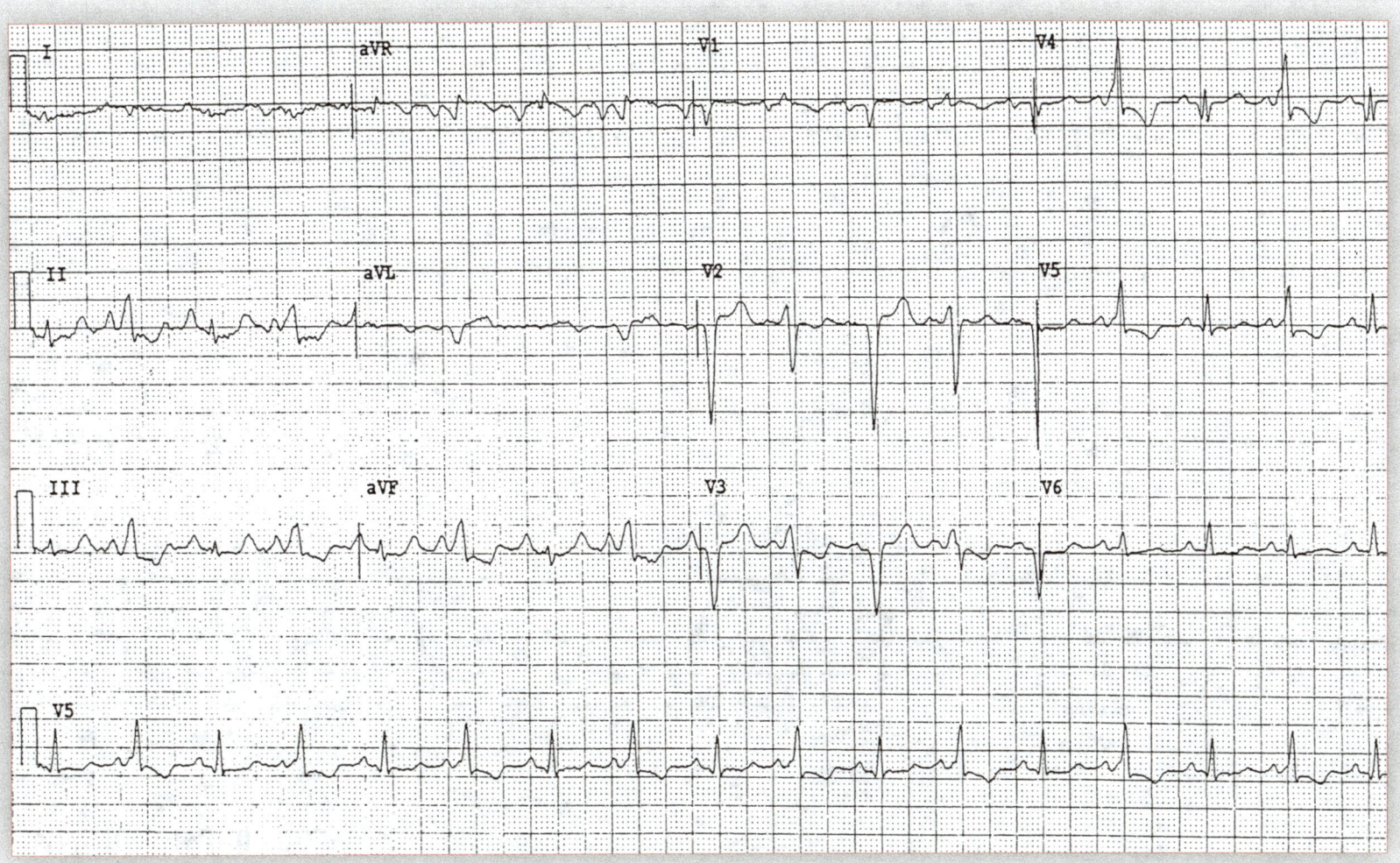

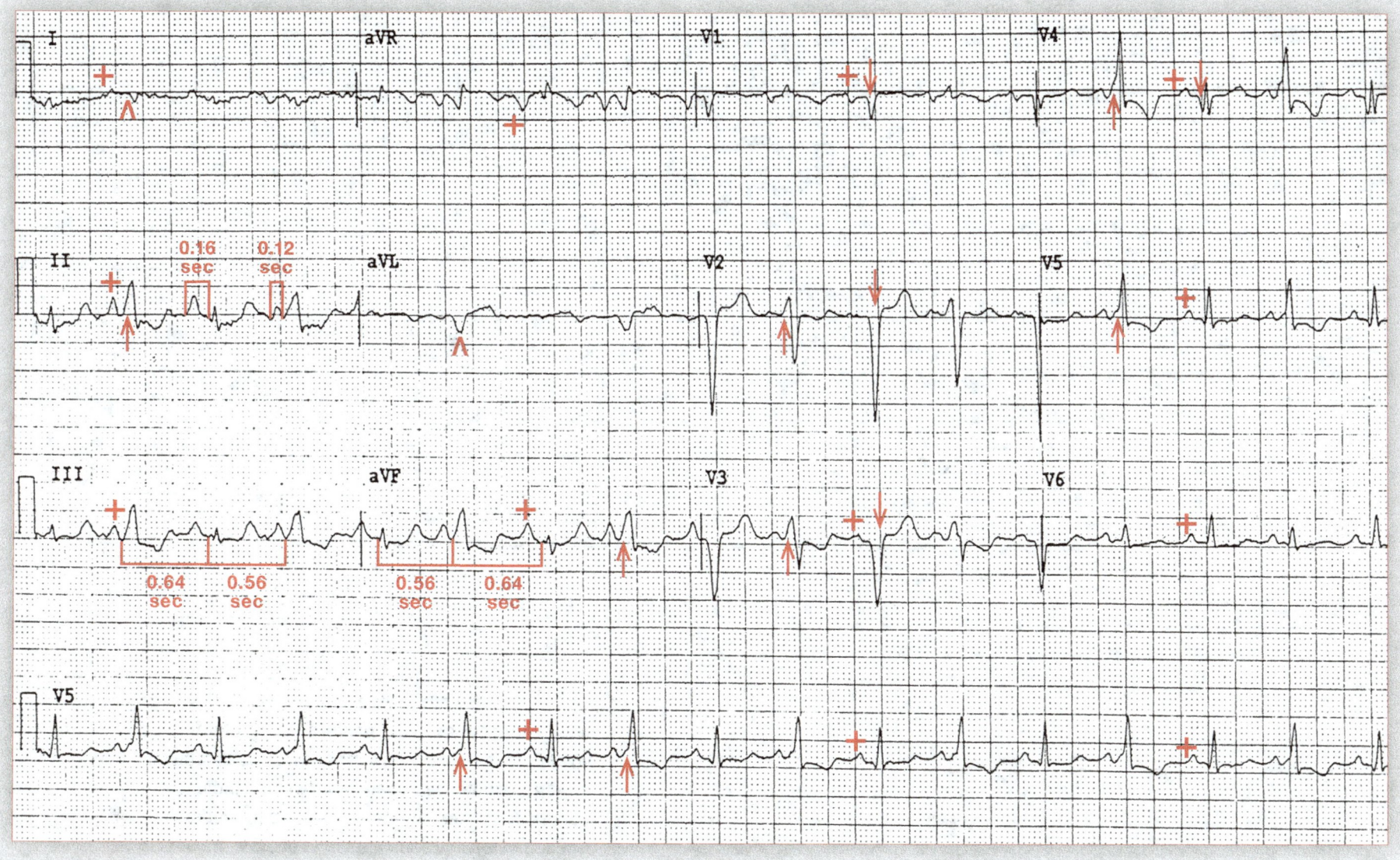

ECG 56 Analysis: Normal sinus rhythm, intermittent Wolff-Parkinson-White pattern, low limb lead voltage, old anterior wall myocardial infarction

There is a slightly irregular rhythm at a rate of 96 bpm. There is a P wave (+) before each QRS complex, and the atrial rate (PP intervals) is regular. The P wave is positive in leads I, II, aVF, and V4-V6. Hence this is a normal sinus rhythm. However, the PR intervals are not constant, alternating between 0.16 and 0.12 second (⊓). As a result, the RR intervals are slightly irregular (ie, 0.56 and 0.64 sec, respectively) (⊔). Therefore, the rhythm is regularly irregular.

The longer PR interval is associated with a QRS complex that has a normal duration (0.08 sec), a normal axis of about 0° (positive QRS complex in lead I and biphasic QRS complex in lead aVF), and low limb lead voltage (defined as a QRS complex amplitude < 5 mm in each limb lead and < 10 mm in each precordial lead). There are QS complexes in leads V1-V3 and a significant Q wave in lead V4 (↓), consistent with an old anterior wall myocardial infarction (MI). The shorter PR interval is associated with a QRS complex with a wide duration (0.16 sec). In addition, this QRS complex has a slurred upstroke of the R wave (↑), accounting for the excess width, which is particularly evident at the base of the QRS complex. This slurred upstroke is called a delta wave and is consistent with the preexcitation pattern of Wolff-Parkinson-White (WPW). Interestingly, the QRS complexes that are wide and preexcited do not have evidence of the old anterior wall MI. This is because there is direct myocardial activation via the accessory pathway and, similar to other situations in which there is direct myocardial activation (ie, left bundle branch block, paced QRS complexes, ventricular complexes), myocardial abnormalities, including a chronic MI, cannot be reliably diagnosed. Therefore, this patient's stress test must be performed with imaging (either nuclear imaging or echocardiography) as the ECG is unreliable at detecting ischemia in the presence of WPW pattern.

There is an alternating pattern of normal QRS complexes and pre-excited QRS complexes, or an intermittent WPW pattern. The QT/QTc intervals are normal (360/450 msec). Although the QRS complexes have a small amplitude in lead I, it appears that there is an initial Q wave in this lead as well as in lead aVL (^, a pseudo lateral wall infarction pattern), with a positive delta wave in lead V1, consistent with a bypass tract located in the left lateral wall.

The presence of intermittent preexcitation generally means that the refractory period of the accessory pathway is relatively long and is not able to conduct at very rapid rates. This implies that if the patient should develop atrial fibrillation, the ventricular response rate would not be very rapid and hence there would be a reduced risk for provoking ventricular fibrillation. ■

Practice ECGs

A 52-year-old man is admitted for an anterior wall ST-segment elevation myocardial infarction (MI), which is treated with angioplasty and stenting of a proximal left anterior descending artery occlusion. After the procedure he is treated with aspirin, clopidogrel, and a β-blocker. On hospital day four, a nurse notices irregular QRS complexes on the patient's telemetry monitor. She checks on the patient, who is sound asleep. The patient has had an uneventful post-intervention course without recurrent chest pain or arrhythmia. The nurse obtains an ECG from the telemetry monitor and asks you to review it.

What is the explanation for the irregular complexes noted on telemetric monitoring?

Is any therapy warranted?

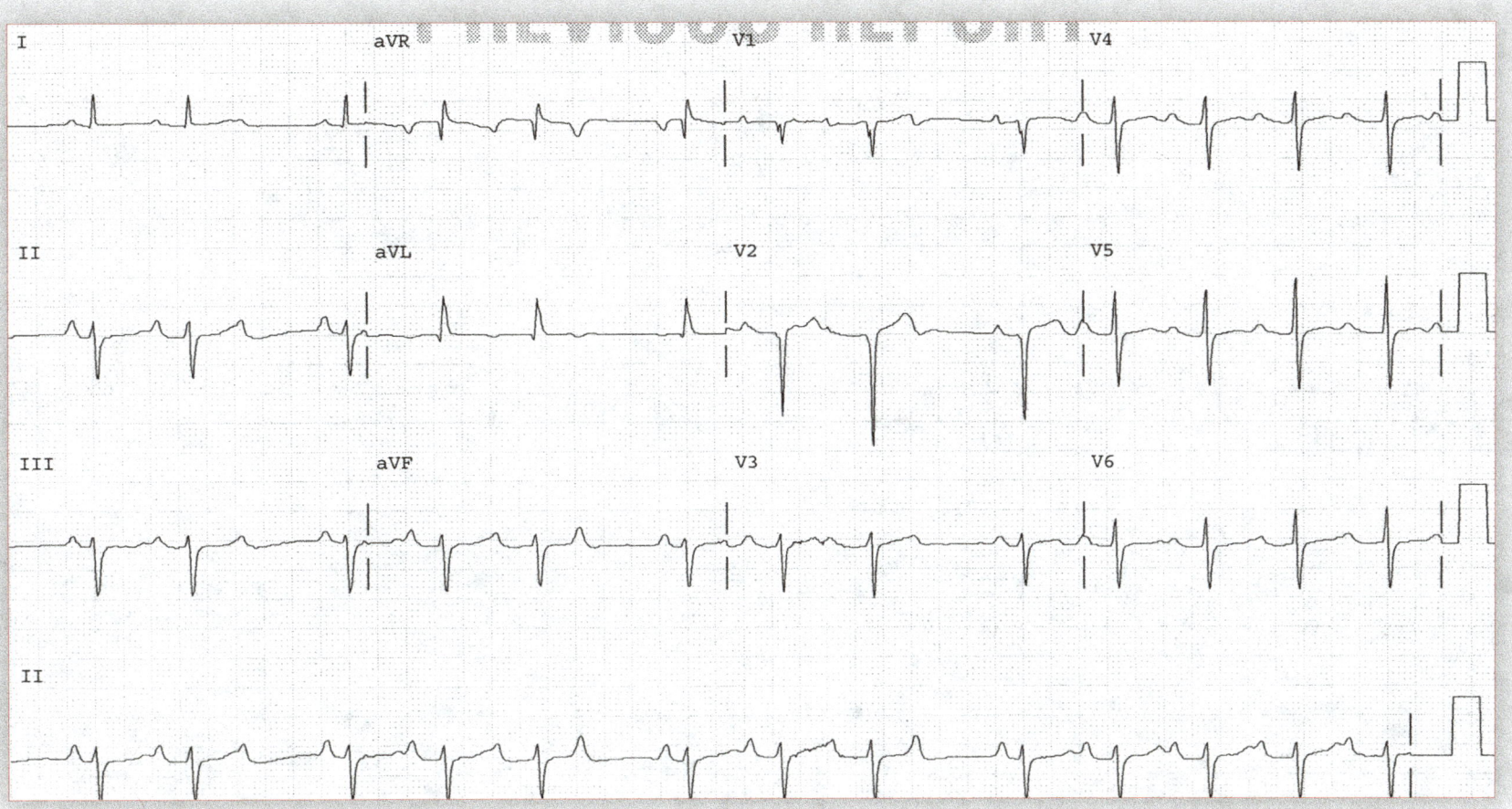

Podrid's Real-World ECGs

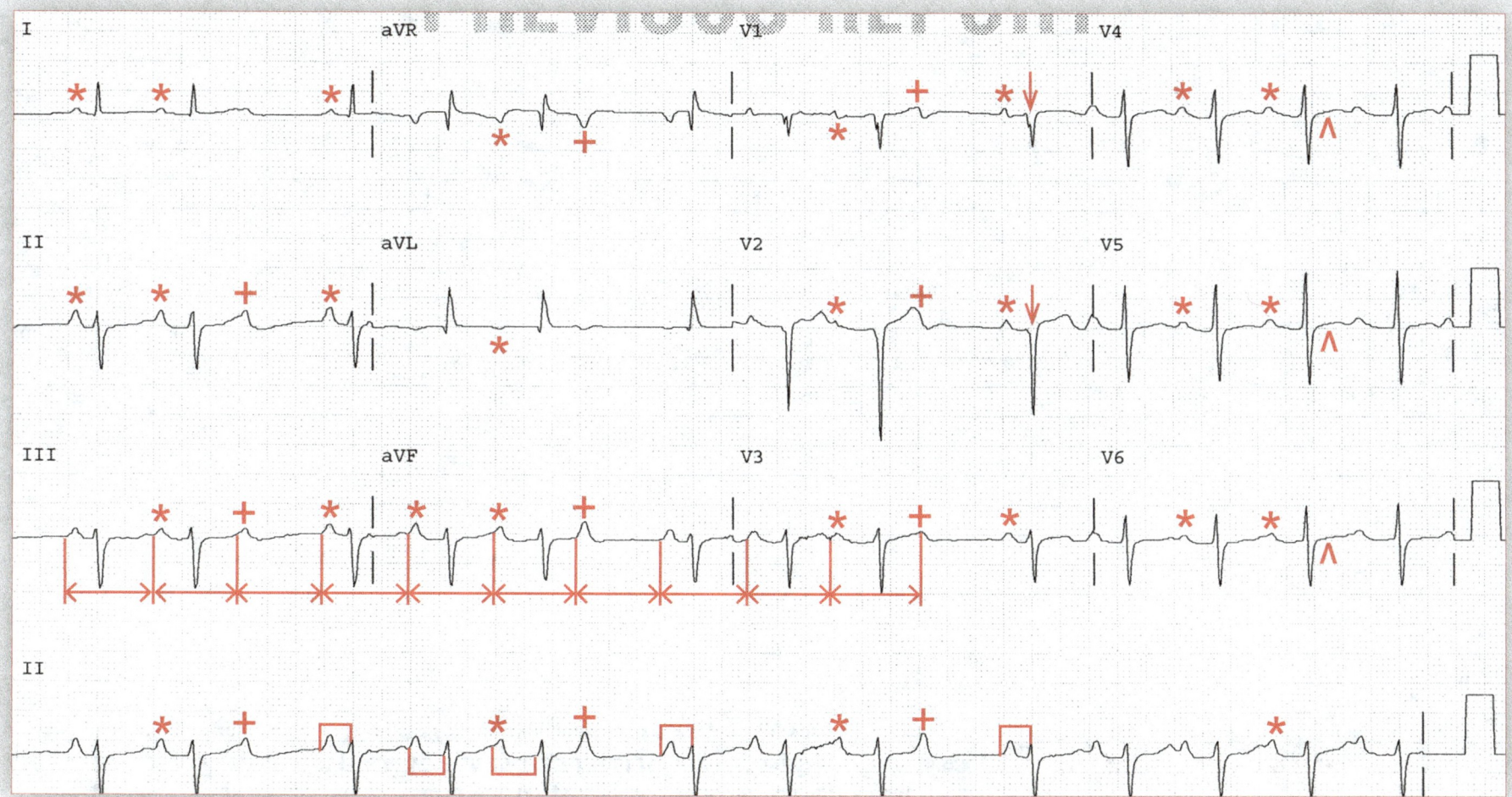

ECG 57 Analysis: Normal sinus rhythm, Mobitz type I second-degree AV block (Wenckebach), left anterior fascicular block, anteroseptal MI, nonspecific T-wave abnormalities

The PP intervals are stable (↔), and the atrial rate is regular at 98 bpm. The P wave (*) is positive in leads I, II, aVF, and V4-V6. Hence this is a normal sinus rhythm. The average ventricular rate is 78 bpm. The QRS complex duration is normal (0.08 sec) and the axis is extremely leftward, between −30° and −90°, consistent with a left anterior fascicular block (positive QRS complex in lead I and negative QRS complex in leads II and aVF with an rS morphology). There is also evidence of an old anteroseptal myocardial infarction (MI; QS complex in leads V1-V2) (↓). Also noted is nonspecific T-wave flattening in the limb leads and in leads V4-V6 (^). The QT/QTc intervals are normal (380/430 msec).

Grouped beating is seen with occasional pauses or long RR intervals. The PR interval (⊓) after each pause is normal at 0.20 second. This is the baseline PR interval. Following this pause there is progressive PR interval lengthening (0.28, 0.32 sec) (⊔) followed by nonconducted P wave (+), which accounts for the pause. This P wave is superimposed on the T wave and not readily apparent. However, by using the PP intervals, it can be seen that the P wave is occurring on time. This is the pattern of Mobitz type I second-degree AV block or Wenckebach. The first group of QRS complexes shows 3:2 Wenckebach, followed by a pattern of 4:3 Wenckebach. The Wenckebach cycle length is even longer at the end of the ECG. Mobitz type I second-degree AV block

(Wenckebach) can be seen during periods of increased vagal tone, such as during sleep. It is indicative of an increased AV nodal refractory period with delayed conduction through the node and is not considered suggestive of AV node injury. Mobitz type I AV block in this case is unlikely related to the patient's recent anterior wall MI. It is, however, commonly seen with an inferior wall MI, generally the result of increased vagal tone as well as edema within the AV junction, around the AV node.

Wenckebach is a conduction abnormality within the AV node. Since the electrophysiologic properties of the AV node are mediated by calcium currents, conduction through this structure is not all or none but can vary depending on changes in nodal properties. The AV node exhibits decremental conduction (ie, conduction through the node prolongs as the heart rate increases). These non-pathologic changes in the speed of AV conduction are usually due to changes in the node's refractory period. It is common for Wenckebach to be noted at night while patients are sleeping. This is likely the result of increased vagal tone in addition to therapy with a β-blocker. In the absence of symptoms, which are unlikely to be present while the patient is sleeping, no therapy is necessary. β-blocker therapy does not need to be withdrawn. Likewise, asymptomatic Wenckebach that occurs during the day does not require therapy. ■

Notes

A 54-year-old woman is admitted to the hospital after she presented to her primary physician with complaints of fatigue. The admission was prompted by an ECG obtained in the clinic. On review, the patient states that 1 week prior to the onset of fatigue she noted an unheralded episode of jaw and chest discomfort that lasted several hours and then resolved. She did not seek any medical care.

What rhythm abnormality is shown?

Based on the ECG, what is the cause of the patient's symptoms over the past week?

What therapy is indicated?

What further testing may be helpful?

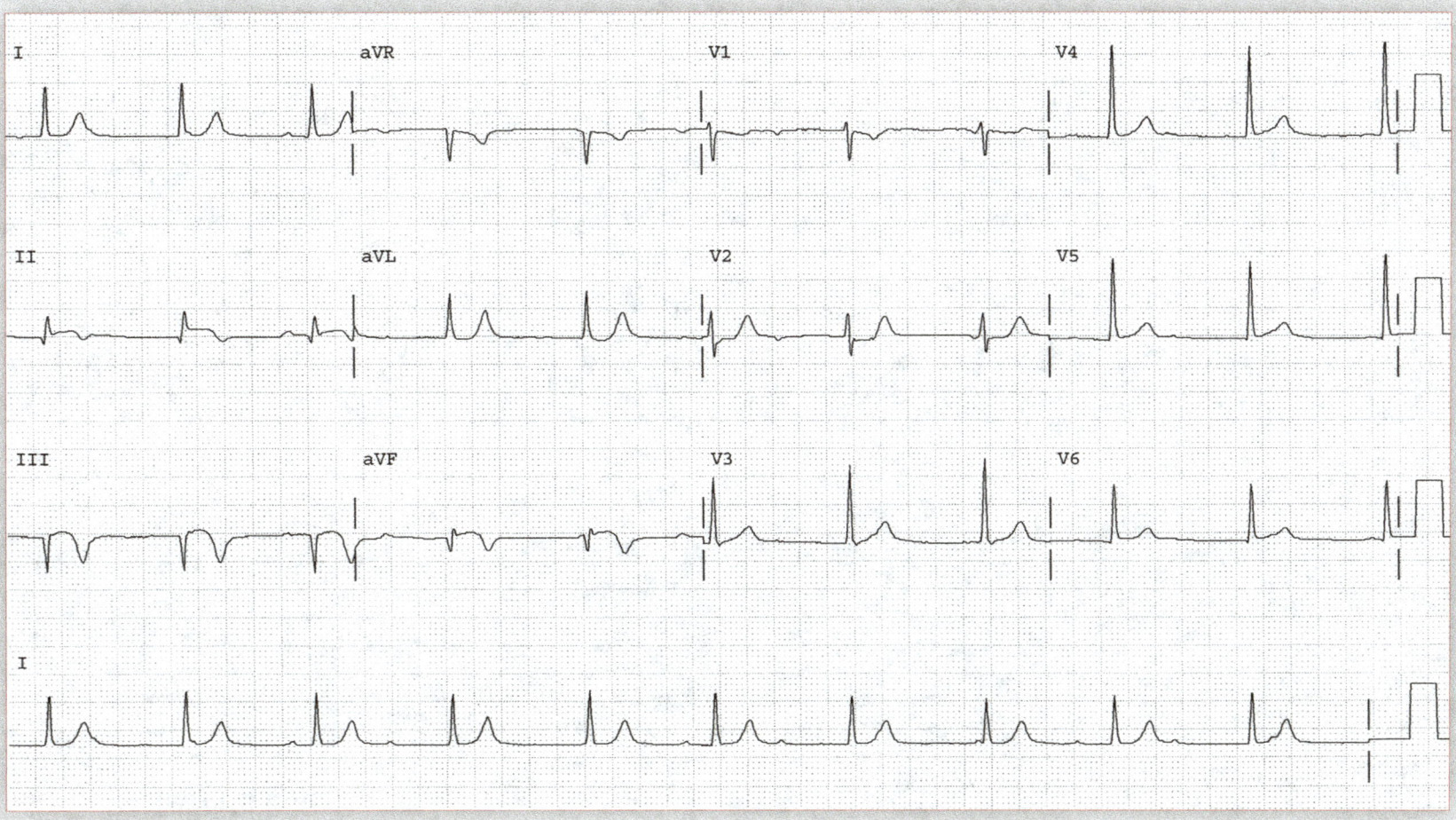

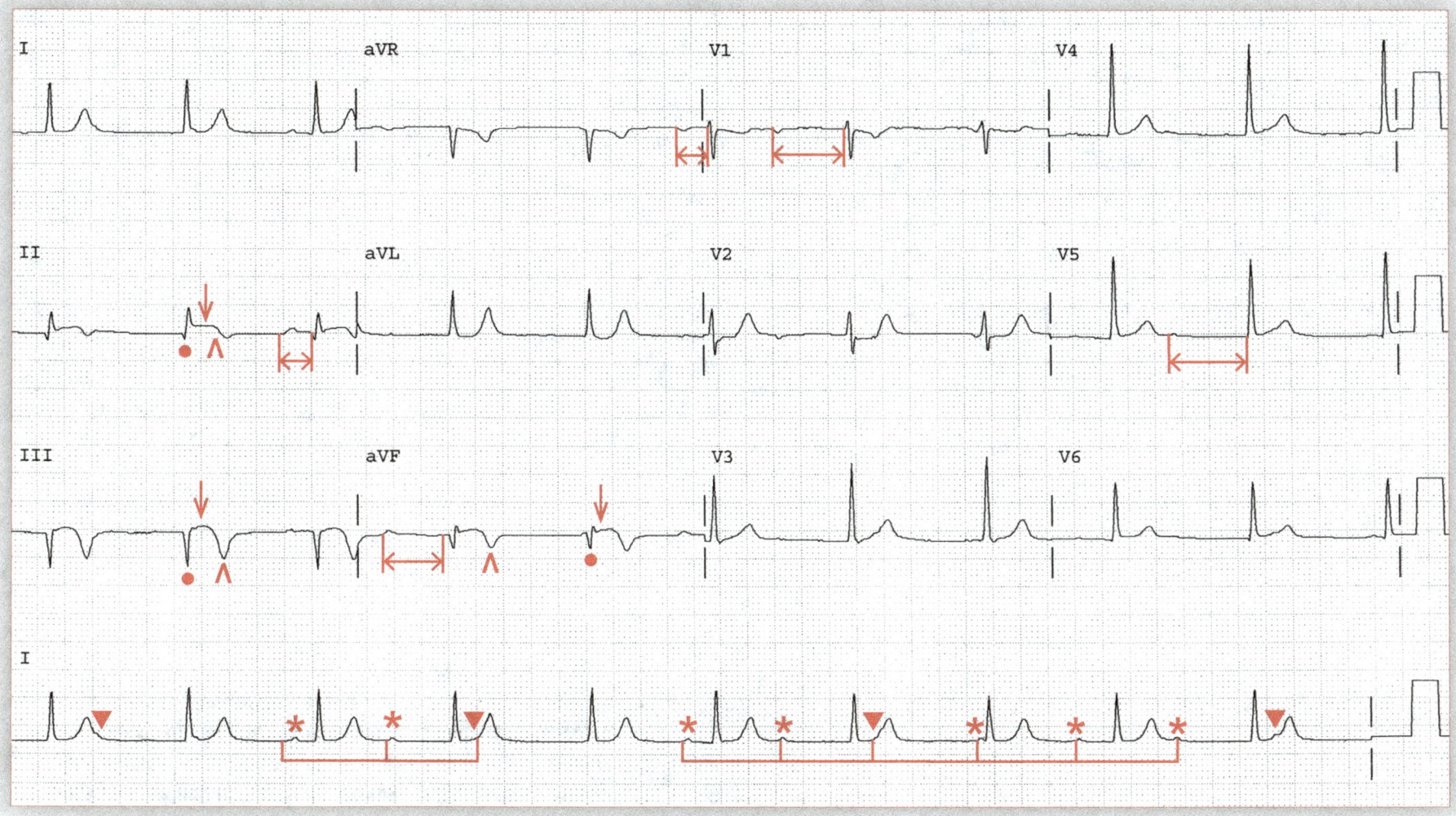

ECG 58 Analysis: Normal sinus rhythm with complete (third-degree) AV block, junctional escape rhythm, acute inferior wall myocardial infarction

There is a regular narrow complex rhythm at a rate of 62 bpm. The QRS complex duration is normal with a normal morphology. There is a physiologic left axis, between 0° and −30° (positive QRS complex in leads I and II and negative QRS complex in lead aVF). The QT/QTc intervals are normal (380/386 msec). Noted are P waves (*) at a rate of 86 bpm. Occasionally the P waves are superimposed on the T waves or the QRS complexes (▼), presenting with bumps on the T waves, which should have a smooth upstroke and downstroke. On occasion a P wave is not seen, being hidden within the QRS complex. The P waves that are seen, however, occur at regular PP intervals (⊔) and are dissociated from the QRS complexes as the PR intervals are variable (↔). Hence AV dissociation is present. Since the atrial rate is faster than the ventricular rate, this is complete heart block with an escape junctional rhythm as the QRS complexes are normal in width and morphology.

Also seen are ST-segment elevations (↓) in leads II, III, and aVF with T-wave inversions (^). These abnormalities are consistent with an acute inferior wall myocardial infarction (MI). The presence of Q waves (●) in these leads indicates that the ECG changes are resolving, confirming that the MI most likely occurred several days before this ECG was obtained, likely a week ago when she experienced chest and jaw pain.

As a result of the inferior wall MI the patient likely had ischemic damage or edema in the AV junctional area. The AV node itself is relatively impervious to ischemia as its electrophysiologic properties are mediated by calcium currents and it is energy and oxygen independent. Thus, AV nodal conduction abnormalities, including complete heart block (with an escape junctional rhythm) are not generally the result of structural damage to the AV node but usually are due to high vagal tone as well as edema in the AV junction around the AV node. Therefore, the conduction abnormalities with an inferior wall MI are usually transient and resolve spontaneously.

The patient will require routine post-MI therapy with aspirin and a statin. β-blocker therapy is important but should not be started until the complete heart block has resolved. Infrequently, the AV block persists, indicating more significant damage to the AV junction. In these cases a pacemaker may be indicated, especially since β-blocker therapy is needed long-term. Evaluation of left ventricular function with an echocardiogram is also warranted. Exercise testing is often performed to establish functional capacity as well as to evaluate other areas of potential ischemia. If symptoms of ischemia recur or if there is evidence of ischemia with exercise testing, anti-ischemic medications (primarily nitrates) would be indicated. Coronary angiography would be indicated if there were recurrent anginal symptoms despite medical therapy or if there were other signs of ongoing ischemia such as hemodynamic instability, heart failure, or ventricular tachycardia. ■

Notes

A 77-year-old woman is admitted to the emergency department after having a pre-syncopal episode. At home, she had become unsteady on her feet and fallen to the ground without loss of consciousness. On arrival, she is conscious but disoriented. Her heart rate is 35 bpm, and her blood pressure 92/60 mm Hg. While she is being stabilized, an ECG is obtained.

What diagnosis is revealed by the ECG?

What is the next step in her management?

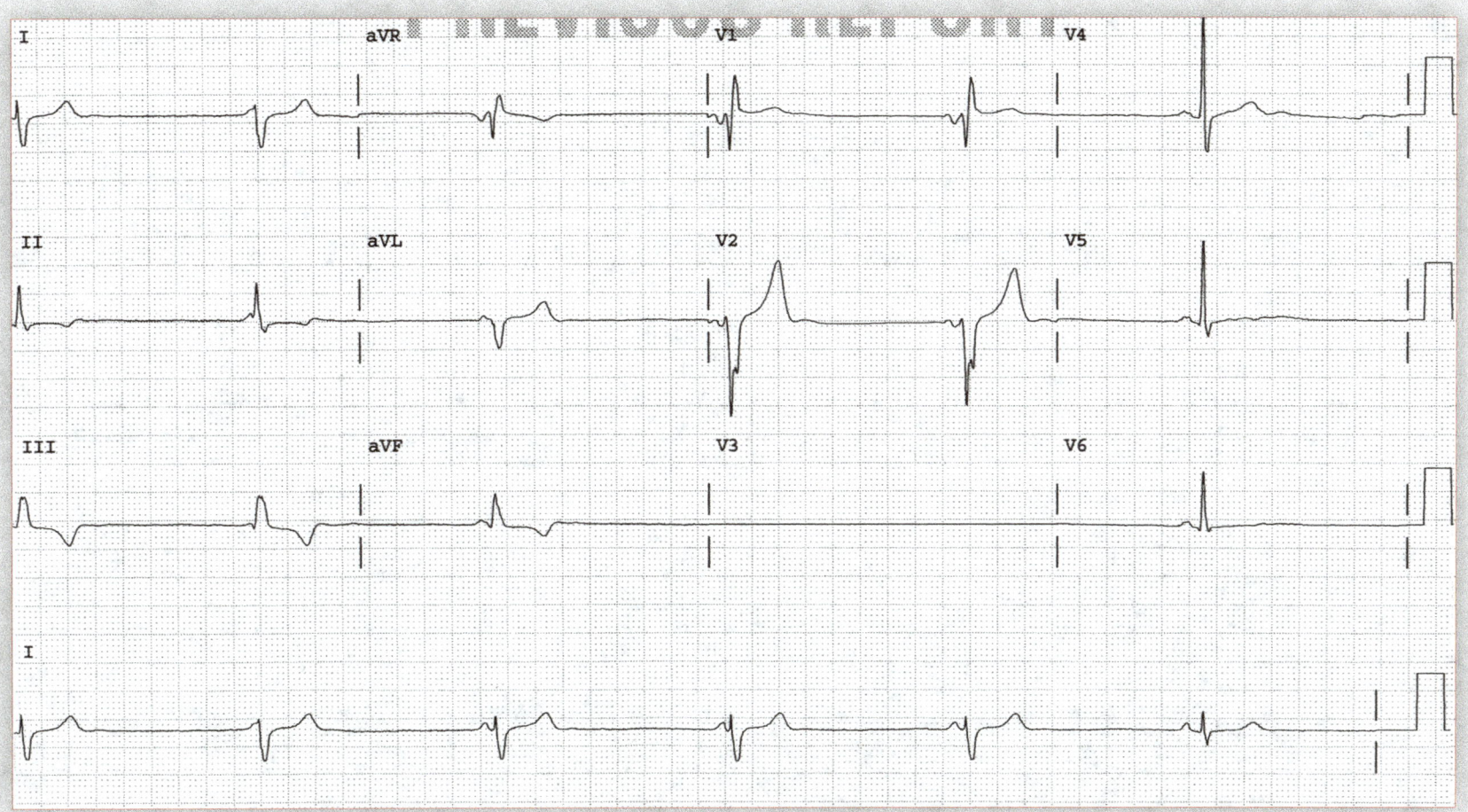

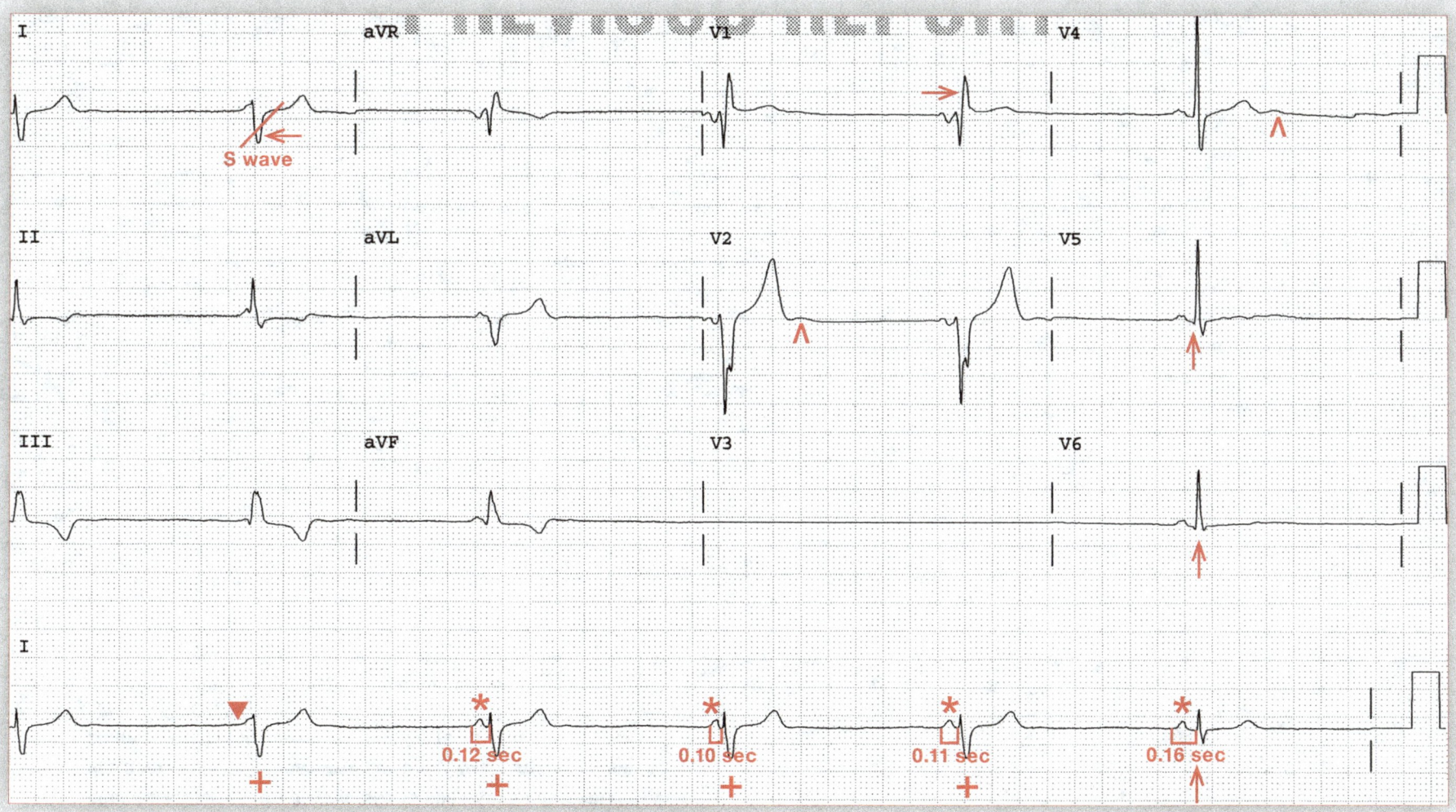

I aVR V1 V4

S wave

II aVL V2 V5

III aVF V3 V6

I

0.12 sec 0.10 sec 0.11 sec 0.16 sec

ECG 59 Analysis: Sinus bradycardia, isorhythmic AV dissociation
with a captured complex, junctional rhythm, left posterior fascicular block,
intraventricular conduction delay to the right ventricle, U waves

The RR intervals are normal at a regular rate of 35 bpm. P waves are seen before each QRS complex (*), with regular PP intervals at a rate of 35 bpm. The P waves are positive in leads I, II, aVF, and V4-V6. Hence this is a sinus rhythm. The PR intervals are not constant (⊔) as they range from 0.10 to 0.12 second. Therefore, AV dissociation is present. The P wave is less obvious before the second QRS complex as it is superimposed on the initial portion of the QRS complex (▼). The atrial and ventricular rates are identical, indicating isorhythmic AV dissociation. AV dissociation may be due to complete heart block, in which the atrial rate is faster than the rate of the QRS complexes, which may be either junctional or ventricular in origin. The location of the escape rhythm is based not on the rate of the QRS complexes but on their morphology. AV dissociation may also be due to an accelerated lower pacemaker (either junctional or ventricular), in which case the atrial rate is slower than the rate of the QRS complexes. When the rate of the P waves and QRS complexes is identical, the term isorhythmic dissociation is applied.

There is a change in the QRS morphology. The first through fifth QRS complexes (+) have a slightly increased duration (0.11 sec) and an intraventricular conduction delay to the right ventricle with a terminal S wave in lead I (←) and an RSR′ morphology in lead V1 (→). The axis is rightward, between +90° and +180° (negative QRS complex in lead I even when the terminal S wave is considered and positive QRS complex in lead aVF). In the absence of any other reason for a right axis (ie, right ventricular hypertrophy, right–left arm lead switch, lateral wall myocardial infarction, dextrocardia, Wolff-Parkinson-White pattern), the diagnosis is a left posterior fascicular block. The last

complex (↑) has a narrow duration (0.08 sec), and there is no right ventricular conduction delay; the axis is no longer rightward as the QRS complex is positive in lead I. There is an on-time P wave before this QRS complex with a PR interval of 0.16 second, which is slightly longer than the previous PR intervals. This suggests that there is intact AV conduction and that this is a captured beat. QRS complexes 1 to 5 are slightly wider and have a right axis, but the initial forces are the same (ie, there is a narrow initial R wave in lead I). Hence these are junctional complexes. Junctional complexes, which originate from an ectopic focus within the AV junction, commonly enter the bundle of His at a slightly different location than the sinus complexes, in which the impulse travels through the AV node. Hence junctional complexes are conducted through the His-Purkinje system slightly differently, resulting in mild differences in axis, amplitude, and occasionally width, with the development of a slight conduction delay. The QT/QTc intervals are normal (500/380 msec). Low-amplitude and normal U waves are also noted in leads V2 and V4 (^).

The presence of a captured complex does not help establish the etiology of the AV dissociation as there could be complete AV block with a captured complex or capture as a result of a slight increase in the sinus rate (not apparent on the ECG), resulting in capture and hence suppression of the junctional focus. Regardless of the etiology of the AV dissociation, the patient appears to have a symptomatic bradyarrhythmia. Unless a reversible etiology is discovered, with resolution of the isorhythmic dissociation and bradycardia (as can occur in vasovagal or neurocardiogenic syncope or other conditions associated with an increased vagal tone), a permanent pacemaker should be considered. ■

Notes

An 81-year-old woman presents to her physician with palpitations, which she has been experiencing intermittently for 1 month. She has not experienced any syncopal or pre-syncopal symptoms and denies exposure to caffeine-containing foods or over-the-counter medications containing a stimulant. A recent thyroid-stimulating hormone (TSH) test was normal. Her physical exam, including vital signs, is unremarkable. As part of her office-based evaluation, an ECG is obtained.

What is your interpretation of the tracing?

Does it suggest a cause for her symptoms?

If so, what therapy might you pursue?

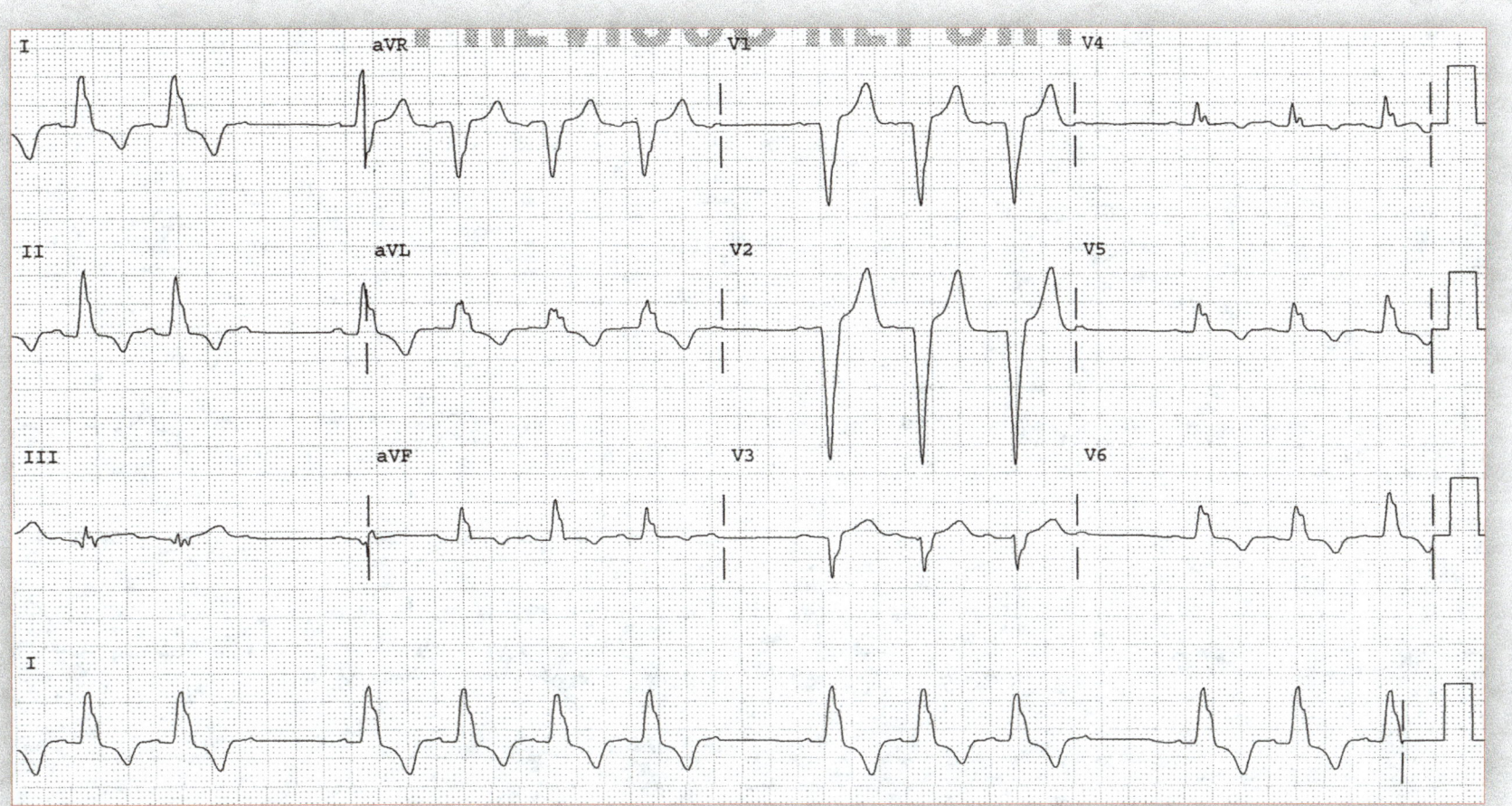

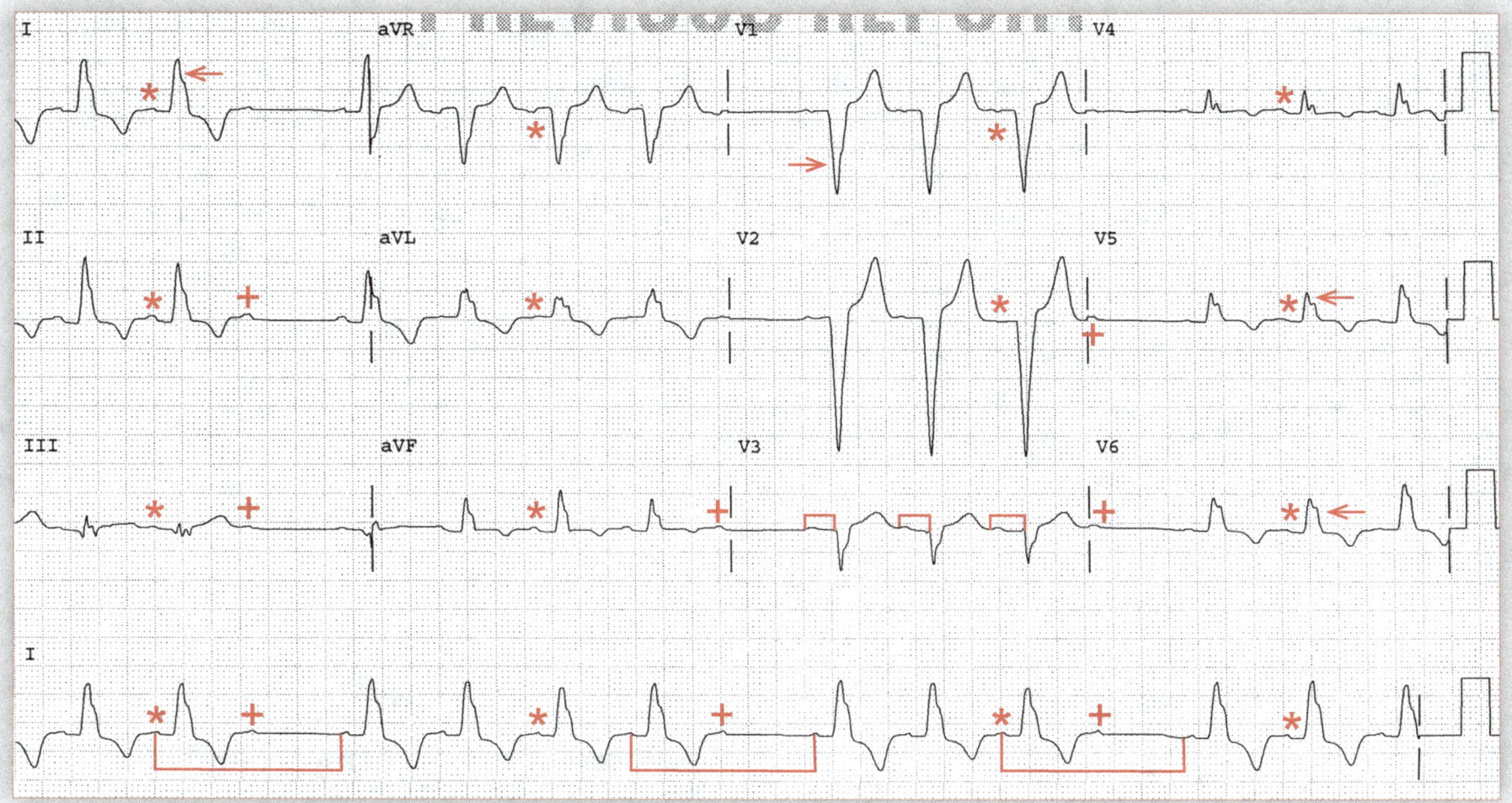

ECG 60 Analysis: Normal sinus rhythm, Mobitz type II second-degree AV block, left bundle branch block

There is a regular atrial rhythm at a rate of 94 bpm. There are P waves (*) before each QRS complex, and they are positive in leads I, II, aVF, and V4-V6. Hence this is normal sinus rhythm. The QRS complex intervals are regularly irregular and grouped beating is present. There are three pauses (⊔), each of which has the same duration (*ie*, twice the underlying sinus rate). The pause is due to a nonconducted, on-time sinus P wave (+); this defines a second-degree AV block. The PR interval (0.18 sec) (⊓) is stable when AV conduction is present. Therefore, this is second-degree AV block, Mobitz type II, which is due to intermittent failure of impulse conduction through the His-Purkinje system. In addition, the QRS complexes are wide (0.16 sec) and have a left bundle branch block pattern (tall, broad R wave in leads I and V5-V6 [←] and a broad QS complex in lead V1 [→]). As both the left anterior and left posterior fascicles are involved, this can be termed bifascicular disease. The QT/QTc intervals are prolonged (440/550 msec) but are normal (360/450 msec) when the increased QRS complex duration is considered.

Mobitz type II second-degree block, when symptomatic or when associated with a widened QRS complex or evidence of bifascicular disease, is an indication for permanent pacemaker implantation as it indicates infra-Hisian disease of the conduction system. When it progresses to complete heart block, Mobitz type II disease is associated with an escape ventricular rhythm that may be slow and associated with symptoms, especially syncope. Even if the rate of the ventricular rhythm is normal, the ventricular focus may be unstable and unpredictable as there is no autonomic control. Hence the ventricular rate may vary widely. The Mobitz type II block, however, is not the cause of this patient's symptoms of palpitations, unless what she means is "skipped beats." The etiology for palpitations needs to be further evaluated. ■

Notes

A 79-year-old woman presents to your urgent care clinic with complaints of 1 day of lightheadedness that came on suddenly and has not resolved. She states that standing makes the lightheadedness worse but denies syncope. On review, she states that preceding this symptom, she had several days of gastroenteritis (with vomiting and diarrhea). These symptoms have largely resolved, but she admits to continued dehydration. Her medical history is notable only for hypertension, for which she takes atenolol. On exam, her vital signs are notable for bradycardia at 44 bpm with an orthostatic fall in her blood pressure. Her cardiopulmonary exam is otherwise normal. Laboratory data are normal except for a blood urea nitrogen level of 46 mg/dL (baseline, 24 mg/dL) and a creatinine level of 1.8 mg/dL (baseline, 1.0 mg/dL). You obtain an ECG.

What abnormalities are shown?

What is the likely etiology?

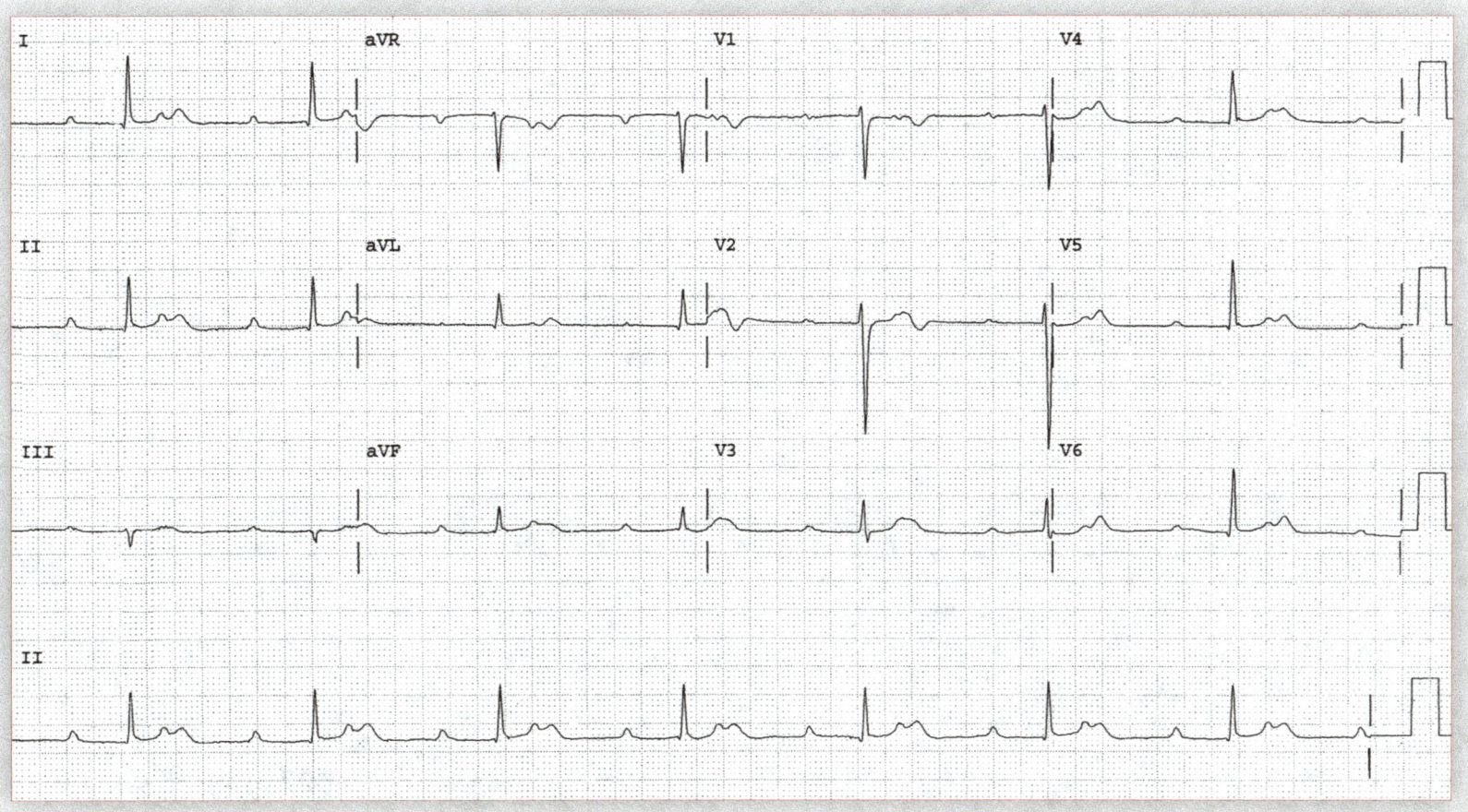

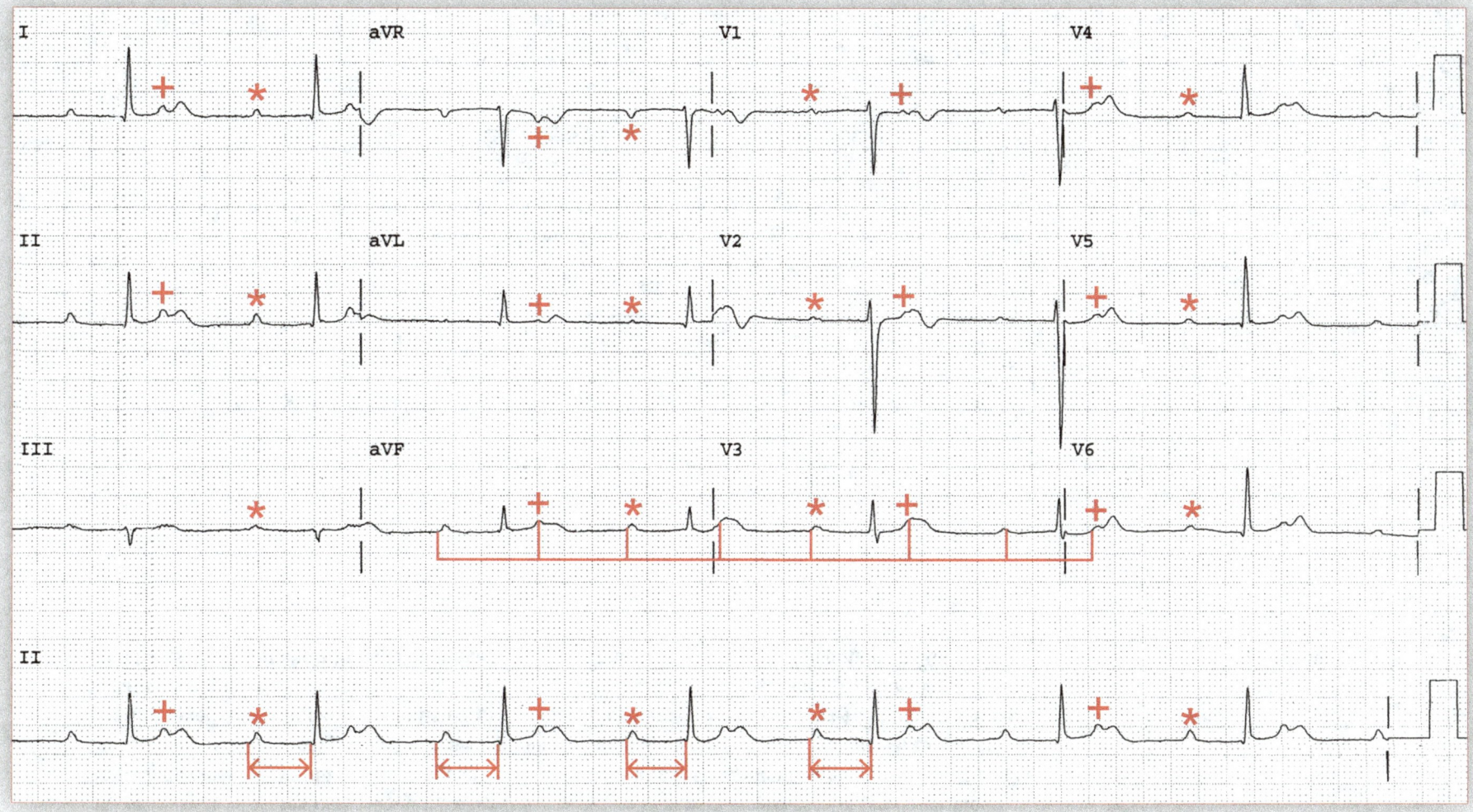

ECG 61 Analysis: Normal sinus rhythm, first-degree AV block (prolonged AV conduction), 2:1 second-degree AV block

The RR intervals are regular at a rate of 44 bpm. A P wave (*) is seen before each QRS complex and the PR interval (↔) is stable at 0.44 second, representing first-degree AV block (prolonged AV conduction). However, a second P wave (+) can be seen at the beginning of the T wave; it is not followed by a QRS complex (*ie*, it is nonconducted). The presence of an occasional nonconducted P wave defines second-degree AV block. The PP intervals are regular (⊔), and hence the atrial rate is stable at 88 bpm. The P wave is positive in leads I, II, aVF, and V4-V6. There is, therefore, a normal sinus rhythm with first- and second-degree AV block present. The second-degree AV block has a pattern of 2:1 conduction. This can be either Mobitz type I or Mobitz type II. The etiology can only be established if there is a change in the pattern of AV conduction (*ie*, there are two or more sequentially conducted P waves). If the PR intervals lengthen progressively, then the diagnosis is a Mobitz type I block; if the PR intervals are constant, it is Mobitz type II.

The QRS complex duration is normal and it has a normal morphology and axis, between 0° and +90° (positive QRS complex in leads I and aVF). The QT/QTc intervals are normal (500/430 msec).

The patient appears to be somewhat dehydrated, with elevated blood urea nitrogen and creatinine levels. This is likely due to the gastroenteritis. The conduction system abnormalities seen on this tracing could be due to an excess effect of β-blocker, as atenolol is a long-acting hydrophilic β-blocker that is cleared from the systemic circulation by the kidneys. This patient's gastroenteritis and dehydration, resulting in pre-renal azotemia, have likely caused an increase in serum atenolol levels and an enhanced β-blocking effect. If this is the cause, then this would be Mobitz type I block, which is an AV nodal conduction abnormality, since the AV node is the structure affected by β-blockade. In contrast, Mobitz type II block is a problem of conduction through the His-Purkinje system, and conduction through this pathway is not affected by β-blockade. Her lightheadedness may be due to continued dehydration from her recent illness or could be the result of her bradycardia. Intravenous fluid infusion to relieve her orthostatic blood pressure response and correct her azotemia is appropriate. If bradycardia worsens or symptoms progress despite intravenous fluid administration, options for immediate treatment of β-blocker toxicity include a catecholamine (*eg*, epinephrine), glucagon, calcium, and possibly insulin plus glucose. As atenolol is a long-acting β-blocker with a half-life of approximately 8 hours and a duration of effect of up to 12 hours with normal renal function and up to 35 hours with marked reduction in renal function, these maneuvers will be short lived. Therefore, if symptoms continue, a catecholamine infusion or placement of a transvenous temporary pacing wire may be required to stabilize the patient until her renal function improves and serum levels of atenolol decrease. ■

Practice Case 62

A 42-year-old man with known pulmonary sarcoidosis is admitted with an episode of unheralded syncope while at home alone. He recovered from the event spontaneously

ECG 62A

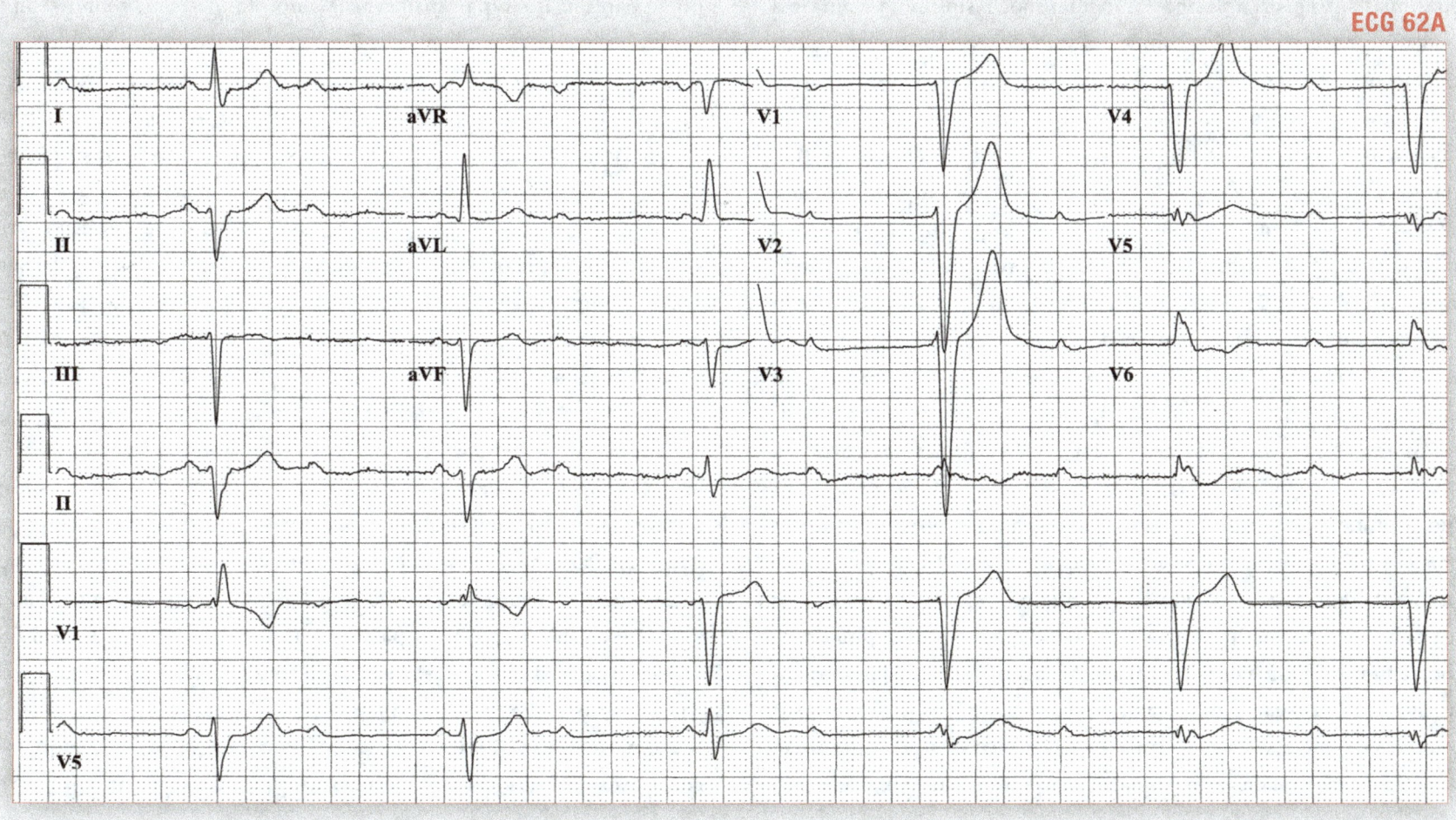

without sequelae and called 911.
His presentation ECG in the emergency
department is shown (62A). A second ECG is
repeated after admission to the hospital (62B).

What abnormalities are depicted?

**What do these abnormalities suggest
about the cause of his syncope?**

ECG 62B

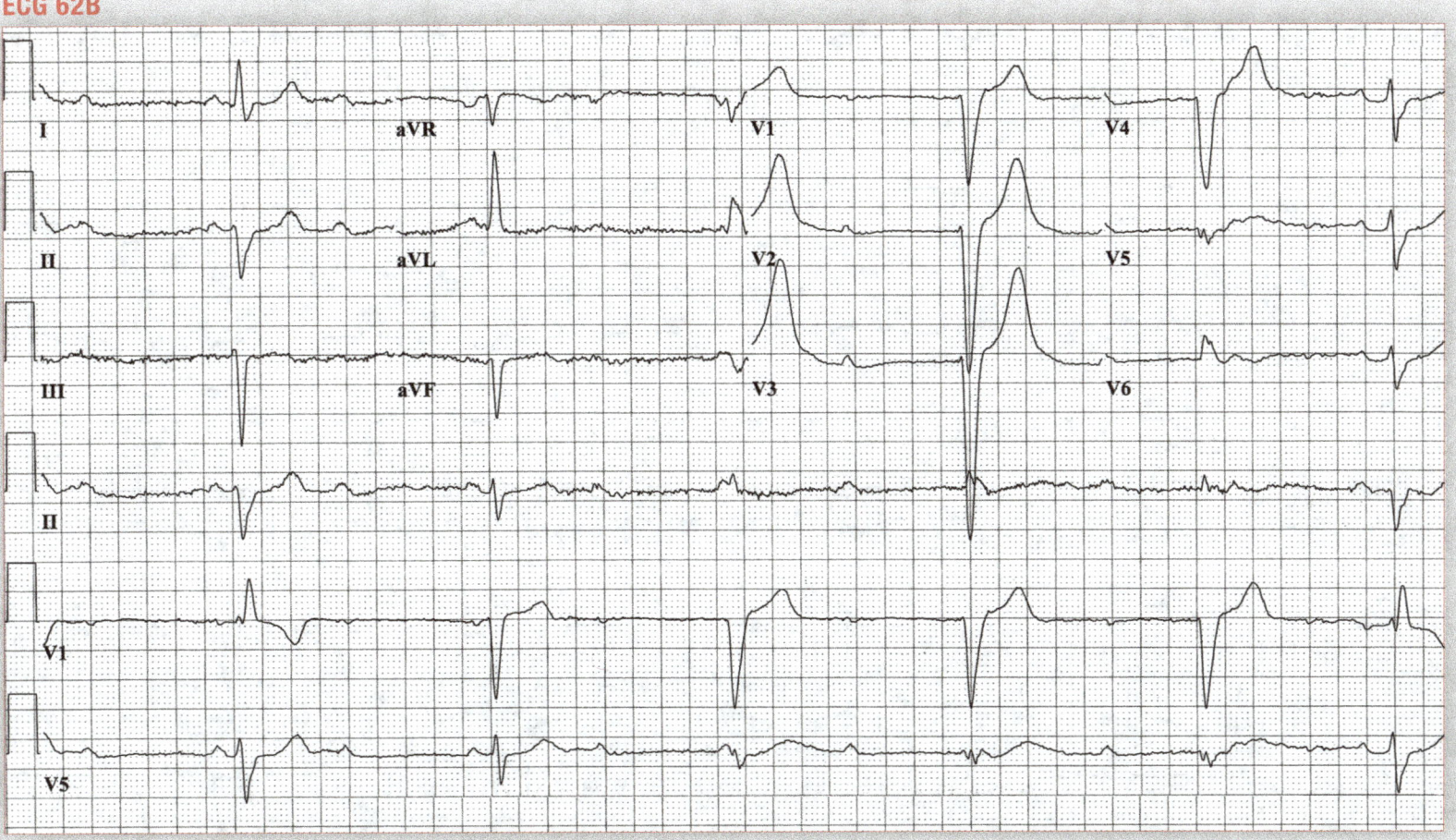

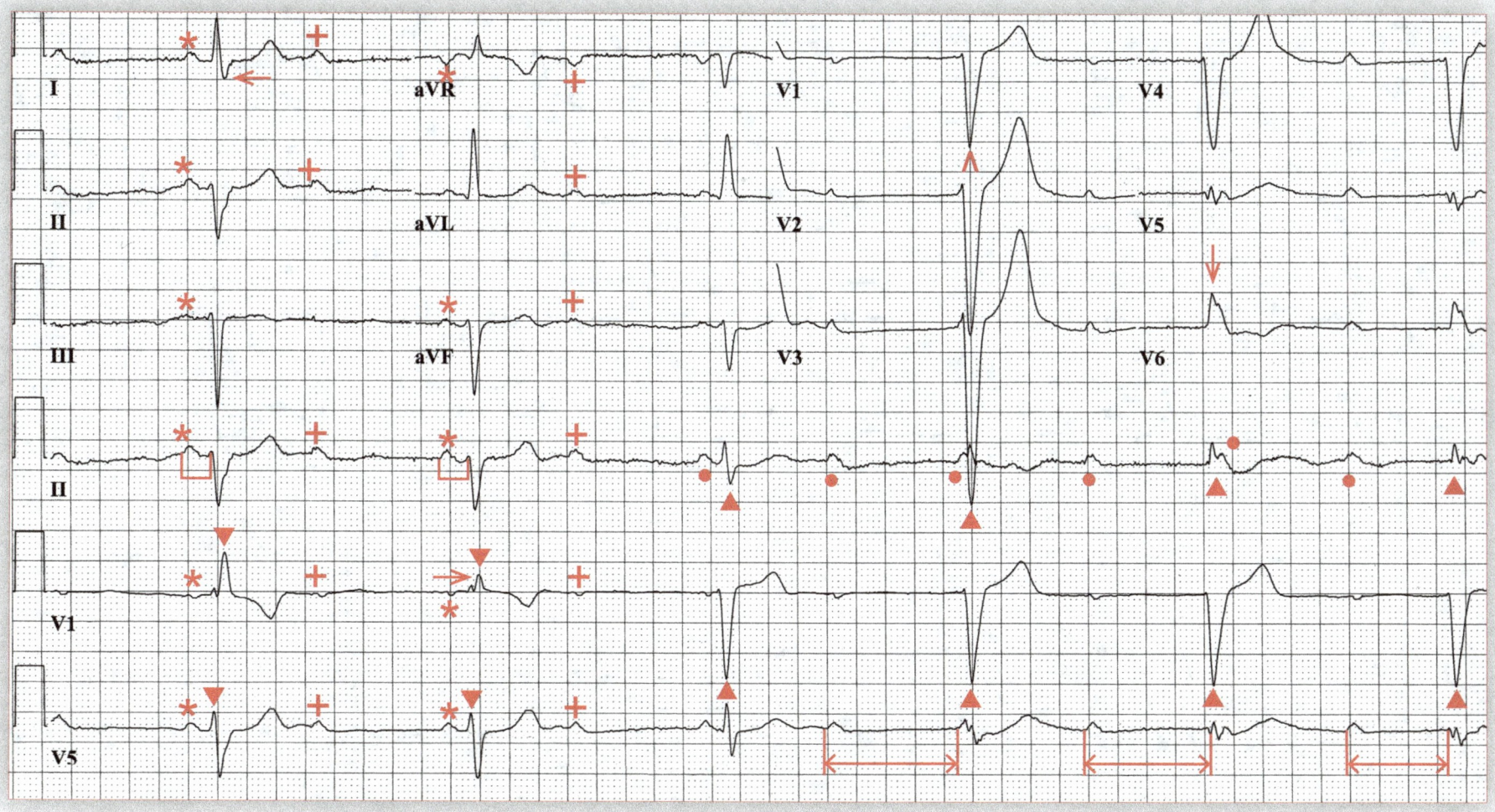

ECG 62A Analysis: Normal sinus rhythm, right bundle branch block (RBBB), left anterior fascicular block (LAFB), 2:1 AV block progressing to complete heart block with an escape ventricular rhythm, trifascicular disease

In **ECG 62A**, the first two QRS complexes (▼), which are at a rate of 34 bpm, have a P wave (*) in front of them with a stable PR interval (⊔) of 0.20 second. The P wave is positive in leads I, II, aVF, and V4-V6, consistent with a normal sinus rhythm. However, an on-time but nonconducted P wave (+) (*ie*, not associated with a QRS complex) is seen after each of these two QRS complexes. Hence the atrial rate is 68 bpm. As every other P wave (+) is nonconducted, this is a second-degree AV block with 2:1 AV conduction.

The first two QRS complexes, which are conducted, have a right bundle branch block (RBBB) pattern (RSR′ morphology in lead V1 [→] and broad S wave in lead I [←]) and a left anterior fascicular block (LAFB), denoted by an extreme left axis, between −30° and −90° (positive QRS complex in lead I and negative QRS complex in leads II and aVF, with an rS morphology). The last four QRS complexes (▲) are at a slightly faster rate (38 bpm) and have a left bundle branch block (LBBB) pattern (deep QS complex in lead V1 [^] and broad R wave in lead V6 [↓]). Noted is atrial activity (●) at a rate of 68 bpm (the same atrial rate as was seen at the beginning of the ECG) with variable PR intervals (↔); this is consistent with AV dissociation. The atrial rate is faster than the ventricular rate and hence this is complete heart block. The QRS complex of the escape rhythm (LBBB morphology) differs from that of the conducted beats (RBBB morphology), and hence this is an escape ventricular rhythm. This indicates that the 2:1 AV block is Mobitz type II and that the block is within the His-Purkinje system. The presence of RBBB and LAFB is diagnostic for bifascicular disease; however, in this case, it can be seen that the complete heart block is associated with an escape ventricular rhythm, indicating disease in the His-Purkinje system. This means that there is conduction disease in the remaining fascicle (*ie*, left posterior fascicle). Therefore, this is trifascicular block.

continues

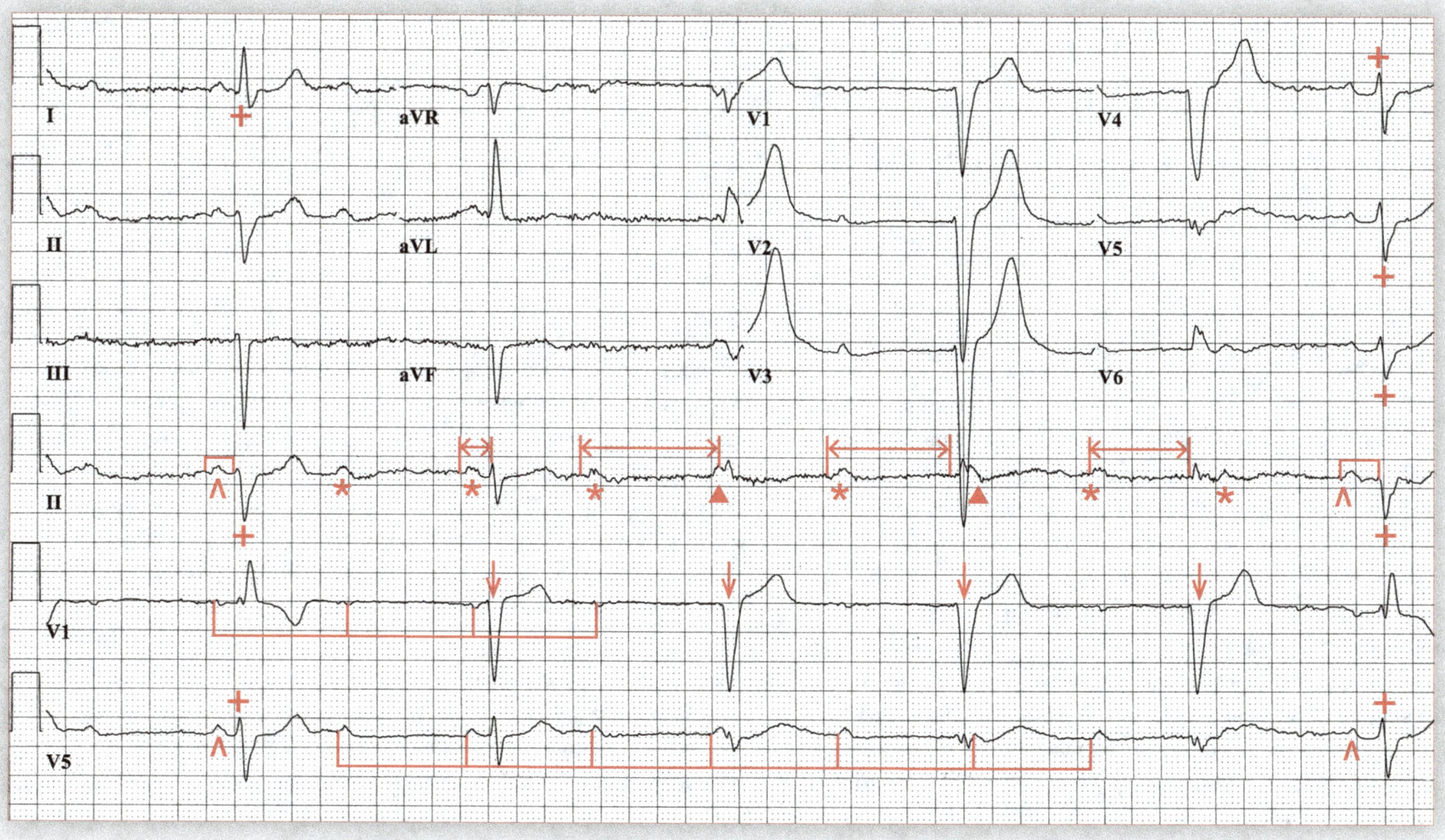

ECG 62B Analysis: Normal sinus rhythm, complete heart block with an escape ventricular rhythm and intermittent capture with complexes having an RBBB and LAFB, trifascicular disease

ECG **62B** shows the same pattern as ECG **62A**. The first and last QRS complexes (+) have an RBBB pattern and there is a P wave (^) before each; the PR intervals preceding them are the same (0.20 sec) (⊓). These complexes are identical to the conducted complexes seen in ECG **62A**. The second, third, fourth, and fifth QRS complexes (↓) have an LBBB pattern at a rate of 36 bpm, similar to the complexes during complete heart block on ECG **62A**. Noted are P waves (*), which have a regular PP interval (⊔) at an atrial rate of 68 bpm. Some of the P waves are not seen because they are superimposed on the QRS complex (▲). However, the P waves that are seen occur at a regular interval (⊔). There is variability of the PR intervals (↔); therefore, AV dissociation is present. As the atrial rate (68 bpm) is faster than the ventricular rate (36 bpm), this is complete AV block with an escape ventricular rhythm. The block is within the His-Purkinje system. However, the first and last QRS complexes (+) are supraventricular in origin and have the same PR interval. Hence they are captured complexes and, therefore, there is complete heart block with intermittent capture. It is not uncommon for there to be intermittent AV conduction (and hence capture) during complete heart block. Indeed, the complete heart block may be transient, with subsequent restoration of intact AV conduction. With the complete heart block and a slow ventricular rate the patient might become symptomatic and even experience syncope. If there is resolution of the complete AV block with resumption of AV conduction, the patient spontaneously recovers; this has been termed Stokes-Adams attacks and is seen with transient complete heart block. ◼

Notes

A 71-year-old woman is admitted to the hospital with a new diagnosis of atrial fibrillation and rapid ventricular response. She was started on verapamil and achieved rate control quickly, eventually spontaneously converting to sinus rhythm. On the day of discharge, an ECG reviewed by the medical resident causes alarm. The resident presents the ECG to you.

What finding on the ECG concerned the house officer?

What would be an appropriate course of action?

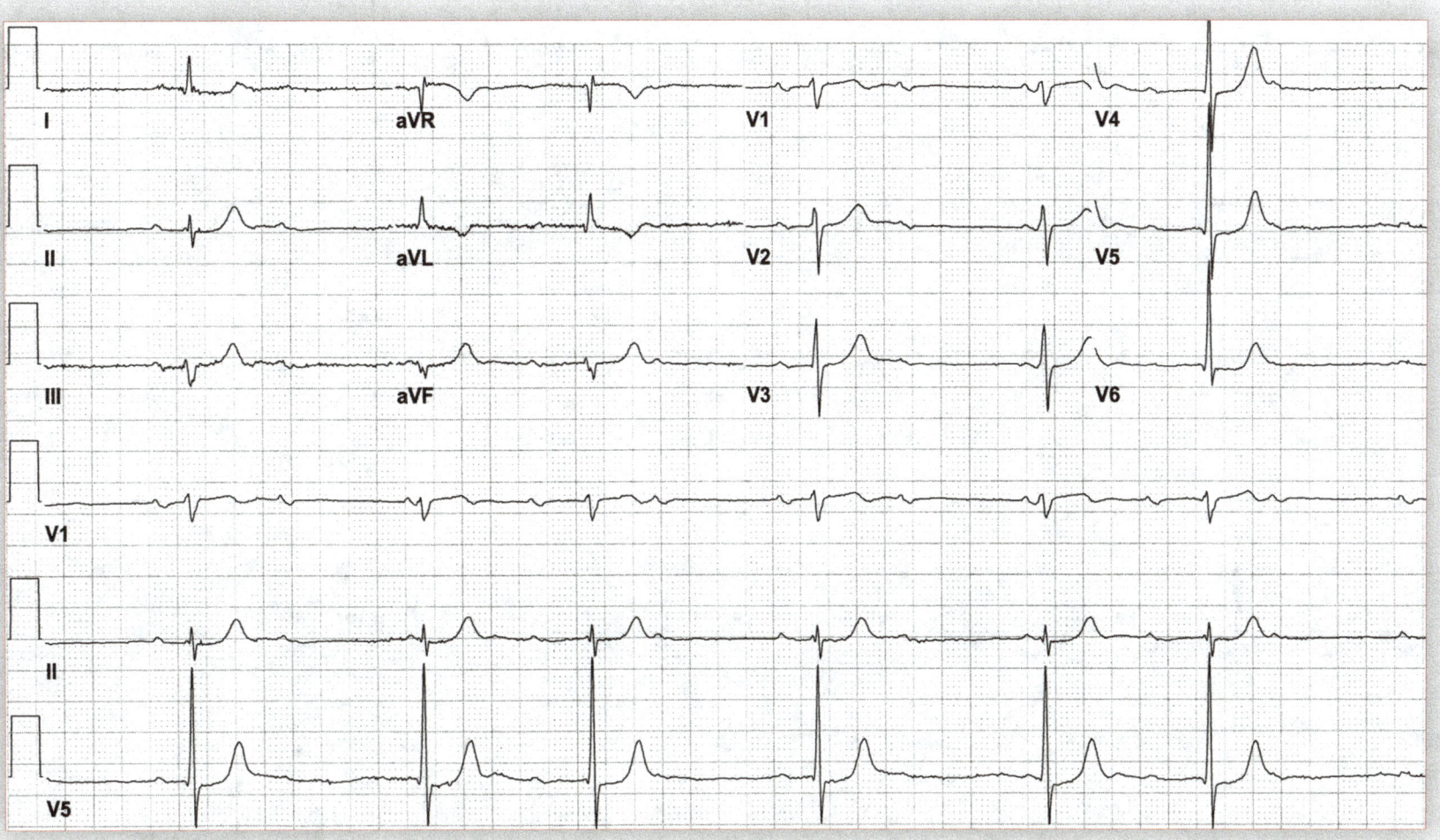

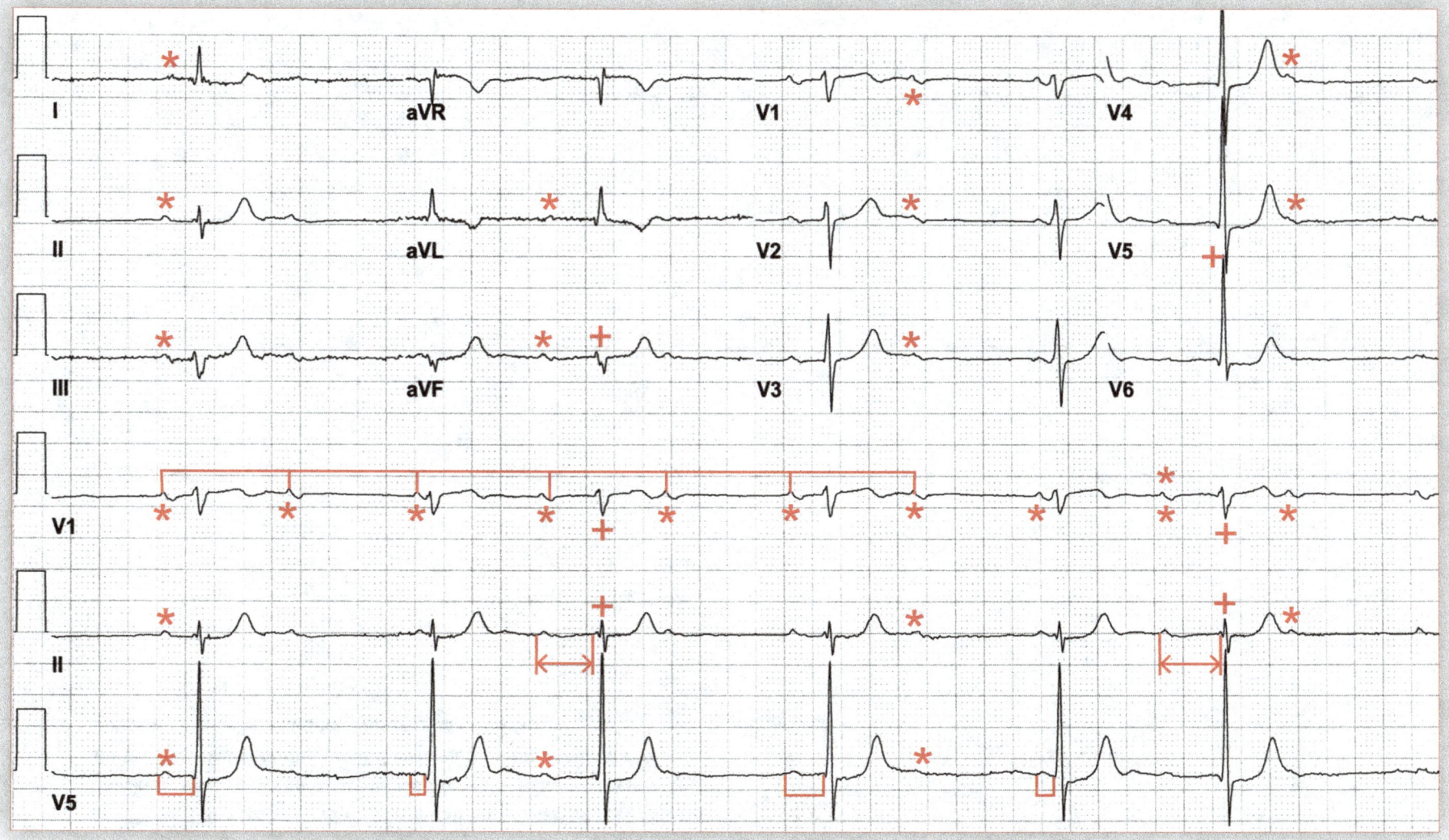

ECG 63 Analysis: Normal sinus rhythm, complete heart block with escape junctional rhythm, intermittent capture, first-degree AV block (prolonged AV conduction)

The rhythm is regularly irregular with long and short RR intervals. The ventricular rate is 42 bpm, although there are two QRS complexes (third and sixth) that are early (+), at a rate of 50 bpm. There are P waves seen (*), and they have a stable PP interval (⊓). The atrial rate is 72 bpm. The P waves are positive in leads I, II, aVF, and V4-V6. Hence this is a normal sinus rhythm. The PR intervals are variable (⊔); hence AV dissociation is present. As the atrial rate is faster than the ventricular rate, this is complete (third-degree) AV block. However, the PR intervals associated with the two early QRS complexes (+) are the same (0.38 sec) (↔). Since these two complexes are early, they are in response to the P waves before them. In addition, the presence of the same PR interval in both cases indicates intact AV conduction. Therefore, these two complexes represent AV conduction with first-degree AV block (prolonged AV conduction). Since the conducted and nonconducted QRS complexes have the same morphology, there is complete heart block with an escape junctional rhythm. Therefore, the AV block is within the AV node. The QRS complexes have a normal duration (0.08 sec) and morphology. There is a left axis, between 0° and −30° (positive QRS complex in leads I and II and negative QRS complex in lead aVF). The QT/QTc intervals are normal (480/400 msec).

It is possible that the complete heart block, which is due to an abnormality of AV nodal conduction, is the result of verapamil. Since verapamil was used for ventricular rate control during atrial fibrillation, this drug is no longer necessary now that sinus rhythm has been restored. Verapamil, a calcium-channel blocker, works only on the AV and sinus nodes, which have their electrophysiologic properties mediated by calcium currents. It has no direct effects on atrial or ventricular myocardium, which have electrophysiologic properties mediated by a fast action potential that is a result of rapid influxes of sodium ion. It is unlikely that the reversion to normal sinus rhythm was related to the verapamil. ■

Notes

A 53-year-old woman with systemic hypertension and resultant mild renal dysfunction is seen by her primary physician. She has not had any new symptoms, and a review of systems is unremarkable. An ECG is obtained as part of her routine evaluation.

What abnormalities are seen?

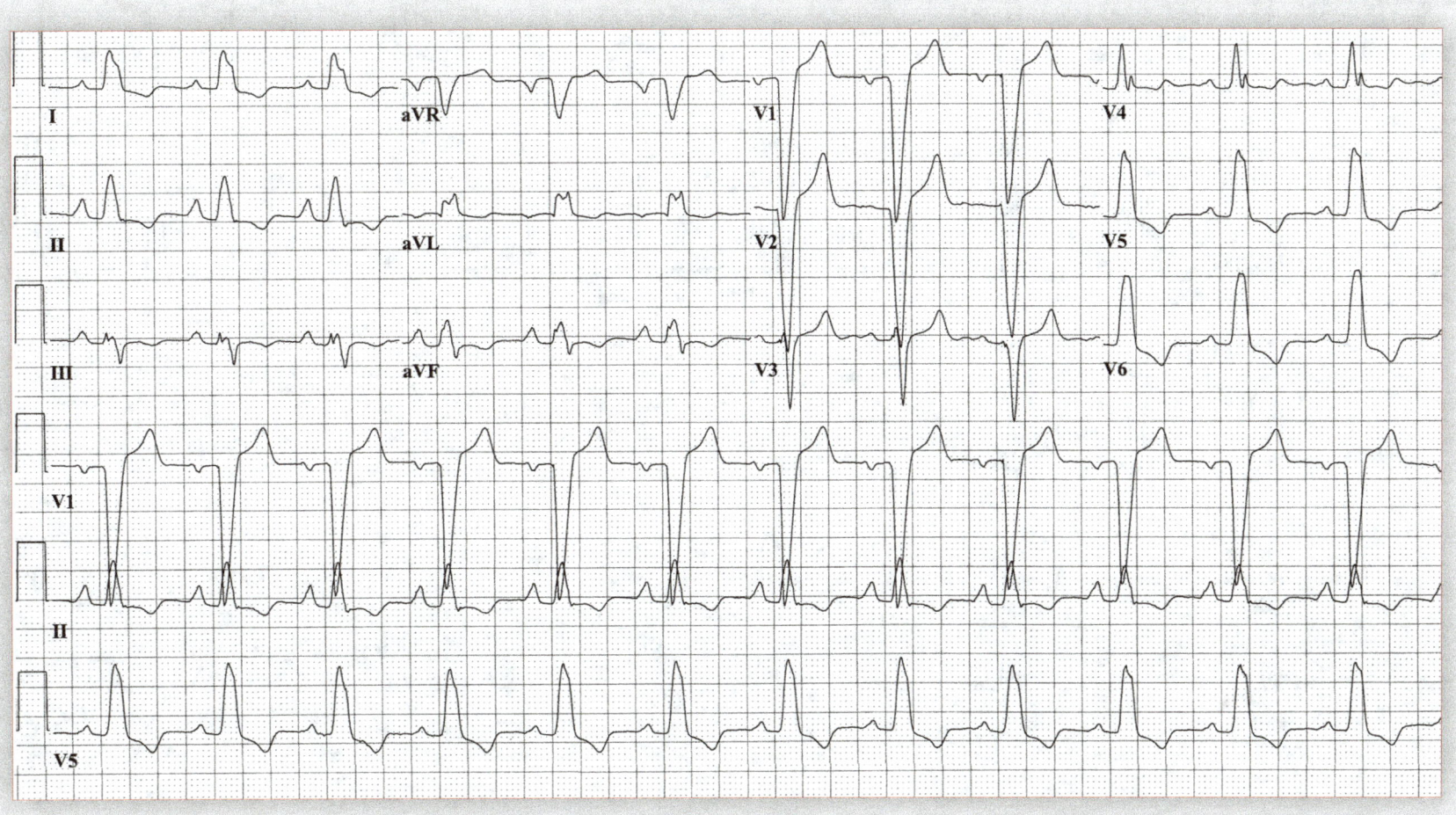

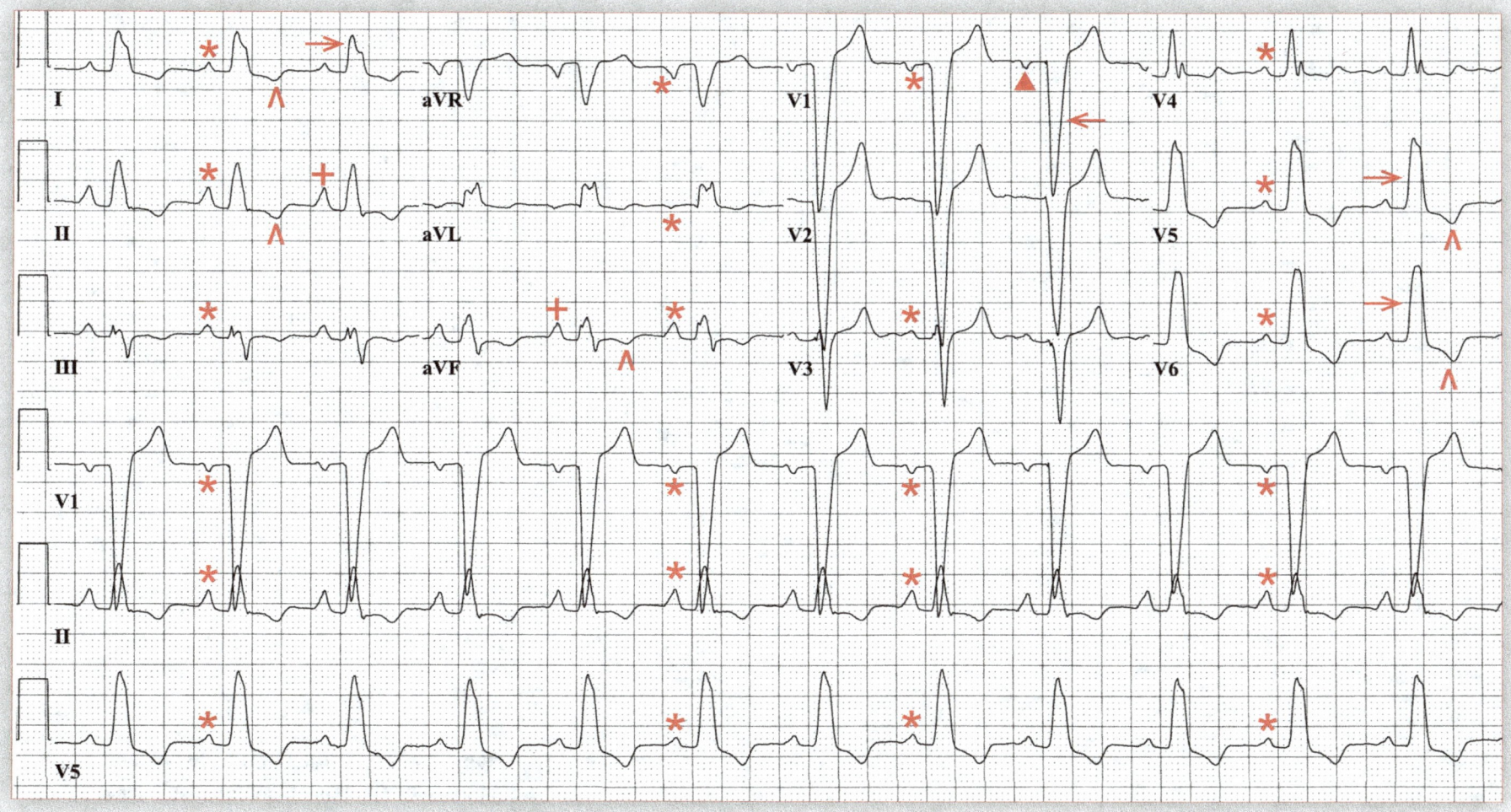

ECG 64 Analysis: Normal sinus rhythm, biatrial hypertrophy (abnormality), left bundle branch block

There is a regular rhythm at a rate of 74 bpm. A P wave (*) is seen before each QRS complex, and the PR interval is constant (0.20 sec). The P wave is positive in leads I, II, aVF, and V4-V6. Hence this is a normal sinus rhythm. The P waves are tall and peaked (+) in leads II and aVF, suggesting right atrial hypertrophy. The presence of a negative P wave (▲) in lead V1 suggests left atrial hypertrophy. These P-wave abnormalities are consistent with biatrial hypertrophy (abnormality). The QRS complex duration is lengthened (0.16 sec), and there is a pattern of a left bundle branch block (broad R wave in leads I and V5-V6 [→] and deep QS complex in lead V1 [←]). Also noted are ST-T wave abnormalities (^) associated with the left bundle branch block. The QT/QTc intervals are prolonged (440/490 msec) but are normal when corrected for the prolonged QRS duration (360/400 msec).

A very common ECG finding in hypertension is left ventricular hypertrophy (LVH). However, in this case, LVH cannot be diagnosed because of the presence of the LBBB. With an LBBB there is direct activation of the left ventricular myocardium, bypassing the normal His-Purkinje system. Hence the diagnosis of left ventricular abnormalities such as LVH cannot be reliably established. An LBBB is often seen with pre-existing LVH due to fibrosis of the septum, which can often affect the His-Purkinje system (especially the left bundle). The presence of LVH can, however, be established with an echocardiogram. In addition, left atrial hypertrophy may develop as a result of the LVH, which is associated with diastolic dysfunction and elevated left ventricular filling pressures. Although the presence of right atrial hypertrophy is uncommon with systemic hypertension, it may occur if there is significant diastolic dysfunction, as may be seen with LVH resulting in pulmonary hypertension and hence elevated right-sided pressures. ■

A 34-year-old man is seen for a physical exam before getting his pilot's license. He denies any current symptoms or any history of symptoms. An ECG is performed as part of his evaluation.

What is your interpretation of his ECG?

What additional evaluation is indicated?

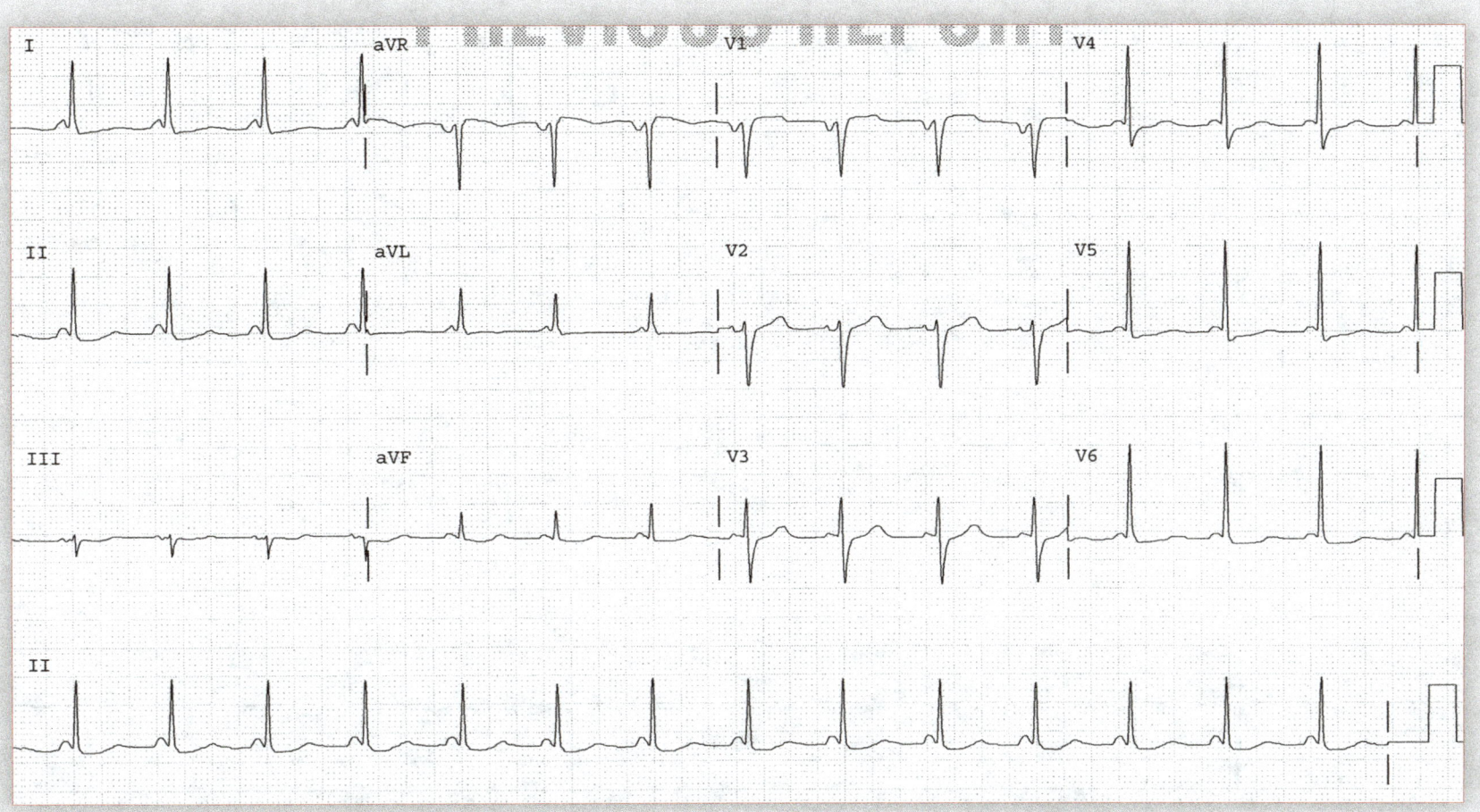

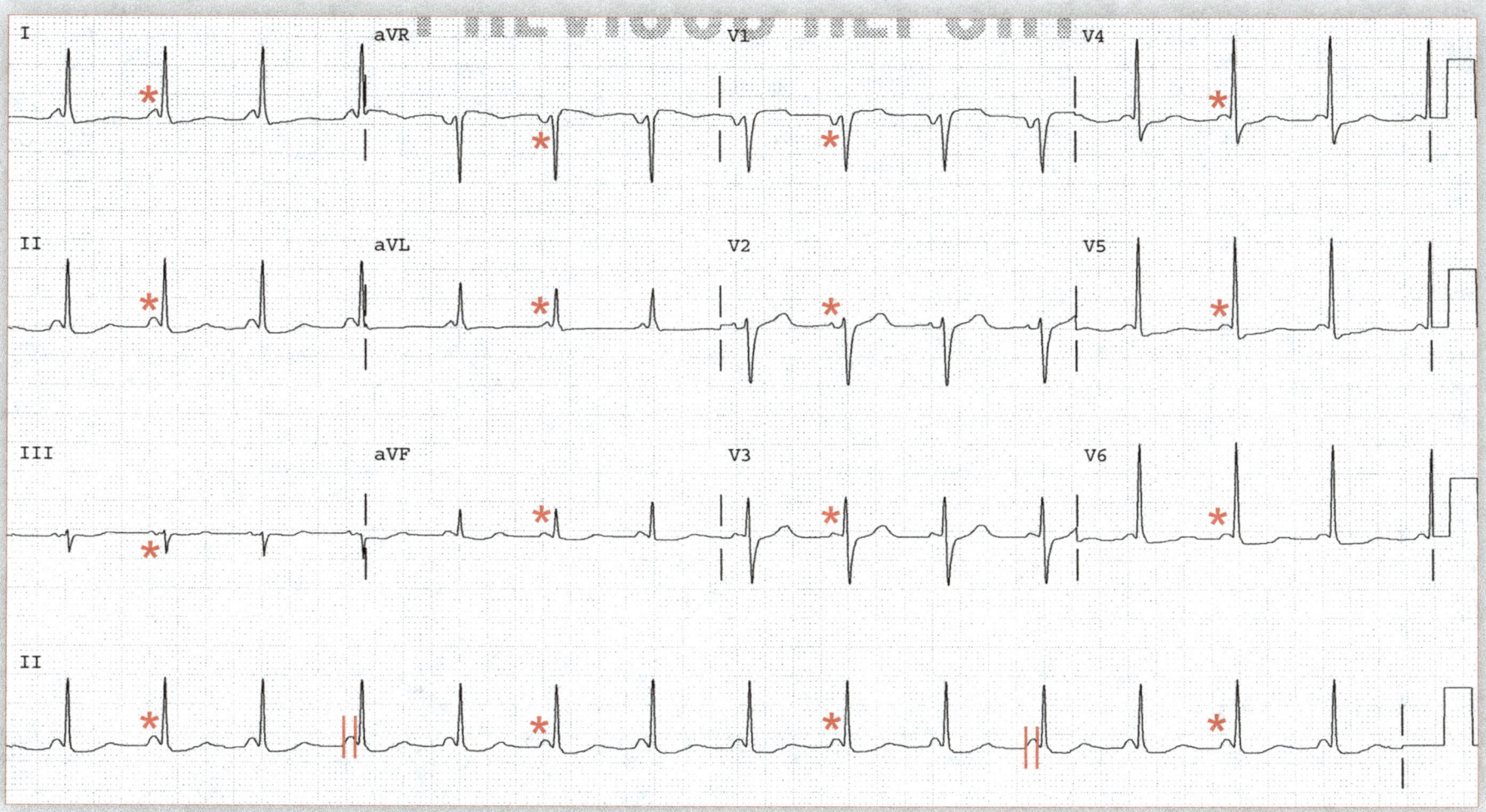

ECG 65 Analysis: **Normal sinus rhythm, short PR interval (enhanced or accelerated AV conduction)**

The rhythm is regular at a rate of 86 bpm. There is a P wave (*) before each QRS complex, and it is positive in leads I, II, aVF, and V4-V6; hence it is a normal sinus rhythm. The PR interval (‖) is constant but short (0.10 sec). The QRS complex is normal in width and morphology. The QT/QTc intervals are normal (380/430 msec).

The normal PR interval ranges from 0.14 to 0.20 second. The PR interval includes the P wave (which reflects atrial depolarization) and the PR segment, which reflects conduction through the AV node and His-Purkinje system. In this case, there is a short PR segment. The major component of the PR segment is AV nodal conduction as the AV node is the site of slowest conduction velocity within the conduction system. A PR interval less than 0.14 second is considered short and indicates either enhanced conduction through the AV node or bypass of the AV node, a result of an accessory pathway. In the case of an accessory pathway, an ECG with a short PR interval and normal QRS complex is due to a pathway called the bundle of James that bypasses the AV node but connects into the bundle of His. This is termed a Lown-Ganong-Levine (LGL) pattern. It is a form of preexcitation syndrome and may be associated with a reentrant arrhythmia called AV reentrant tachycardia. This patient does not have any history of arrhythmia and has no symptoms suggestive of arrhythmia. He has an LGL pattern, but not LGL syndrome. Hence no additional evaluation or therapy is warranted. ■

Practice Case 66

A 55-year-old man with a strong family history of cardiac disease presents to the clinic for a routine physical. He states that most of the male members of his family have had pacemakers

ECG 66A

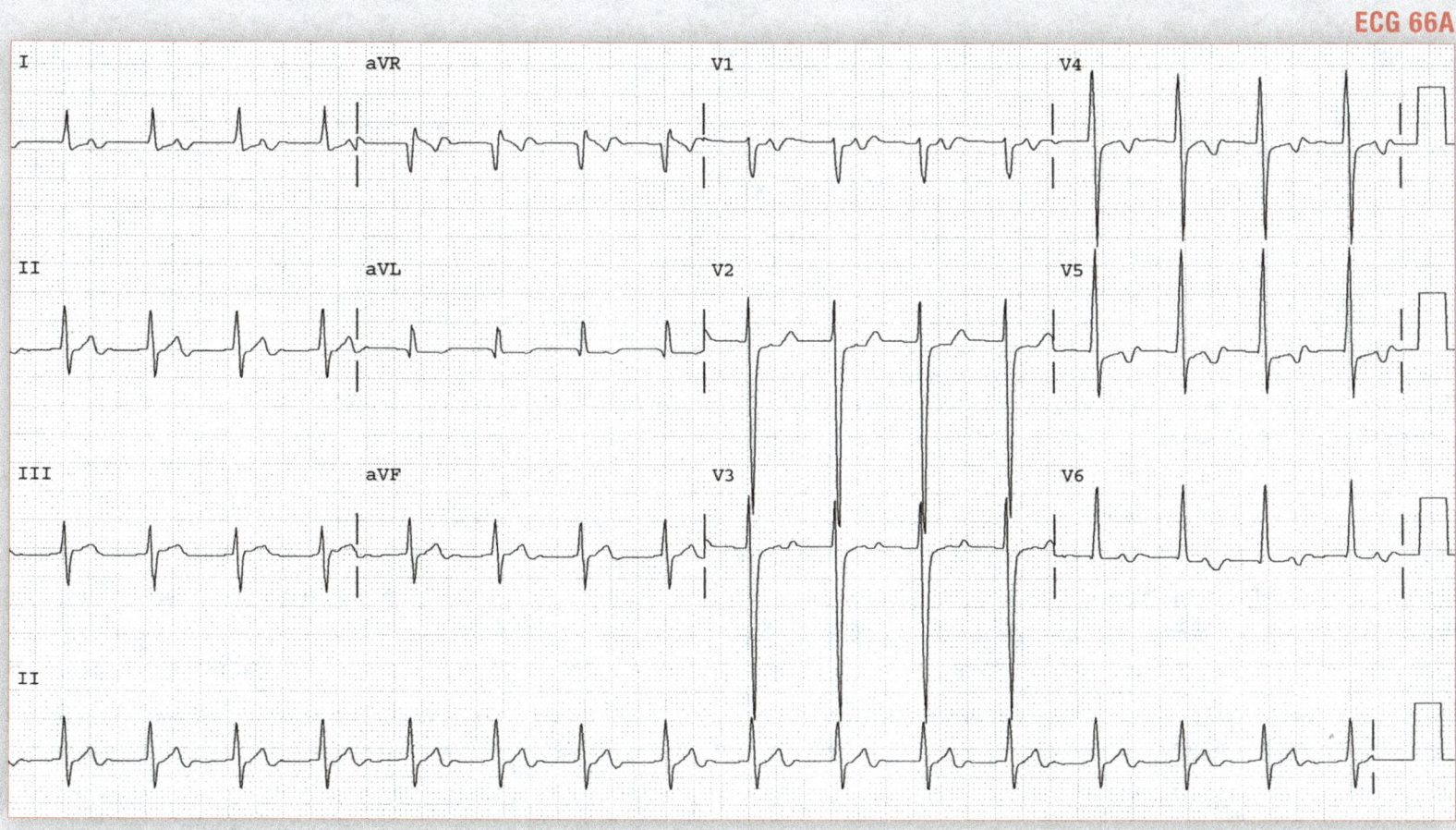

implanted in their fifth to sixth decade of life.
His review of systems is negative. Given his family
history of cardiac disease, a routine ECG is performed
(66A) and is compared with a previous ECG (66B).

What abnormality is present?

Is there any change in the ECGs?

Is any therapy warranted?

ECG 66B

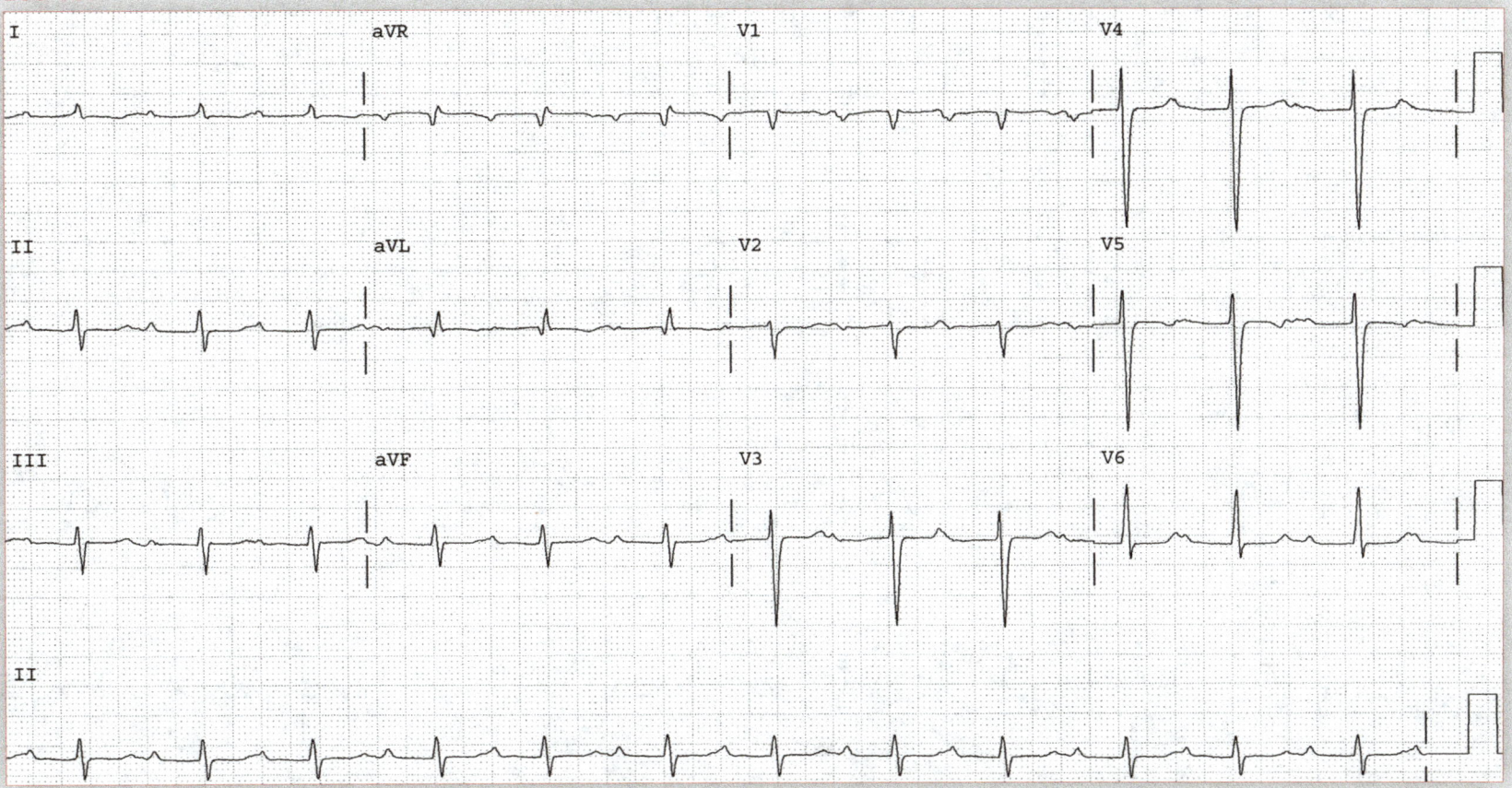

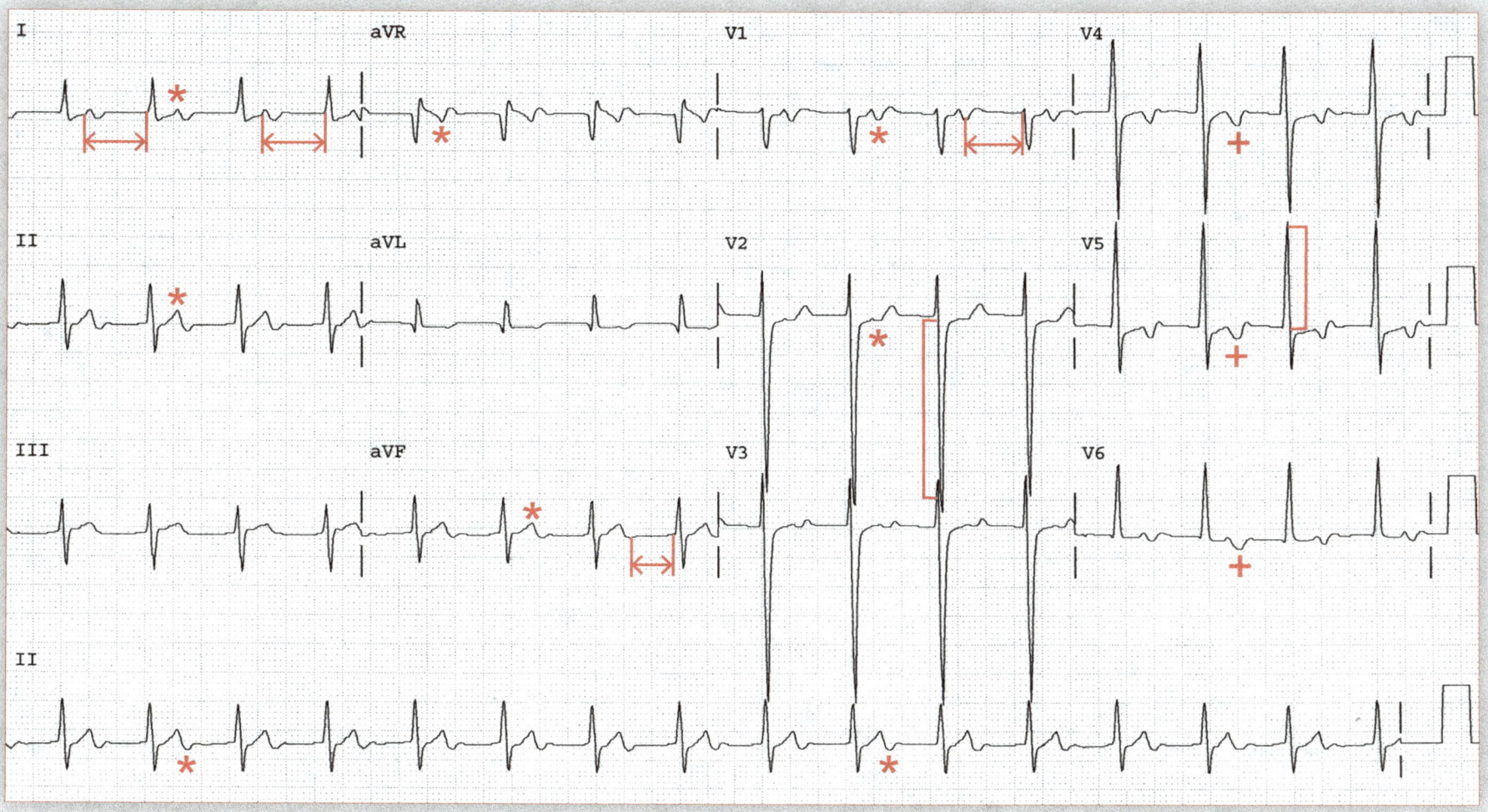

ECG 66A Analysis: Sinus tachycardia, short RP tachycardia, nonspecific T-wave abnormalities, left ventricular hypertrophy

ECG **66A** shows a regular rhythm at a rate of 100 bpm; hence this is a tachycardia. The QRS complex duration is normal (0.08 sec) and there is a normal morphology and axis, between 0° and +90° (positive QRS complex in leads I and aVF). The depth of the S wave in lead V2 is 30 mm ([ ), and the R-wave amplitude in lead V5 is 17 mm ( ]), for a total of 47 mm. This meets one of the criteria for left ventricular hypertrophy (LVH; S-wave depth in lead V1 or V2 + R-wave amplitude in lead V5 or V6 ≥ 35 mm). Apparent T-wave abnormalities (+) are seen in leads V4-V6; these are likely secondary to LVH. The QT/QTc intervals are normal (320/410 msec).

P waves are not obvious, but abnormal waveforms are seen in the ST segments in leads I and V1-V3 that are suggestive of superimposed P waves (*). This is, therefore, short RP tachycardia with a long PR interval (0.42 sec) (↔). The etiology for short RP tachycardia includes sinus tachycardia with first-degree AV block (prolonged AV conduction), atrial tachycardia, ectopic junctional tachycardia (with a retrograde P wave), atrial flutter with 2:1 AV block, typical AV nodal reentrant tachycardia (*ie*, slow-fast), or AV reentrant tachycardia (associated with preexcitation or an accessory pathway). It appears that the P waves are positive in lead aVF, eliminating any arrhythmia with retrograde P waves (*ie*, ectopic junctional tachycardia, AV nodal reentrant tachycardia, or AV reentrant tachycardia). A second atrial waveform is not seen, and hence this is not atrial flutter with 2:1 AV block. It is not certain whether the P waves are positive or negative in leads I and V4-V6 as the negative T-wave abnormalities might be due to P waves. Thus this is either sinus or atrial tachycardia. *continues*

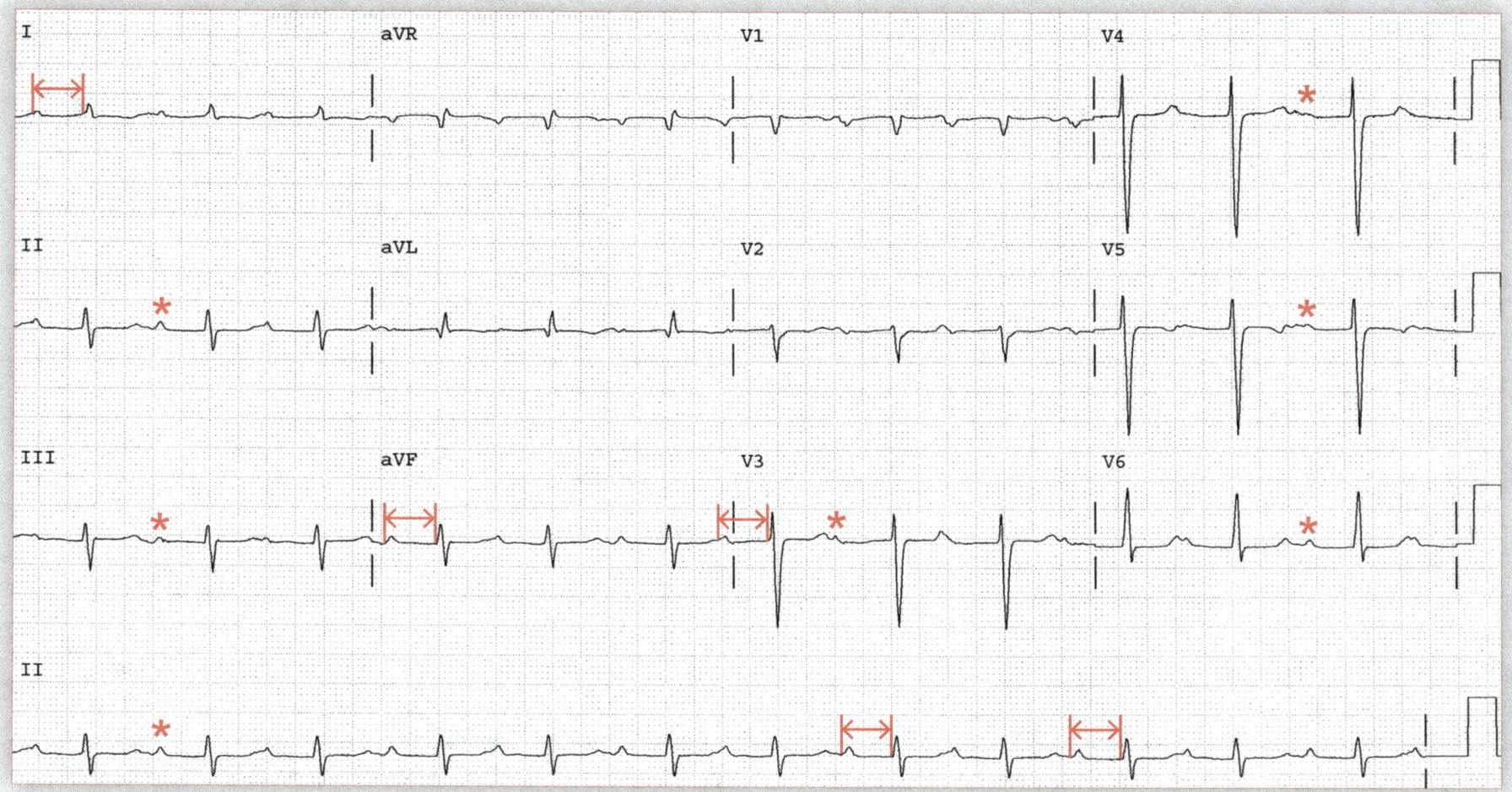

**ECG 66B Analysis: Normal sinus rhythm, first-degree AV block
(prolonged AV conduction), nonspecific T-wave abnormalities**

ECG **66B** shows a regular rhythm at a rate of 72 bpm. The QRS complex duration, morphology, and axis are identical to those seen in ECG **66A**. The QT/QTc intervals are also the same. Positive or upright P waves (*) are now obviously seen before some of the QRS complexes in leads I, II, aVF, and V3-V6. The PR interval is constant at 0.38 second (↔). Therefore, this is a normal sinus rhythm with first-degree AV block (prolonged AV conduction). The P waves are obvious on this ECG because the sinus rate is slower than in ECG **66A**. The PR interval in ECG **66B** is very similar to the interval seen in ECG **66A** (↔) between the abnormal waveform and the subsequent QRS complex. Therefore, this abnormal waveform is a superimposed P wave, as a result of the more rapid heart rate, and it is not apparent as a distinct waveform. The fact that the PR interval as measured on

ECG **66B** is very similar to the interval on ECG **66A** confirms that the short RP tachycardia is sinus tachycardia with first-degree AV block.

When the sinus rate increases in the setting of first-degree AV block, the P wave may become superimposed on the preceding ST segment or T wave; hence the P wave may not be obvious. However, the ST segment and T-wave upstroke and downstroke should be smooth. Any notching or bumps in the ST segment or on the T waves should raise suspicion for superimposed P waves. In this situation, it may be useful to slow the sinus rhythm, which can be accomplished by enhancing vagal tone, as with carotid sinus pressure or Valsalva maneuver. In addition, P waves should be sought if there is any pause in the RR intervals, as may occur with a premature complex. ■

Practice Case 67

A 34-year-old man presents to his primary physician for a routine exam. He is about to embark on his third triathlon, for which he has been actively training for over a year. A thorough review of systems is negative.

ECG 67A

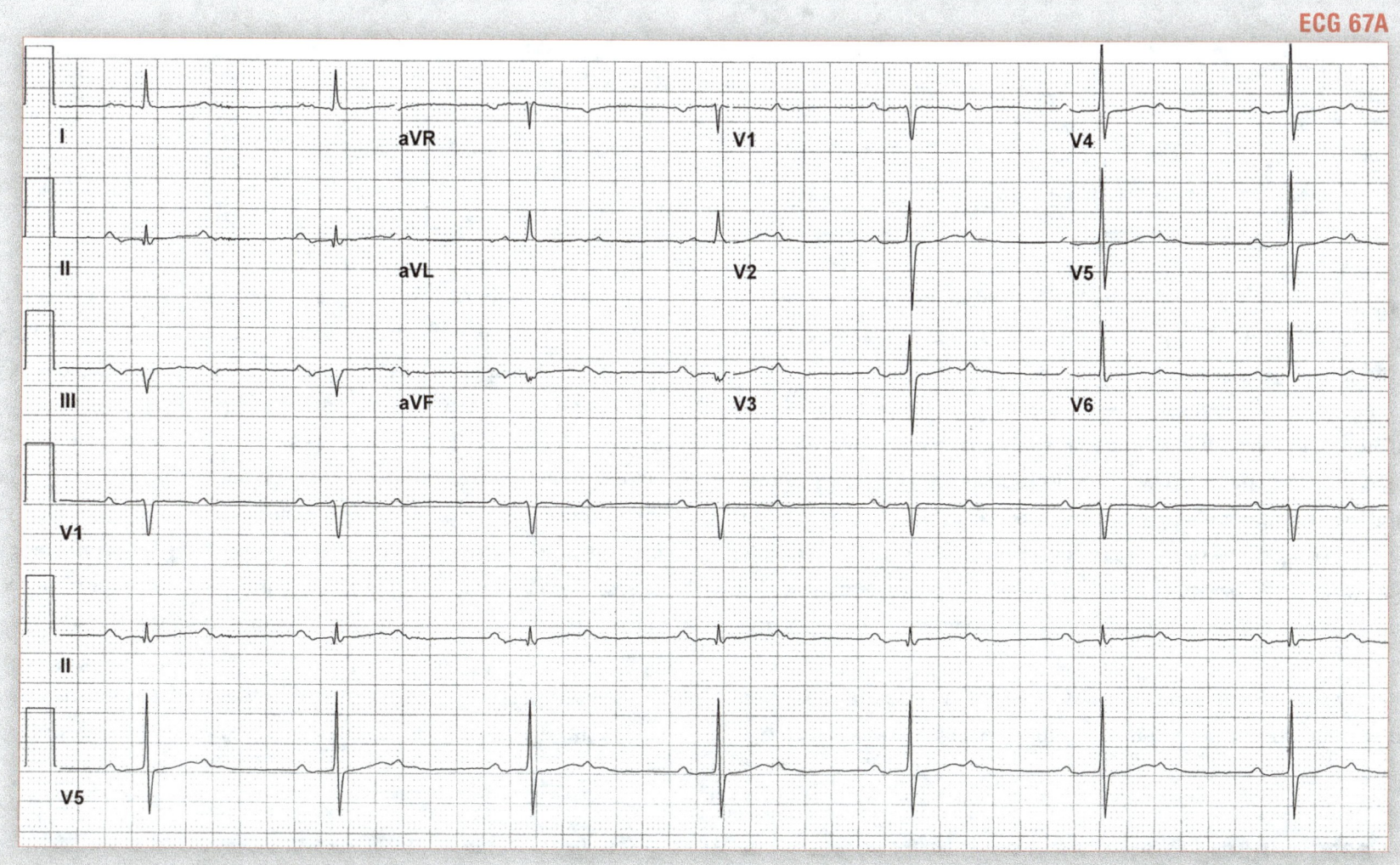

The patient has no known medical diagnoses. As part of the evaluation, the physician obtains an ECG (67A). The physician requests that the patient return the next day for follow-up, and a second ECG is obtained (67B).

What conduction abnormalities are noted on ECG 67A?

What is the likely cause?

What further diagnostic information does the second ECG (67B) provide?

ECG 67B

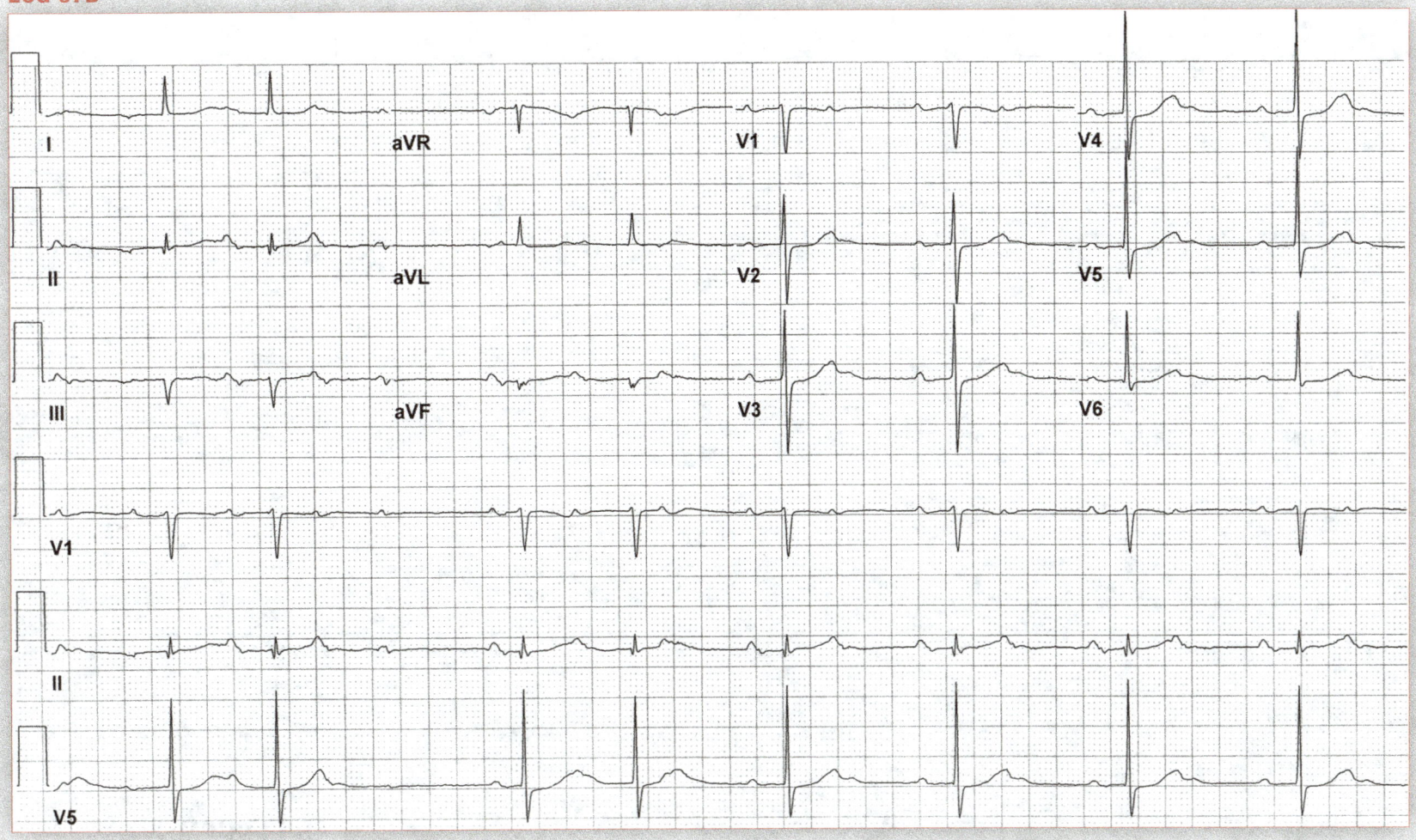

Podrid's Real-World ECGs

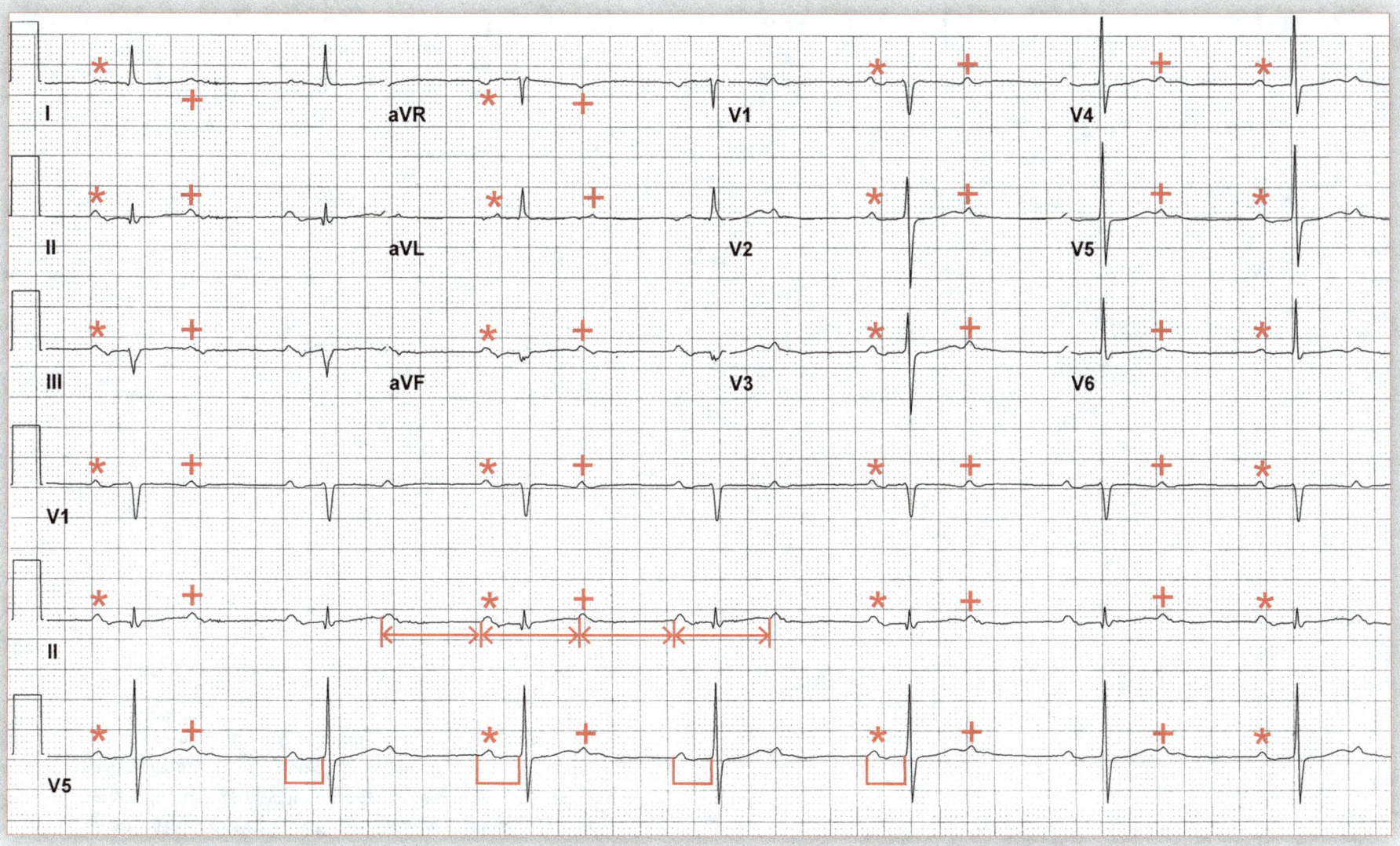

ECG 67A Analysis: Normal sinus rhythm, first-degree AV block (prolonged AV conduction), 2:1 second-degree AV block, low limb lead voltage

ECG 67A shows P waves (*,+) that have a regular PP interval (↔) at a rate of 84 bpm. There is a second P wave after each QRS complex (+). This second P wave is nonconducted. There are P waves (*) before each QRS complex, and they are positive in leads I, II, aVF, and V4-V6. Hence this is a normal sinus rhythm. The presence of occasional non-conducted P waves defines second-degree AV block. When the P wave is conducted the PR interval (⊔) is constant, although prolonged at 0.28 second; hence there is also a first-degree AV block (prolonged AV conduction). As every other P wave is nonconducted there is a second-degree AV block with 2:1 conduction; this may be either Mobitz type I or Mobitz type II. The ventricular rate is 42 bpm.

The QRS complex duration is normal (0.08 sec), and there is low voltage in the limb leads (< 5 mm in each limb lead). There is a physiologic left axis, between 0° and −30° (positive QRS complex in leads I and II and negative QRS complex in lead aVF). The QT/QTc intervals are normal (460/384 msec).

continues

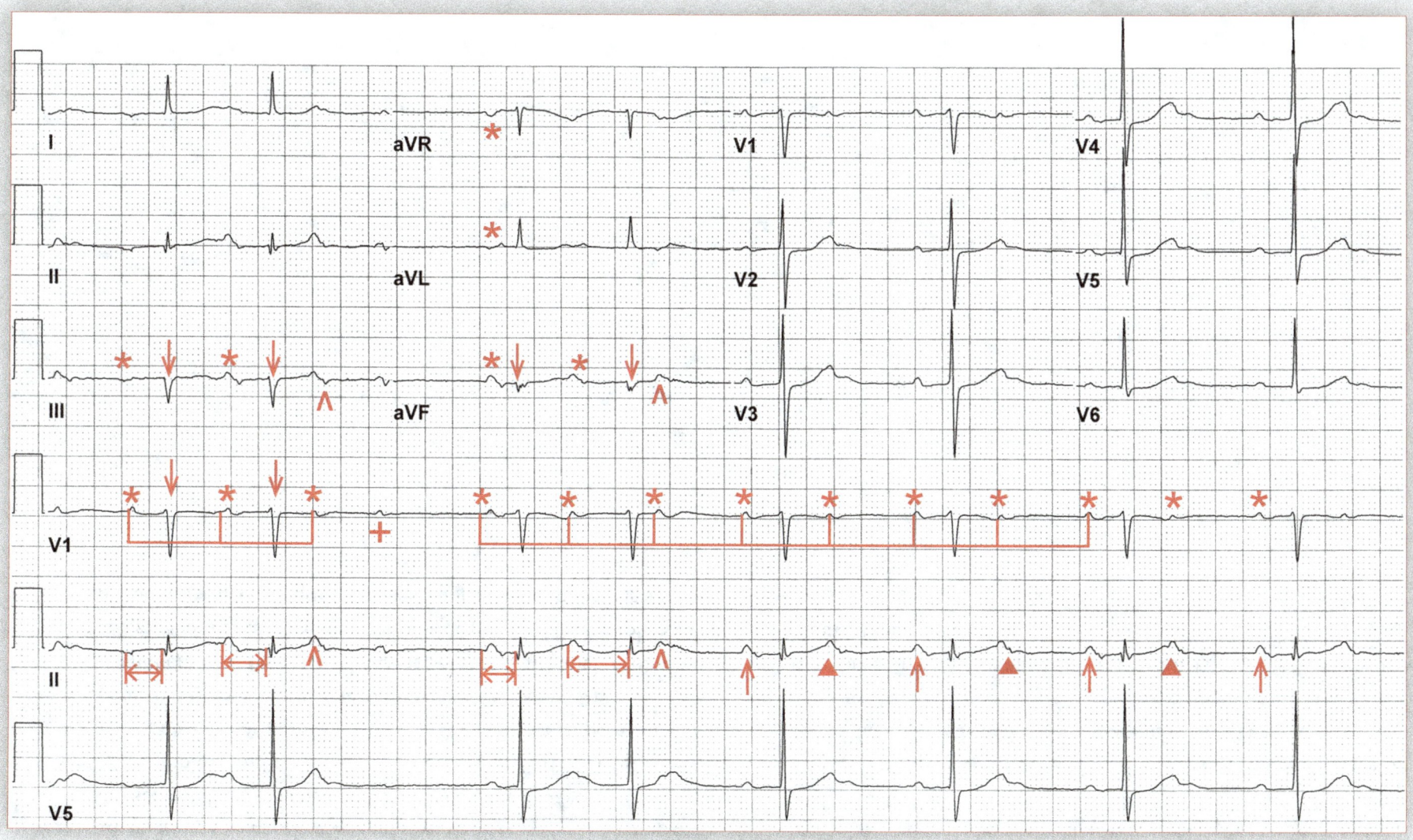

ECG 67B Analysis: Normal sinus rhythm, first-degree AV block (prolonged AV conduction), Mobitz type I second-degree AV block (Wenckebach), premature atrial complex

In **ECG 67B** the rhythm is irregularly irregular. There are P waves (∗) occurring at a regular rate of 96 bpm (⊔). The P waves are positive in leads I, II, aVF, and V4-V6. Hence this is a normal sinus rhythm. However, the fourth P wave (+) is early and has a different morphology. Hence this is a premature atrial complex. Complexes 1 through 4 (↓) are preceded by a P wave, but there is progressive lengthening of the PR interval from 0.28 second (which is the baseline PR interval and is identical to that in **ECG 67A**) to 0.36 second (↔). The P wave following the second and fourth QRS complexes (∧) is nonconducted. Hence this is a pattern of 3:2 Wenckebach. The QRS complexes that follow (complexes 5–8) are regular at a rate of 46 bpm. Each QRS complex is preceded by a P wave (↑) with a PR interval of 0.28 second, similar to the PR intervals of the first complex of the Wenckebach cycles and identical to those in **ECG 67A**. However, after each QRS complex there is another P wave (▲) that is not conducted. Hence this is second-

degree heart block with 2:1 AV conduction, similar to the pattern seen in **ECG 67A**.

As there is 3:2 Wenckebach along with 2:1 AV block, the 2:1 AV block is also Wenckebach or Mobitz type I. Hence the conduction abnormality on both ECGs is second-degree AV block, type I or Wenckebach.

Highly conditioned athletes and well-conditioned people in general demonstrate ECG markers of high vagal tone, including sinus bradycardia, first-degree AV block (prolonged AV conduction), and Mobitz type I second-degree AV block. These are not pathologic entities in these subjects. The physiologic effect of conditioning is enhanced vagal tone. Indeed the athletic heart functions more efficiently at a slower heart rate and with a greater stroke volume. ■

A 56-year-old woman with known familial dilated cardiomyopathy presents to the emergency department having suffered an episode of syncope while dining with friends in a restaurant. She regained consciousness spontaneously and relates that she felt lightheaded before the episode. She has never had an event like this in the past but states that her primary doctor has told her that her ECG is "not normal." Her vital

ECG 68A

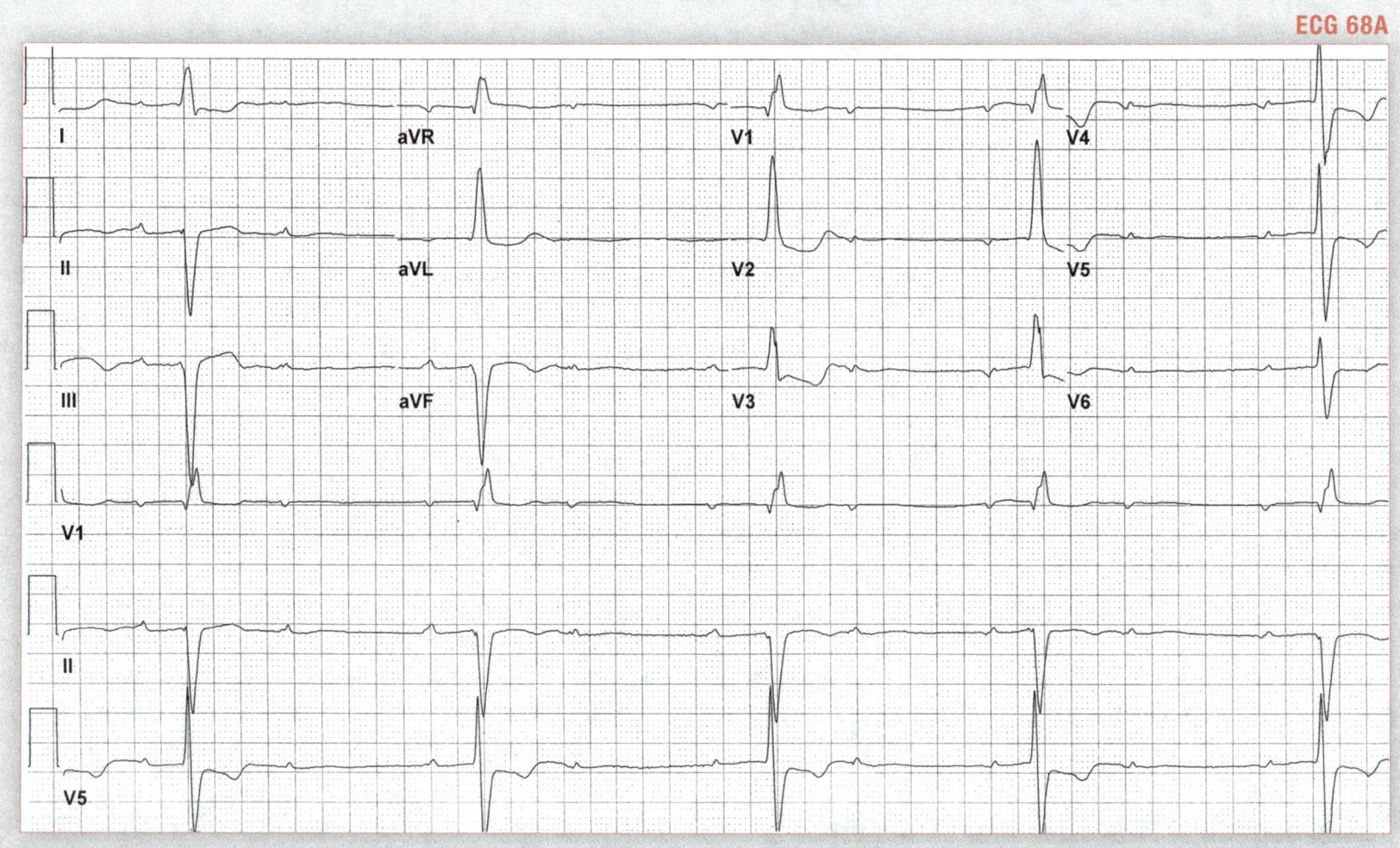

I   aVR   V1   V4

II   aVL   V2   V5

III   aVF   V3   V6

V1

II

V5

signs are notable for an apical heart rate of 30 bpm. Her physical exam is notable for clear lung fields, a jugular venous pressure of 7 cm H$_2$O, a diffuse and displaced point of maximal impulse, and an S3 gallop with a grade I/VI apical holosystolic blowing murmur. Her abdominal, extremity, and neurologic exams are normal. An ECG is obtained (68A). She is admitted to the hospital for further evaluation, and a second ECG (68B) is obtained the following day.

What abnormality is depicted on ECG 68A?

What further information does ECG 68B provide?

What therapy is indicated?

ECG 68B

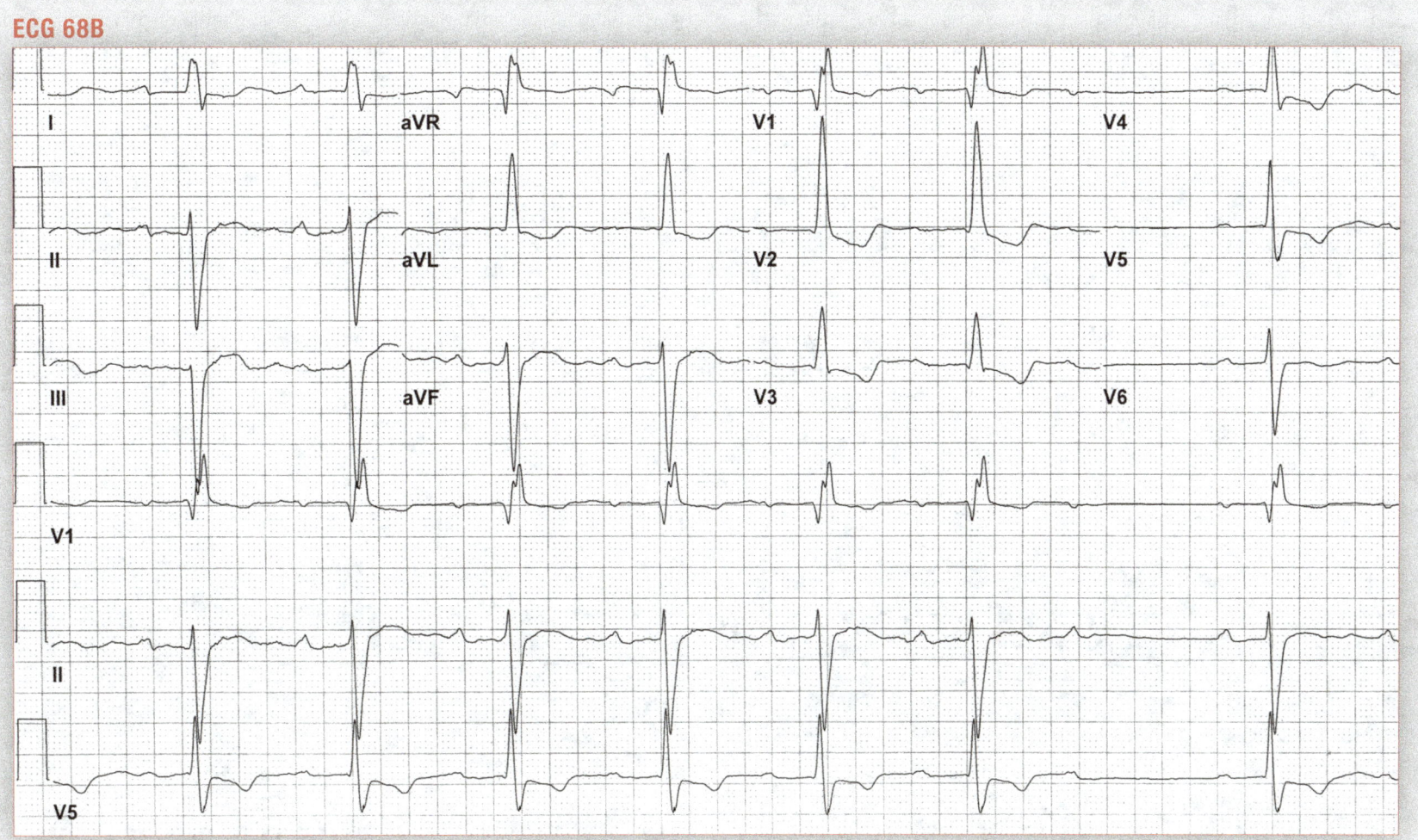

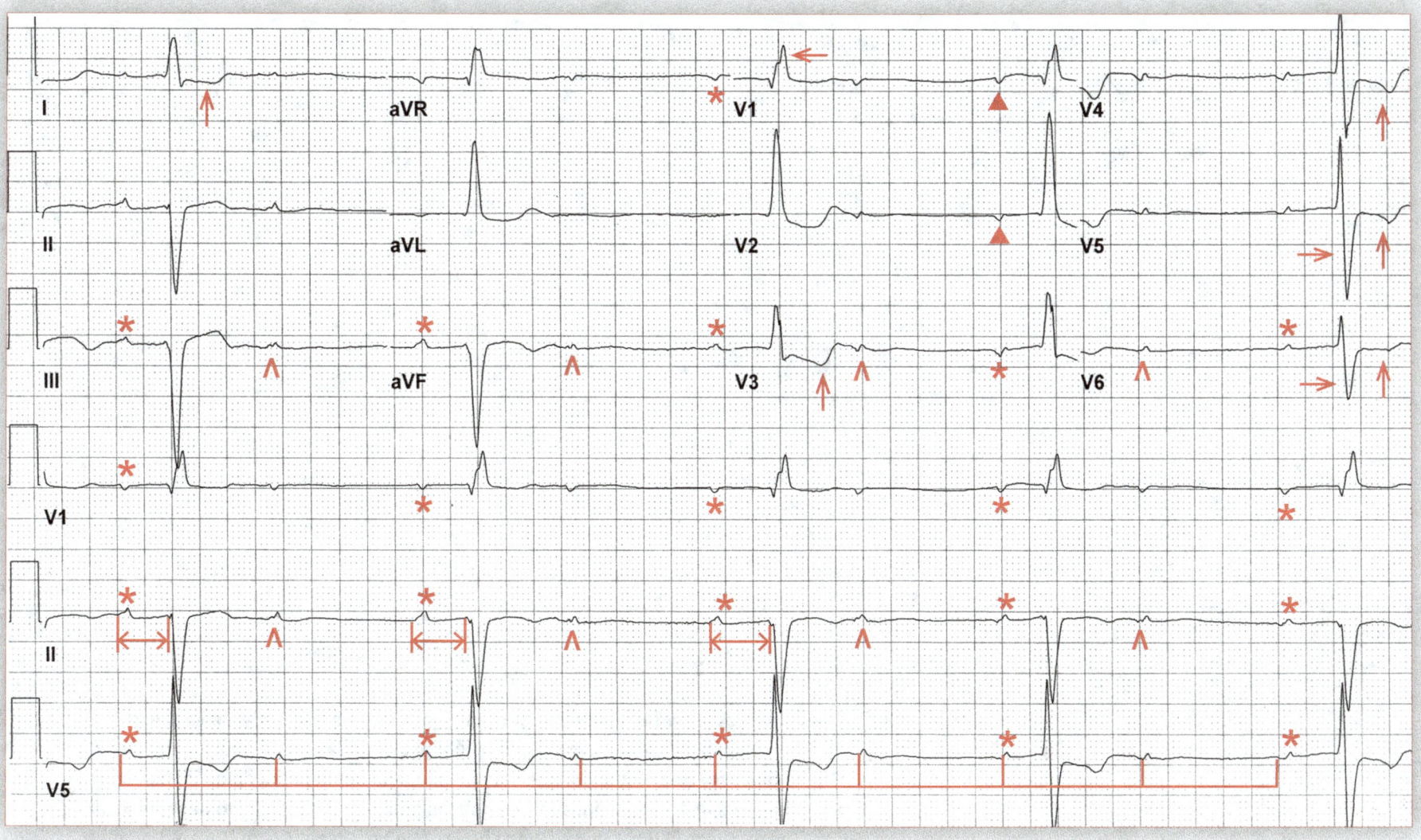

ECG 68A Analysis: Sinus bradycardia, left atrial hypertrophy, first-degree AV block (prolonged AV conduction), 2:1 second-degree AV block, left anterior fascicular block (LAFB), right bundle branch block (RBBB), nonspecific ST-T wave abnormalities

In **ECG 68A**, there is a regular rhythm at a rate of 28 bpm. The QRS complexes are wide (0.16 sec) and have a right bundle branch block (RBBB) pattern (tall R wave in lead V1 [←] and broad terminal S wave in leads V5-V6 [→]). The axis is extremely leftward, between −30° and −90° (positive QRS complex in lead I and negative QRS complex in leads II and aVF, with an rS morphology). This is, therefore, left anterior fascicular block (LAFB). Hence there is bifascicular block.

The QT/QTc intervals are normal (580/400 msec and 500/340 msec when accounting for the widened QRS complex). There are also ST-T wave changes (↑) noted in leads I and V3-V6. There are P waves (*) before each QRS complex, and they are positive in leads I, II, aVF, and V4-V6. The PR interval (↔) is prolonged at 0.40 second and is stable. Hence there is first-degree AV block (prolonged AV conduction).

This has often been called trifascicular disease; however, the location of the conduction slowing accounting for the prolonged PR interval (*ie*, AV nodal or His-Purkinje) cannot be established from this ECG. Hence trifascicular disease cannot be established with certainty. There is a second on-time but nonconducted P wave (^) (*ie*, unassociated with a QRS complex) after each QRS complex. The PP intervals are constant (⊔) at an atrial rate of 56 bpm; hence this is sinus bradycardia. There is also second-degree AV block with a 2:1 conduction pattern. This may be Mobitz type I or Mobitz type II. The presence of 2:1 AV block does not help establish trifascicular disease. The presence of other conduction abnormalities (RBBB, LAFB, and first-degree AV block) does not help establish the etiology of the second-degree AV block. In addition, the P waves in leads V1-V3 are primarily negative (▲), consistent with left atrial hypertrophy.　　*continues*

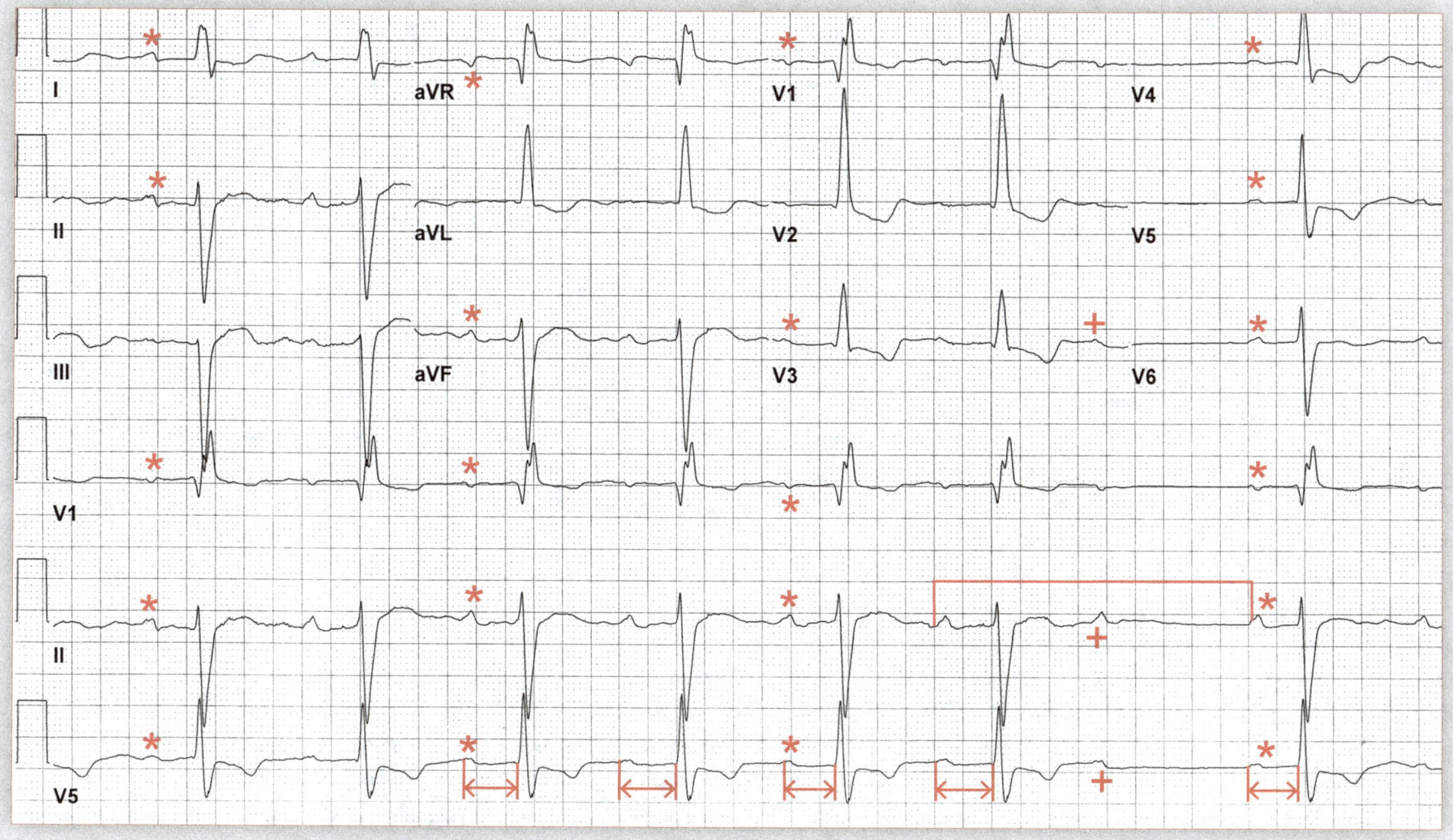

ECG 68B Analysis: Sinus bradycardia, left atrial hypertrophy, first-degree AV block (prolonged AV conduction), Mobitz type II second-degree AV block, LAFB, RBBB, trifascicular block disease

In **ECG 68B,** the QRS morphology, duration, and axis are the same as in **ECG 68A.** The QT/QTc intervals and ST-T wave abnormalities are also the same. There is a regular atrial rhythm at a rate of 54 bpm. The P wave is positive in leads I, II, aVF, and V4-V6; hence this is sinus bradycardia. There is a P wave (*) before each QRS complex and the PR interval (↔) is stable at 0.40 second, similar to the PR interval of the conducted complexes in **ECG 68A.** There is a pause seen (⊓) with an on-time but nonconducted P wave (+). The pause is equal to two RR intervals. All the PR intervals are constant, including those before and after the pause. This is Mobitz type II second-degree AV block. Therefore, the 2:1 AV block seen in **ECG 68A,** obtained the previous day, is also Mobitz type II. As Mobitz type II block is due to disease within the His-Purkinje system, it is now established that the patient has evidence of trifascicular disease; and the pause (*ie,* Mobitz type II) is the result of intermittent block in the left posterior fascicle, which is the only part of the conduction system that is responsible for AV conduction to the ventricles.

The patient displays a degree of AV block that warrants pacemaker implantation. Depending on her degree of heart failure and left ventricular dysfunction, more advanced therapies such as cardiac resynchronization as well as implantation of a cardiac defibrillator may be considered. ■

A 48-year-old diabetic man with atrial fibrillation on digoxin has a history of viral gastroenteritis and polyuria. As his oral intake was poor due to gastroenteritis, he stopped taking his insulin for several days. He is brought to the hospital by his wife, who noted that he was confused and at times obtunded. On exam, his mucous membrane are very dry. His blood pressure is 90/60 mm Hg, and his heart rate is 40 to 50 bpm. His respiratory rate is rapid with deep inspirations.

His consciousness is waxing and waning, and he is barely rousable. Laboratory values include the following: blood urea nitrogen 65 mg/dL, creatinine 2.3 mg/dL, serum sodium 156 mmol/L, serum potassium 3.0 mEq/L, and serum bicarbonate 16 mmol/L. The serum glucose level is 760 mg/dL. Blood gases show a pH of 7.24, normal PO_2, and PCO_2 of 25 mm Hg. A diagnosis of ketoacidosis is made, and the patient is treated appropriately. An ECG is obtained.

What is the abnormality on the ECG?

What is a possible cause?

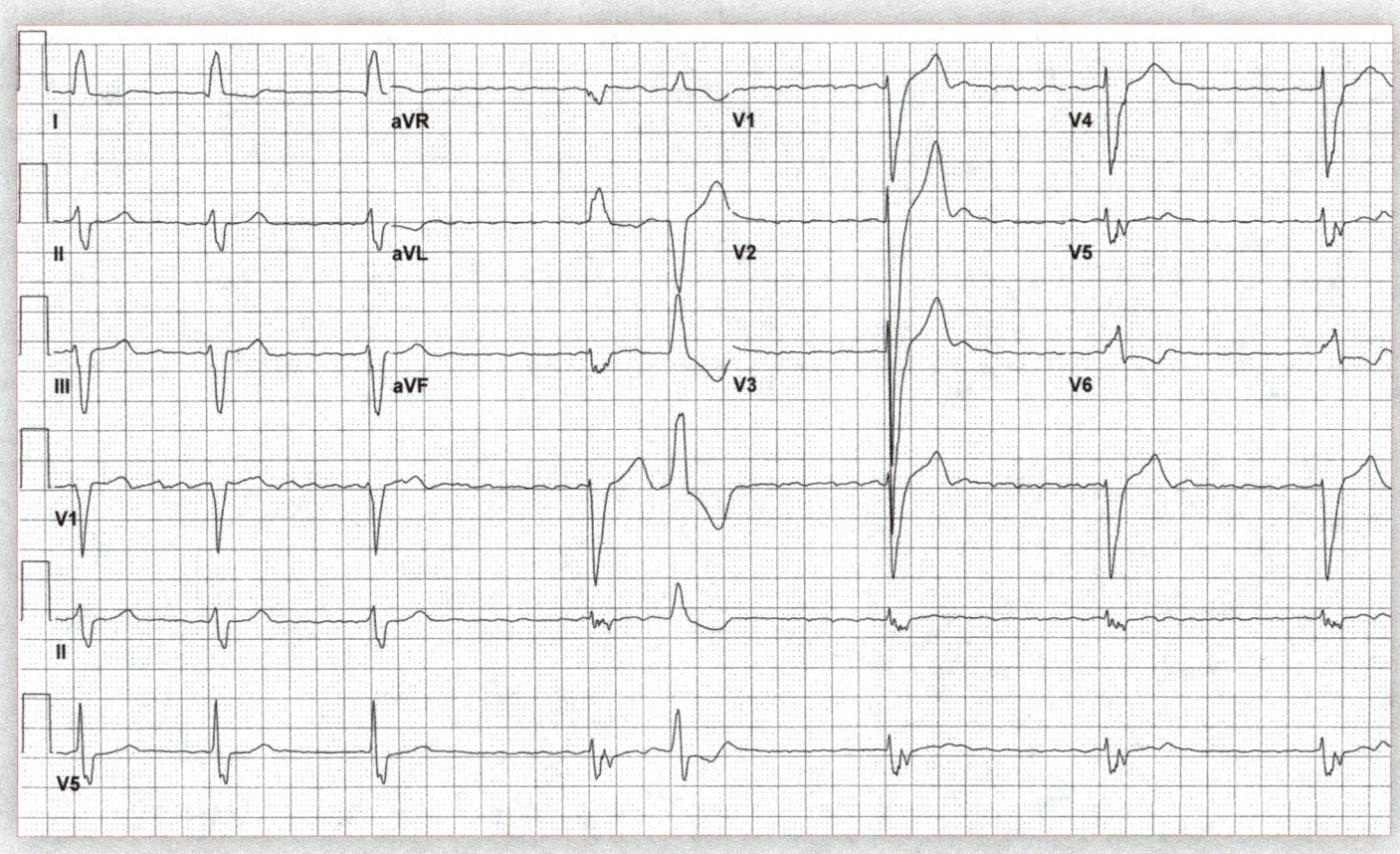

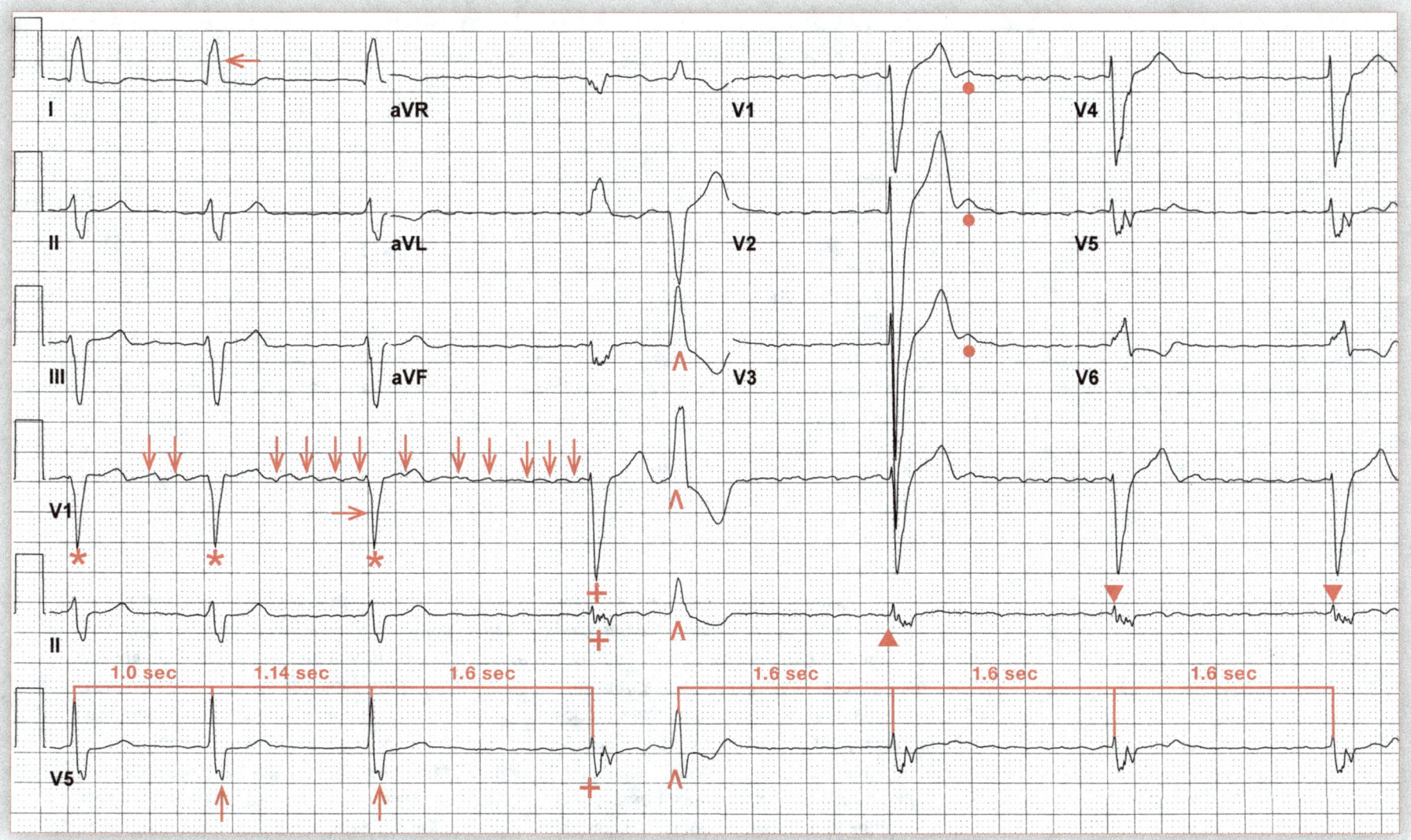

ECG 69 Analysis: Atrial fibrillation with intermittent complete AV block and an escape
ventricular rhythm, intraventricular conduction delay, premature ventricular complex, U waves

The underlying rhythm is atrial fibrillation; there is no organized atrial activity and fibrillatory waves are seen, particularly in lead V1 (↓). The fibrillatory waves are irregular in morphology, amplitude, and interval. The RR intervals of the first three complexes (∗) are irregular (1.0 and 1.14 sec, with rates of 48–60 bpm), and hence they are the result of intact AV nodal conduction that occurs irregularly due to the atrial fibrillation. The QRS complex is wide (0.14 sec) and has a morphology resembling a left bundle branch block, with a broad R wave in lead I (←) and a QS complex in lead V1 (→). However, there is also a normal and narrow R wave and a prominent S wave in lead V5 (↑), reflecting terminal forces being directed from left to right. This is not seen with a left bundle branch block but rather is more consistent with a right bundle branch block. Hence the QRS complexes have an intraventricular conduction delay. The QT/QTc intervals are slightly prolonged (480/450 msec), although they are normal when the prolonged QRS complex duration is considered (420/400 msec).

Noted is that the fourth QRS complex (+) occurs after a longer RR interval (↔) (1.6 sec, rate 38 bpm). Following this complex is a very wide and abnormal QRS complex (complex 5), which is a premature ventricular complex (^). The RR interval from the premature ventricular complex to the next QRS complex (complex 6) (▲) as well as the RR intervals of the last two QRS complexes (7 and 8) (▼) are the same (RR interval 1.6 sec, rate 38 bpm) and are identical to the RR interval between complexes 3 (∗) and 4 (+). Hence there is regulation of these RR intervals during atrial fibrillation, which indicates the presence of complete AV block. The fourth, sixth, seventh, and eighth

QRS complexes have a wider duration (0.18 sec) and a morphology (in leads II and V5) that is different from the first three QRS complexes. These are, therefore, escape ventricular complexes. Also noted after the ventricular complexes in leads V1-V3 are prominent U waves (●), suggesting hypokalemia, although prominent U waves may also be seen with significant bradycardia.

This patient has ketoacidosis, precipitated by a viral infection as well as the discontinuation of insulin. He is very dehydrated due to the ketoacidosis (associated with polyuria) as well as poor oral intake. Renal insufficiency (due to prerenal azotemia) has likely led to an increase in serum digoxin levels, resulting in signs of digoxin toxicity. Although this can result in complete AV block, it would be associated with an escape junctional rhythm. In this case, the escape rhythm is ventricular, meaning that the complete heart block results from a conduction abnormality within the His-Purkinje system. Although digoxin toxicity is usually associated with conduction block within the AV node and hence a junctional escape rhythm, very high levels may also suppress conduction within the His-Purkinje system, resulting in an escape ventricular rhythm. It is also likely that the His-Purkinje conduction abnormality is the result of the acidosis and other metabolic derangements. Appropriate therapy includes correcting the ketoacidosis and electrolyte abnormalities, as well as withholding digoxin until renal function recovers. If the complete AV block resolves, permanent pacing is not indicated. Persistence of complete heart block means that there is permanent His-Purkinje conduction disease and in this situation permanent pacing would be indicated. ■

Notes

A n ECG from an asymptomatic
42-year-old man is shown.

What abnormalities are noted?

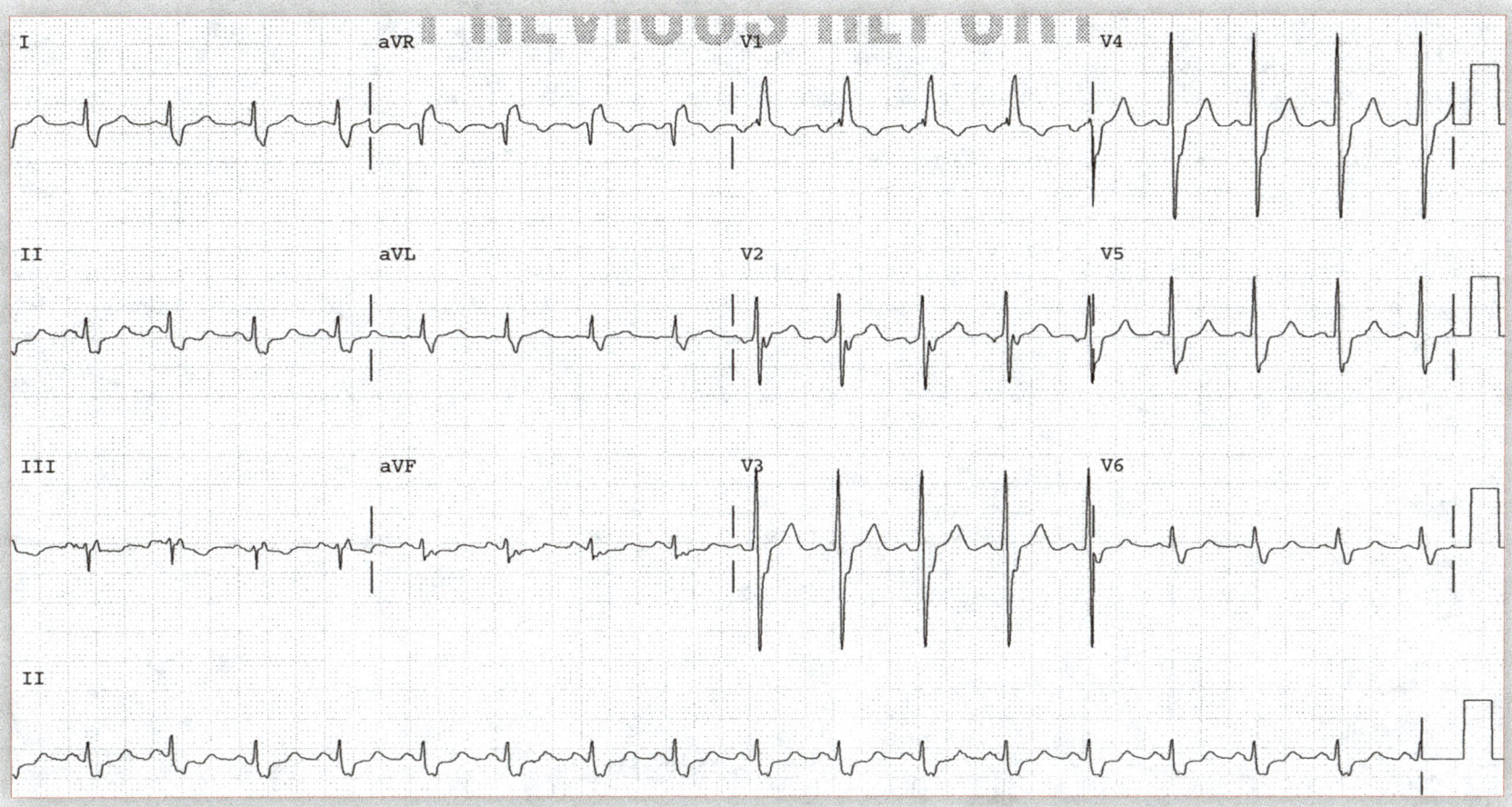

Podrid's Real-World ECGs

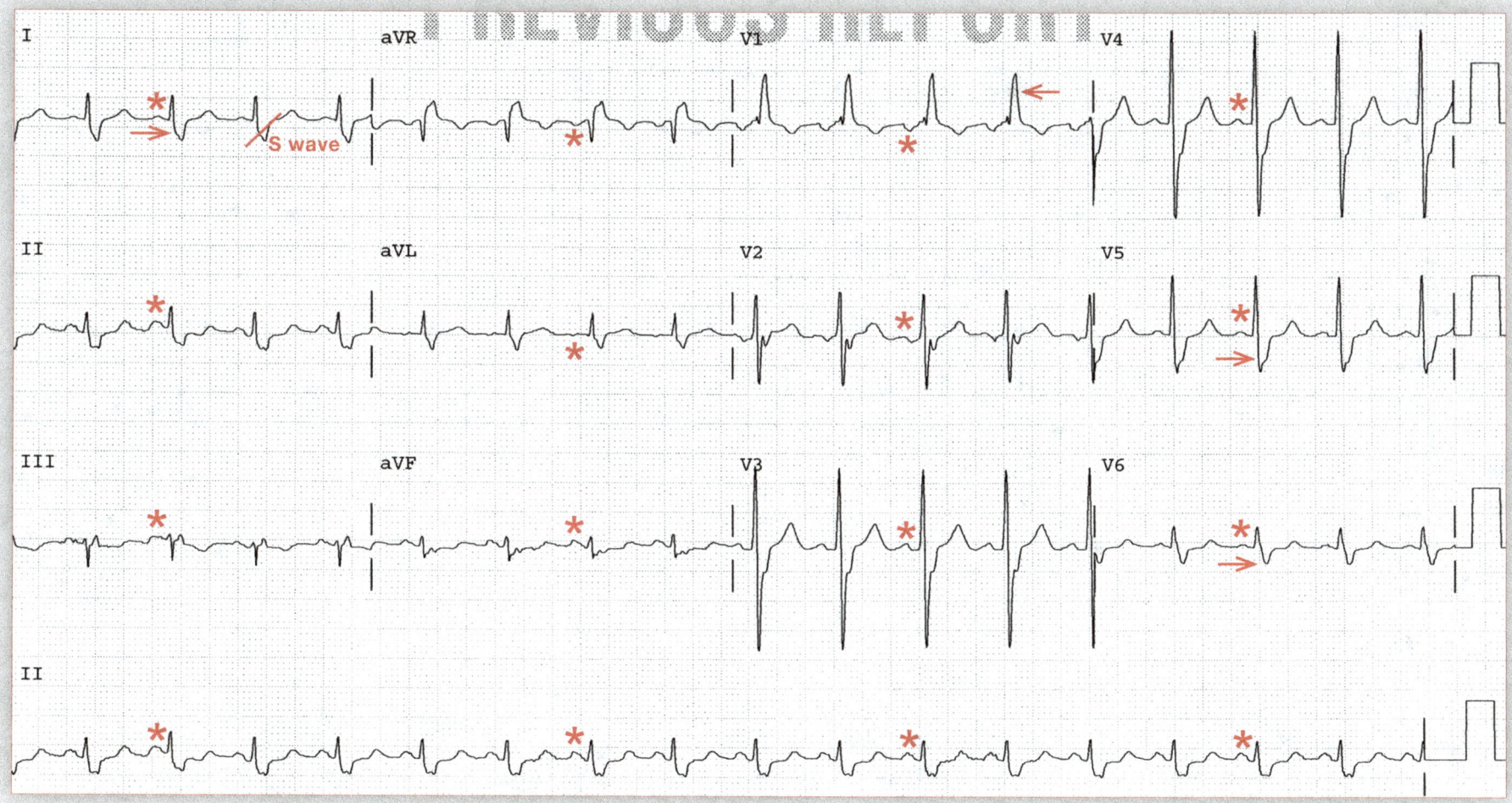

PREVIOUS REPORT

ECG 70 Analysis: Sinus tachycardia, right bundle branch block

There is a regular rhythm at a rate of 100 bpm. There is a P wave (*) before each QRS complex and the PR interval is stable (0.16 sec). The QRS complex duration is prolonged (0.14 sec), and there is an RSR′ morphology (←) in lead V1 and a broad S wave (→) in leads I and V5-V6. This is a pattern of a right bundle branch block. The QT/QTc intervals are prolonged (360/465 msec) but are normal when the prolonged QRS complex duration is considered (300/388 msec). Although the axis appears to be rightward, this is a result of the broad S wave in lead I.

Since axis determination is based on left ventricular forces, the S wave (representing right ventricular activation) should not be considered.

An isolated right bundle branch block is not uncommon in the normal population and generally is not indicative of any underlying cardiac abnormality. In the absence of any symptoms that point to a cardiac problem, no further evaluation or therapy is necessary. ■

Practice Case 71

An 89-year-old man with a history of paroxysmal atrial fibrillation, for which he takes warfarin, is admitted to the neurosurgical intensive care unit after presenting with a traumatic fall and large intracerebral hemorrhage. His admission ECG (71A) is interpreted as

ECG 71A

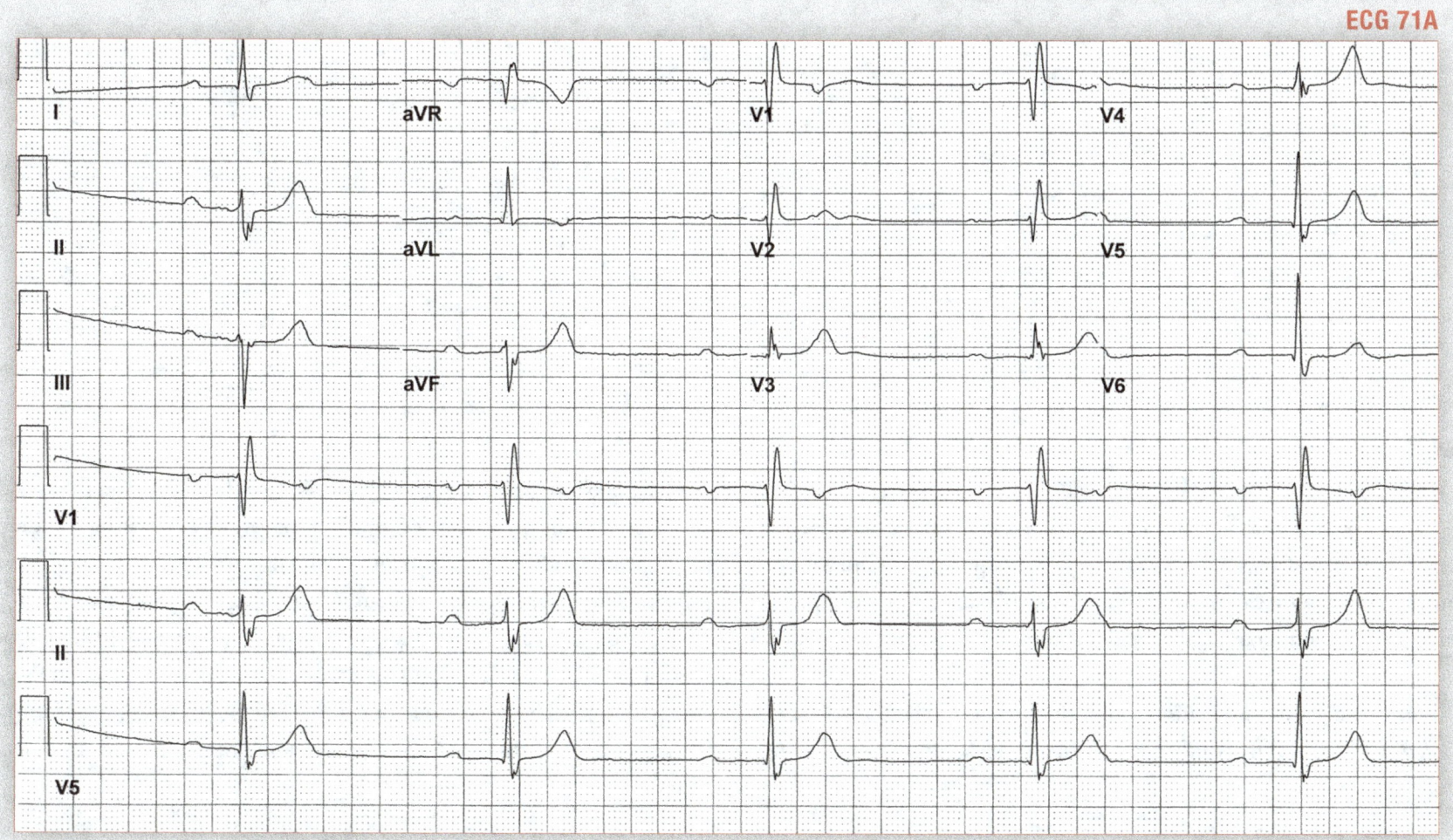

sinus bradycardia. The following day during rounds, an astute medical student notices that the patient's PR interval is different on the lead II telemetry than the previous day. An ECG is obtained (71B) and the primary neurology team requests your interpretation.

What are the findings on the initial ECG (71A)?

How does the follow-up ECG (71B) assist in the diagnosis?

ECG 71B

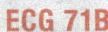

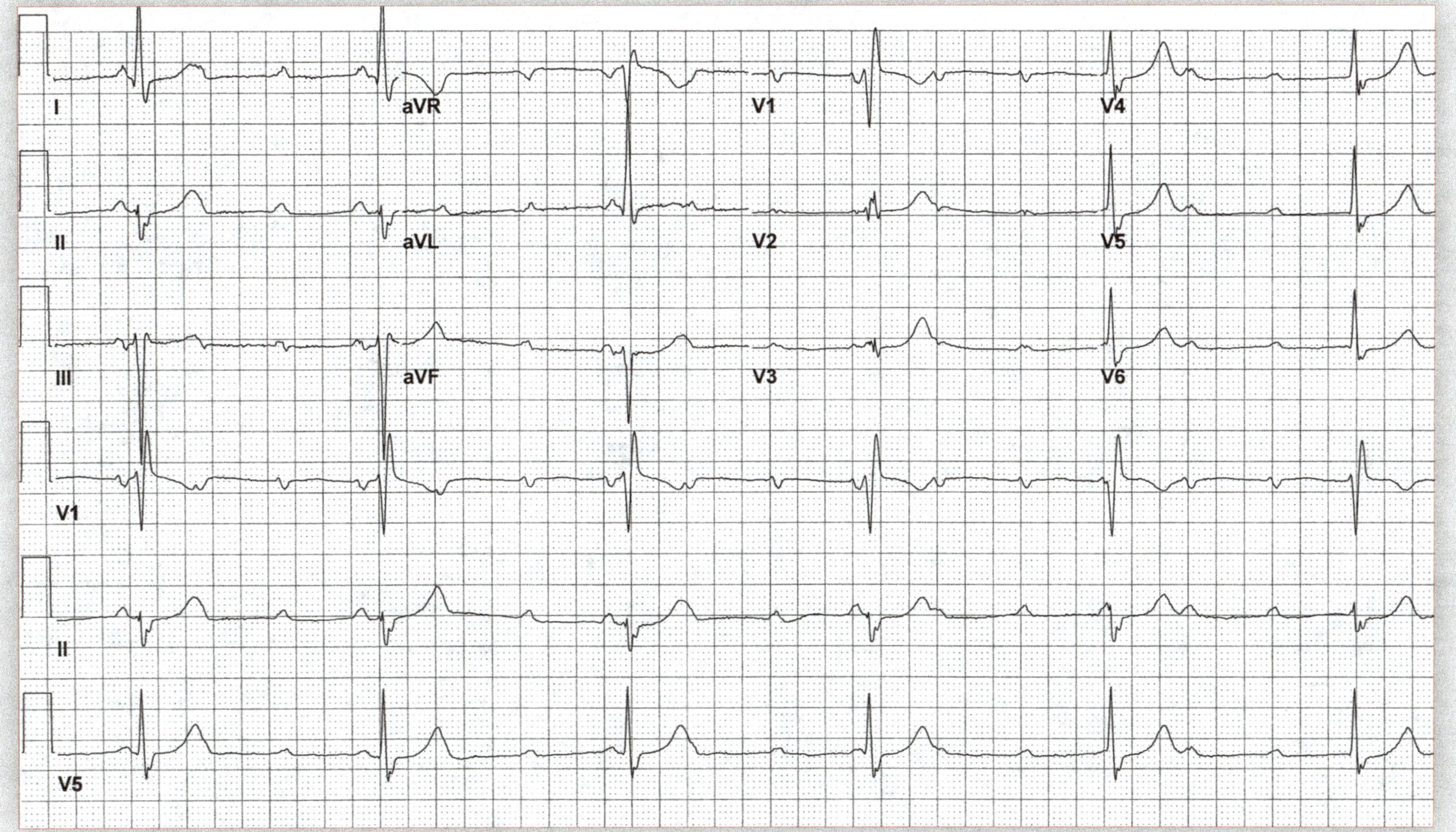

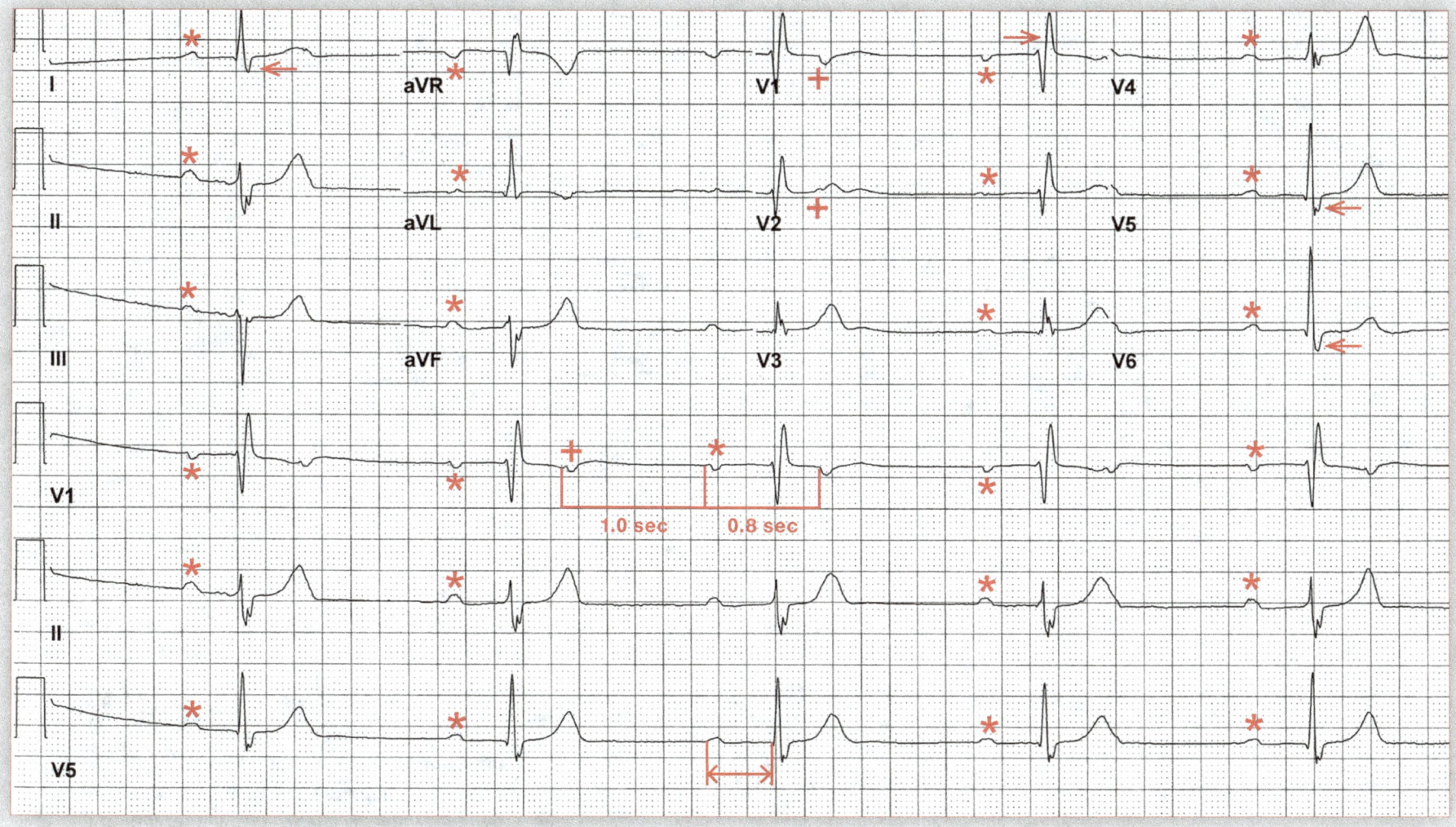

ECG 71A Analysis: Sinus rhythm with ventriculophasic arrhythmia, first-degree AV block (prolonged AV conduction), second-degree AV block with 2:1 conduction, right bundle branch block, left anterior fascicular block

ECG 71A shows a regular rhythm at a rate of 32 bpm. There are P waves (*) before each QRS complex and the PR interval is stable (↔) but prolonged (0.44 sec), defining a first-degree AV block. Noted in leads V1-V2 is a second, nonconducted P wave (+) that has the same morphology as the conducted P wave. The atrial rate is 64 bpm. Hence every other P wave is conducted, indicating second-degree AV block with 2:1 AV conduction. The PP intervals (atrial rate) are not regular; the PP interval around the QRS complex is shorter (0.8 sec) than the PP interval without a QRS complex (1.0 sec). This represents ventriculophasic arrhythmia. Ventriculophasic arrhythmia can be seen whenever there is 2:1 AV block or complete heart block. Although the exact mechanism is not clear, it is hypothesized that the shortened PP interval around the QRS complex can be a result of enhancement of sinus node rate with ventricular contraction due to pulsatile blood flow through the sinus node artery, which increases sinus node automaticity; increased stretch on the right atrium, which increases sinus

node automaticity; or alteration of carotid sinus outputs (baroreceptor changes) related to the stroke volume with ventricular contraction. It is a normal physiologic occurrence.

The QRS complexes are widened (0.14 sec) and there is a pattern of right bundle branch block (RBBB; RSR′ morphology in lead V1 [→] and broad S wave in leads I and V5-V6 [←]). The axis is extremely leftward, between −30° and −90° (positive QRS complex in lead I and negative QRS complex in leads II and aVF with an rS morphology), defining a left anterior fascicular block (LAFB).

Even though there is a first-degree AV block (prolonged AV conduction) and bifascicular disease (RBBB and LAFB), this cannot be called trifascicular disease as it is not certain whether the first-degree AV block is the result of AV nodal disease or His-Purkinje disease (*ie*, whether the 2:1 AV block is Mobitz type I or Mobitz type II).

continues

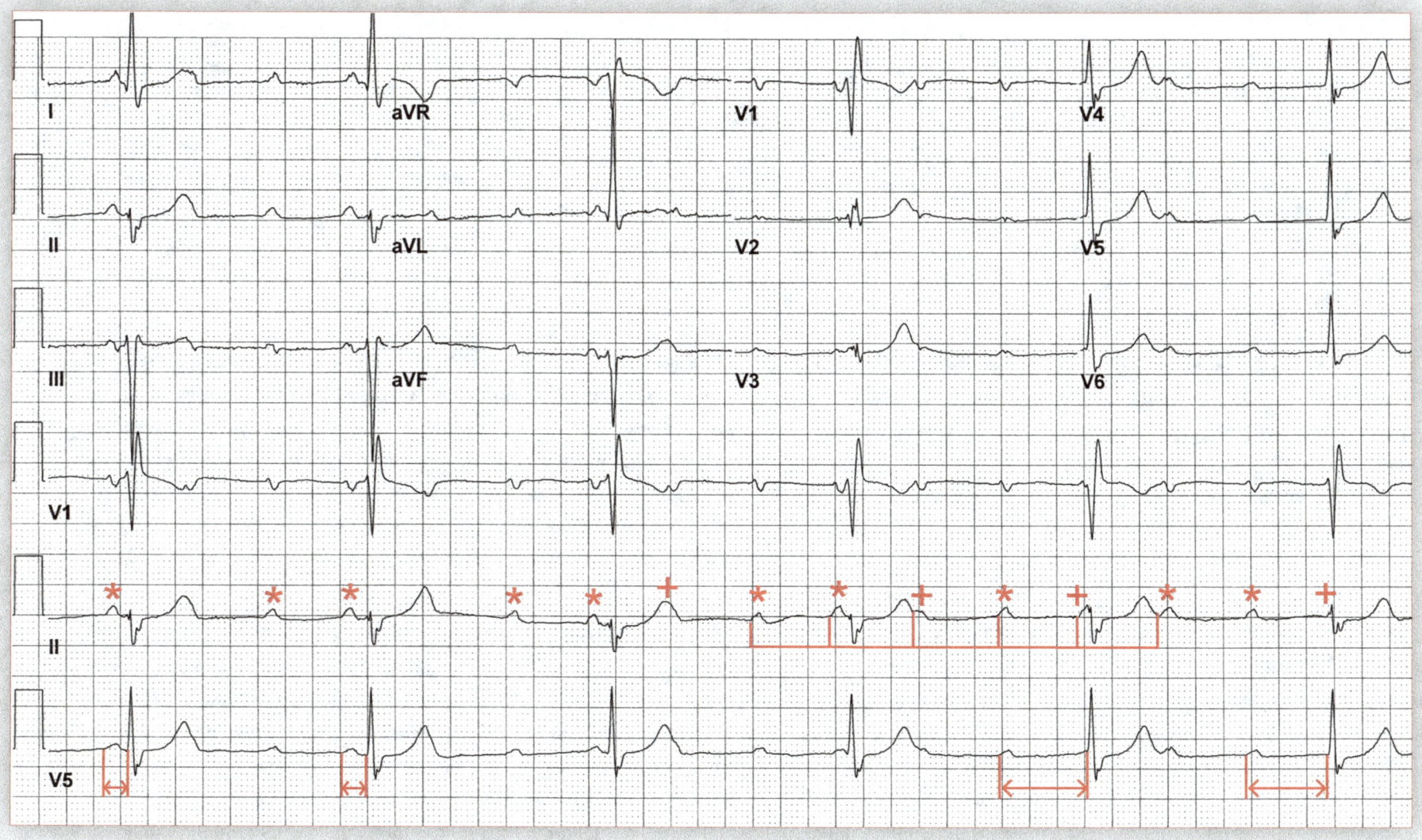

ECG 71B Analysis: Sinus tachycardia, complete heart block, junctional escape rhythm

ECG 71B shows a regular rhythm at a rate of 34 bpm. There are P waves (*) at a regular rate of 100 bpm (⊔), although some of the P waves are not obvious as they are superimposed on the QRS complex or T wave (+). The P waves are positive in leads I, II, aVF, and V4-V6. Hence this is sinus tachycardia. The PR interval (↔) is inconsistent and always different than the baseline PR interval (0.44 sec as seen on ECG 71A), indicating AV dissociation. The atrial rate is faster than the ventricular rate, which is diagnostic for complete heart block. In contrast, an atrial rate that is slower than the ventricular rate would indicate an accelerated lower focus (*ie*, junctional or ventricular). The QRS complex has an RBBB and LAFB, identical in morphology and axis to the QRS complexes seen in ECG 71A; hence the escape rhythm is junctional and the 2:1 AV block is a Mobitz type I. This confirms the fact that trifascicular disease was not present but that the first-degree AV block with 2:1 AV conduction is the result of AV nodal disease (Mobitz type I).

AV block is seen in approximately 10% of patients with intracerebral hemorrhage as well as in patients with acute ischemic stroke. Although AV block in the context of cerebral infarction portends a worse prognosis, it does not seem to be an independent predictor of mortality in cerebral hemorrhage. Despite the baseline conduction abnormalities, the development of complete heart block is associated with a stable junctional escape, so pacemaker implantation may be avoided as AV block is likely a transient complication of the acute neurologic process rather than a progression of the underlying conduction system disease. ■

Notes

A 65-year-old man with known hereditary hemochromatosis presents with palpitations. He is otherwise well. A review of systems is unremarkable, and his vital signs are normal. However, the following are noted on physical exam: a normal cardiac point of maximal impulse with an irregular rhythm and an S4 gallop, bronzing of the skin, and small testes. Laboratory values include a normal thyroid-stimulating hormone level, a transferrin saturation of 80%, and mild transaminitis. An ECG is obtained.

What abnormalities are noted?

What therapy is indicated?

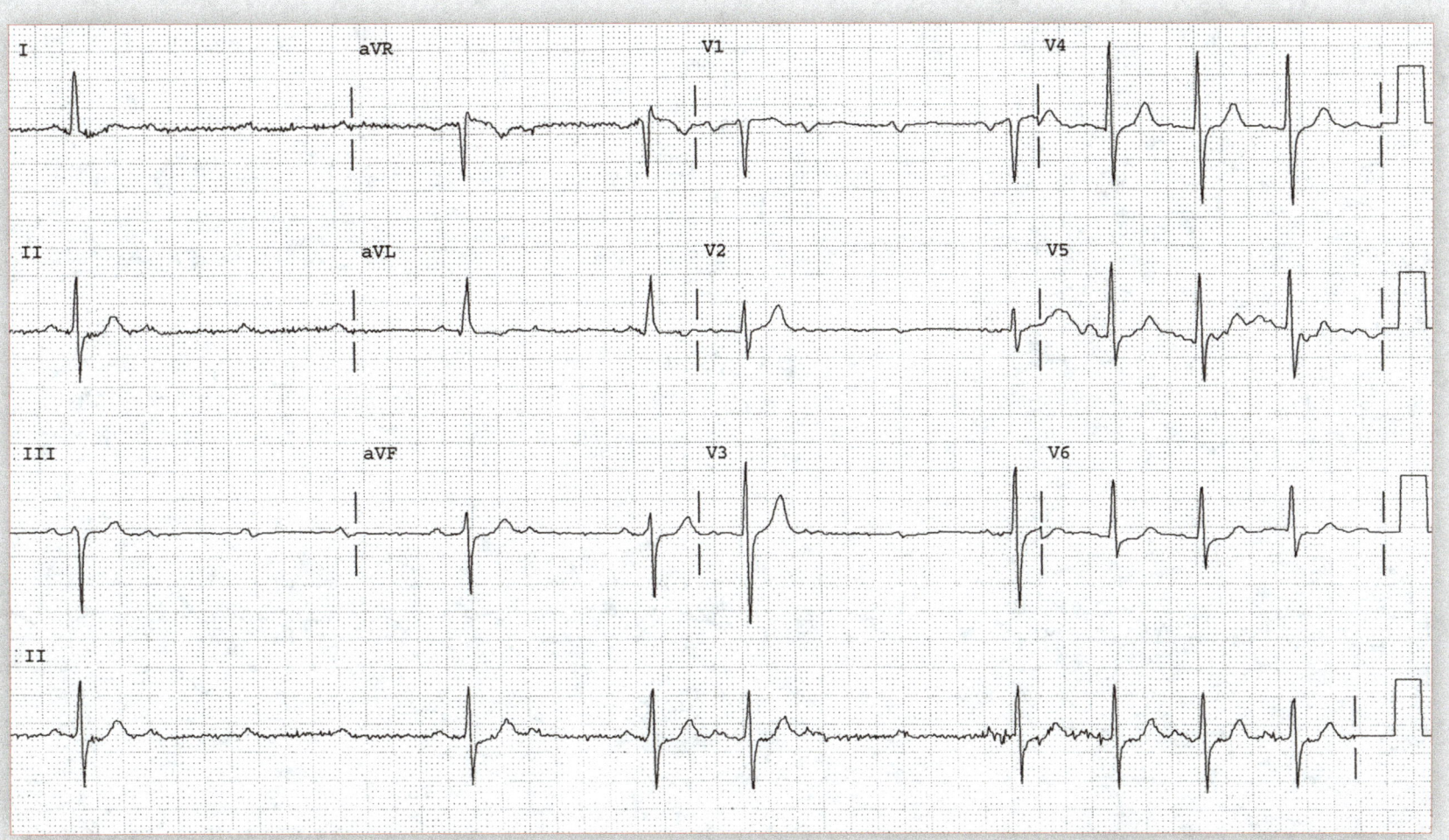

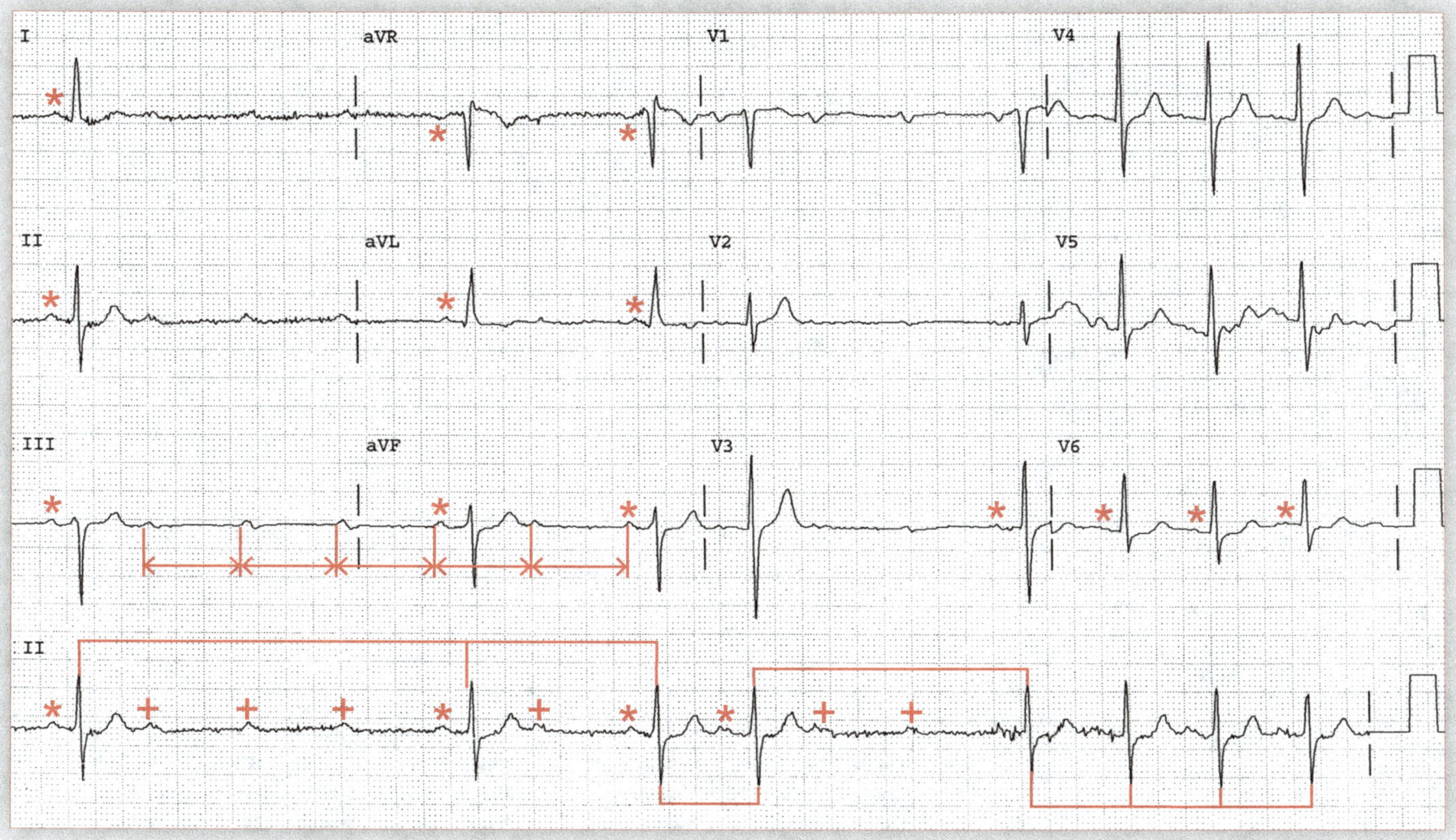

ECG 72 Analysis: Normal sinus rhythm, first-degree AV block (prolonged
AV conduction), Mobitz type II second-degree AV block (high-degree AV block)

The rhythm is irregular, although a pattern can be seen (all of the short intervals are the same [⊔]); hence the rhythm is regularly irregular. The QRS complexes are normal in duration (0.08 sec) and morphology. There is a left axis, between 0° and −30° (positive QRS complex in leads I and II and negative QRS complex in lead aVF). The QT/QTc intervals are slightly prolonged (380/455 msec). P waves (*) are seen before each QRS complex, with a stable PR interval (0.22 sec). There are additional P waves seen (+) with a stable PP interval and an atrial rate of 86 bpm (↔). The P waves are positive in leads I, II, aVF, and V4-V6. Hence there is a normal sinus rhythm with first-degree AV block (prolonged AV conduction). The RR intervals between the third and fourth QRS complexes and between the last four QRS complexes are similar (⊔); the ventricular rate is 86 bpm. There are three pauses or long RR intervals seen (⊓). During these pauses there are on-time, nonconducted P waves (+) (ie, three nonconducted P waves during the first pause, one during the second pause, and two sequential nonconducted P waves during the third pause). The presence of two or more sequential nonconducted P waves is seen with Mobitz type II second-degree AV block; with Mobitz type I block only one nonconducted P wave is seen. The presence of two or more nonconducted P waves is often called high-degree AV block.

Patients with hemochromatosis may develop conduction defects due to the underlying genetic mutation or the infiltrative cardiomyopathy. The iron deposition is associated with features of restrictive cardiomyopathy or dilated cardiomyopathy. This patient does not manifest physical exam findings of depressed left ventricular function or heart failure. However, the S4 gallop may point to a disorder of left ventricular relaxation in the context of cardiac iron deposition. An echocardiogram is warranted. Given Mobitz type II heart block, particularly with multiple nonconducted P waves and a slow ventricular rate, pacemaker implantation is indicated. Phlebotomy and/or chelation therapy is indicated as well, which in some cases can reverse left ventricular dysfunction. The effect of these therapies on conduction system disease is unknown. ◼

Notes

A 68-year-old woman with ischemic cardiomyopathy requests an urgent appointment with her cardiologist for lightheadedness, dyspnea, and fatigue over the past 24 hours. Upon evaluation, her heart rate is noted to be 32 bpm, and her blood pressure is 98/60 mm Hg. Her exam shows clear lung fields, a jugular venous pressure of 8 cm H_2O, a 2-cm laterally displaced cardiac point of maximal impulse, normal cardiac sounds without gallops, and a soft blowing systolic murmur at the apex. Her abdominal and extremity exams are normal. An ECG is obtained.

What ECG abnormality explains her symptoms?

What therapy is indicated?

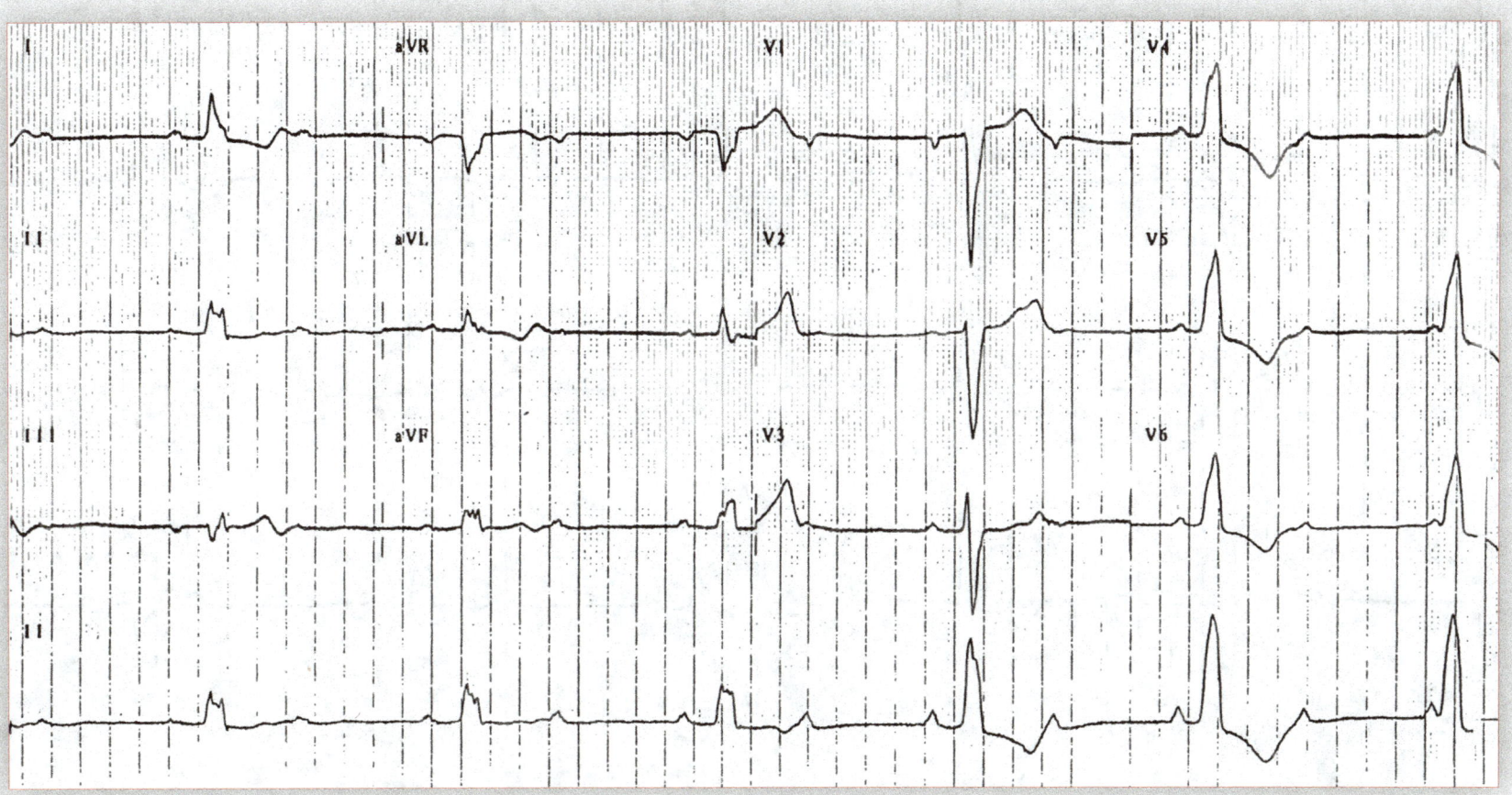

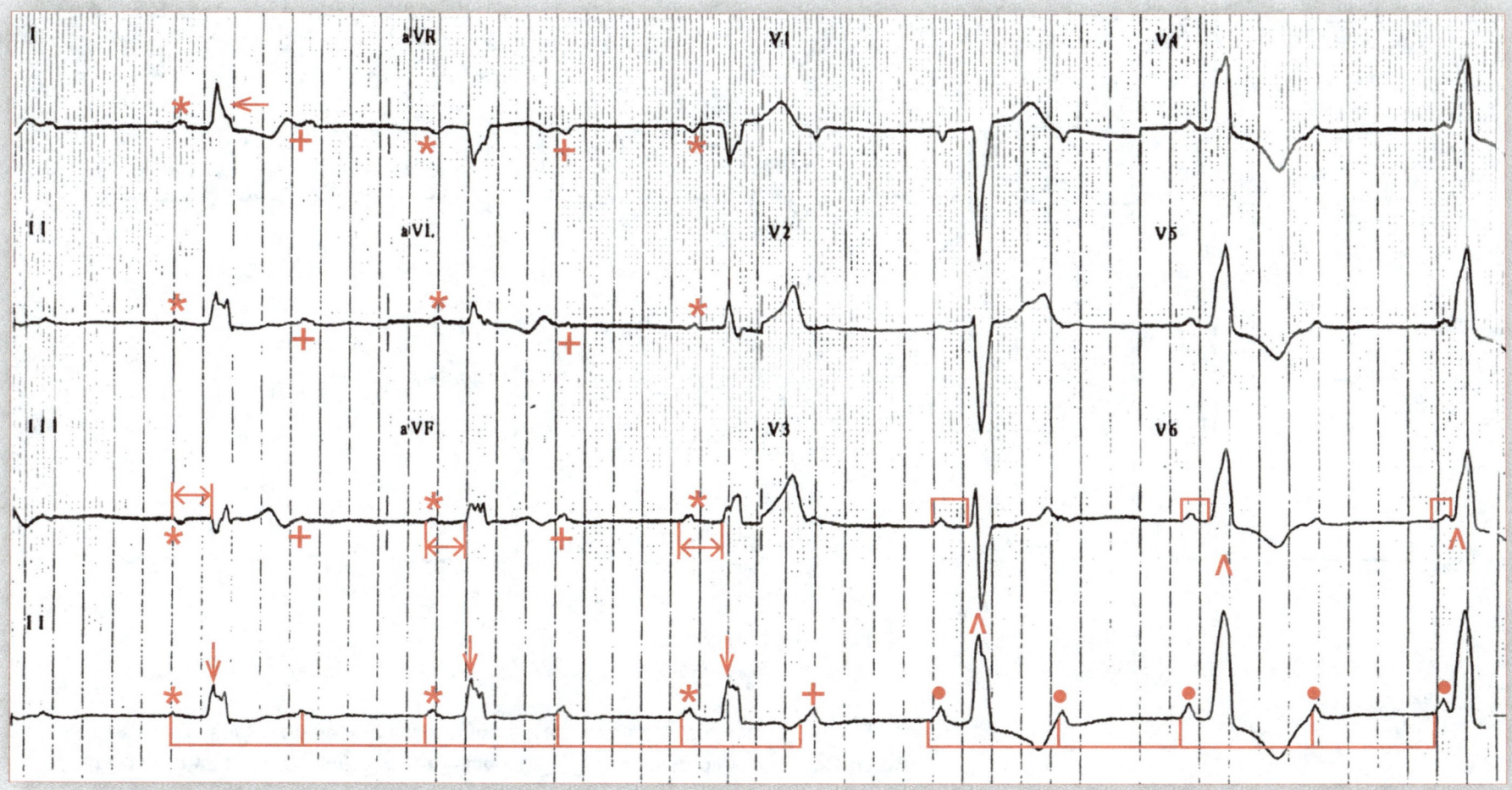

ECG 73 Analysis: Normal sinus rhythm, left bundle branch block, first-degree AV block (prolonged AV conduction), 2:1 second-degree AV block progressing to complete heart block, escape ventricular rhythm

The initial portion of the ECG (first three QRS complexes [↓]) shows a regular rhythm at a rate of 32 bpm. P waves are seen before each of the first three QRS complexes (*) and the PR interval (↔) is constant (0.24 sec), indicating first-degree AV block (prolonged AV conduction). There are also on-time but nonconducted P waves after each of these QRS complexes (+). Therefore, there is a stable atrial rate (⊔) of 64 bpm. The P wave is positive in leads I, II, aVF, and V4-V6; hence the rhythm is sinus. As every other P wave (+) is nonconducted, this is second-degree AV block with 2:1 AV conduction; the second-degree block may be either Mobitz type I or Mobitz type II. Hence there is first- and second-degree AV block.

The QRS complex is wide (0.16 sec) and has a left bundle branch block (LBBB) pattern (broad R wave in lead I [←]). The QT/QTc intervals are normal (560/410 msec and 480/350 msec when the prolonged QRS complex duration is considered). The presence of an LBBB is considered bifascicular disease. Along with the first-degree AV block and second-degree AV block with 2:1 conduction, a diagnosis of trifascicular disease may be considered. However, it is not clear whether the first- and second-degree AV block is due to an AV nodal or His-Purkinje conduction abnormality. A diagnosis of trifascicular disease can only be made if the abnormality is in the His-Purkinje system. A change in the pattern of conduction would be necessary to establish the etiology for the 2:1 AV block.

In the second portion of the ECG (*ie*, the last three QRS complexes [^]), there is a change in the pattern. P waves are seen (●) and the atrial rate is the same (⊔) (64 bpm), but the ventricular rate is 36 bpm and there is now AV dissociation with a variable PR interval (⊓). In addition, the QRS complex morphology has changed, although the complexes still have an LBBB pattern. This is now complete heart block with an escape ventricular rhythm. Hence, the 2:1 AV block was Mobitz type II, related to conduction problems within the His-Purkinje system. This indicates that indeed trifascicular disease is present.

At this time, the patient should be stabilized and temporary pacemaker insertion considered as this is a ventricular escape rhythm that is potentially unstable and unreliable, resulting in wide variability in rate. Permanent pacemaker implantation is warranted thereafter. Provided there are no signs of active ischemia, more advanced device therapy for heart failure may be considered. Depending on the patient's left ventricular ejection fraction, an implantable cardioverter-defibrillator may be considered. As the patient's QRS complex is wide with an LBBB, cardiac resynchronization therapy may also be considered if the patient has systolic dysfunction and heart failure symptoms persist despite medical therapy. ■

Practice Case 74

A 77-year-old man is admitted to the hospital with syncope heralded by lightheadedness. On admission, an ECG is obtained (74A). During his first night in the hospital, the patient's heart

ECG 74A

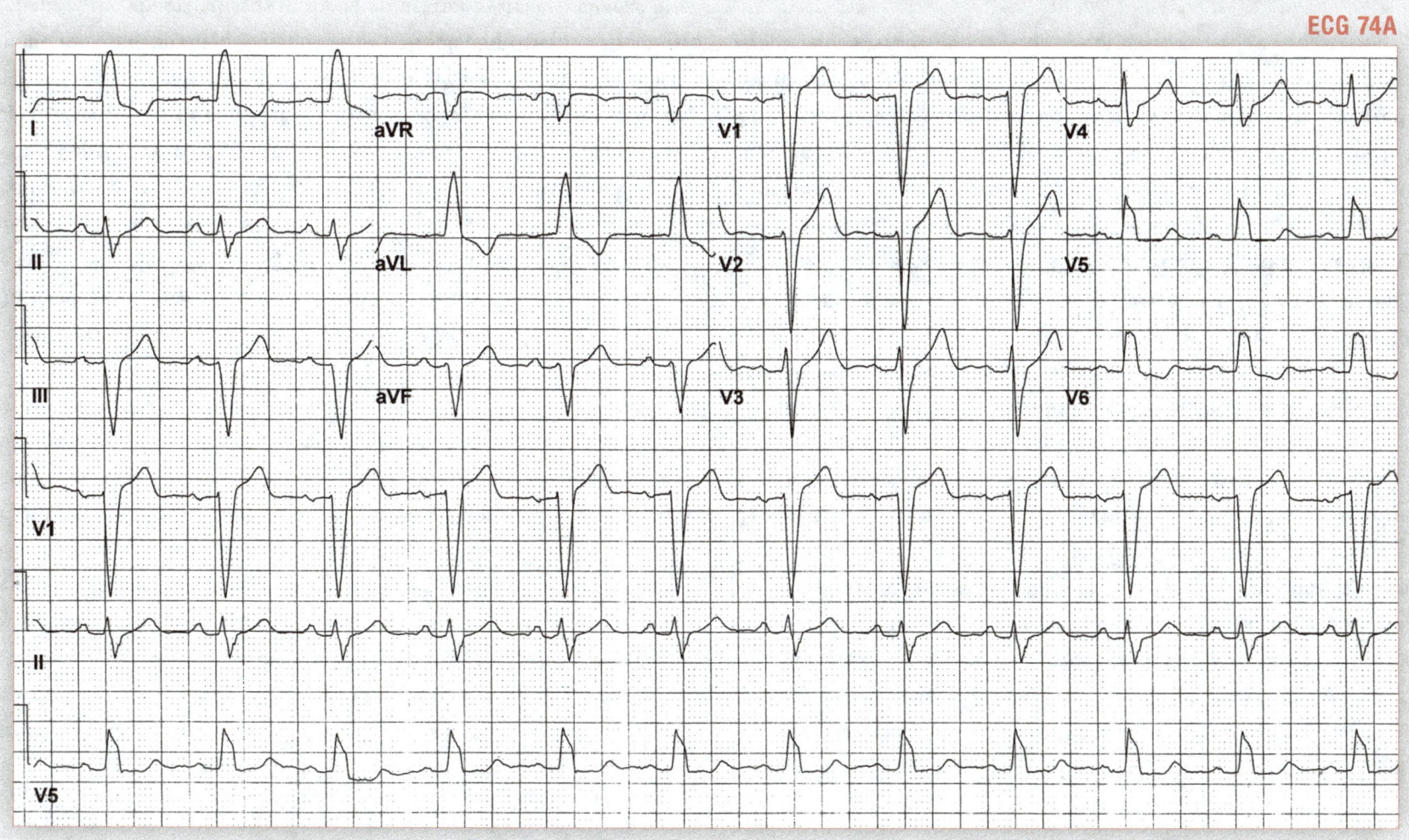

rate slows and the medical resident notes a change in the appearance of his tracing on the telemetry monitor. She obtains a second ECG (74B).

What abnormalities are evident?

What accounts for the change noticed by the resident?

What therapy is warranted?

ECG 74B

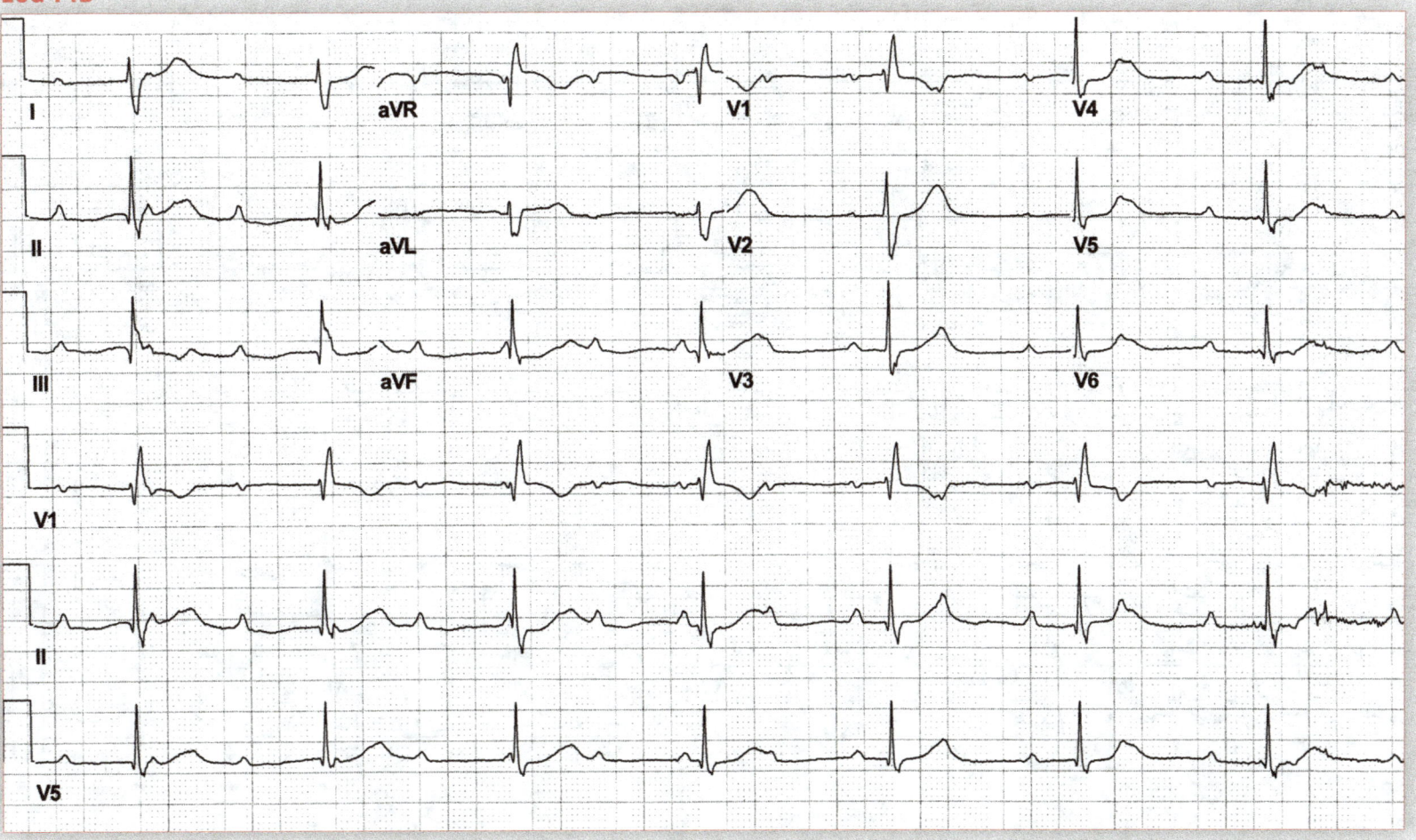

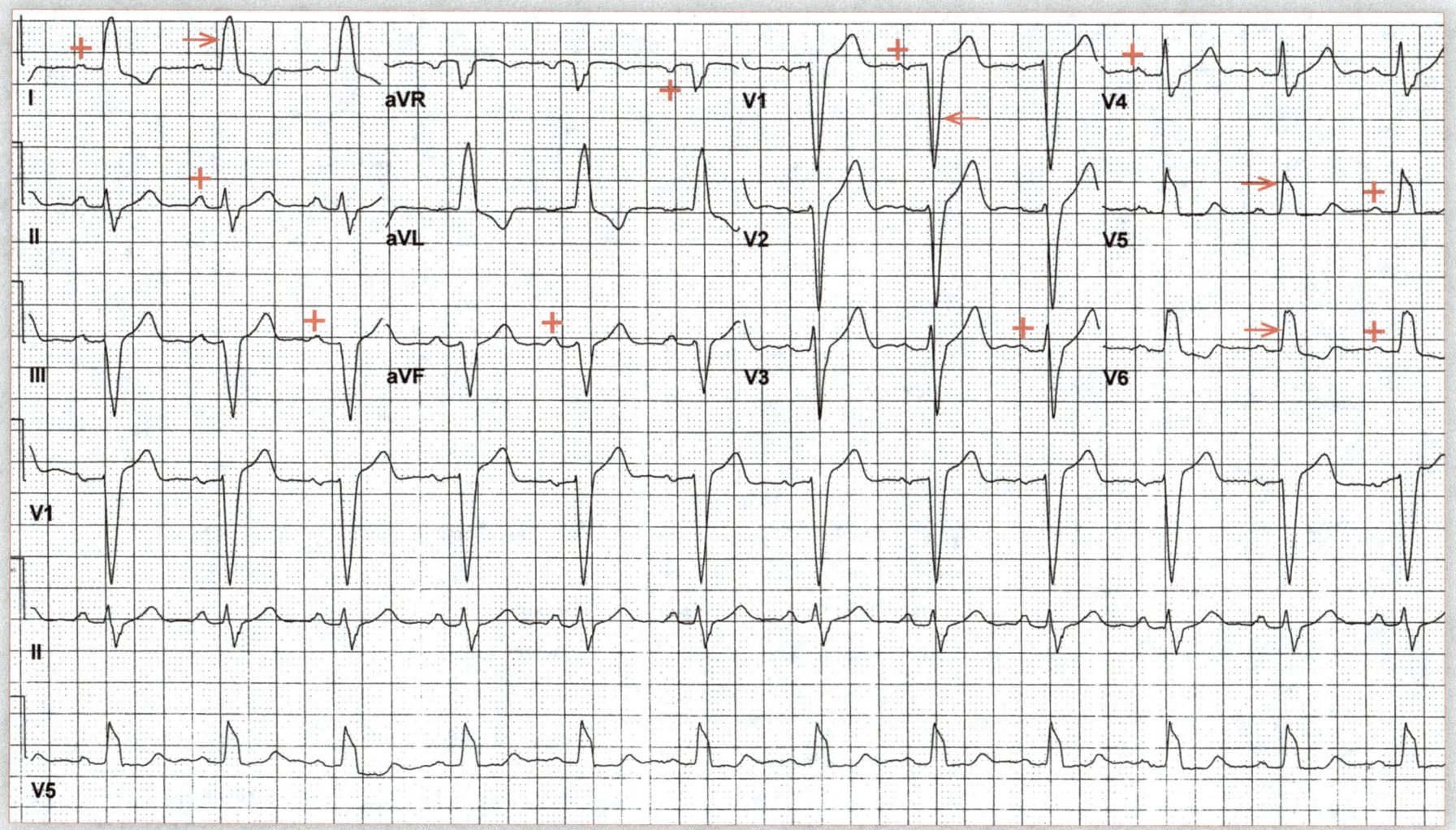

ECG 74A Analysis: Normal sinus rhythm, left bundle branch block

In **ECG 74A**, there is a regular rhythm at a rate of 76 bpm. A P wave (**+**) precedes each QRS complex, and the PR interval is stable (0.20 sec). The P waves are positive in leads I, II, aVF, and V4-V6. Hence this is a normal sinus rhythm. The QRS complex duration is prolonged (0.16 sec), and the morphology is that of a left bundle branch block (LBBB; broad R wave in leads I and V5-V6 [→] with a deep QS complex in lead V1 [←]). The QT/QTc intervals are prolonged (440/495 msec) but are normal when the increased QRS complex duration is considered (360/405 msec).

continues

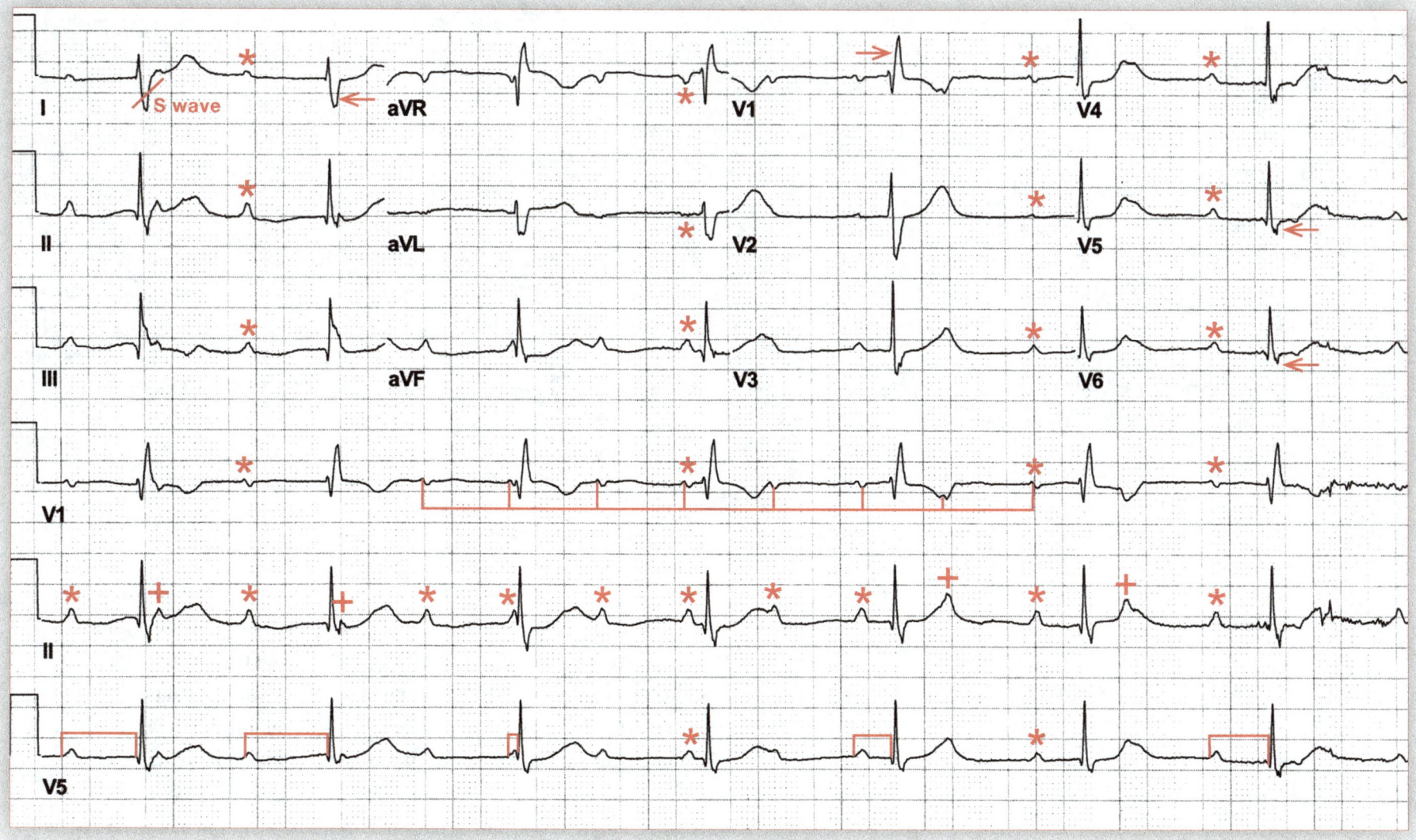

ECG 74B Analysis: Normal sinus rhythm, AV dissociation/complete heart block, escape junctional rhythm with right bundle branch block and left posterior fascicular block

ECG 74B shows regular RR intervals at a rate of 42 bpm. P waves (*) can be seen, occurring at regular PP intervals (⊔) and an atrial rate of 90 bpm. Some of the P waves are not obvious as they are super-imposed on the QRS complex or located in ST segments or T waves (+). The P waves are positive in leads I, II, aVF, and V4-V6. Hence this is a normal sinus rhythm. The PR intervals are not constant (⊓) and are variable, indicating AV dissociation. Since the atrial rate is faster than the ventricular rate, this is complete (third-degree) AV block. The QRS complexes are wide (0.16 sec), and they have a typical right bundle branch block (RBBB) morphology (RSR′ morphology in lead V1 [→] and broad S wave in leads I and V5-V6 [←]). The axis is rightward, between +90° and +180°. The QRS complex is negative in lead I (even when the terminal S wave is ignored) and positive in lead aVF. As there is an rS morphology in lead I, this is a left posterior fascicular block (LPFB). Since the QRS complexes are supraventricular in morphology (typical RBBB with normal initial forces), this is an escape junctional rhythm with an RBBB and LPFB. The complete AV block is the result of block within the AV node.

However, there has been a marked change in the QRS morphology in ECG 74B compared with ECG 74A: During sinus rhythm there is an LBBB, and with complete heart block the escape junctional rhythm has an RBBB and an LPFB. This indicates the presence of bi-bundle branch block or trifascicular disease in addition to disease within the AV node.

As this patient has significant conduction system disease, this represents a potentially unstable condition. Although the presence of complete heart block with an escape junctional rhythm may not require perma-nent pacing in the absence of symptoms, he does present with a history of syncope and lightheadedness, which warrants permanent pacemaker implantation. He also has evidence of trifascicular disease with symp-toms, another indication for permanent pacemaker insertion. ■

Notes

A 31-year-old man presents to the emergency department with a complaint of palpitations associated with lightheadedness.

What abnormality is depicted?

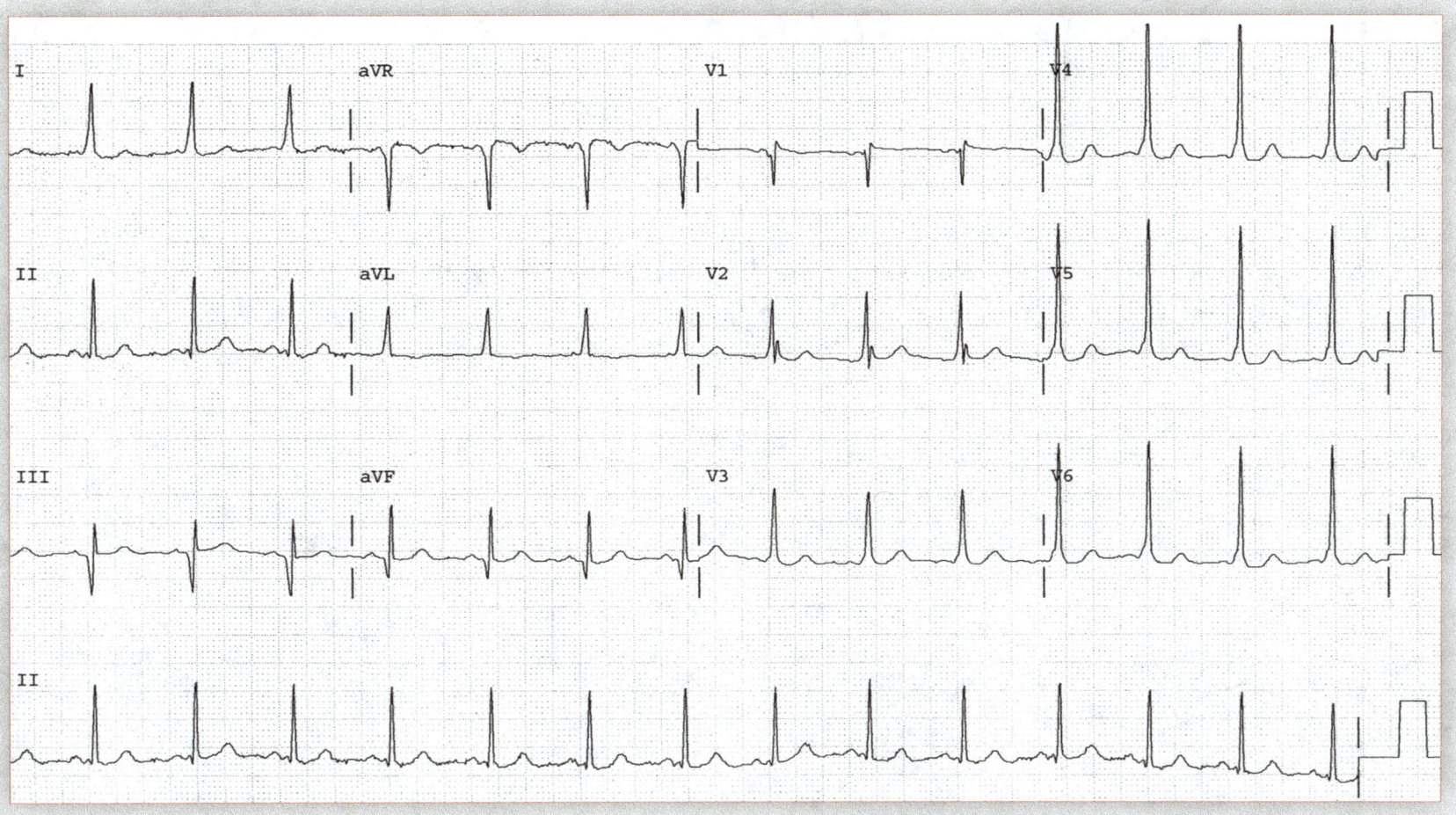

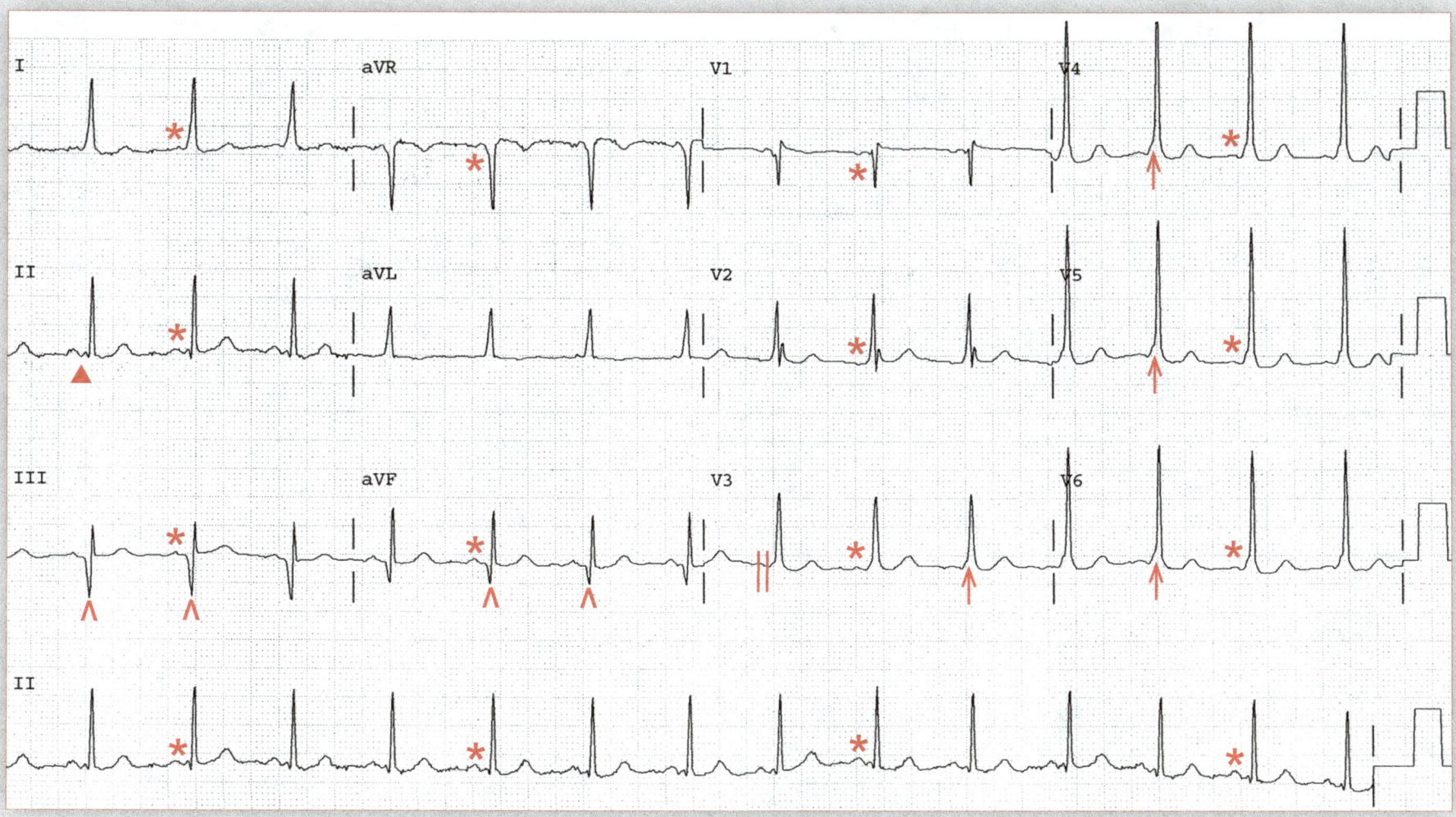

ECG 75 Analysis: Normal sinus rhythm, Wolff-Parkinson-White pattern

There is a regular rhythm at a rate of 86 bpm. There is a P wave (*) before each QRS complex, and the PR interval is constant but short (0.12 sec) (‖). The QRS complex duration appears to be normal in the limb leads (0.08 sec) but prolonged in the precordial leads (0.14 sec). Noted in precordial leads V2-V6 is a widening of the base of the QRS complex, resulting from a slurred upstroke or a delta wave (↑), that accounts for the QRS widening. A delta wave with short PR interval defines Wolff-Parkinson-White pattern.

The apparent absence of a delta wave, short PR interval, and widened QRS complex in the limb leads are due to the fact that the delta wave is isoelectric in these leads and hence not obvious. In lead II the waveform seen immediately after the P wave (▲) is indeed the delta wave. The Q waves in leads III and aVF (^) are also delta waves, although the Q waves could be confused with an inferior wall myocardial infarction. This is a pseudo-infarction pattern and indicates that the accessory pathway is in the posteroseptal wall. In Wolff-Parkinson-White pattern there is direct myocardial activation via the accessory pathway and hence ventricular abnormalities cannot be reliably diagnosed. It is important to note that the delta wave and short PR interval may, therefore, not be obvious in every lead.

The presence of symptoms of palpitations and lightheadedness is strongly suggestive of an arrhythmia. In patients with Wolff-Parkinson-White pattern on the ECG, the presence of symptoms suggesting an arrhythmia requires an evaluation. This should start with ambulatory or more extended monitoring. Many such patients undergo electrophysiologic testing to establish whether any supraventricular arrhythmia can be provoked. If so, radiofrequency ablation of the accessory pathway is often performed. Many such patients undergo radiofrequency ablation even if no arrhythmia is documented. ■

A 69-year-old man with a history of coronary artery disease presents to his cardiologist for a routine visit. He has no complaints except for brief episodes of lightheadedness that occur sporadically throughout the day. He has continued to take his medications, which include a β-blocker, aspirin, an angiotensin-converting enzyme inhibitor, and a long-acting nitrate. An ECG is obtained.

What does the ECG show?

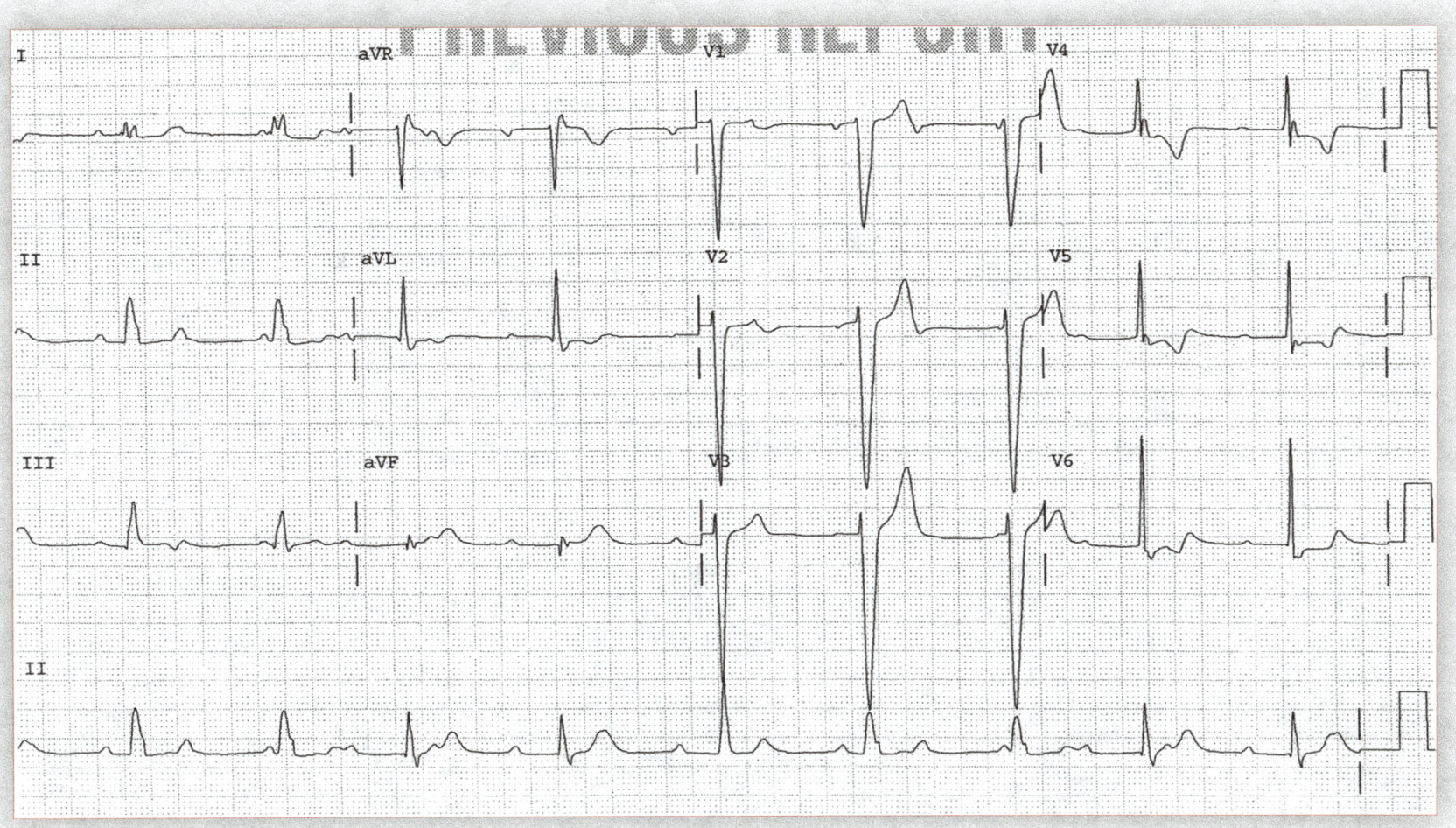

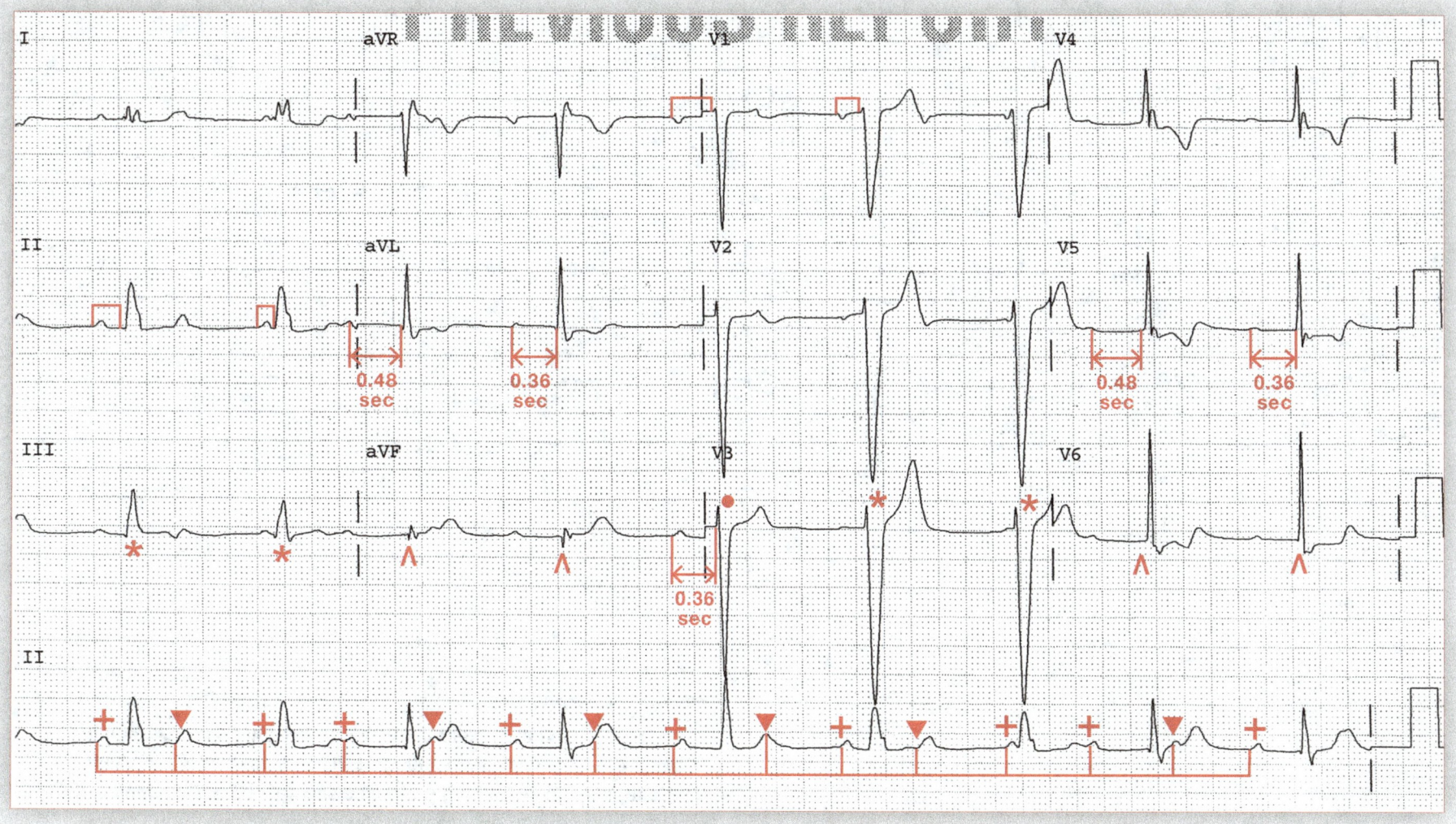

ECG 76 Analysis: Normal sinus rhythm, first-degree AV block (prolonged AV conduction),
Mobitz type II second-degree AV block, third-degree (complete) AV block,
escape ventricular complexes, fusion complex, retrograde concealed conduction

There is an irregular rhythm at an average rate of 54 bpm; however, there are P waves (+) with a regular PP interval (⊔) at an atrial rate of 96 bpm, although some of the P waves are within the T waves and ST segments (▼). The P waves are positive in leads I, II, aVF, and V4-V6. Hence there is an underlying normal sinus rhythm. The QRS complexes have several different morphologies. QRS complexes 1, 2, 6, and 7 (*) have a prolonged duration (0.16 sec), while complexes 3, 4, 8, and 9 (^) have a normal duration (0.10 sec). The fifth QRS complex (●) has a morphology that is different than both the wide and narrow QRS complexes, although it also resembles both of them; the duration of this QRS complex is 0.12 sec. The wide QRS complexes are associated with PR intervals that are variable (⊓), indicating AV dissociation. As the atrial rate is faster than the ventricular rate, complete or third-degree AV block is present. The QT/QTc intervals of these QRS complexes are normal (400/380 msec).

The PR intervals before the third and eighth QRS complexes, which are narrow and occur earlier with a shorter RR interval, are the same (0.48 sec) (↔). Hence these are conducted and the QRS complex is thus the native complex. The PR intervals before the fourth, fifth, and ninth QRS complexes (0.36 sec) (↔) are also the same, meaning that these narrow complexes are also captured. Thus, there is complete heart block with intermittent AV conduction or capture. However, the PR interval of the first captured QRS complexes (complexes 3 and 8) is slightly longer (0.48 sec) than that of the subsequent captured QRS complexes (4 and 9) (0.36 sec). This is due to retrograde concealed conduction. That is, the preceding QRS complexes (2 and 7), which are ventricular in origin, have produced retrograde (ventriculoatrial) conduction into the AV node but do not completely conduct through the node; rather they partially penetrate the node (*ie*, they are concealed within the node), rendering it partially refractory. As a result, the next P wave is conducted at a slower rate and hence a slightly longer PR interval. Therefore, the PR interval (0.36 sec) before the fourth and ninth QRS complexes represents the baseline PR interval.

The fifth QRS complex has a morphology that resembles both the narrow and wide QRS complexes. The PR interval before this complex is the same as the PR interval before the fourth and ninth QRS complexes (0.36 sec; *ie*, the baseline PR interval). Therefore, this is a fusion complex, resulting from an impulse conducted through the AV node–His-Purkinje system that fused with the impulse coming from the ventricle. Fusion complexes reflect the presence of AV dissociation.

Finally, the narrow QRS complexes are associated with a pattern of 2:1 AV conduction (2:1 AV block); that is, every other P wave is nonconducted. Therefore, this is second-degree AV block with 2:1 AV conduction. As the escape rhythm is ventricular, the 2:1 AV block is the result of Mobitz type II second-degree AV block. ■

Practice Case 77

A 72-year-old woman presents to her primary care physician with complaints of palpitations. These episodes, which have become more frequent over the past several months, are unheralded and sometimes wake her from sleep. She has noted lightheadedness

ECG 77A

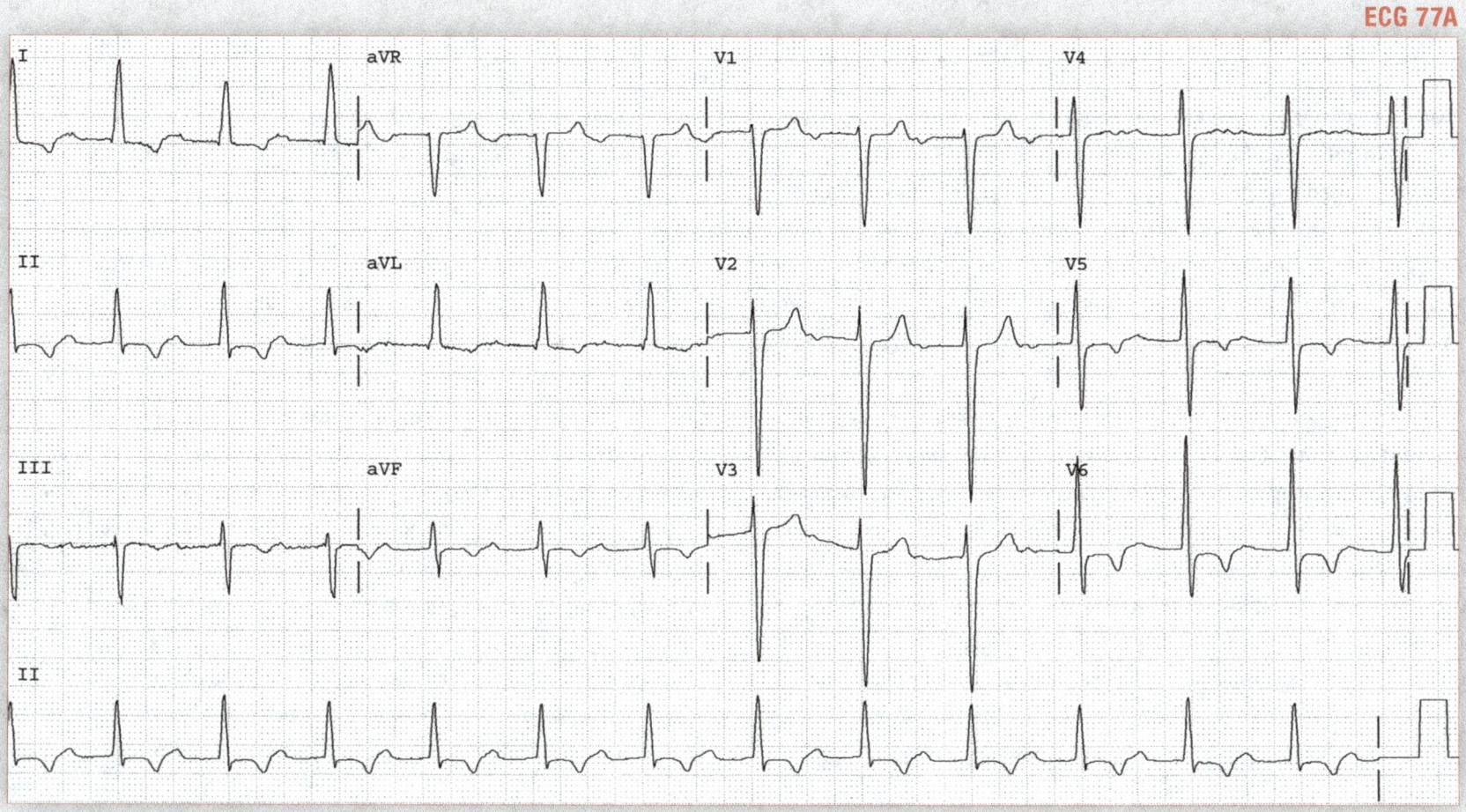

on one occasion but has never lost consciousness. Her physician obtains an ECG during the initial portion of the visit (77A). She was asymptomatic at the time. During the interview, she notes the abrupt onset of palpitations. The physician obtains another ECG (77B).

What rhythm does ECG 77A show?

Is a conduction abnormality present?

Is therapy indicated based on the finding in ECG 77B?

ECG 77B

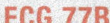

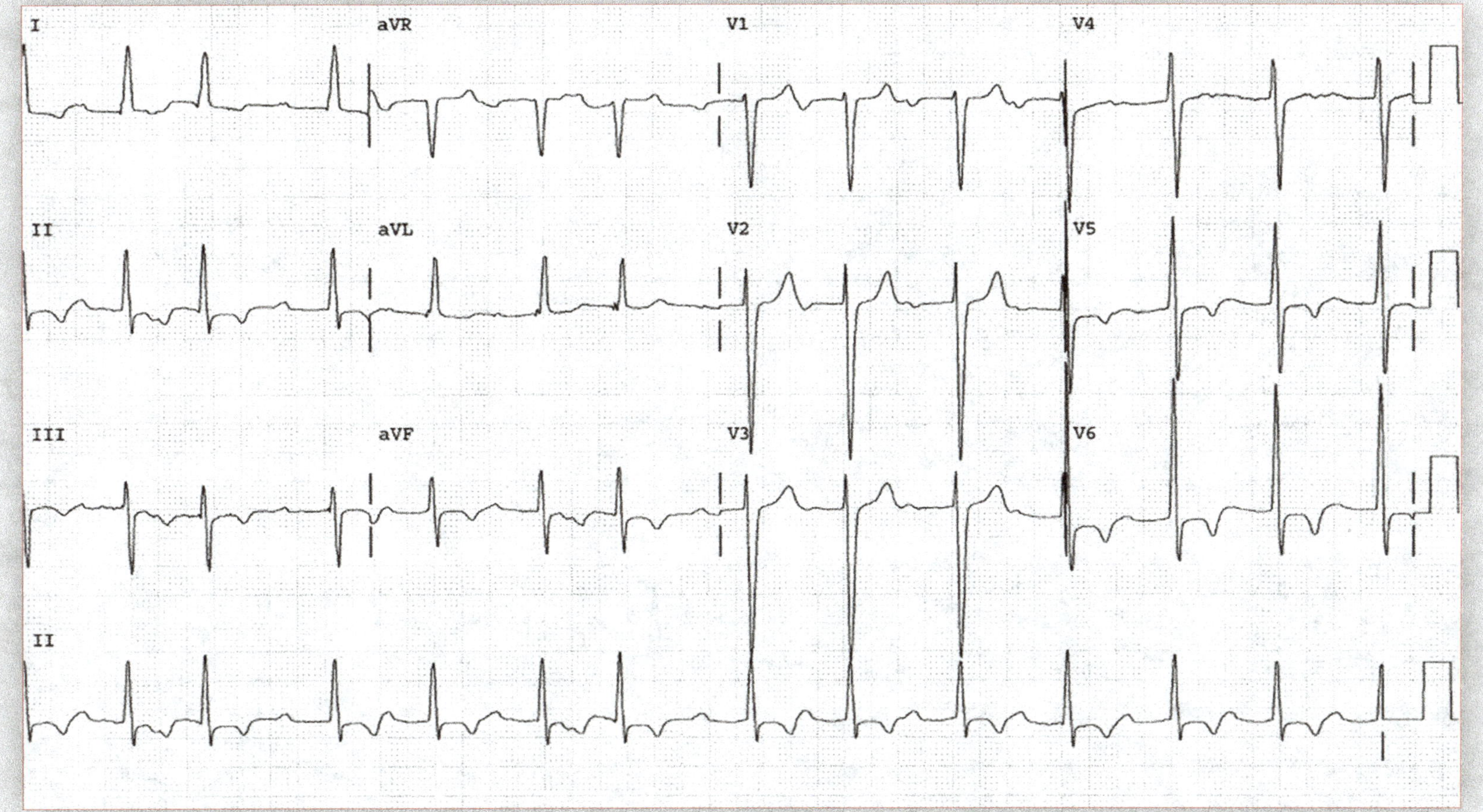

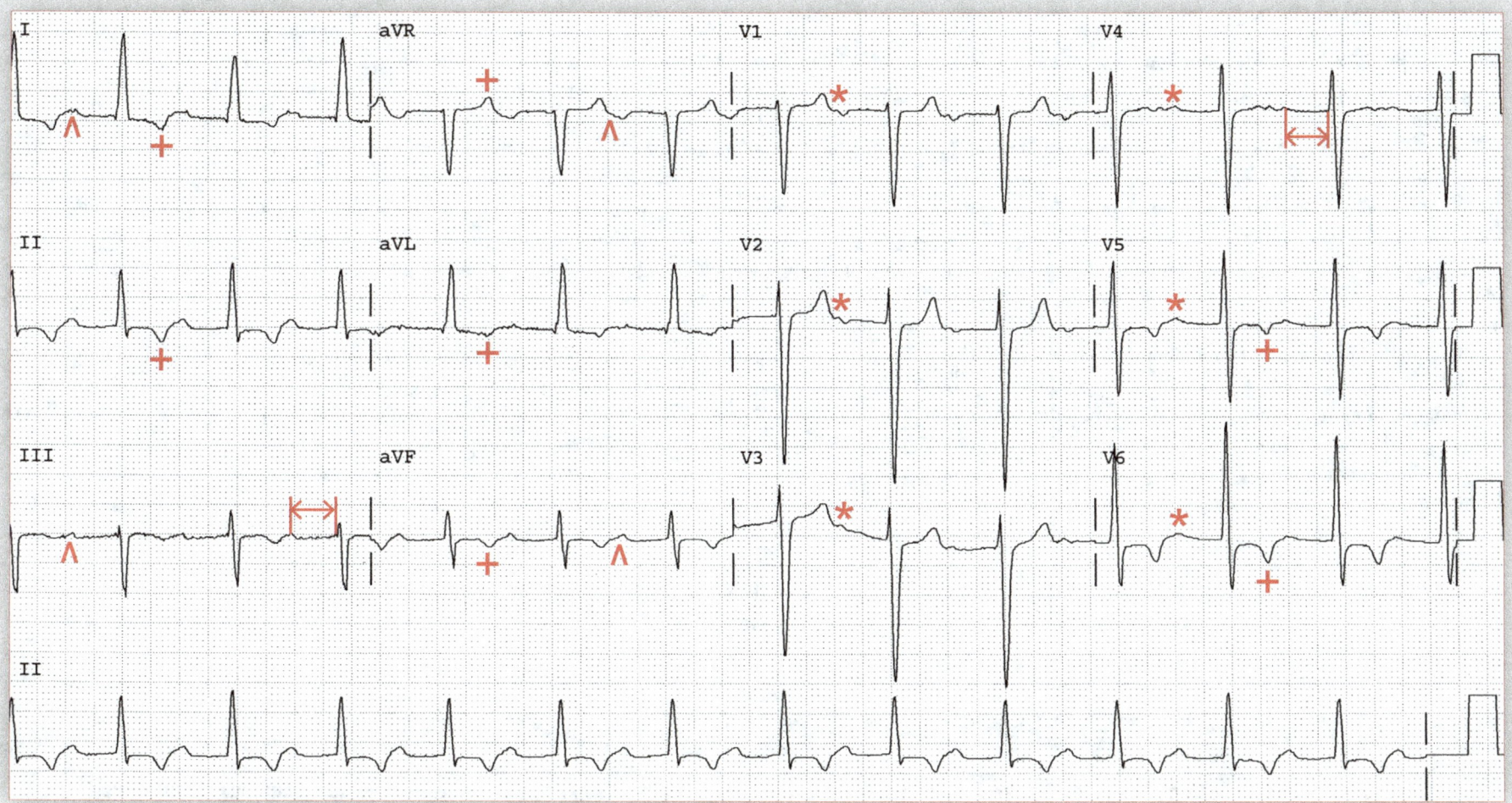

ECG 77A Analysis: Normal sinus rhythm, first-degree AV block (prolonged AV conduction), nonspecific T-wave abnormalities

In **ECG 77A**, there is a regular rhythm at a rate of 78 bpm. The QRS complex duration is normal (0.10 sec) and there is a normal morphology and axis, between 0° and +90° (positive QRS complex in leads I and aVF). The QT/QTc intervals are normal (380/430 msec). There are diffuse T-wave abnormalities (+) that are nonspecific. P waves are not obviously seen in most of the leads; however, there is a small waveform noted after the T wave in leads V1-V6 (*). On closer inspection this waveform can also be seen in the limb leads (^), altering the end of the T wave. This is the P wave and the PR interval is 0.36 second (↔), indicating a first-degree AV block (prolonged AV conduction).

continues

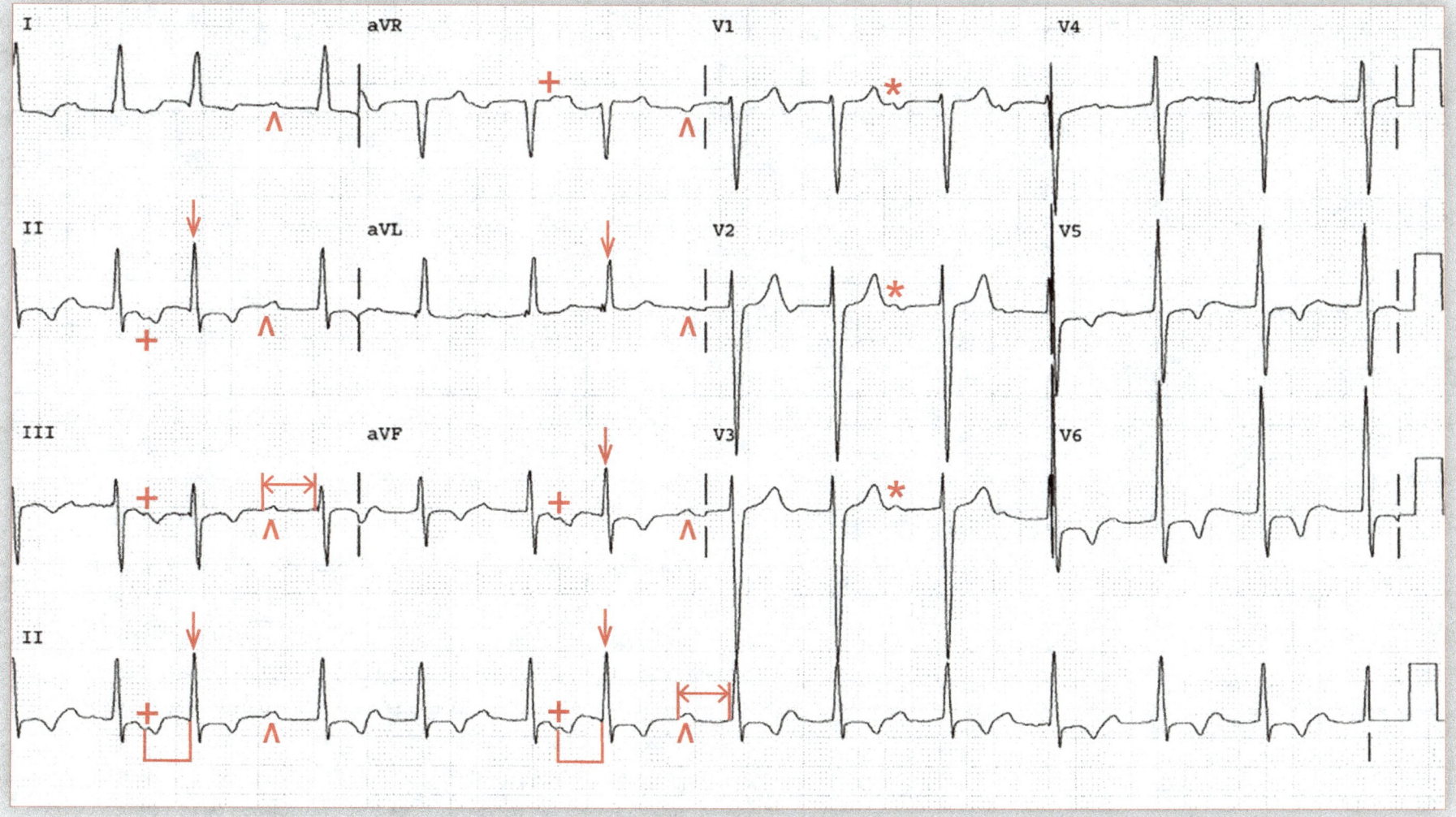

ECG 77B Analysis: Normal sinus rhythm, premature atrial complexes, first-degree AV block (prolonged AV conduction), nonspecific T-wave abnormalities

The rate in **ECG 77B** is 80 bpm, but the rhythm is regularly irregular as a result of two premature QRS complexes (second and sixth) (↓) that are followed by pauses. The QRS complex duration, morphology, and axis are the same as in **ECG 77A**, as are the QT/QTc intervals. Diffuse T-wave abnormalities are also noted and are the same as in **ECG 77A**. As with **ECG 77A**, small waveforms noted at the end of the T wave in leads V1-V3 are suggestive of P waves (*). The second and sixth QRS complexes are premature (↓), and in leads II, III, and aVF small P waves (+) can be seen in the T waves preceding these two QRS complexes; the PR interval is 0.30 second (⊔). These are, therefore, premature atrial complexes. After the premature beat there is a pause that allows the sinus P wave to be seen clearly (^), confirming the presence of a normal sinus rhythm with a first-degree AV block and a PR interval of 0.36 second (↔). This is the same PR interval as that measured on **ECG 77A**. Importantly, P waves that are not obvious (as a result of first-degree AV block and tachycardia) may be seen superimposed on the T wave or after a pause or long RR interval, as was seen after the premature atrial complex.

It appears that the palpitations are the result of premature atrial complexes. These premature complexes are common, benign, and generally do not require therapy. However, in the presence of associated symptoms, medical therapy with a β-blocker, calcium-channel blocker, or anti-arrhythmic drug can be attempted. ■

Practice Case 78

A 76-year-old man with an underlying cardiomyopathy, believed to be the result of excessive alcohol use, presents to the emergency department with complaints of intermittent lightheadedness associated with shortness of breath. An ECG is obtained (78A), but no specific diagnosis is provided. He is scheduled for a

ECG 78A

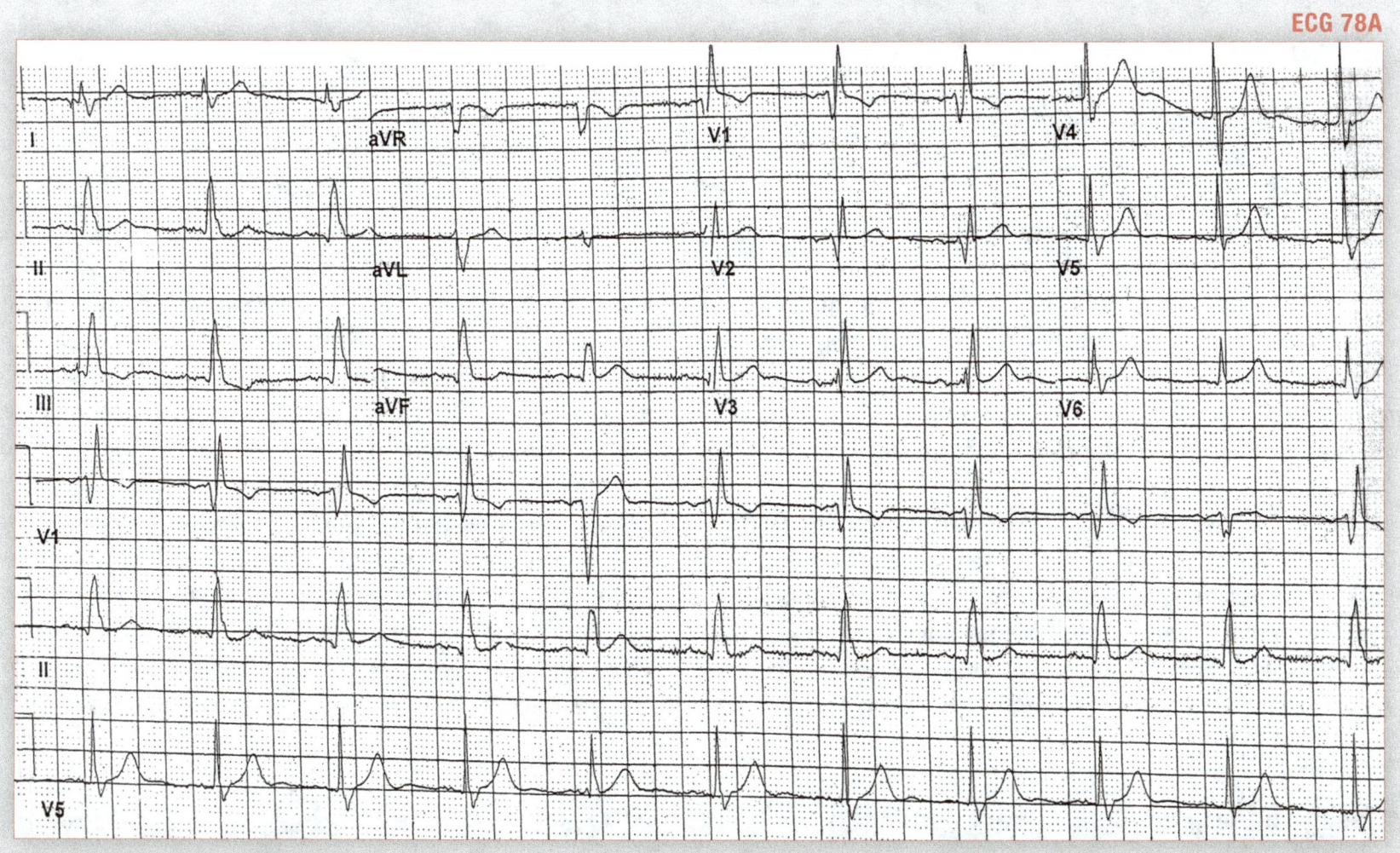

Holter monitor and referred to a cardiologist for further evaluation. The Holter monitor does not show any abnormality, but he had no symptoms while wearing it. When the man sees a cardiologist, he states that he has been experiencing lightheadedness that began the previous day. An ECG is obtained (ECG 78B).

Are there any findings of concern on ECG 78A?

What does ECG 78B show?

What therapy is indicated?

ECG 78B

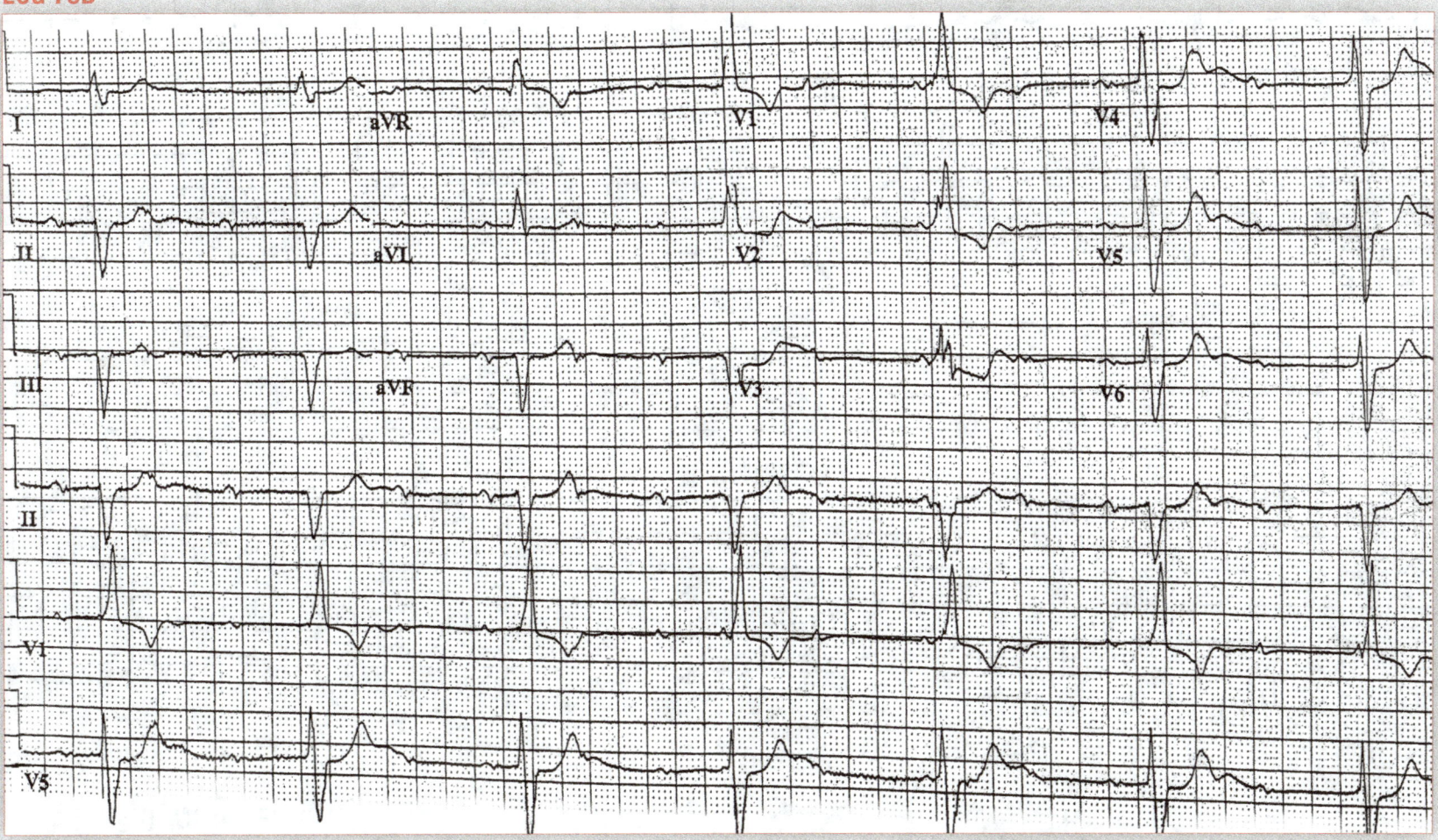

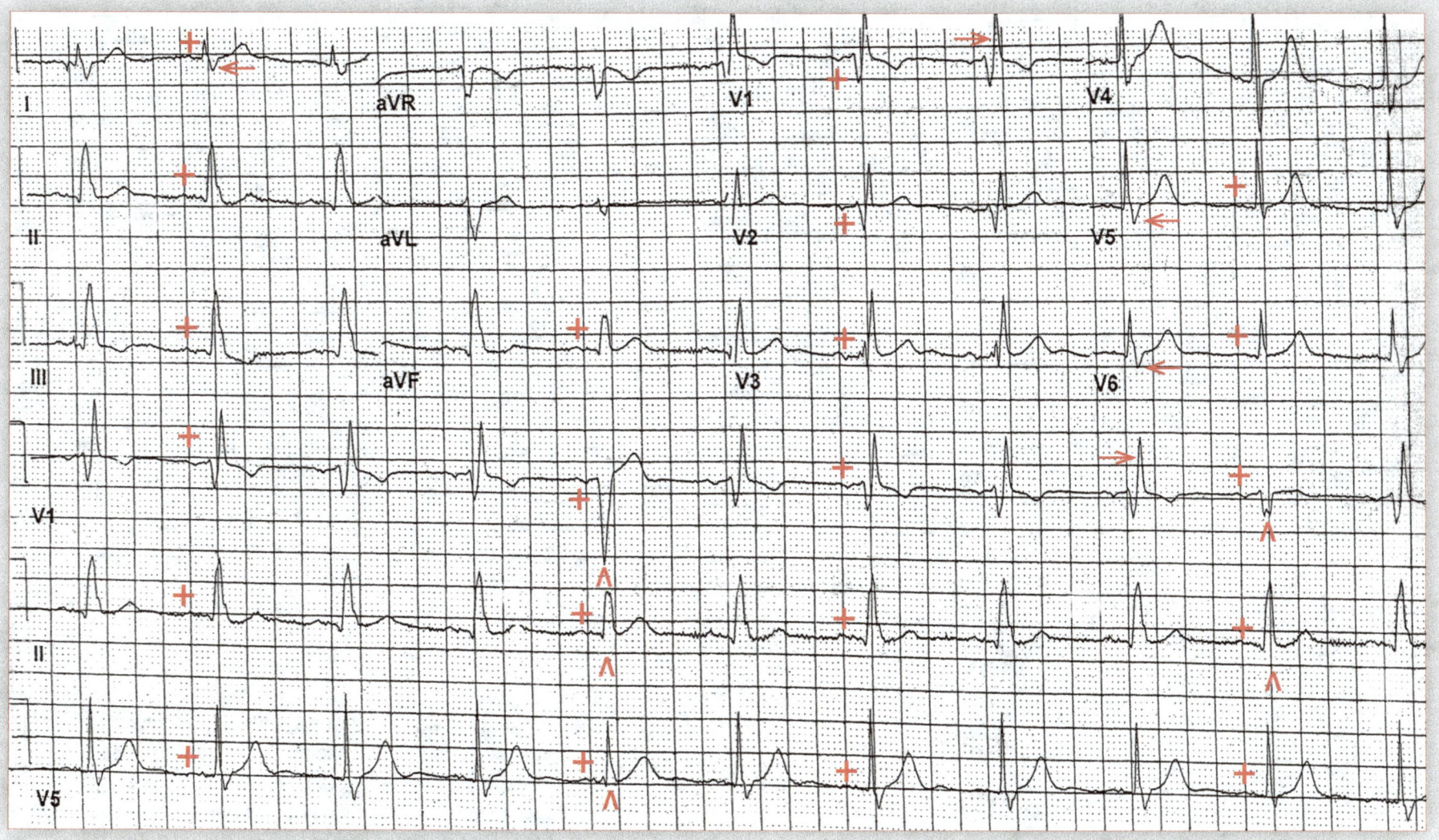

ECG 78A Analysis: Normal sinus rhythm, bi-bundle branch block (alternating right and left bundle branch block), trifascicular disease

ECG 78A shows a regular rhythm at a rate of 64 bpm. There is a P wave (+) before each QRS complex with a stable PR interval (0.20 sec). The P waves are positive in leads I, II, aVF, and V4-V6. Hence there is a normal sinus rhythm. The QRS complex duration is increased (0.14 sec), and all but two QRS complexes (5 and 10) (^) have a right bundle branch block morphology with an RSR' morphology in lead V1 (→) and broad terminal S waves in leads I and V5-V6 (←). The axis is normal, between 0° and +90° (positive QRS complex in leads I and aVF). The QT/QTc intervals are normal (400/410 msec and 340/350 msec when the prolonged QRS complex duration is considered). However, the fifth and 10th QRS complexes (^) have the same duration (0.14 sec) but a different morphology; they have a left bundle branch block morphology with a QS complex in lead V1 and a broad R wave in lead V5. The P wave and PR intervals before these complexes are the same as before all the other QRS complexes. Hence there is evidence of block in both the right and left bundles. This is termed bi-bundle branch block; it can also be termed trifascicular disease.

The presence of trifascicular disease or bi-bundle branch block, which indicates the presence of diffuse conduction disease involving the entire ventricular conduction system, increases the risk for complete heart block; this will be associated with an escape ventricular rhythm because an escape rhythm can only originate from below the His-Purkinje system (ie, the ventricular myocardium). The patient's symptoms of lightheadedness and shortness of breath are likely due to intermittent complete heart block with an escape rhythm that is slow.

continues

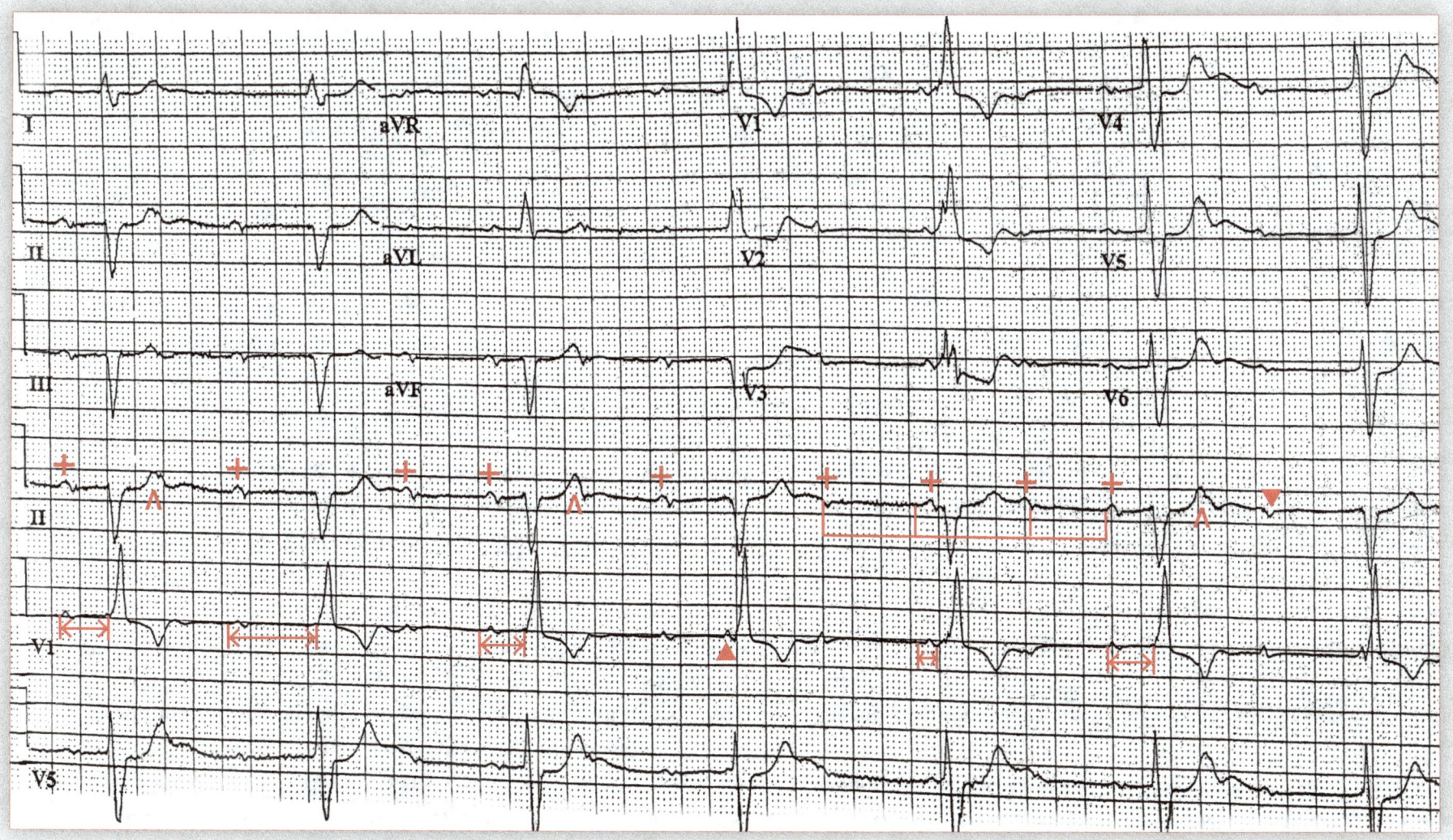

ECG 78B Analysis: Normal sinus rhythm, complete heart block, escape ventricular rhythm, nonconducted (blocked) premature atrial complex

In **ECG 78B**, obtained while the patient was symptomatic, there is a regular rhythm at a rate of 40 bpm. P waves are seen (+), although some of the P waves are not obvious as they are within the QRS complexes or on the T waves (^). When the P waves are seen, however, the PP interval is constant (⊔) at an atrial rate of 98 bpm. The last P wave (▼) is early and has a different morphology: it is a premature atrial complex that is nonconducted. Another premature P wave can be seen immediately before the fourth QRS complex (▲). There is no relationship between the P waves and the QRS complexes (*ie*, the PR intervals are variable; ↔). Therefore, AV dissociation is present. As the atrial rate is faster than the ventricular rate, this is complete heart block (or third-degree AV block).

The QRS complexes are wide (0.16 sec), and their morphology is unlike that of the QRS complexes in **ECG 78A** (*ie*, they have neither a typical right or left bundle branch block morphology). Hence these are ventricular complexes.

As would be expected in the presence of bi-bundle branch block, the development of complete heart block is associated with an escape ventricular rhythm. The slow escape ventricular rhythm is very likely the cause of the patient's symptoms. Hence the insertion of a permanent pacemaker is indicated. ■

Practice Case 79

A 75-year-old woman presents to the emergency department with dizziness and headache. Her blood pressure is noted to be 220/100 mm Hg. The exam is otherwise unremarkable except for a slow heart rate. An ECG is obtained (79A). She is admitted to the hospital for severe

ECG 79A

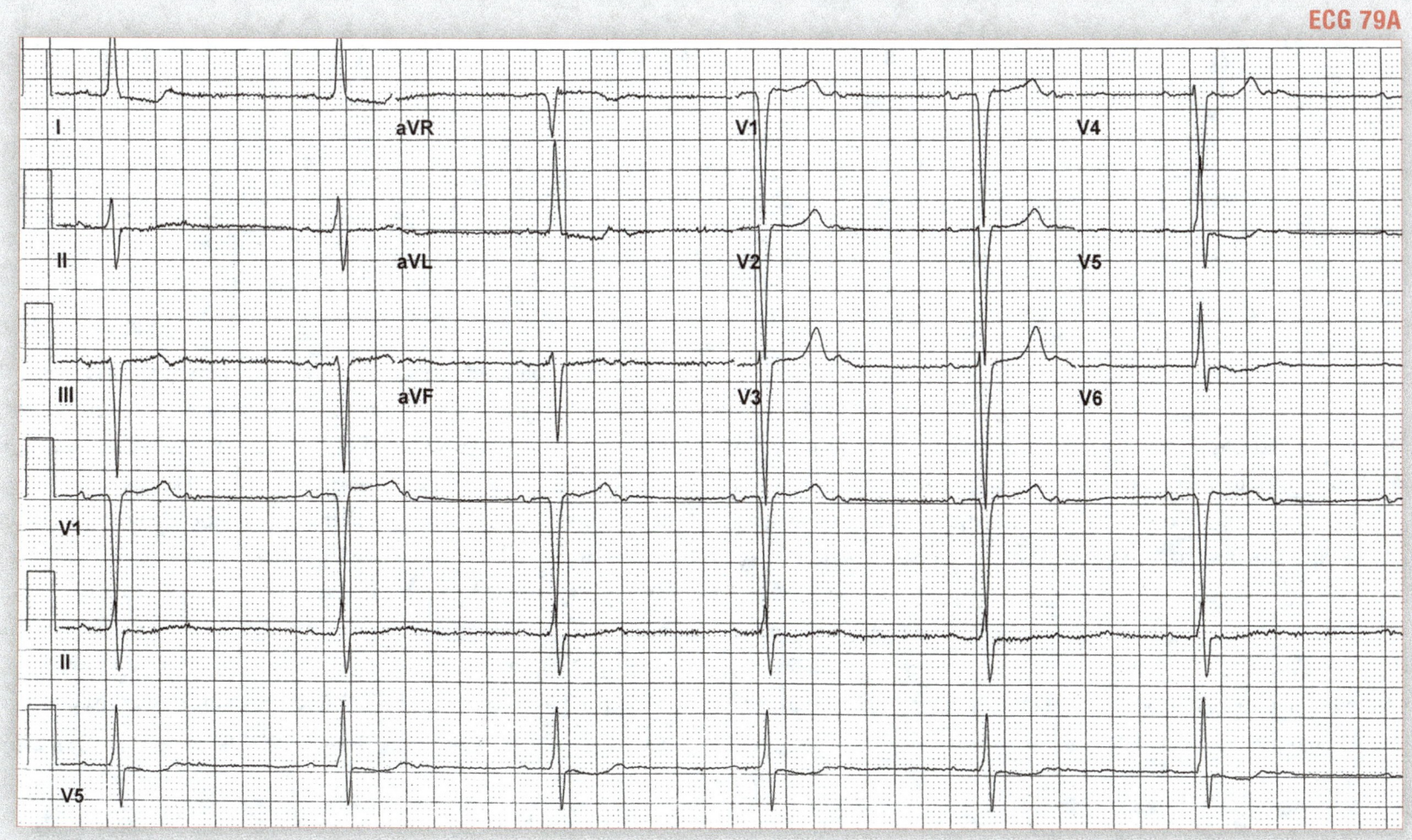

hypertension and initiated on therapy with an angiotensin-converting enzyme (ACE) inhibitor, calcium-channel blocker, and β-blocker. After therapy her blood pressure is 140/80 mm Hg, and her pulse remains slow. However, telemetry shows a change and another ECG is obtained (79B).

What accounts for the slow heart rate?

What therapy is necessary?

ECG 79B

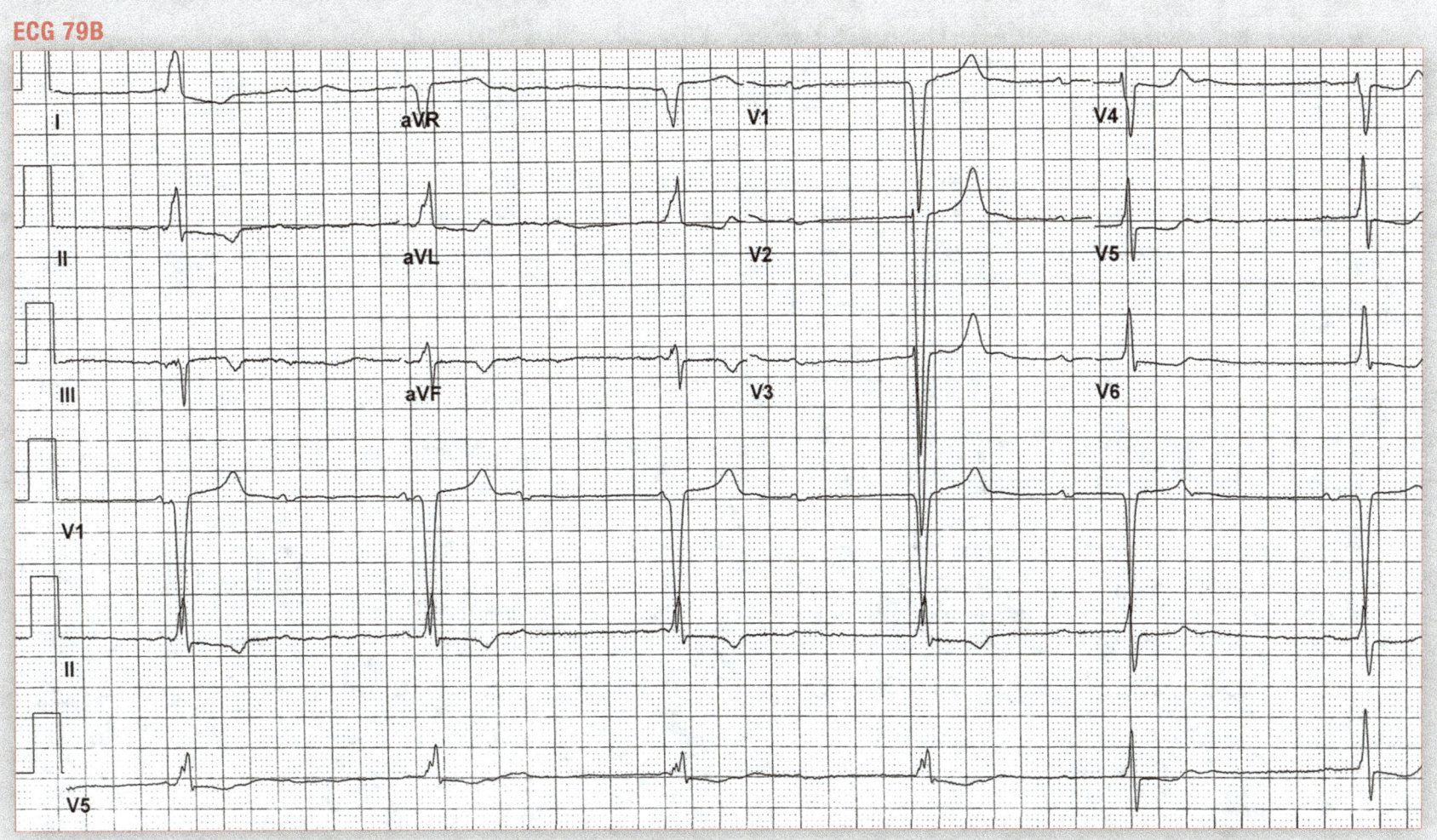

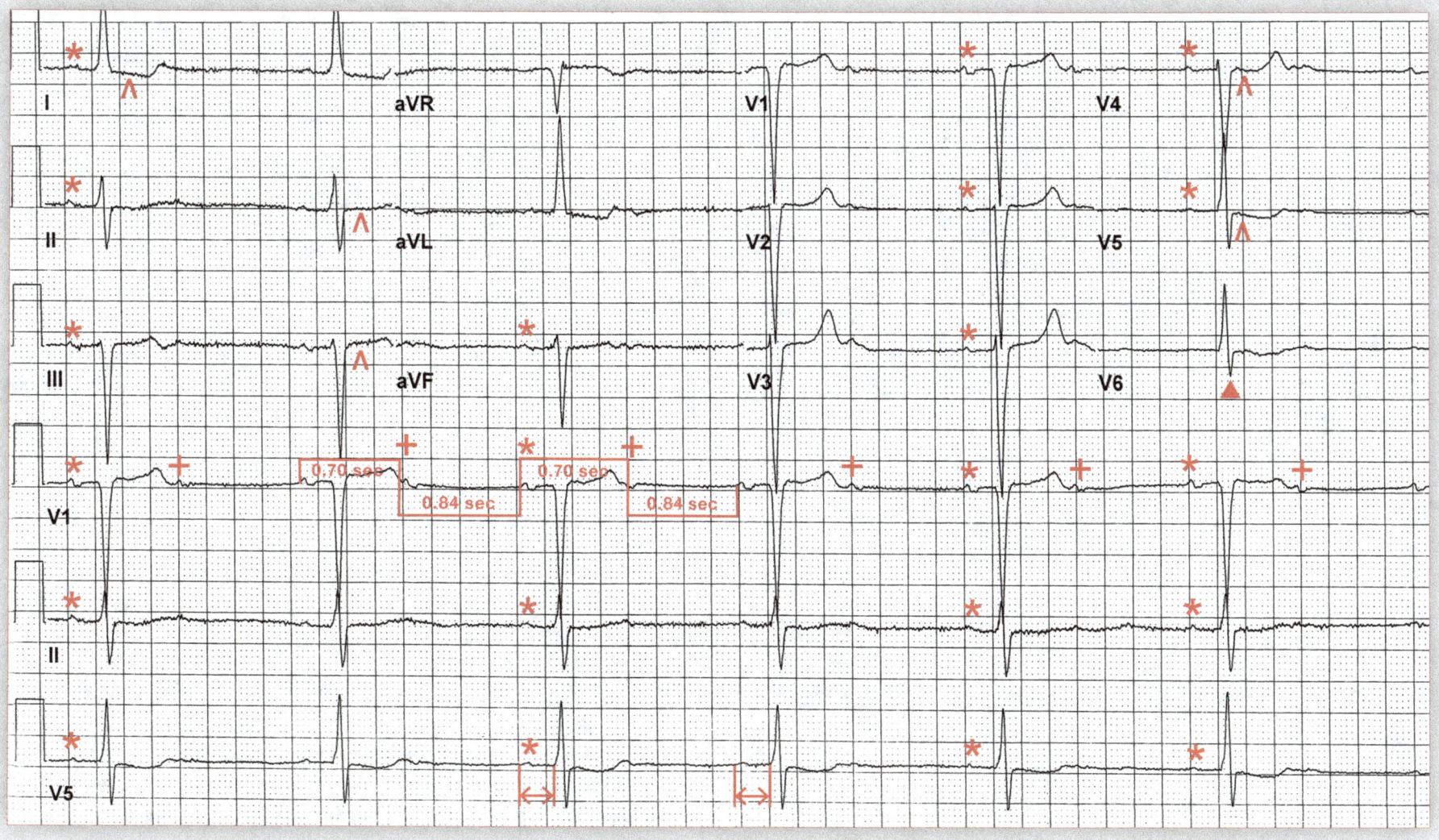

ECG 79A Analysis: Normal sinus rhythm with ventriculophasic arrhythmia, first-degree AV block (prolonged AV conduction), 2:1 second-degree AV block, intraventricular conduction delay

ECG 79A shows regular RR intervals at a rate of 36 bpm. There is a P wave (*) before each QRS complex with a stable PR interval (↔) of 0.24 second (first-degree AV block or prolonged AV conduction). A second P wave (+) can be seen after each QRS complex. This P wave is nonconducted. The presence of an occasional nonconducted P wave defines second-degree AV block, and there is a pattern of 2:1 AV conduction. The atrial rate is not constant, and the PP interval surrounding the QRS complex (⊓) is shorter (0.70 sec) than the PP interval without a QRS complex (⊔) (0.84 sec). This represents ventriculophasic arrhythmia. This finding can be seen whenever there is 2:1 AV block or complete heart block. Ventriculophasic arrhythmia is due to enhanced sinus node impulse generation resulting from ventricular contraction. This may be the result of increased sinus nodal artery pulsatile blood flow with ventricular contraction; stretching of the right atrium with ventricular contraction, resulting in an increase in sinus node automaticity; or baroreceptor changes resulting from the stroke volume occurring with ventricular contraction.

The QRS complexes are wide (0.11 sec) but are not wide enough to be a full left bundle branch block (LBBB; *ie*, they are not ≥ 0.12 sec). They do not demonstrate a pattern of a right bundle branch block nor do they have a typical LBBB pattern as there is a terminal S wave in lead V6 (▲) representing terminal forces in a left-to-right direction, which cannot be seen with an LBBB. Hence this is an intraventricular conduction delay (IVCD). There are nonspecific ST-T wave changes (^). The axis is leftward, between 0° and −30° (positive QRS complex in lead I, biphasic QRS complex in lead II, and negative QRS complex in lead aVF). The QT/QTc intervals are 500/390 msec (460/360 msec when corrected for the prolonged QRS complex duration).   *continues*

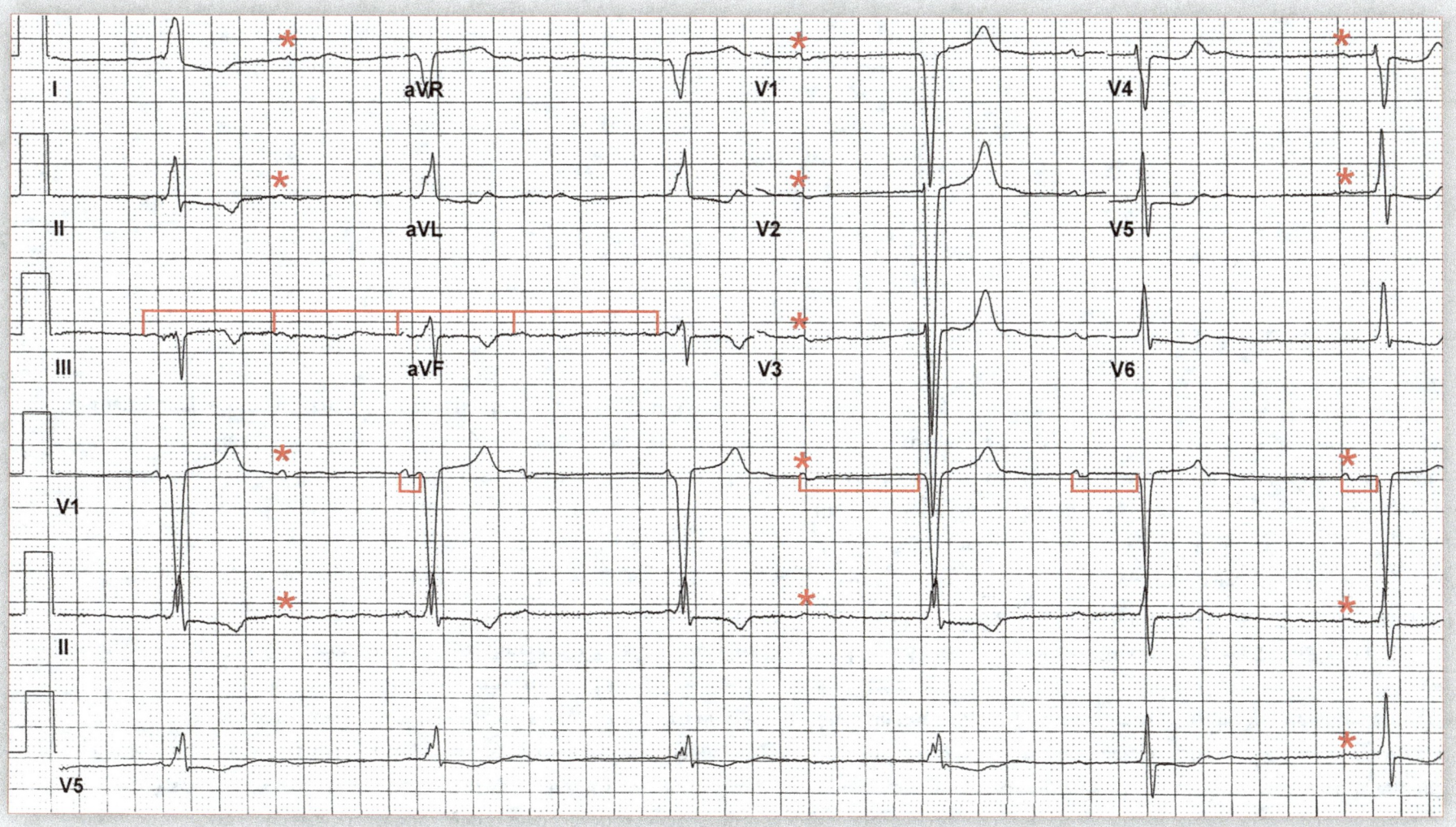

ECG 79B Analysis: Normal sinus rhythm, complete AV block, escape junctional rhythm

In ECG 79B, there are regular RR intervals at a rate of 34 bpm. The atrial rate is constant (⊓) at 72 bpm, and the P waves (*) are positive in leads I, II, aVF, and V4-V5. The PR interval (⊔) is not constant, and AV dissociation is present. AV dissociation with an atrial rate faster than the ventricular rate indicates complete heart block. The escape rhythm has a widened QRS complex (0.11–0.12 sec) that is almost identical in morphology to that seen in ECG 79A; hence this is an escape junctional rhythm. The slight difference in the QRS morphology of these junctional complexes when compared with the sinus complexes is due to the fact that the junctional complex originates from an ectopic focus within the AV junction and the impulse it generates enters the bundle of His at a different location when compared with the sinus impulse, which is conducted through the AV node. The difference in conduction pathway through the His-Purkinje system will result in a slightly different morphology, axis, or amplitude.

The etiology of the conduction problem with 2:1 AV conduction can be established when complete heart block develops; the origin of the escape rhythm indicates whether the block is within the AV node or is infra-Hisian (*ie*, within the His-Purkinje system). If the escape QRS complex is narrow or similar to the conducted QRS complexes, the 2:1 AV block is Mobitz type I due to conduction abnormality within the AV node. An escape QRS complex that is wide and abnormal is consistent with a ventricular focus and hence the 2:1 AV block is Mobitz type II with infra-Hisian disease. If ECG 79B were the only tracing available, it would be uncertain whether the escape rhythm was junctional with an underlying IVCD or a ventricular rhythm. In this situation an invasive electrophysiologic study would be required to determine the locus of the block. However, as ECG 79A is available and shows that the conducted complexes have the same morphology as the dissociated complexes in ECG 79B, it is clear that this is an escape junctional rhythm.

The 2:1 AV block is a result of underlying AV nodal disease. Severe hypertension can result in a decrease in sympathetic tone and an increase in vagal tone mediated through the baroreceptors and, therefore, can contribute to AV nodal conduction abnormalities. The repeat ECG shows complete heart block with an escape junctional rhythm that is possibly a result of β-blocker therapy in the presence of underlying AV nodal disease. The first step would be to discontinue the β-blocker. If conduction improves, then no further therapy is indicated. However, if complete heart block persists, indicating structural disease of the AV node, then a permanent pacemaker is indicated. ■

A 25-year-old woman with persistent cardiomyopathy following a pregnancy 6 months ago presents to her primary care physician with complaints of intermittent palpitations. Episodes are unheralded and without any other associated symptoms.

She denies dyspnea. Of note, symptoms started 1 week ago, approximately 2 weeks after she self-discontinued her β-blocker. She states that she "doesn't need those pills anymore." An ECG is obtained during one of her episodes of palpitations.

What is the cause of the patient's symptoms?

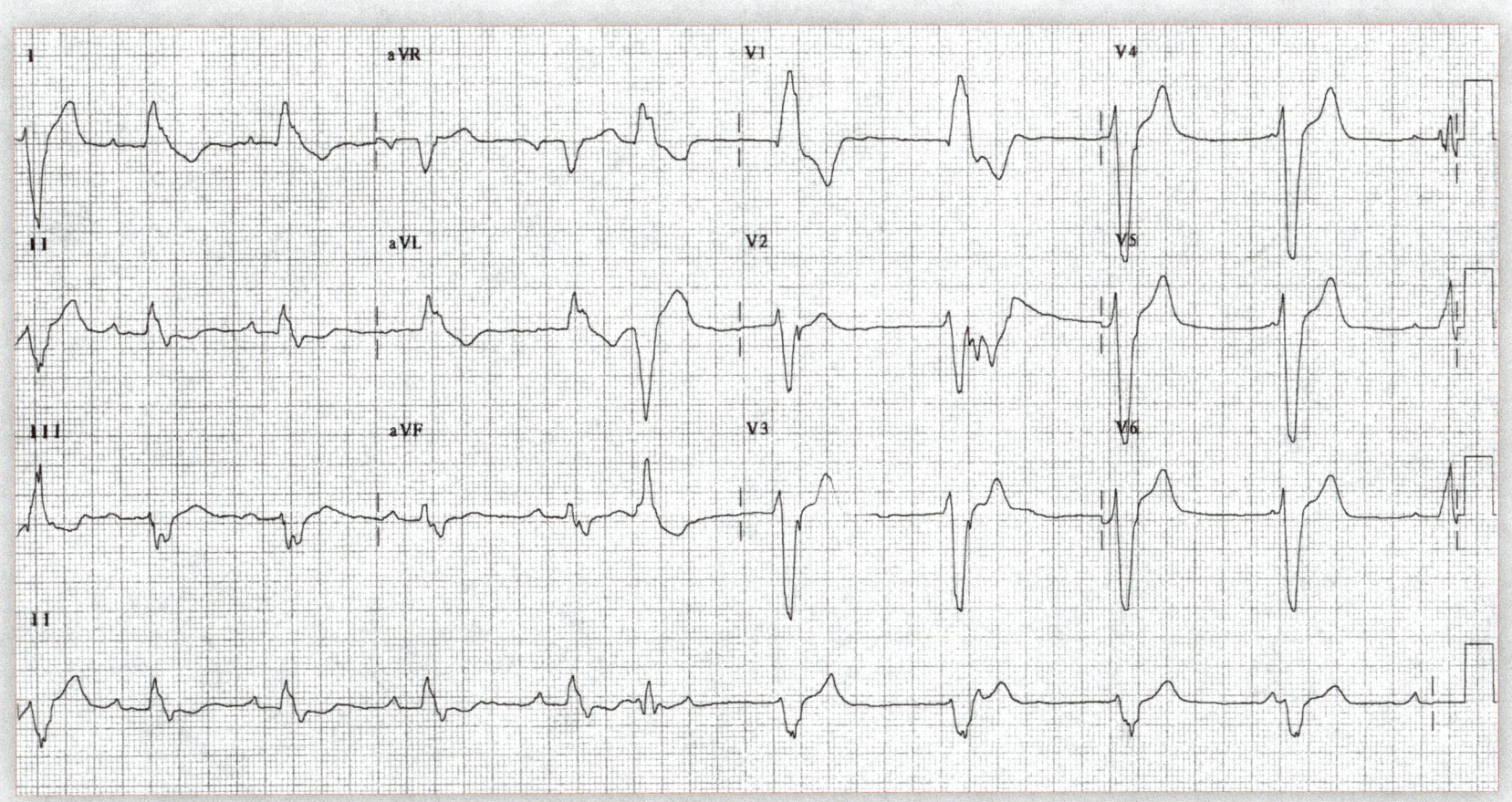

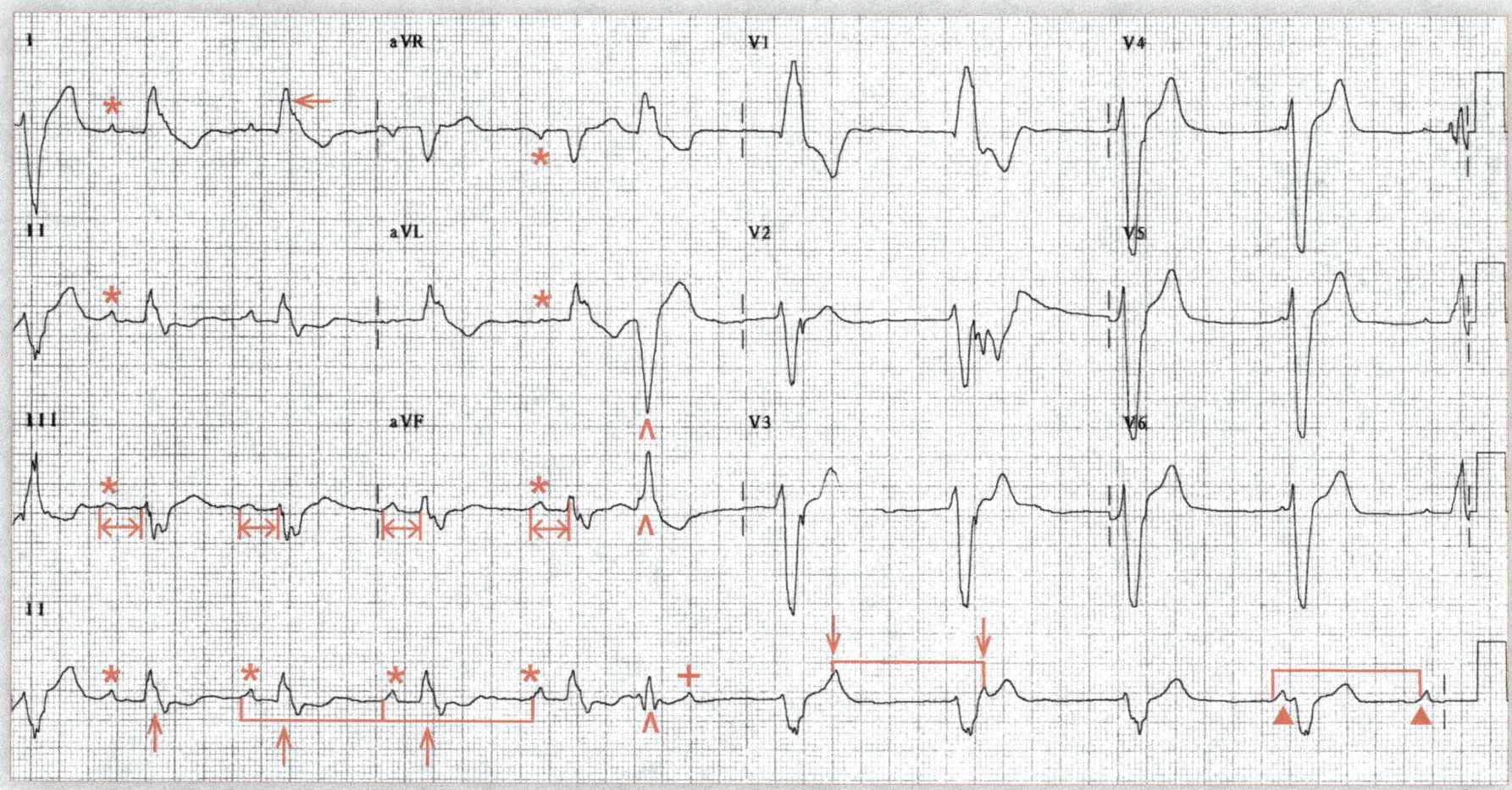

ECG 80 Analysis: Normal sinus rhythm, first-degree AV block (prolonged AV conduction), left bundle branch block, premature ventricular complex, complete heart block with ventricular escape, trifascicular disease

There is a regular rhythm at a rate of 62 bpm. There is a P wave (*) before the first four QRS complexes (↑) with a constant PR interval of 0.24 second (↔) (first-degree AV block or prolonged AV conduction). The P waves are positive in leads I, II, aVF, and V4-V6. Hence there is a normal sinus rhythm. The QRS complex is widened at 0.18 second, and it has a left bundle branch block pattern (broad R wave in lead I [←]). A single premature ventricular complex (^) is followed by an on-time, nonconducted sinus P wave (+); thereafter, the QRS complexes are wider (0.20 sec), have a different morphology, and occur at a regular rate of 50 bpm. There are still sinus P waves at a regular interval (⊓) and a rate of 62 bpm (▲,↓), although on occasion they are not obvious because they are superimposed on QRS complexes, ST segments, or T waves (↓). There is no relationship between the P waves and QRS complexes, although the PP interval remains constant when the P waves are seen (⊓). Therefore, there is AV dissociation and, as the atrial rate is faster (62 bpm) than the ventricular rate (50 bpm),

there is complete heart block with an escape ventricular rhythm. Thus the patient's symptoms are the result of the slow ventricular rhythm and not related to the discontinuation of β-blocker. A permanent pacemaker is warranted.

The patient has bifascicular disease given the presence of a left bundle branch block (*ie*, disease of the left anterior and left posterior fascicles). Diagnosing trifascicular block requires evidence of disease in the remaining fascicle. The presence of first-degree AV block (with the LBBB) is not sufficient to diagnose trifascicular block since the first-degree AV block could be due to disease of either the His-Purkinje system (*ie*, of the remaining fascicle) or the AV node. However, the ECG also demonstrates complete heart block with a ventricular escape rhythm. Since the escape rhythm comes from the ventricle (and is not junctional), this implicates disease of the His-Purkinje system. Therefore, trifascicular disease can be established in this patient. ■

Notes

A **48-year-old man with idiopathic dilated cardiomyopathy is undergoing routine evaluation** by his cardiologist. An ECG is obtained.

What abnormalities are noted?

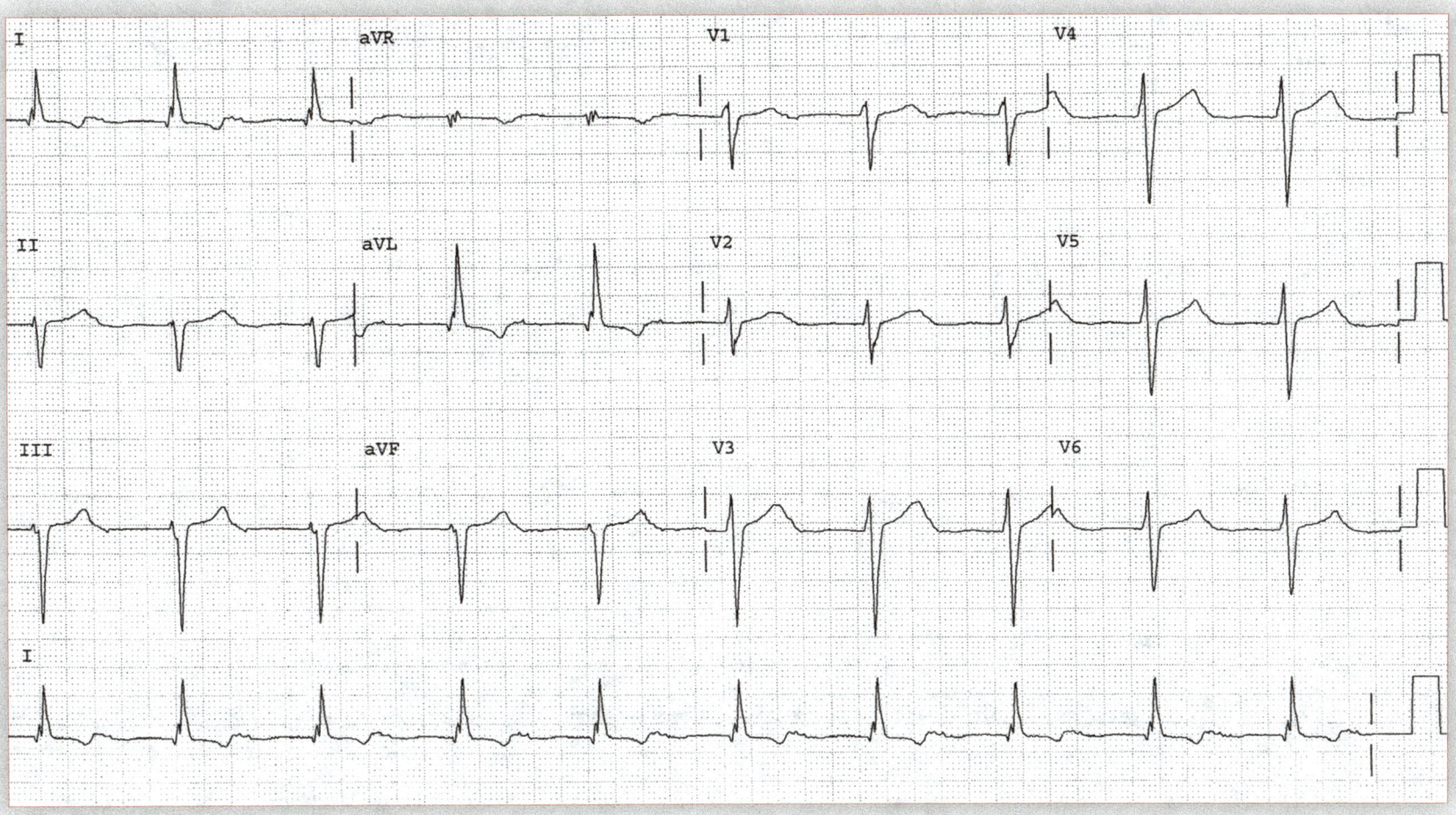

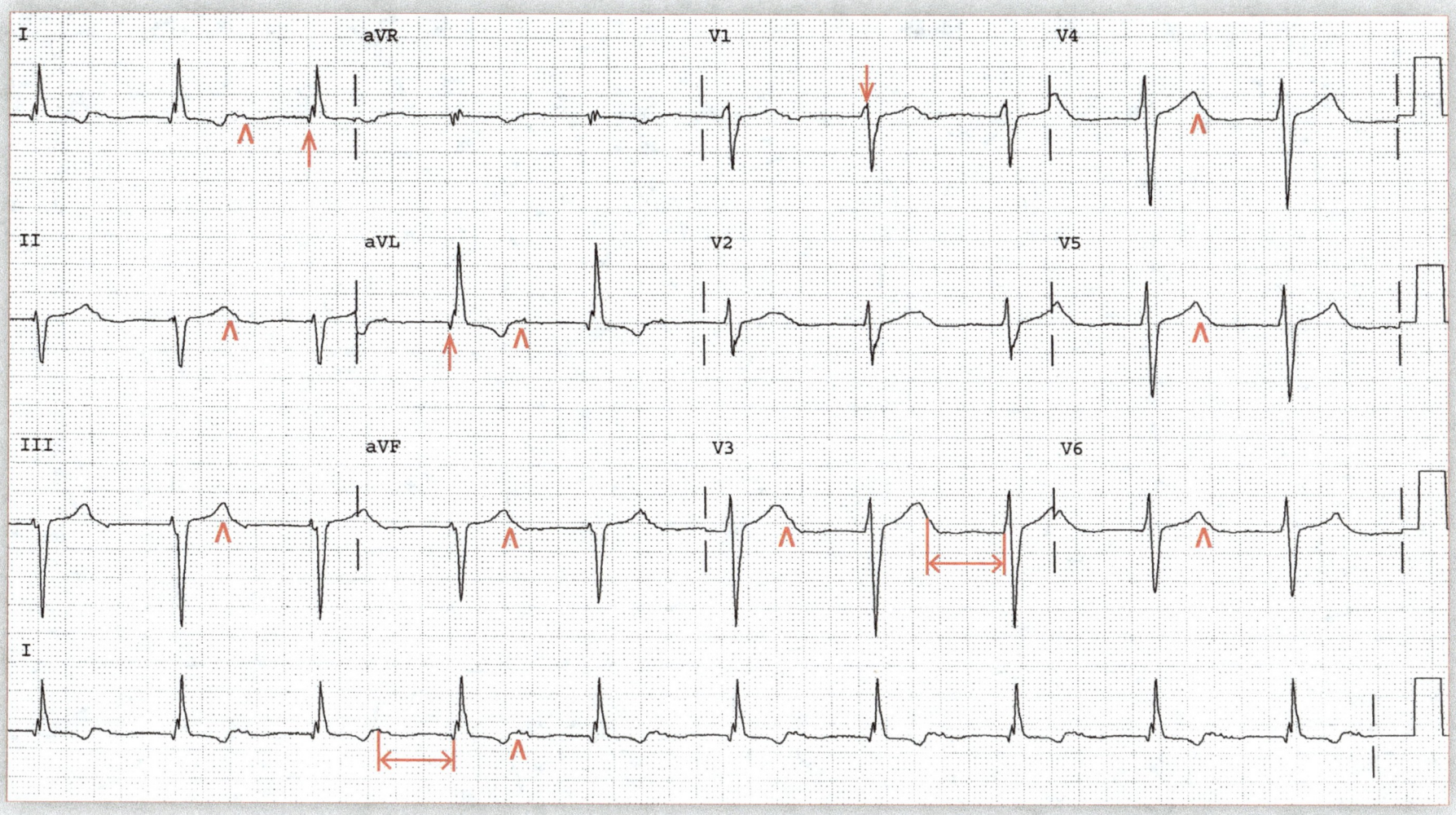

ECG 81 Analysis: Normal sinus rhythm, first-degree AV block (prolonged AV conduction), left anterior fascicular block, intraventricular conduction delay, long QT interval

There is a regular rhythm at a rate of 60 bpm. There is a P wave (^) before each QRS complex that can be seen superimposed on the end of the T wave (resulting in a notching of the downslope of the T wave); this is seen primarily in leads I, II, III, aVL, and V3-V6. The P wave is positive in leads I, II, and V4-V6. Hence this is a normal sinus rhythm. There is a stable but prolonged PR interval (↔) (0.56 sec), indicating first-degree AV block or prolonged AV conduction. The QRS complex duration is prolonged (0.12 sec). Although the morphology of the QRS complex looks like a left bundle branch block (LBBB), there is a septal Q wave in leads I and aVL (↑) and an initial septal R wave in lead V1 (↓). Septal Q waves cannot be present with an LBBB as the septal branch (which innervates the septum in a left-to-right direction, accounting for the septal waveforms) comes from the left bundle. Hence this is an intraventricular conduction delay (IVCD).

The axis is extremely leftward, between −30° and −90° (positive QRS complex in lead I and negative QRS complex in leads II and aVF). The QRS complexes have an rS morphology in leads II and aVF. No Q wave is noted; therefore, the left axis is not the result of an inferior wall myocardial infarction. Hence this represents a left anterior fascicular block (LAFB). As this is not an LBBB, diagnosing an LAFB is possible. In the presence of an LBBB, an LAFB is not an appropriate diagnosis, since there is no conduction through either of the fascicles coming from the left bundle (*ie*, left anterior and left posterior fascicles). An LAFB does not prolong the QRS complex duration; therefore, the IVCD is an independent finding. The QT/QTc intervals are prolonged (500/500 msec) but are only slightly prolonged when the QRS complex duration is considered (460/460 msec).

Idiopathic dilated cardiomyopathy is often associated with conduction system disease due to the diffuse myocardial fibrosis that can occur. Although an LBBB may be seen, it is also common to see a nonspecific IVCD as a result of diffuse fibrosis of the left ventricle associated with slowing of His-Purkinje conduction. An LAFB is also commonly seen. The first-degree AV block may be due to AV nodal disease or possibly underlying disease of the right bundle branch as well as the left posterior fascicle (*ie*, trifascicular disease). There is no way on this surface ECG to establish the etiology for the first-degree AV block. ■

A 42-year-old man is admitted to the hospital with a non–ST-segment elevation myocardial infarction. He is rendered pain free with institution of medical therapy and is admitted to the step-down unit. During his initial hours of hospitalization, he remains stable, but a change in his QRS complexes is noted on telemetry. An ECG is obtained.

What abnormality is noted?

What further action is warranted based on this ECG?

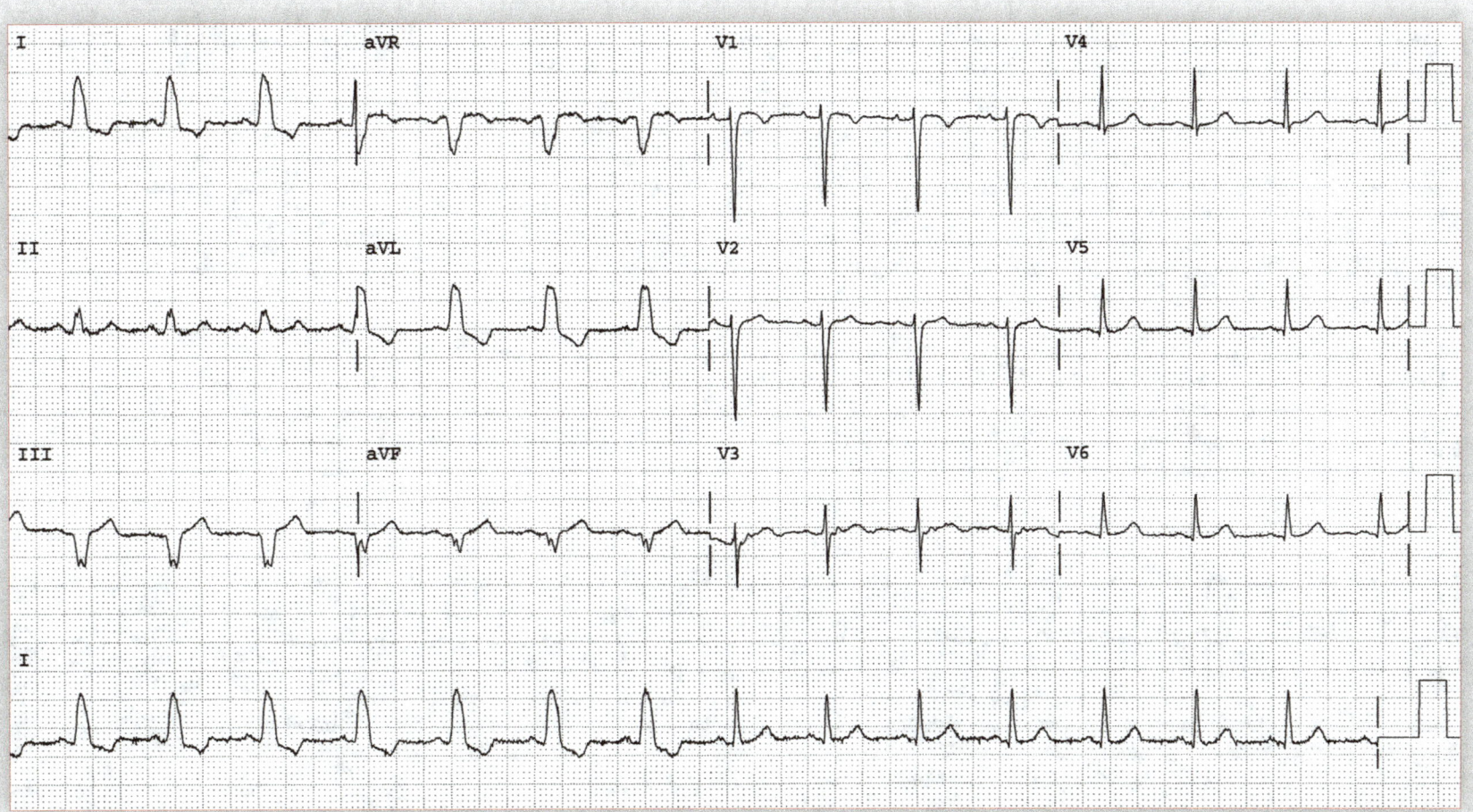

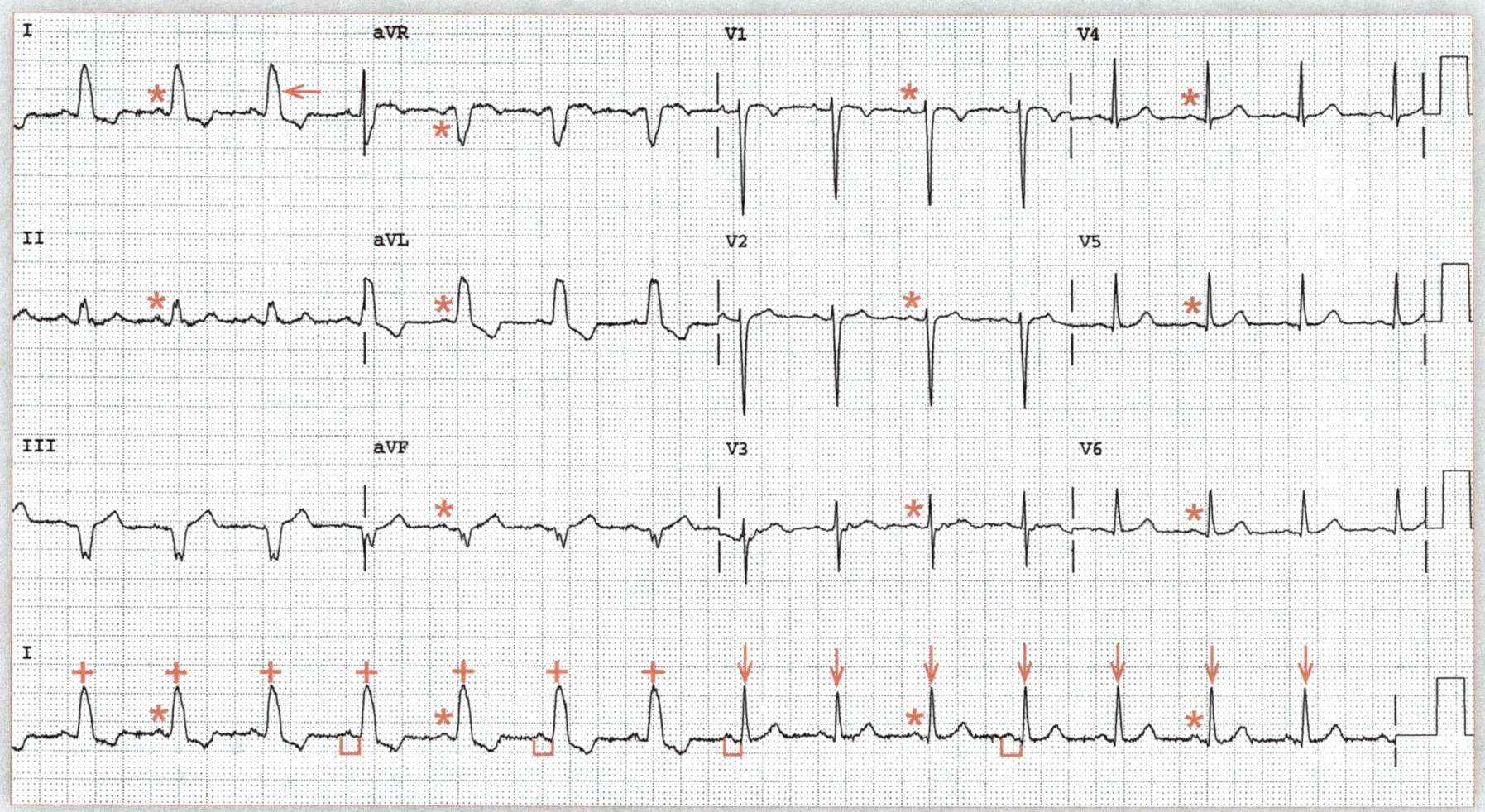

ECG 82 Analysis: Normal sinus rhythm, rate-related or intermittent left bundle branch block

The rhythm is regular at a rate of 86 bpm. There is a P wave (*) before each QRS complex and the PR interval is constant at 0.16 second (⊔). The P waves are positive in leads I, II, aVF, and V4-V6. Hence this is a normal sinus rhythm. The first seven QRS complexes are wide (+) (0.14 sec) and have a left bundle branch block (LBBB) morphology (broad R wave in lead I [←]), while the last QRS complexes (↓) are narrow and have a normal duration and morphology. This is an intermittent LBBB. Although the RR intervals of the wide and narrow QRS complexes appear to be the same, there are likely subtle differences, with the RR interval of the complexes with LBBB being slightly shorter. Hence this may represent a rate-related LBBB. The QT/QTc intervals of the narrow QRS complexes are normal (360/430 msec), and the QT/QTc intervals of the complexes with an LBBB are prolonged (400/480 msec) but are normal when the widened QRS complex duration is considered (340/410 msec).

The emergence of a rate-related LBBB in a patient with a myocardial infarction (ST-segment elevation or non–ST-segment elevation) suggests that there has been injury to the interventricular septum. Damage to the conduction system in this area can lead to fascicular block or even a bundle branch block. The rate-related LBBB is not a manifestation of ongoing ischemia, as the patient was at this point asymptomatic and there are no acute ECG changes after the resolution of the LBBB. This conduction abnormality is the result of damage due to the myocardial infarction. While the LBBB is intermittent or rate related at this point, it is possible that a permanent or persistent LBBB will develop in the future. ■

Notes

A 71-year-old woman is admitted with unheralded syncope. She states that she is not taking any cardiac medications. An ECG is obtained on admission.

What abnormalities are noted?

What pathology is suggested?

What therapy is warranted?

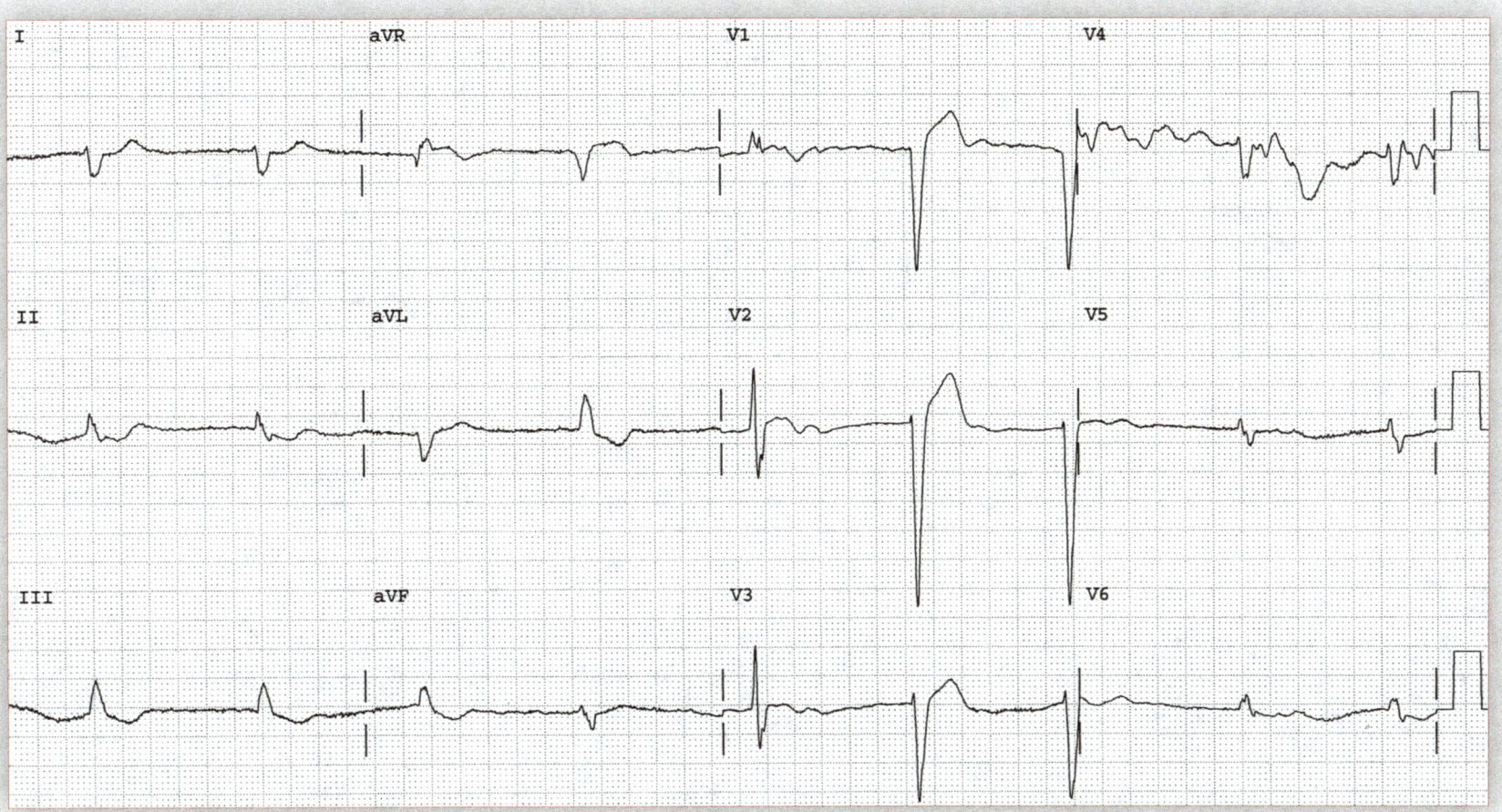

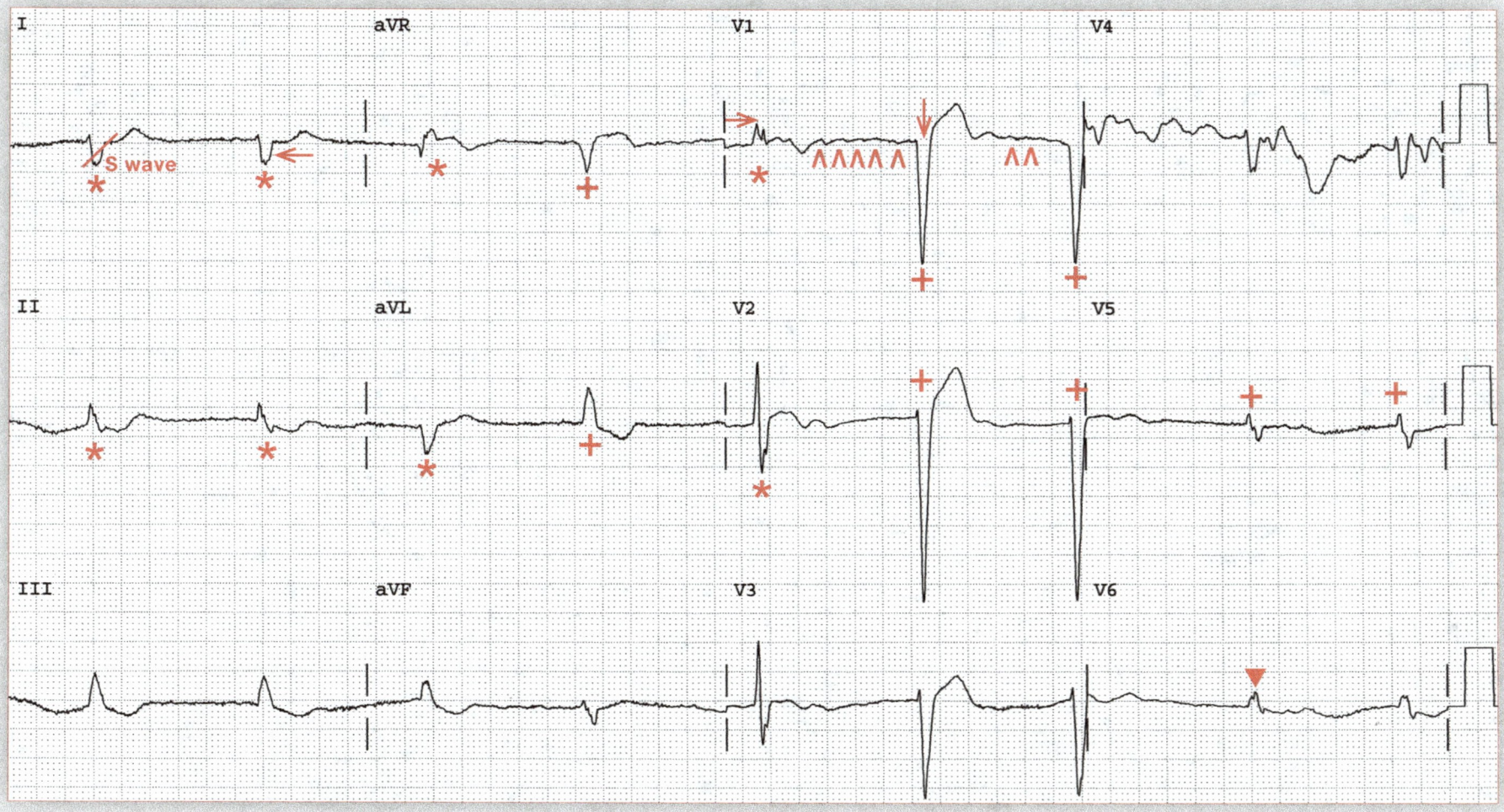

ECG 83 Analysis: Atrial fibrillation with slow ventricular response, intermittent left and right bundle branch block, bi-bundle branch block

The rhythm is slow and irregularly irregular at an average rate of 56 bpm. There are no P waves seen, but there is evidence of fibrillatory waves, seen best in lead V1 (^). The first three QRS complexes (*) and the fifth complex (*) are wide (0.12 sec) and have a right bundle branch block morphology (broad R wave in lead V1 [→] and broad S wave in lead I [←]). The axis is rightward, between +90° and +180°. There is a negative QRS complex in lead I even when considering the broad terminal S wave, which is due to the right bundle branch block. This is consistent with a left posterior fascicular block (negative QRS complex in lead I and positive QRS complex in lead aVF). In contrast, the fourth and sixth through ninth QRS complexes (+), which are also wide (0.12 sec), have a left bundle branch block morphology (broad QS complex in lead V1 [↓] and broad R wave in lead V6 [▼]). The QT/QTc intervals are prolonged (480/464 msec) but are normal when the increased QRS complex duration is considered (440/425 msec).

The alternating right and left bundle branch block pattern indicates conduction block in both bundles and is termed bi-bundle branch block, which may also be called trifascicular disease. In addition, the patient has atrial fibrillation with a slow ventricular response rate in the absence of taking an AV nodal blocking agent. This represents high-grade conduction system disease (of the AV node and His-Purkinje system) and warrants permanent pacemaker implantation as the syncope was very likely due to transient complete heart block with an escape ventricular rhythm. ■

Notes

An ECG from a 32-year-old man with
familial cardiomyopathy is shown.

What abnormalities are depicted?

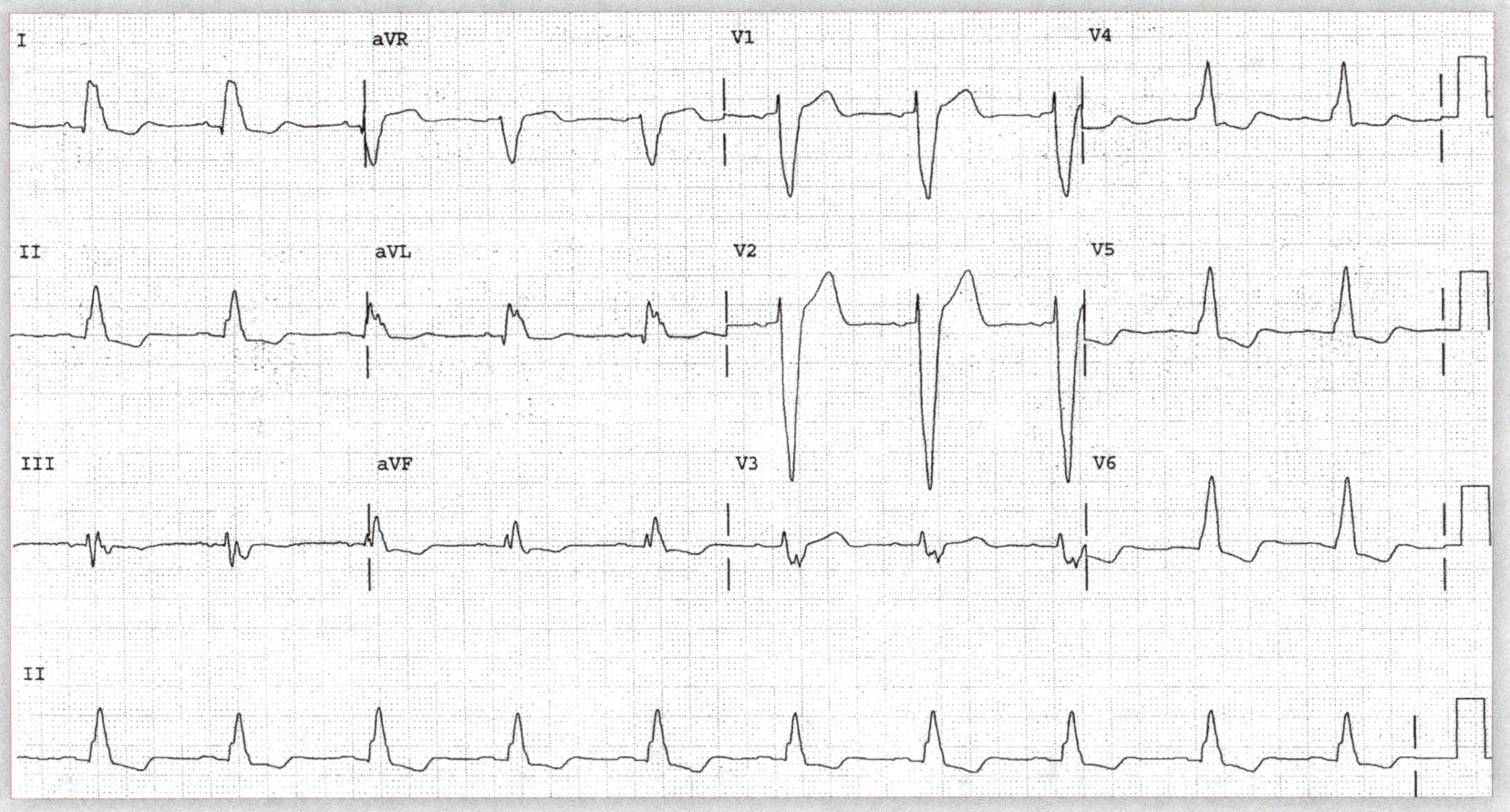

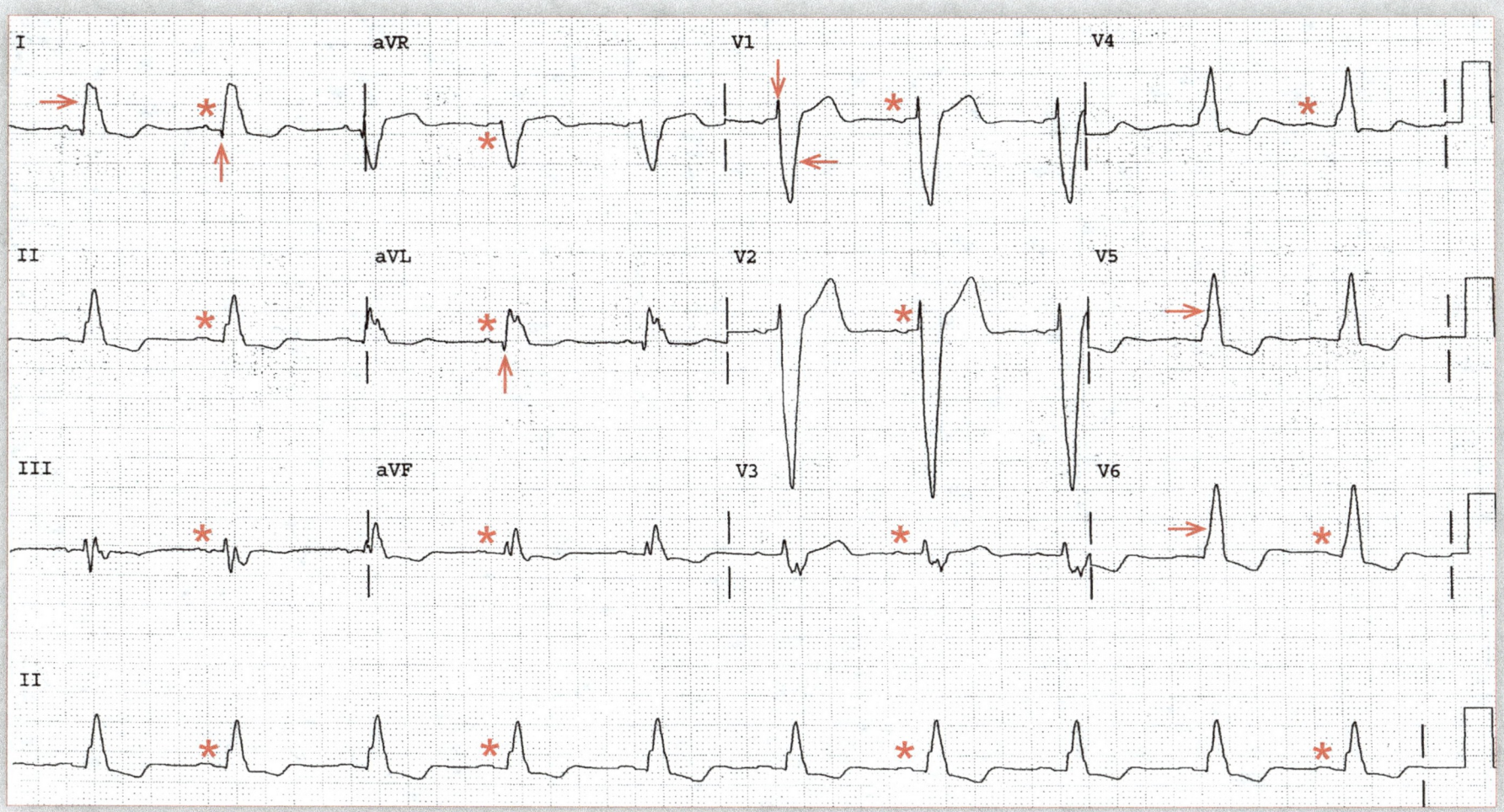

ECG 84 Analysis: Normal sinus rhythm, intraventricular conduction delay

There is a regular rhythm at a rate of 62 bpm. There is a P wave (*) before each QRS complex with a consistent PR interval (0.20 sec). The QRS complex duration is prolonged (0.18 sec). Although the morphology resembles that of a left bundle branch block (LBBB; broad R wave in leads I [→] and V5-V6 and deep S wave in lead V1 [←]), there are septal Q waves (↑) in leads I and aVL and a septal R wave (↓) in lead V1. Septal forces cannot be seen with an LBBB as the septal (median) fascicle, which innervates the interventricular septum in a left-to-right direction (accounting for the initial septal Q waves in leads I, aVL, and V5-V6 and the septal R wave in lead V1), comes from the left bundle. Thus with an LBBB there is no initial septal activation. Hence this is not an LBBB but is an intraventricular conduction delay (IVCD). The QT/QTc intervals are prolonged (520/530 msec) but are normal when corrected for the increased QRS complex duration (420/430 msec).

With an LBBB, activation of the left ventricle is not via the normal His-Purkinje system but rather occurs directly through the ventricular myocardium, and hence the activation sequence is abnormal. Abnormalities of the left ventricular myocardium cannot be diagnosed reliably with an LBBB. In contrast, the presence of an IVCD indicates that left ventricular activation is occurring via the normal conduction system but is diffusely slowed. Since the impulse travels along the normal His-Purkinje system, abnormalities that affect the left ventricle can be identified (*eg*, axis shift, acute and chronic myocardial infarction, ischemia, left ventricular hypertrophy, pericarditis). Commonly a wide QRS complex is the result of an underlying cardiomyopathy and is due to diffuse myocardial fibrosis and therefore marked slowing of impulse conduction. There is in fact a correlation between the left ventricular ejection fraction and the QRS complex duration with an IVCD. ■

Notes

A 30-year-old woman with known congenital heart disease and significant left-to-right shunting that has now progressed to Eisenmenger's syndrome presents for a routine physical exam. Her only complaint is that of intermittent palpitations. Her ECG is shown.

What is the abnormality?

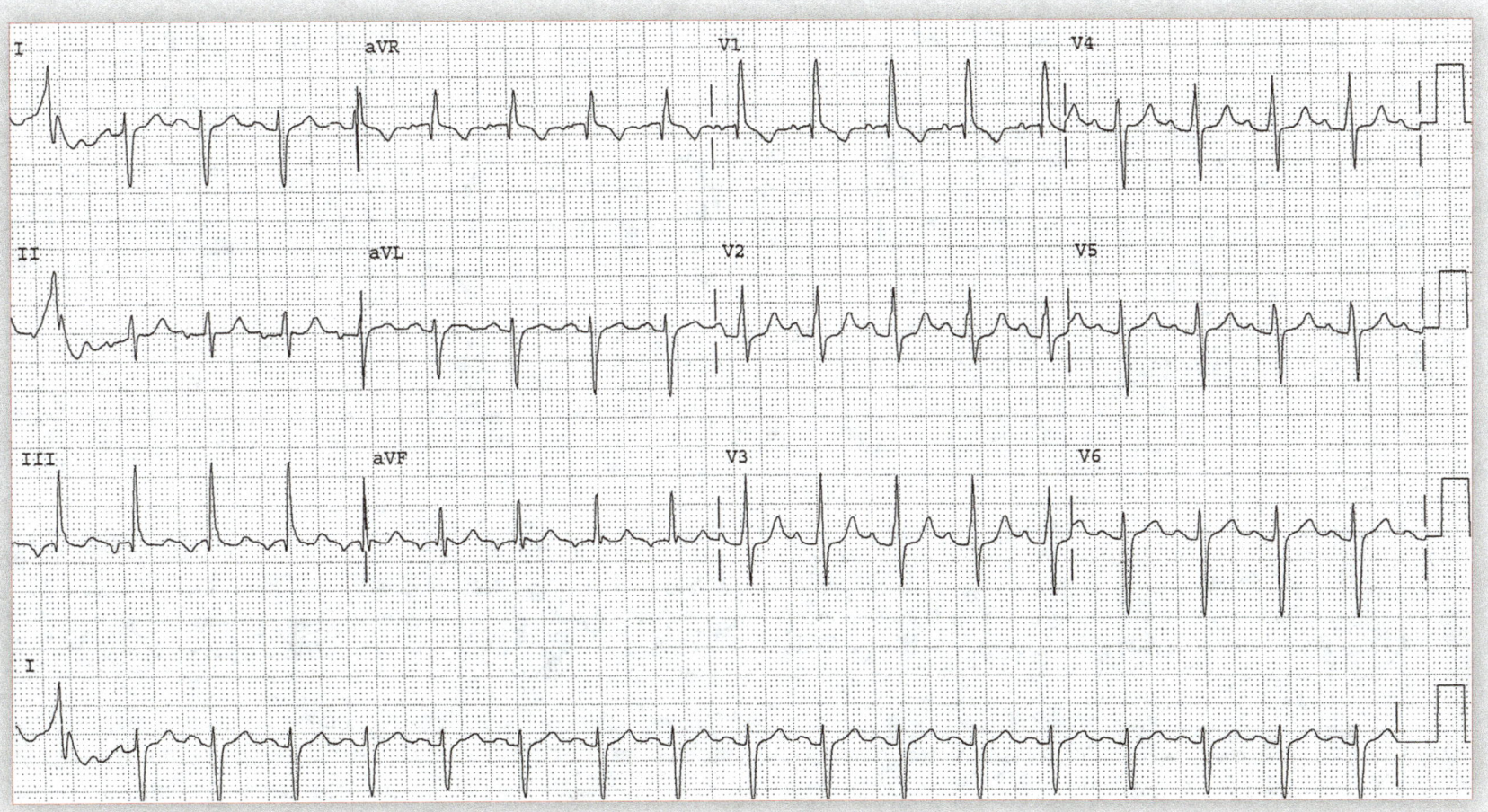

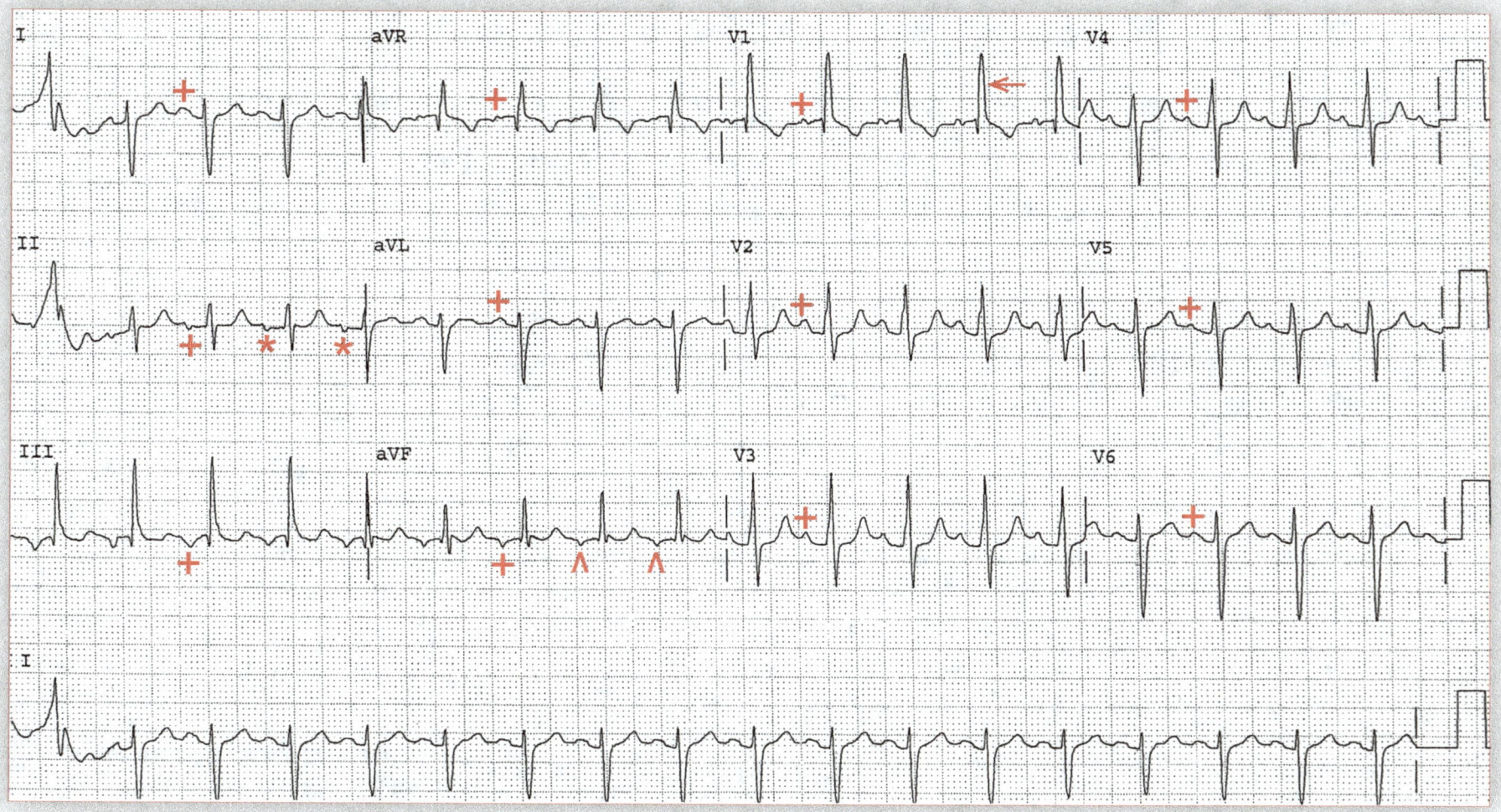

ECG 85 Analysis: Atrial tachycardia, right ventricular hypertrophy, right axis

There is a regular rhythm at a rate of 110 bpm. There is a P wave (+) before each QRS complex with a stable PR interval (0.20 sec). The P wave is upright in leads I and V4-V6. However, it is negative in lead aVF (^) and biphasic in lead II (*), indicating that the rhythm is not sinus but rather originates from the low atrium (*ie*, negative P wave in lead aVF). Hence this is atrial tachycardia. The QRS complex duration is normal (0.10 sec). However, there is a tall R wave in lead V1 (12 mm) (←) and an R/S ratio in leads V5-V6 < 1 (*ie*, the S wave is deeper than the R-wave height). These are criteria for right ventricular hypertrophy. The axis is rightward, between +90° and +180° (negative QRS complex in lead I and positive QRS complex in lead aVF). In this case, the right axis is due to right ventricular hypertrophy and not a left posterior fascicular block.

Patients with congenital heart disease who have significant left-to-right shunting can develop severe pulmonary arterial hypertension and subsequent right ventricular hypertrophy (RVH). RVH is often associated with a shift in the electrical axis to the right, as is seen in this ECG. With the development of significant pulmonary arterial hypertension and RVH, the shunting becomes right to left, and this is Eisenmenger's syndrome. Atrial tachycardia is often seen in this condition, reflecting abnormalities of the right atrium. As the atrial tachycardia results from an ectopic focus, the rate of the tachycardia may vary and fast rates may account for the patient's palpitations.

Notes

A 72-year-old man with known multivessel coronary disease presents for routine follow-up. He has stable New York Heart Association class II heart failure. He has no new complaints. His vital signs and physical exam are normal. As part of his evaluation, an ECG is obtained.

What abnormalities are noted?

Is any additional evaluation or therapy necessary?

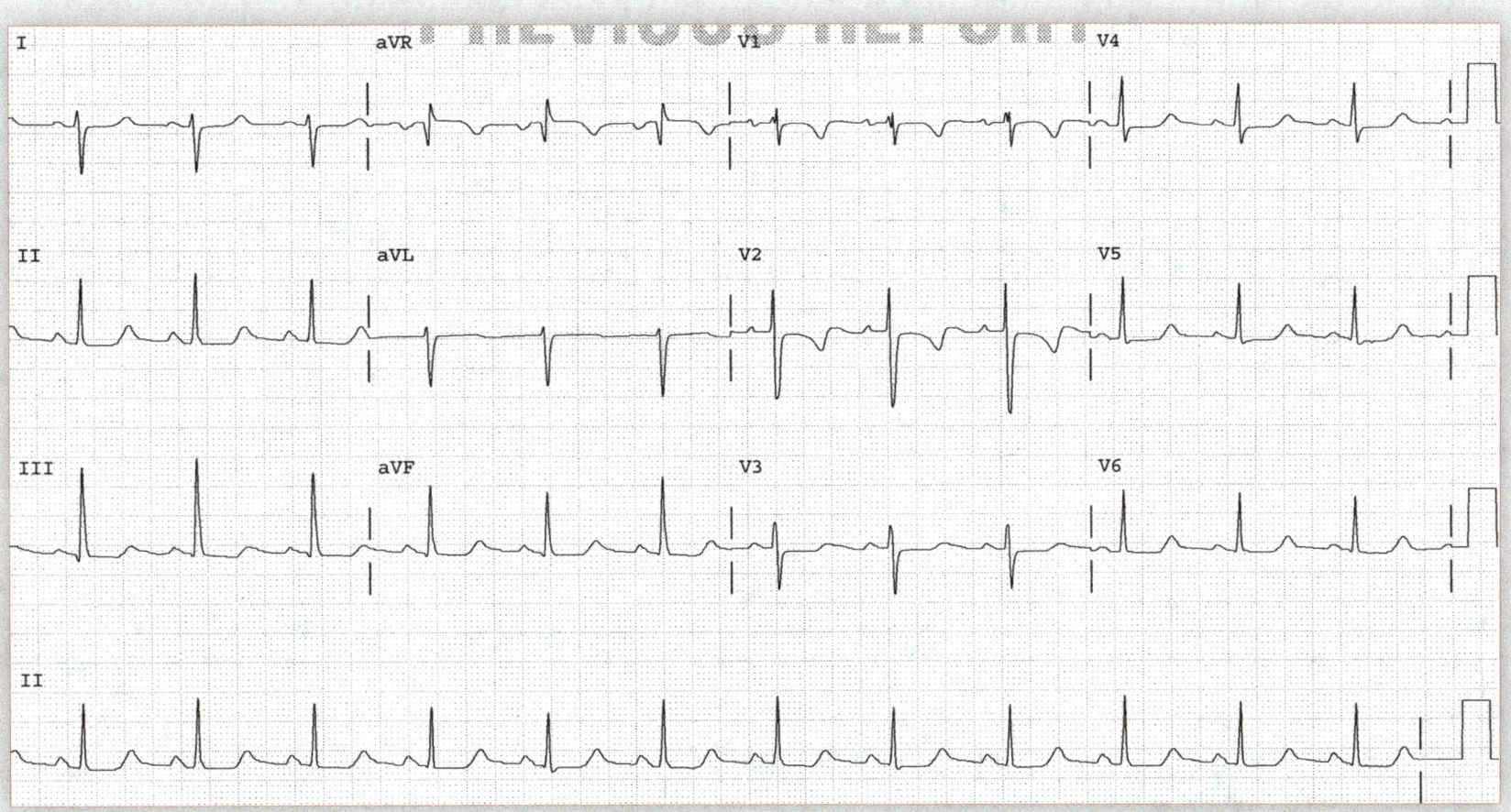

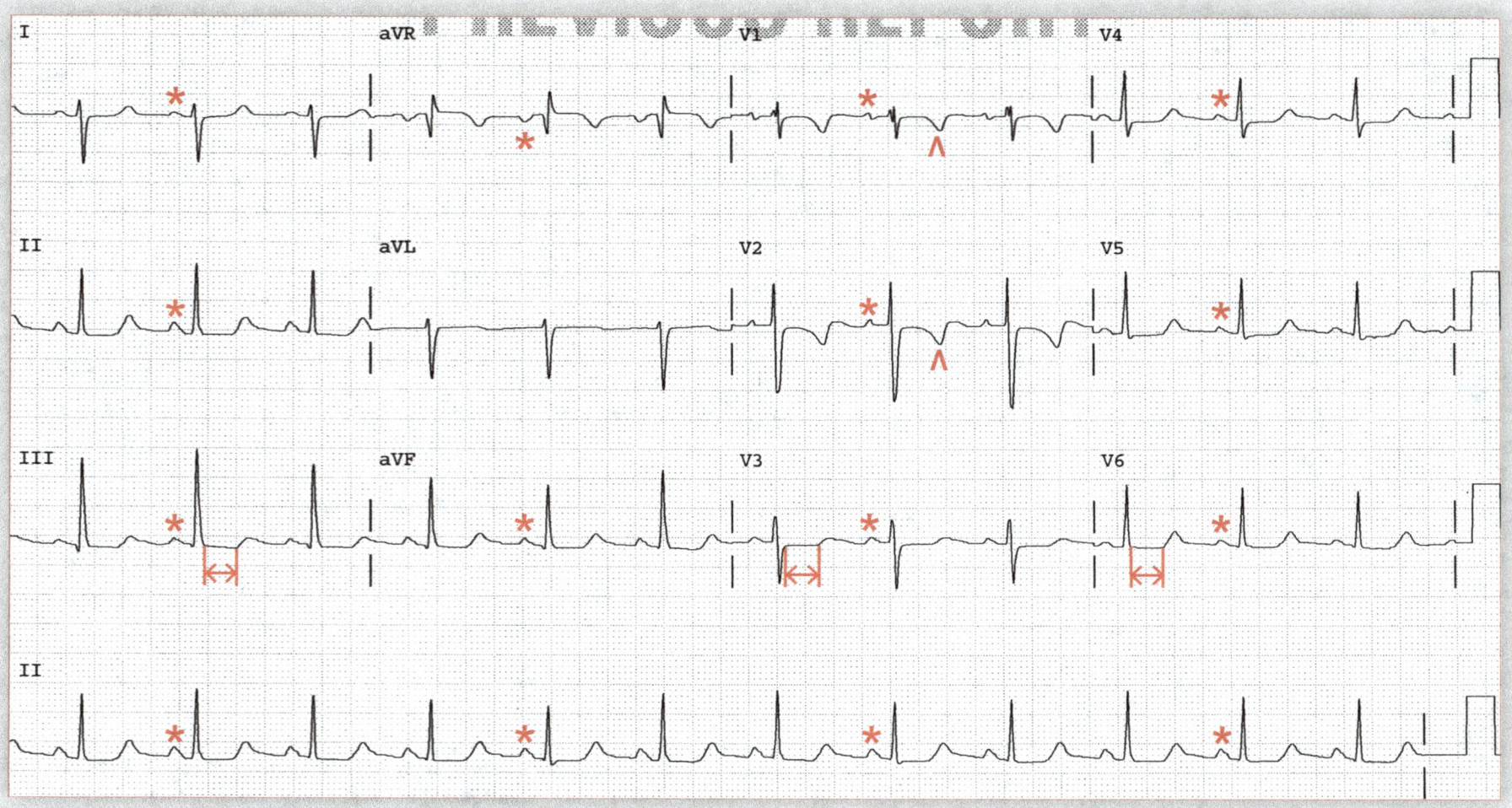

ECG 86 Analysis: Normal sinus rhythm, left posterior fascicular block, long QT interval (delayed repolarization), nonspecific T-wave abnormality

The rhythm is regular at a rate of 74 bpm. There is a P wave (*) before each QRS complex, and the PR interval is stable at 0.20 second. The P waves are positive in leads I, II, aVF, and V4-V6. Hence this is a normal sinus rhythm. The QRS complex duration (0.08 sec) and morphology are normal. The QRS complex is negative in lead I (rS morphology) and positive in lead aVF. Hence the axis is rightward, between +90° and +180°. In the absence of any other cause for a right axis (*ie*, right ventricular hypertrophy, lateral wall myocardial infarction, dextrocardia, right–left arm lead switch, Wolff-Parkinson-White pattern), the etiology for this is a left posterior fascicular block (LPFB). The QT/QTc intervals are prolonged (440/490 msec) as a result of a long ST segment (↔). This is termed delayed repolarization and suggests the presence of hypocalcemia or hypomagnesemia. In addition, there is T-wave inversion (^) in leads V1 (which is normal) and V2. In the absence of any specific symptoms, the T-wave abnormality is nonspecific.

The concept of the hemiblock, or fascicular block, was put forth by Rosenbaum and colleagues in 1970. The definition of a fascicular block was based only on the electrical axis of the heart in the frontal plan. An LPFB was defined as a right QRS axis, between +90° and +180°. The left posterior fascicle is a broad, fan-shaped extension of the main left bundle that spreads along the inferoposterior aspect of the left ventricle. Since it is broad and diffuse, an LPFB is not common and is seen far less often than a left anterior fascicular block. No additional evaluation or therapy for the LPFB is necessary. However, the long QT interval suggests either low calcium or magnesium levels. These levels should be checked and, if low, repleted. ■

A 17-year-old who is trying out for his high school basketball team presents for a routine physical exam. He denies any symptoms or past medical conditions. As part of the screening, an ECG is obtained and he is told that he is not eligible to try out for the team.

What is the abnormality of concern?

Is additional testing warranted?

Should he be permitted to try out for the team?

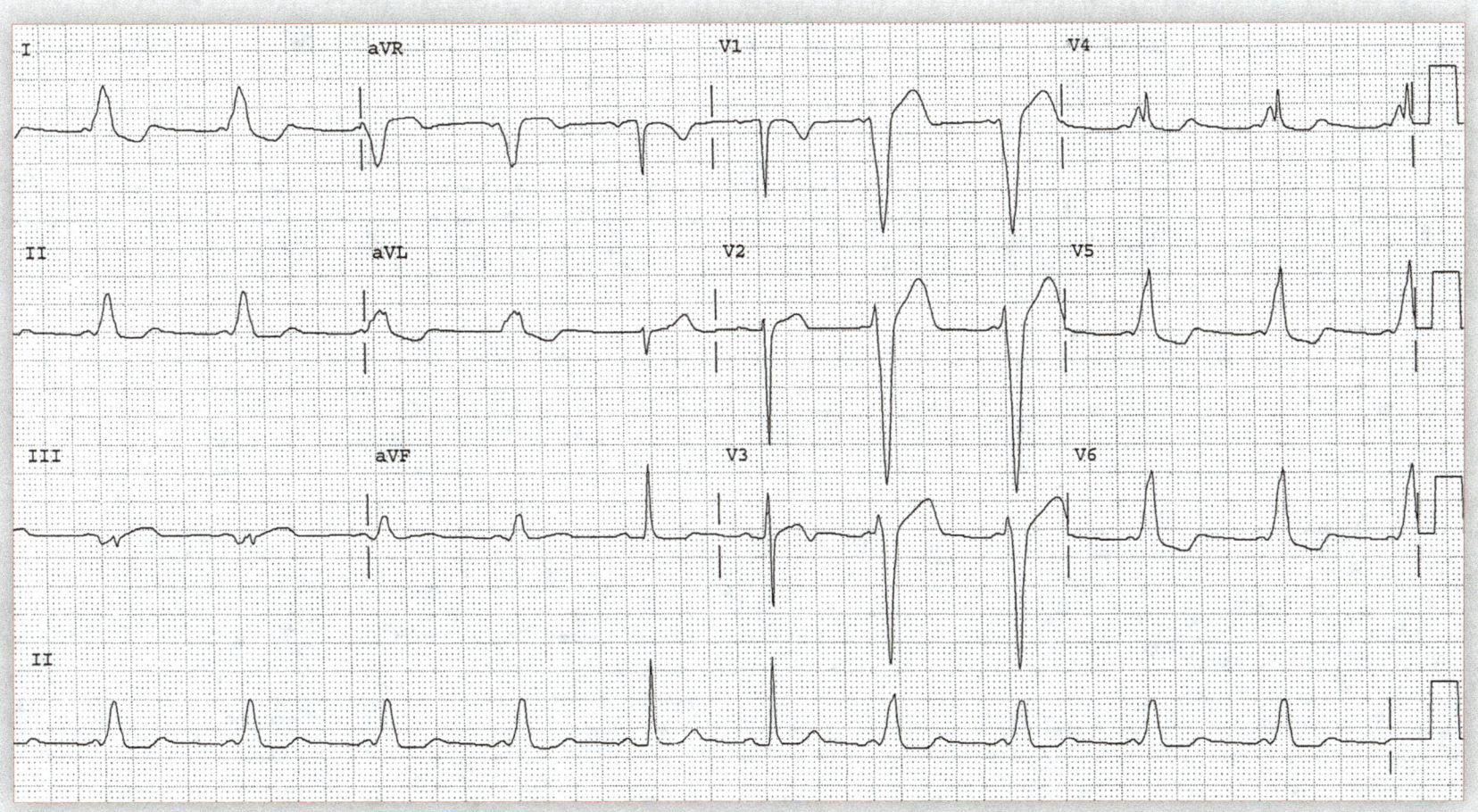

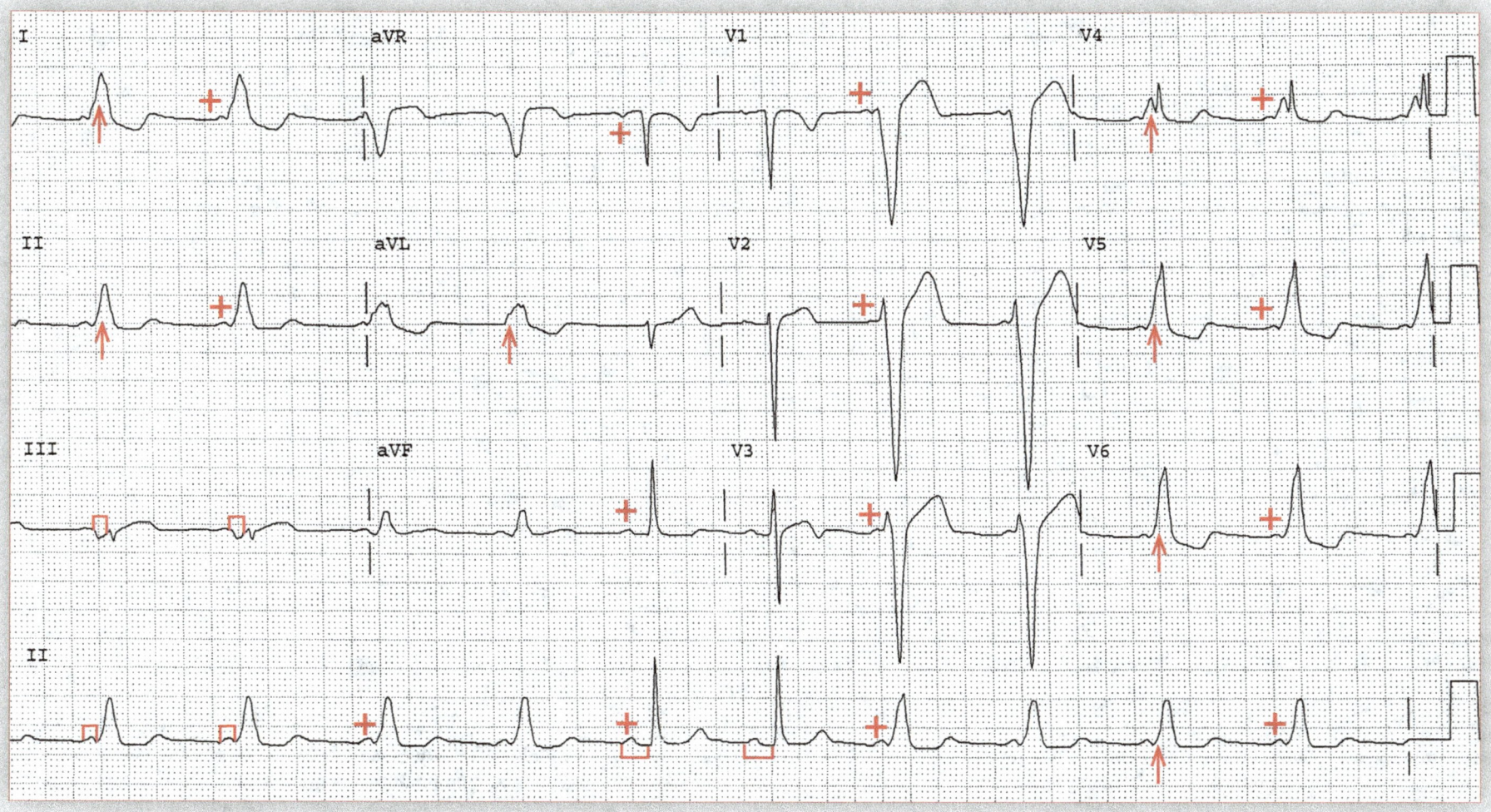

ECG 87 Analysis: **Normal sinus rhythm, intermittent preexcitation (Wolff-Parkinson-White pattern)**

There is a regular rhythm at a rate of 68 bpm. There are P waves (+) before each QRS complex, and they are positive in leads I, II, aVF, and V4-V6. Hence this is a normal sinus rhythm. There are two different PR intervals (0.12 sec [⊓] and 0.20 sec [⊔]). There are also two different QRS complex morphologies. Complexes 1 to 4 and 7 to 10 are wide with a duration of 0.16 second; these complexes are associated with the short PR interval (0.12 msec). They are wide as a result of a slowed upstroke (↑). A wide QRS complex with a sinus P wave and a short PR interval is the hallmark of preexcitation (*ie*, a Wolff-Parkinson-White [WPW] pattern). The slowed upstroke is the result of a delta wave, which is quite prominent in this patient. The delta wave is due to initial myocardial activation via the accessory pathway that occurs before ventricular activation via the normal AV node–His-Purkinje system (hence preexcitation). As a result of preexcitation, abnormalities of the left ventricle cannot be diagnosed and hence no further analysis of the QRS complex is possible. The fifth and sixth QRS complexes have a normal duration (0.08 sec) and morphology. They have a normal PR interval (0.20) msec. They likely have a normal axis, between 0° and +90° (positive QRS complex in leads II and aVF).

These are, therefore, normal complexes due to ventricular activation via the normal conduction system. Therefore, there is an intermittent WPW pattern. The QT/QTc intervals of the preexcited complexes are prolonged (460/490 msec) but are normal when the prolonged QRS complex duration is considered (400/425 msec). The QT/QTc intervals of the non-preexcited QRS complexes are normal (400/425 msec).

The presence of an intermittent WPW pattern generally means that the accessory pathway has a relatively long refractory period. In this situation the accessory pathway is not likely to conduct impulses rapidly. Importantly, should atrial fibrillation develop, it is not likely that it would be associated with very rapid impulse conduction to the ventricles. The rapid ventricular activation during atrial fibrillation is the mechanism for sudden death in these patients. As he has never had any symptoms to suggest an arrhythmia, there is no reason for any additional electrophysiologic evaluation in this asymptomatic young patient and there is no reason to prevent him from partaking in sports. Indeed, only about 10% of patients with a WPW pattern on the ECG have documented arrhythmia. ■

A 71-year-old man is undergoing treadmill testing. His complaint is that of decreasing exercise tolerance and fatigue. He has no known medical diagnoses and does not take any medications. His physical exam is notable only for a resting heart rate of 58 bpm. His baseline ECG is notable only for a first-degree AV block. Presented is his ECG during peak exercise.

What abnormality is noted?

What therapy is indicated?

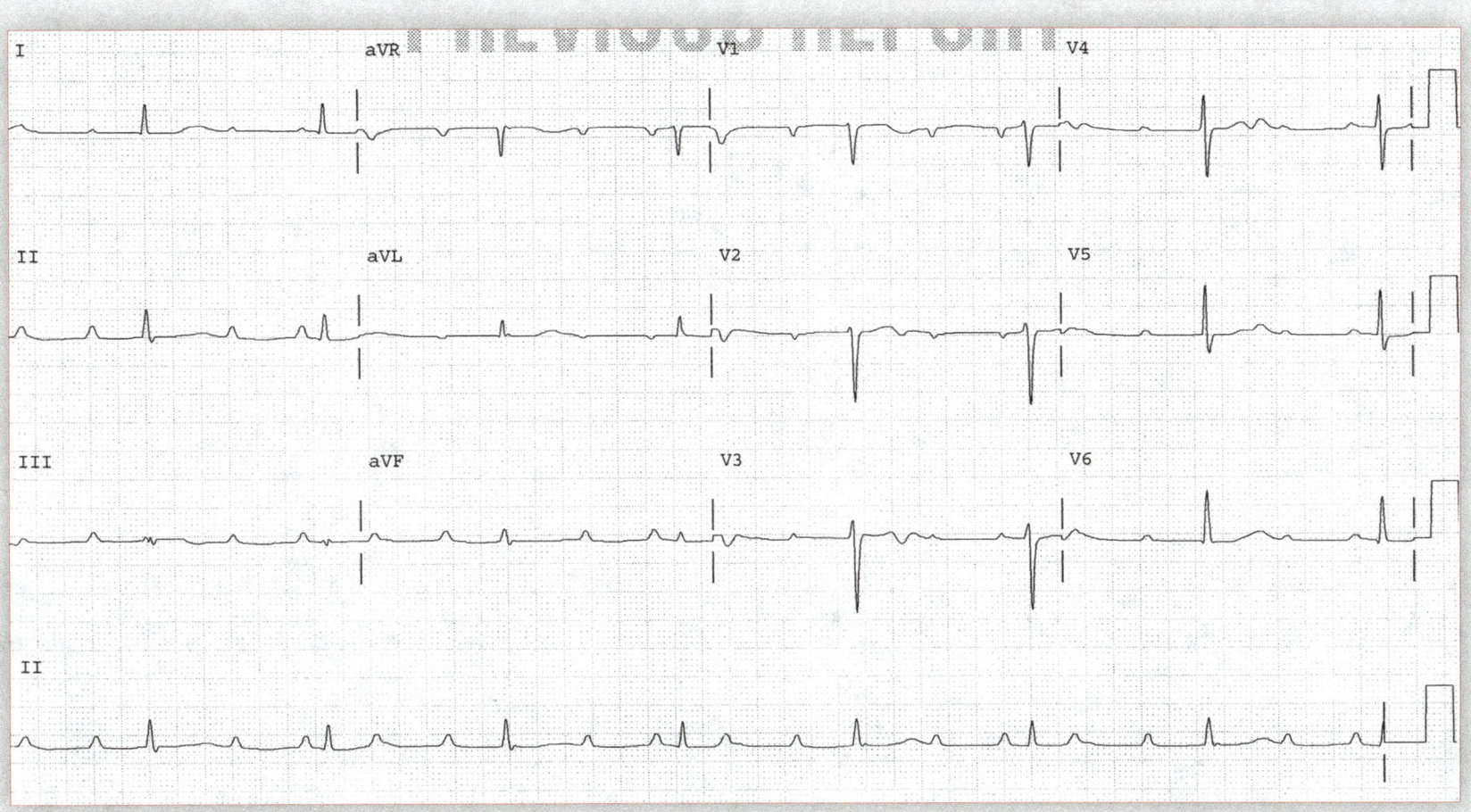

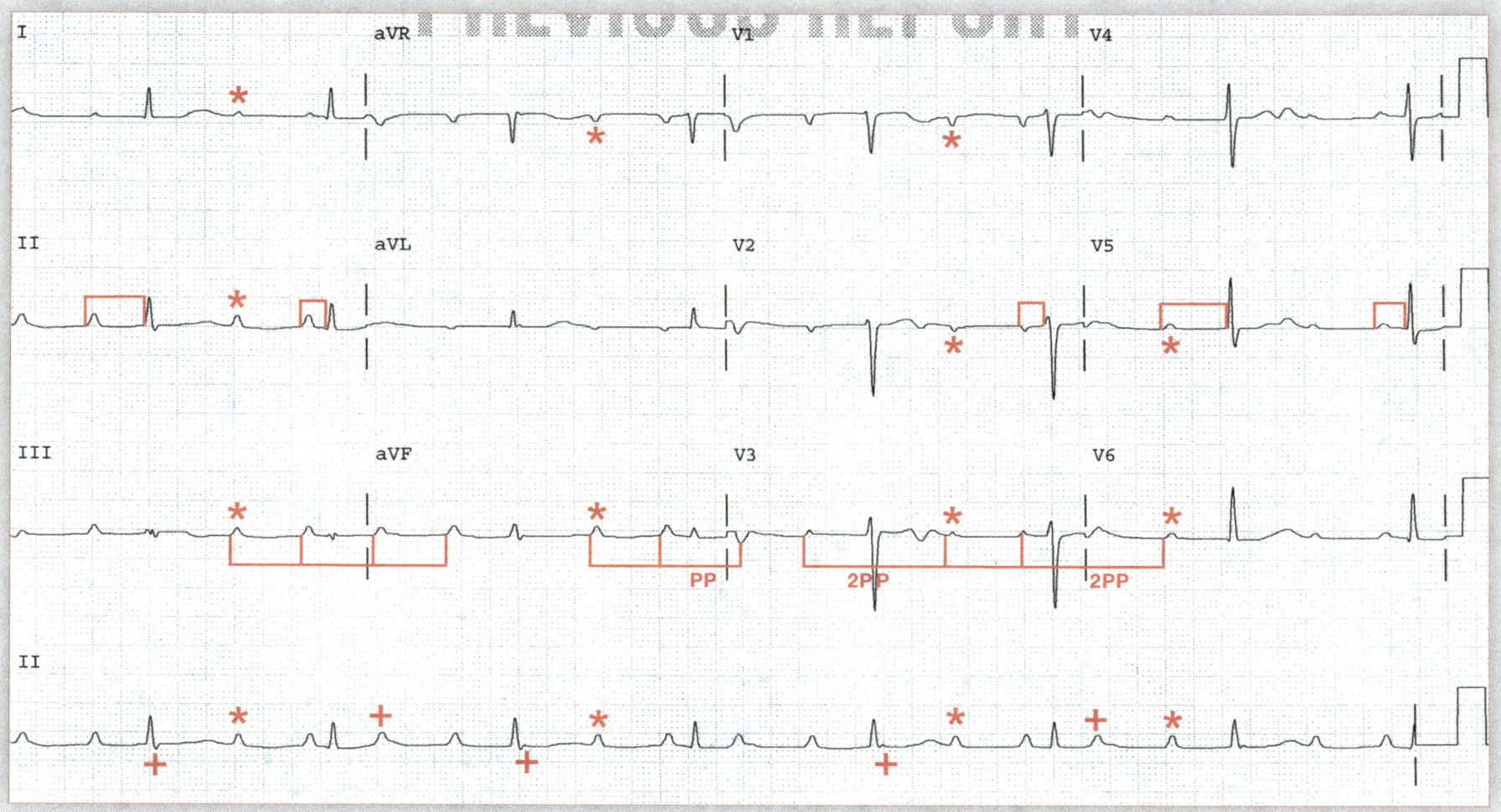

ECG 88 Analysis: Sinus tachycardia, complete heart block, escape junctional rhythm, low limb lead voltage

There are regular RR intervals at a rate of 46 bpm. There are P waves (*) with a regular PP interval (⊔) at a rate of 124 bpm. Although there are occasional P waves that are not seen because they are simultaneous with the QRS complex or T wave (+) (the measured PP interval when the P wave is not seen is thus equivalent to two PP intervals), the PP interval remains regular. The P waves are positive in leads I, II, aVF, and V4-V6. Hence this is sinus tachycardia. The PR intervals are variable (⊓); thus AV dissociation is present. The QRS complex duration is normal (0.08 sec) and it has a normal morphology and axis, between 0° and +90° (positive QRS complex in leads I and aVF). The QT/QTc intervals are normal (520/440 msec).

There is low voltage in the limb leads (< 5 mm in each lead). The atrial rate is faster than the ventricular rate. Hence this is complete heart block with an escape junctional rhythm. The site of the block is the AV node.

In patients with early disease of the AV node, the node may show signs of disease prior to the onset of complete heart block only in the context of increased stimulation. During exertion, as the sinus node rate rises, the normal AV node will conduct at a commensurate increased rate with a shortening of the PR interval (on average 5 msec for each 10-beat increase in sinus rate). The diseased AV node may not be able to conduct impulses at an elevated rate, leading to progressive prolongation of the PR segment and even complete heart block, as in this patient. With the complete AV block the escape junctional rhythm may have an inappropriately slow rate if there is intrinsic junctional disease. This is one form of "chronotropic incompetence." Although his sinus rate increases appropriately, he develops complete AV block and a junctional escape rhythm with a rate that does not increase appropriately in response to exercise and increased catecholamines. This is likely the cause of this patient's exertional intolerance. Implantation of a dual-chamber pacemaker that is programmed to function as a P-wave–synchronous or P-wave–activated ventricular pacemaker should alleviate the symptoms. ■

Notes

A 72-year-old woman with longstanding hypertension, treated only with a β-blocker, undergoes a routine physical exam. During the exam, an irregular radial pulse is noted and an ECG is obtained.

What abnormality on the ECG explains the physical exam findings?

What consequences of the patient's hypertension are evident on the tracing?

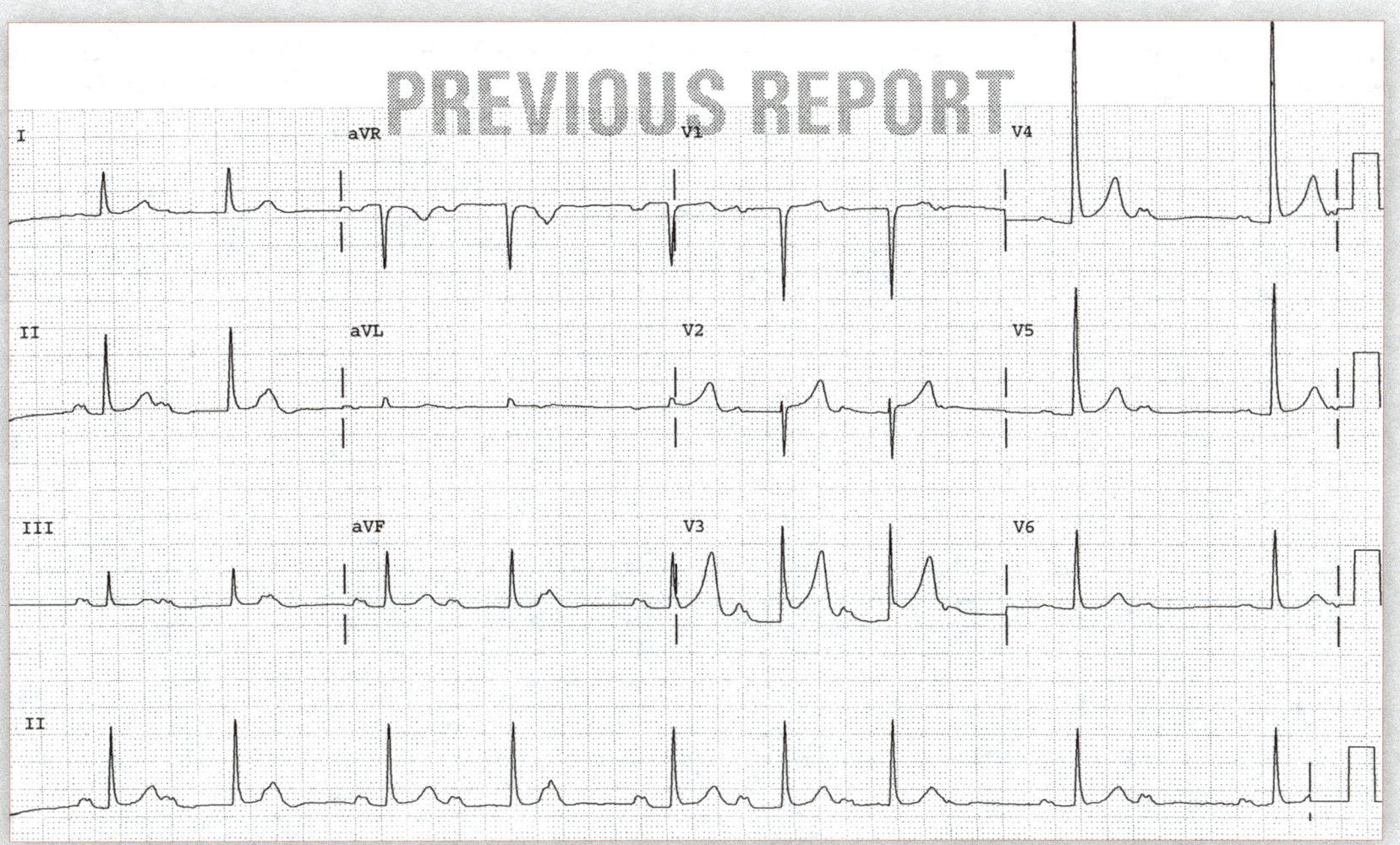

Podrid's Real-World ECGs

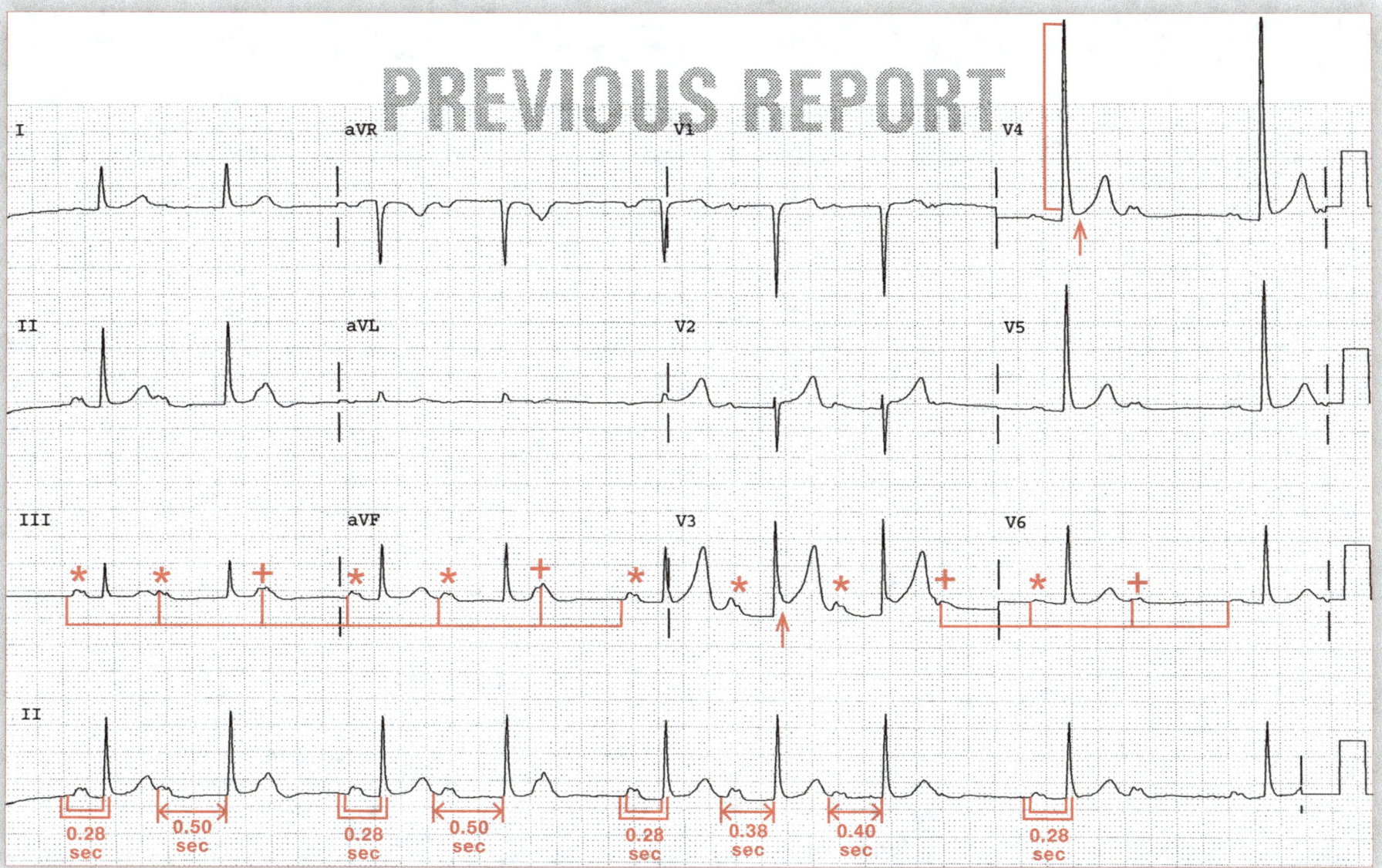

PREVIOUS REPORT

ECG 89 Analysis: Normal sinus rhythm, P mitrale (left atrial hypertrophy or abnormality), first-degree AV block (prolonged AV conduction), Mobitz type I second-degree AV block (Wenckebach), left ventricular hypertrophy, normal early repolarization

There are P waves (*), and the PP interval is fairly regular (⊔) at a rate of 88 bpm. Occasionally, the P wave is superimposed on the T wave or is immediately after the T wave (+). The P waves are positive in leads I, II, aVF, and V4-V6. Hence there is a normal sinus rhythm. In addition, the P waves are abnormal; they are broad and notched in leads II, aVF, and V3-V5 (ie, P mitrale due to left atrial hypertrophy). The QRS complexes (at an average rate of 54 bpm) are regularly irregularly with a variable pattern. There is grouped beating with a pause that is the result of on-time but nonconducted P waves (+), which as stated above are occasionally superimposed on the T wave, altering the morphology. There are P waves before each QRS complex, but the PR interval (⊔,↔) is prolonging from a baseline of 0.28 second to 0.50 second. The PR interval (⊔) after the pause represents the baseline PR interval (ie, 0.28 sec). Therefore, there is first-degree AV block (prolonged AV conduction). Second-degree heart block is also present (occasional nonconducted P wave), and the pattern of progressive PR interval prolongation is diagnostic for Mobitz type I or Wenckebach second-degree AV block. The pattern of AV block is variable, however, and there is 2:1, 3:2, and 4:3 conduction present.

The QRS complex duration is normal (0.08 sec) and there is a normal axis, between 0° and +90° (positive QRS complex in leads I and aVF). The QRS complex amplitude is increased, especially in lead V4 (38 mm) ([ ), and this meets one of the criteria for left ventricular hypertrophy (ie, S-wave depth or R-wave amplitude in any precordial lead ≥ 25 mm). The J-point and ST-segment elevation (↑) seen in leads V3-V4 represents early repolarization, frequently seen with left ventricular hypertrophy. The QT/QTc intervals are normal (440/420 msec).

Longstanding elevation in ventricular and, by extension, atrial pressures results in left ventricular and left atrial hypertrophy, which are evident on the surface ECG in this case. These structural alterations may result in conduction abnormalities as the specialized cardiomyocytes and their intracellular connections that comprise the conduction system are injured and fibrose over time. In addition, the β-blocker alters AV nodal conduction and may be a contributing factor to the occurrence of Wenckebach. Although Wenckebach usually occurs with a fixed pattern of AV block, there may be variable AV block present. ■

Notes

An 85-year-old man presents to the emergency department because of chest discomfort that occurred about 1 hour before presentation and lasted for 35 minutes. He states that the chest discomfort was similar to what he experienced before his heart attack 5 years ago. His physical exam is unremarkable. Vital signs are stable.

Cardiac biomarkers are obtained and they are negative. He is admitted to the hospital to "rule out" a myocardial infarction (MI) and for observation. Laboratory tests and cardiac biomarkers obtained 4 and then 8 hours later are unremarkable. His admission ECG is shown.

Did he have a previous MI?

If so, what is the location of the infarction?

What other abnormalities are seen?

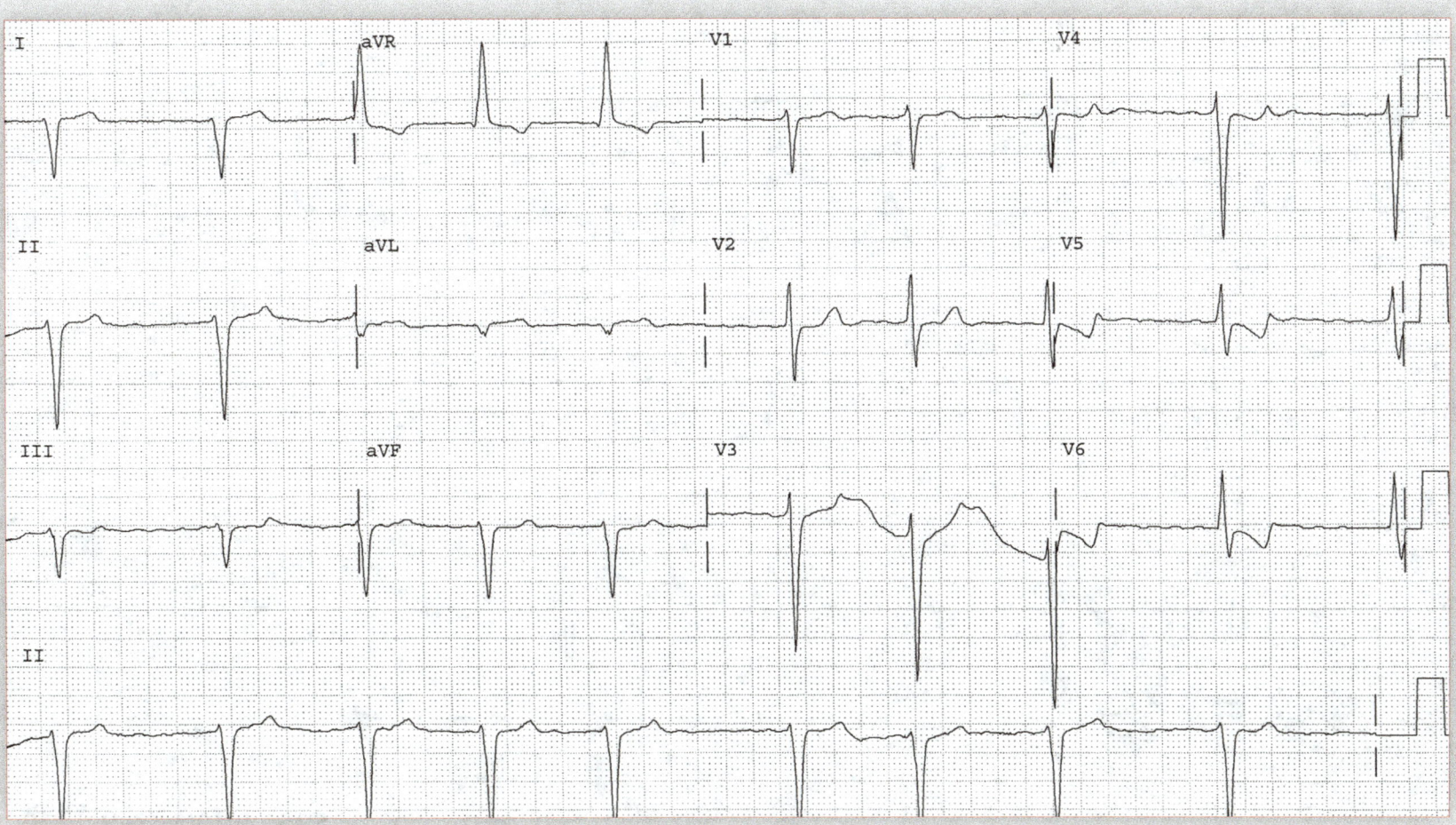

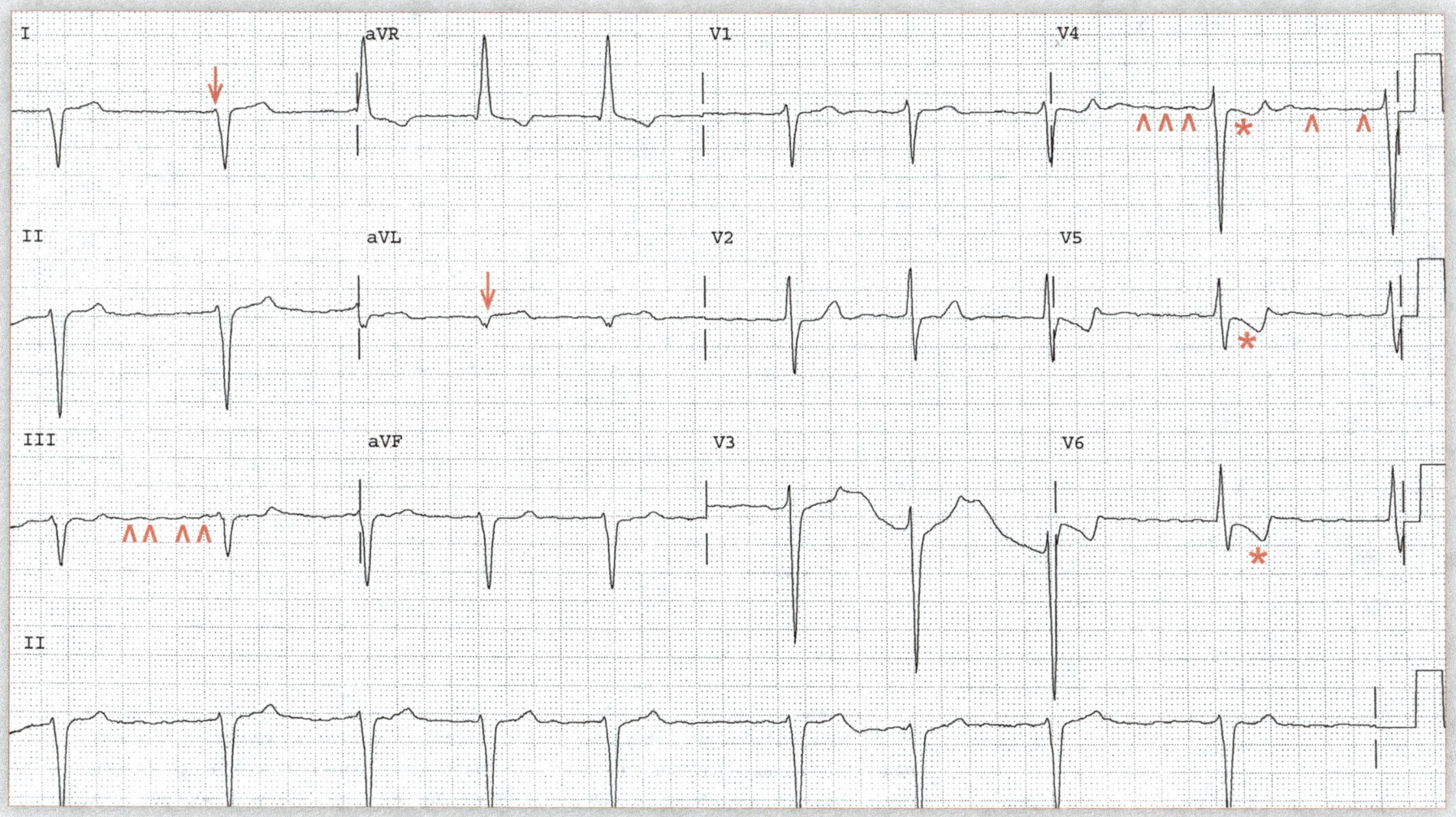

ECG 90 Analysis: Atrial fibrillation, indeterminate axis due to an old lateral wall MI and left anterior fascicular block, intraventricular conduction delay, nonspecific ST-T wave changes

The rhythm is irregularly irregular, and there is no organized atrial activity or P waves. The average ventricular rate is 60 bpm. Occasional low-amplitude undulations can be seen (^). Hence this is atrial fibrillation. The QRS complex duration is almost 0.12 second, but there is no pattern of a left or right bundle branch block. Hence this is an intraventricular conduction delay. The QT/QTc intervals are normal (420/420 msec). There are nonspecific ST-T wave changes in leads V4-V6 (*). The axis appears to be indeterminate, between –90° and +/-180° (negative QRS complex in leads I and aVF). However, the initial waveform in leads I and aVL is a Q wave (QS morphology) (↓), and hence this is an old lateral wall myocardial infarction (MI). The presence of an rS complex in lead I would suggest an axis shift (to the right) due to a conduction abnormality. In contrast, a QS or Qr complex in lead I is the result of a lateral wall MI and does not represent a conduction problem accounting for the axis shift. If this QRS complex is not considered, the axis is actually extremely leftward, between –30°

and –90° (negative QRS complex in leads II and aVF; both have an rS morphology), this is termed a left anterior fascicular block. Hence this patient has a left anterior fascicular block and an old lateral wall MI, which together give the appearance of an indeterminate axis.

When there is a supraventricular rhythm, the presence of an indeterminate axis will only occur when there are two coexisting abnormalities, as there is no conduction pattern through the normal His-Purkinje system that will produce this axis. Conditions associated with an indeterminate axis, in addition to what is present in this patient, include right ventricular hypertrophy with an inferior wall MI or a left anterior fascicular block, a left posterior fascicular block associated with an inferior wall MI, or both an inferior and lateral wall MI. Another situation in which there is an indeterminate axis is a right–left arm lead switch associated with a left anterior fascicular block or an old inferior wall myocardial infarction. ■

Notes

A 78-year-old man presents to his physician with dyspnea on exertion and general fatigue for the past several weeks. He states that his symptoms have been variable, with days of profound fatigue with minimal exertion and days of full energy. A review of systems is otherwise unremarkable, and the patient specifically denies angina as well as orthopnea. An ECG is obtained as part of his evaluation.

What abnormalities on the ECG might explain his symptoms?

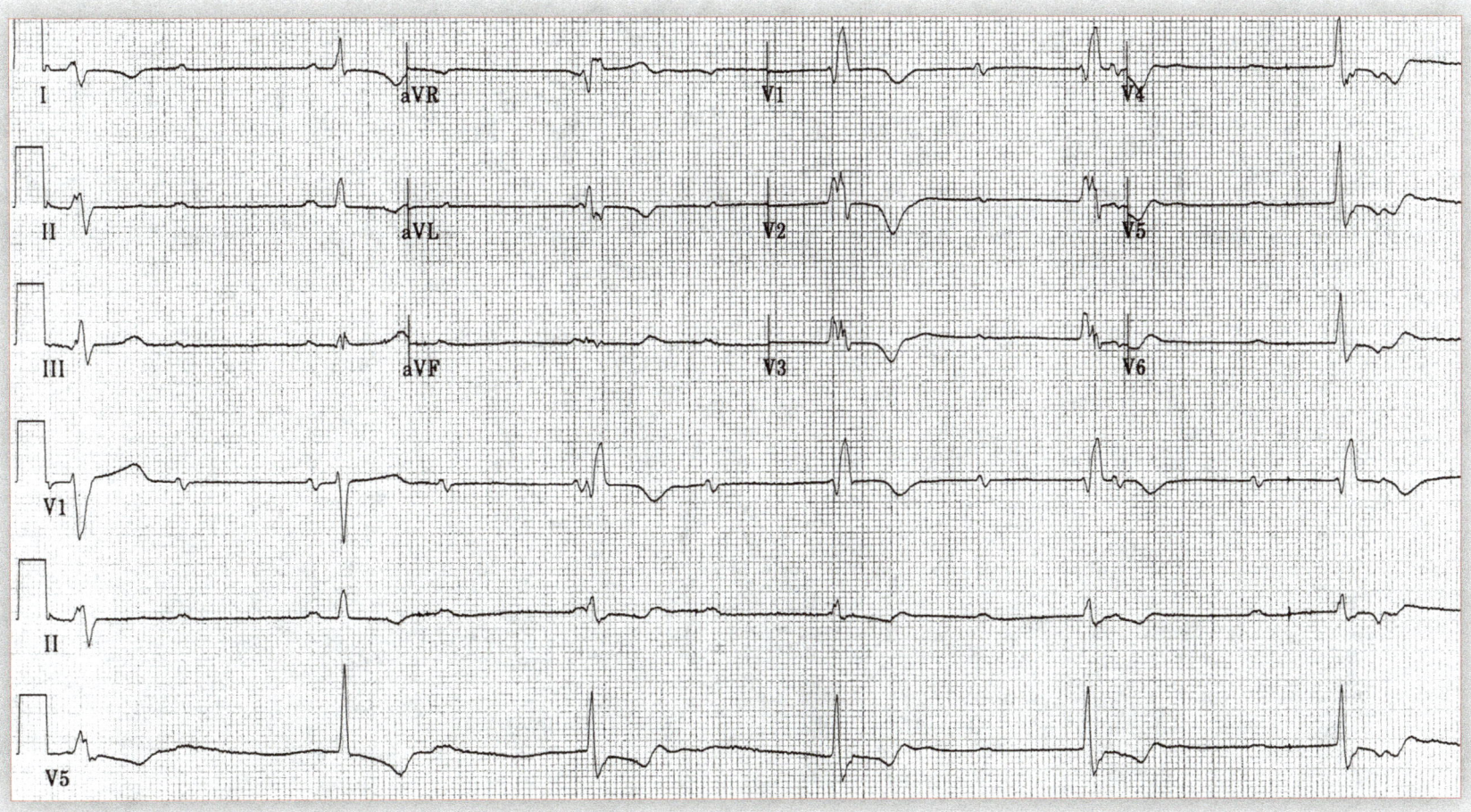

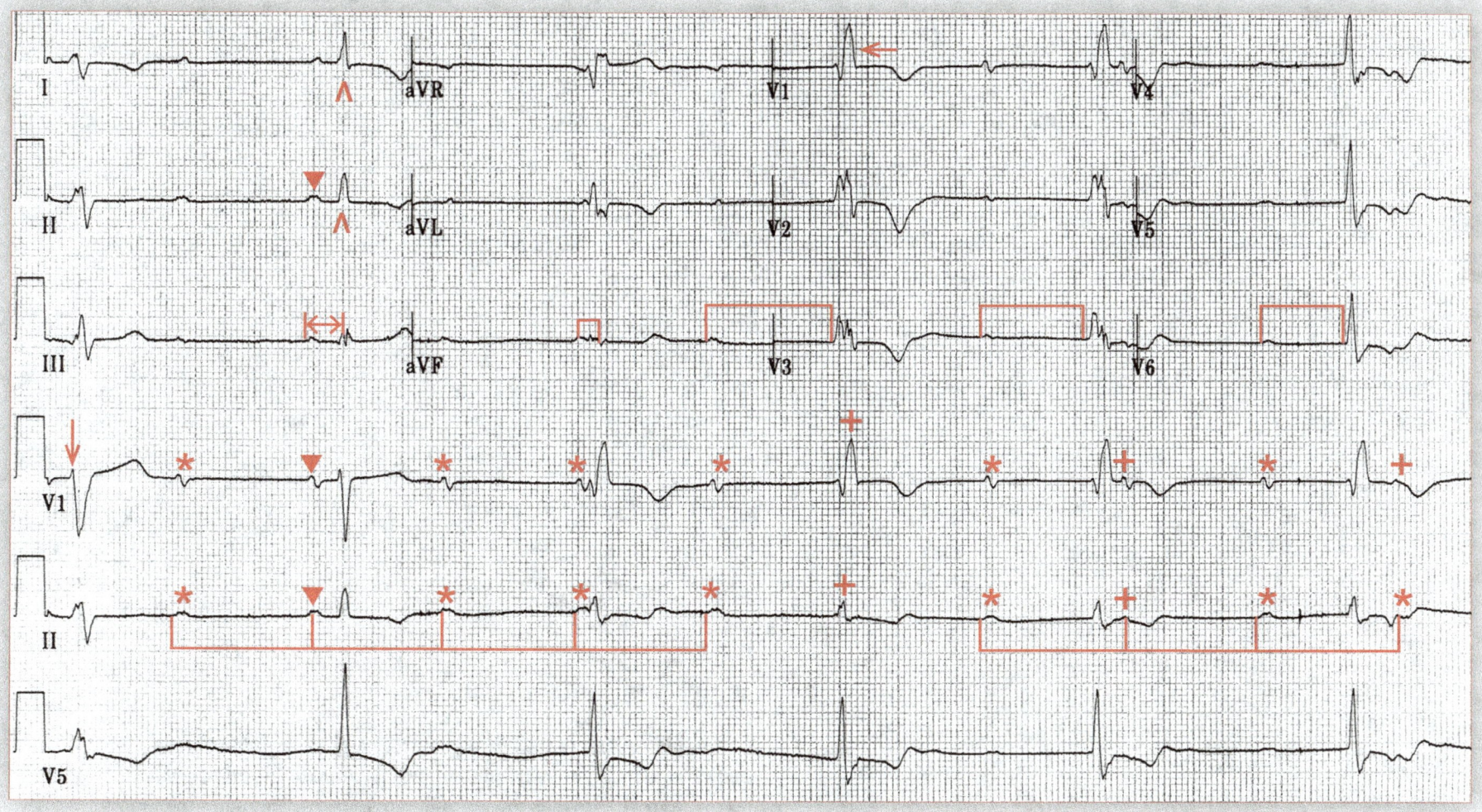

ECG 91 Analysis: Normal sinus rhythm, third-degree (complete) heart block, escape ventricular rhythm, intermittent capture

There are regular RR intervals at a rate of 34 bpm. Regular P waves (*) are seen with a stable PP interval (⊔) at a rate of 64 bpm. Some of the P waves are not obvious because they are superimposed on the QRS complex, in ST segments, or on T waves (+). However, P waves that are seen are at a regular interval (⊔). The P waves are positive in leads I, II, aVF, and V4-V6; hence there is an underlying normal sinus rhythm at a rate of 64 bpm. The PR intervals are variable (⊓), indicating AV dissociation. The atrial rate is faster than the ventricular rate; hence there is complete (third-degree) AV block. The QRS complexes are wide (0.14 sec) and have an unusual right bundle branch block pattern (RSR′ morphology in lead V1 [←] but no broad S wave in lead I). The second complex (^) has a normal duration (0.08 sec) and morphology. There is an on-time sinus P wave (▼) preceding this complex with a PR interval of 0.20 second (↔). This is a conducted complex and it has a normal morphology that is different than that of the dissociated QRS complexes. This confirms the fact that the dissociated QRS complexes are ventricular; hence the escape rhythm is ventricular. Not uncommonly, complete heart block may be associated with intermittent capture, or indeed the complete heart block itself may be intermittent. The first QRS complex (↓) is also wide but has a morphology that is different from the dissociated QRS complexes that are ventricular. This is also a ventricular complex that is from a different location within the left ventricle.

Ventricular escape rhythms are inherently unstable as they are an unprotected focus within the ventricular myocardium. Hence there is no control over the rate at which this ventricular focus can stimulate the ventricle; the rate may vary widely, from very slow to fast, depending on sympathetic tone and circulating catecholamines. This is in contrast to supraventricular rhythms, in which the ventricular response rate is controlled by the rate of conduction through the AV node. Escape ventricular rhythms also signify disease of the His-Purkinje conduction system. Hence complete heart block with a ventricular escape rhythm is an indication for pacemaker implantation, even if the patient is asymptomatic. In this patient, the escape ventricular rhythm, although quite bradycardic, did not result in pre-syncope or syncope. However, during times of even minimal exertion, this escape ventricular rhythm may not mount an appropriate heart rate response or increase in stroke volume and may not be able to supply the cardiac output required to meet demand, resulting in dyspnea and fatigue. This phenomenon of a limitation in cardiac output by bradycardia has been referred to as chronotropic incompetence. ■

A 50-year-old woman with known idiopathic first-degree AV block is seen by her cardiologist for a routine appointment. Her condition has been stable for years. The patient states that she has been feeling well overall and only notes some mild dysmenorrhea for which she recently began taking an herbal supplement. It seems to have helped. On physical exam, the heart rate is 46 bpm, consistent with prior assessments. Her exam is otherwise normal. An ECG is obtained.

What abnormalities are evident?

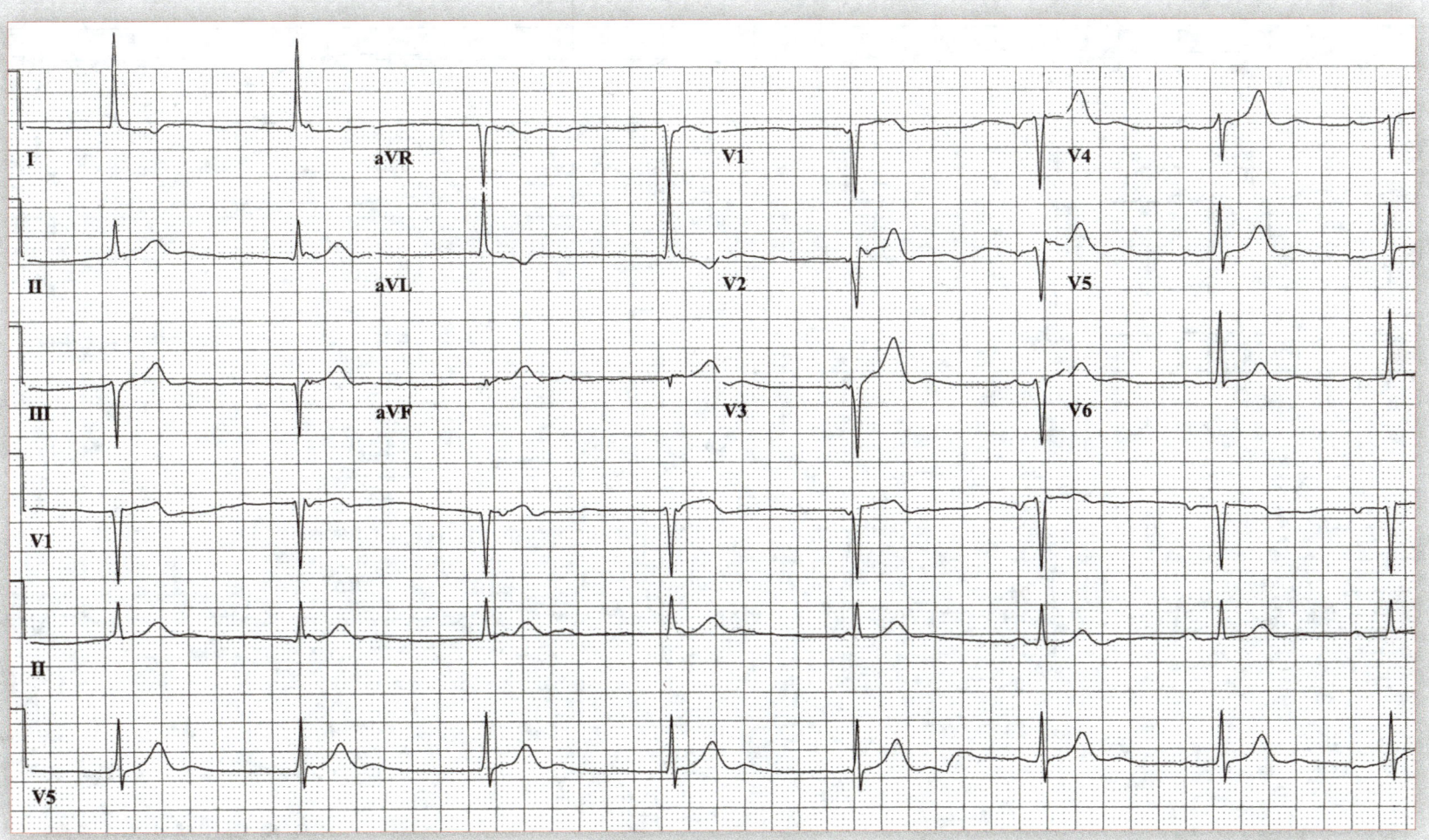

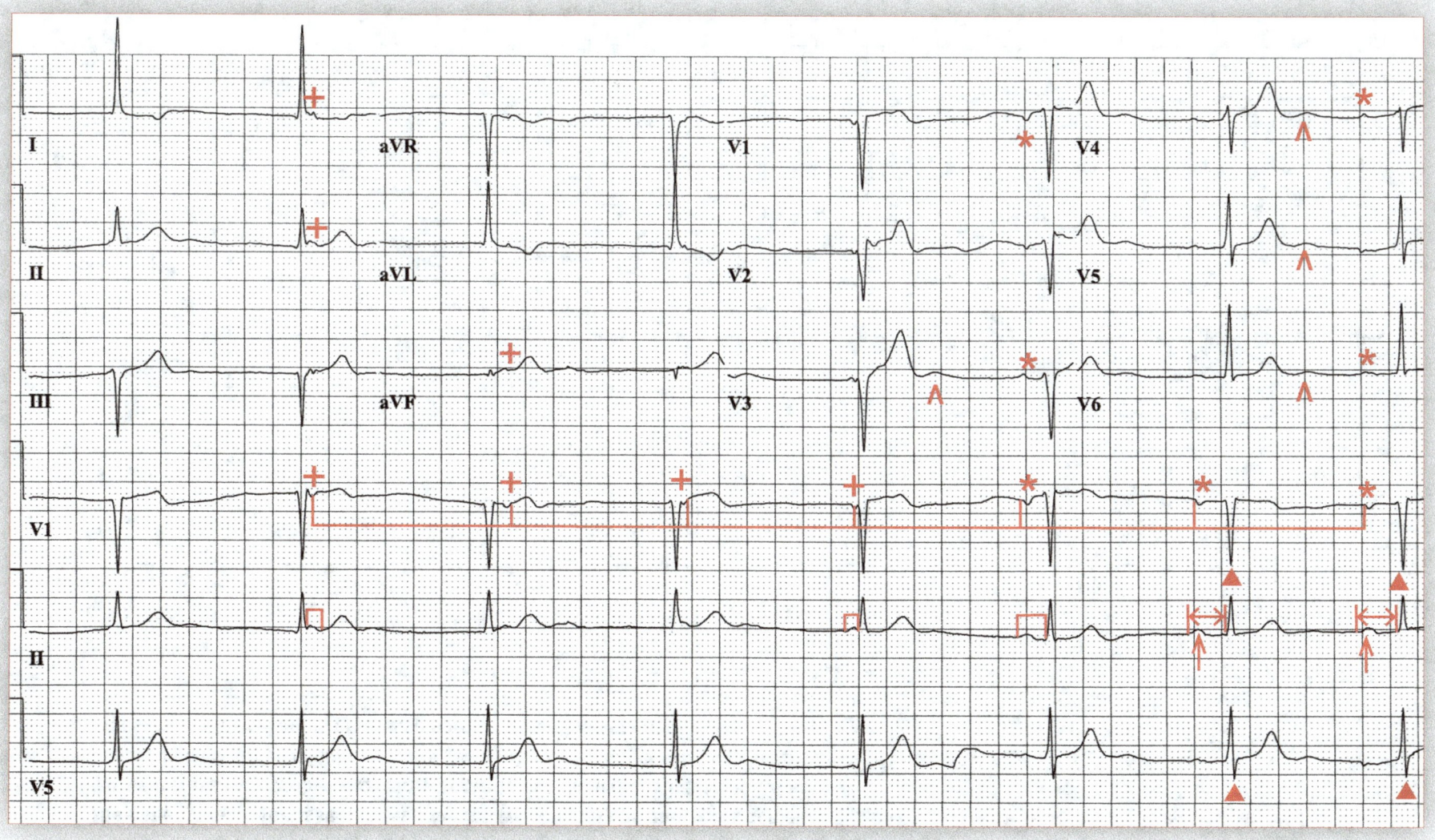

ECG 92 Analysis: Sinus bradycardia, complete heart block with junctional escape rhythm, intermittent AV conduction (capture) with first-degree AV block (prolonged AV conduction), U waves

There are regular RR intervals at a rate of 46 bpm. The QRS complexes have a normal duration (0.08 sec) and morphology. They have a left axis, between 0° and −30° (positive QRS complex in leads I and II and negative QRS complex in lead aVF). The QT/QTc intervals are normal (420/370 msec). There are low-amplitude U waves in leads V3-V6 (^). U waves are seen most commonly in leads V1-V3 and are unusual in the lateral precordial leads; their presence may be due to the bradycardia, although they may also suggest hypokalemia.

There are P waves (+,*) with a fairly constant PP interval (⊔) at a rate of 50 bpm. Some of the P waves are less obvious, being superimposed on the QRS complex or within the ST segment (+). The P waves are positive in leads I, II, aVF, and V4-V6. Hence they are sinus P waves and the underlying rhythm is sinus bradycardia. There is no consistent relationship between the P waves and the QRS complexes (*ie*, variable PR intervals [⊓]), and hence AV dissociation is present. The atrial rate is faster than the ventricular rate; therefore, there is complete (third-degree) AV block. As the QRS complex duration and morphology are normal, these are supraventricular complexes and, therefore, there is an escape junctional rhythm. The last two QRS complexes (7 and 8) (▲), which have the same morphology as the others, are early and they

are occurring at a rate of 50 bpm. There is an on-time P wave before each of these complexes (↑) with a stable PR interval (↔) (0.28 sec). This indicates that they are captured and hence sinus complexes with a first-degree AV block (prolonged AV conduction). Overall, this ECG demonstrates complete (third-degree) AV block with an escape junctional rhythm and intermittent capture. Since the escape rhythm is junctional, the cause for the complete heart block is disease within the AV node.

Certain herbal preparations contain compounds that can inhibit cardiac conduction by altering autonomic tone. Passion flower and chamomile may have β-adrenergic–blocking effects. Cohosh, used for dysmenorrhea, exhibits enhanced vagal effects. Interactions between unregulated herbal and "natural" supplements and medications as well as underlying organic disease must be considered. In this case, the patient's conduction disease, evidenced by marked first-degree AV block when AV conduction is intact, may have been exacerbated by the vagal effects of her new herbal medication, resulting in a complete heart block at the level of the AV junction. Fortunately, she has no infra-Hisian disease and the AV junctional escape rhythm is intact. ■

Notes

A 72-year-old man who has no previous cardiac history presents to the emergency department with severe pleuritic chest pain. His lung exam is unremarkable. Laboratory values are all within normal limits. An ECG is obtained. As there is a concern about a pulmonary embolism, he undergoes angiography, which is unremarkable. He is admitted to the hospital for further workup.

What does the ECG show?

Based on the ECG, is any further evaluation warranted?

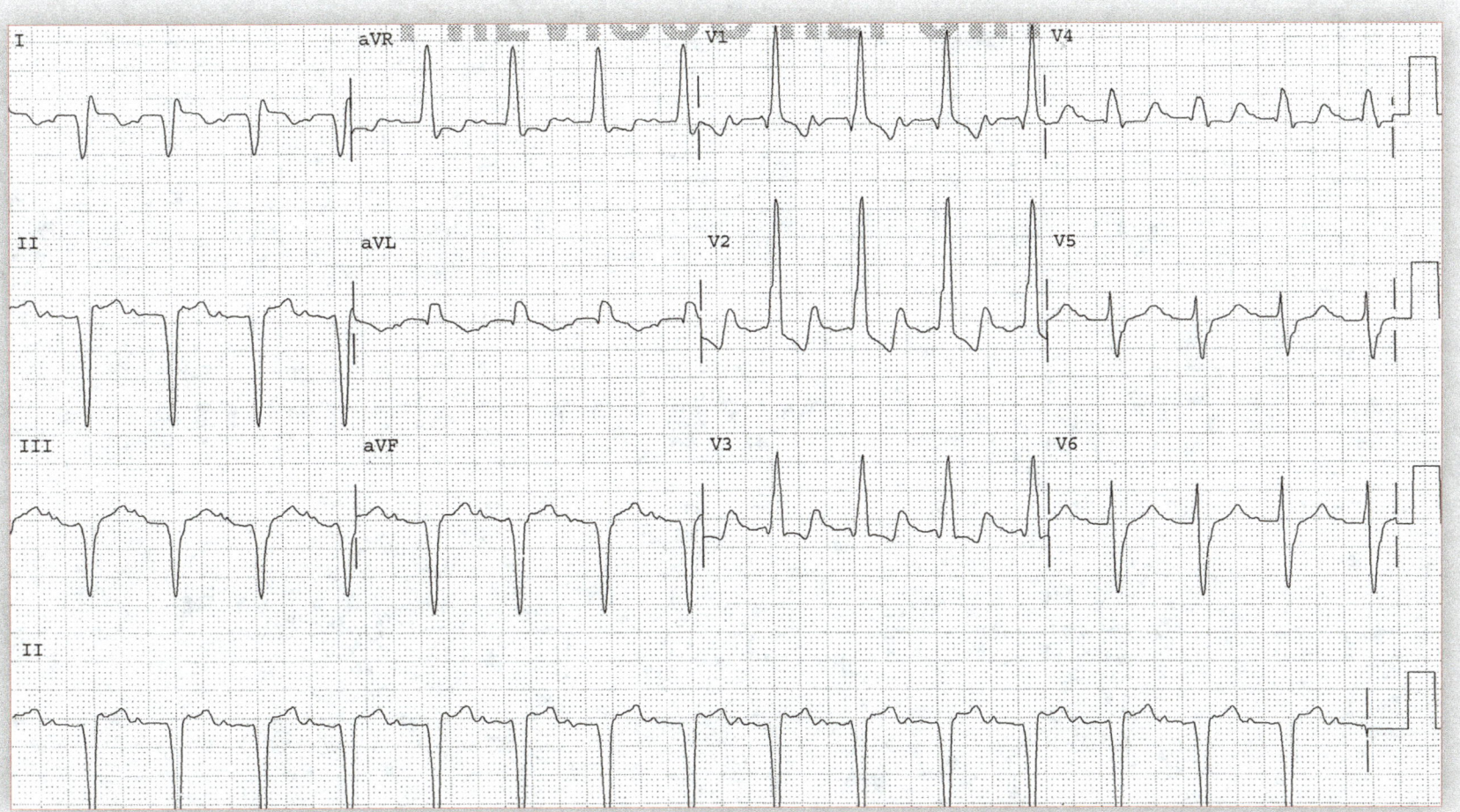

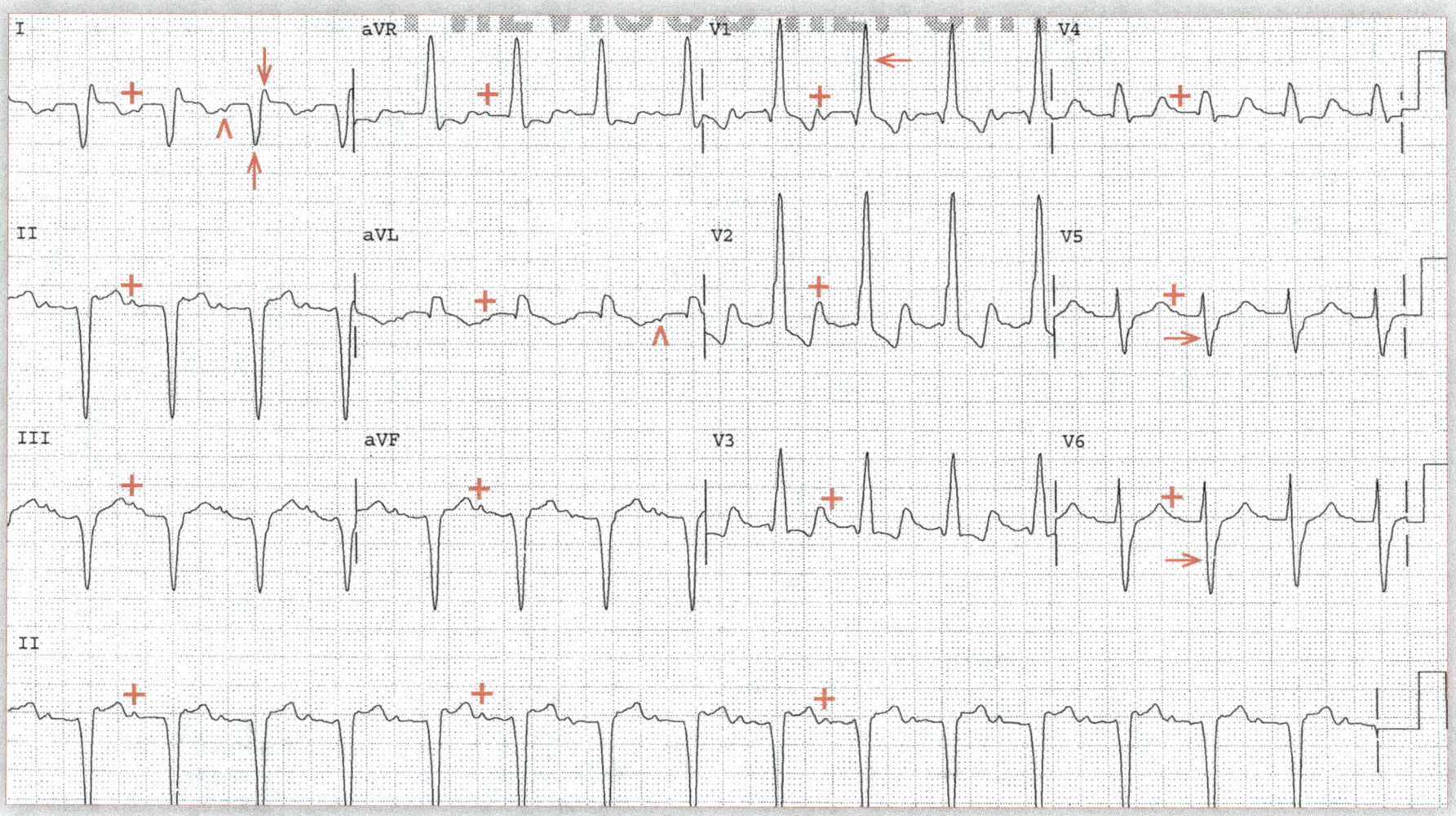

ECG 93 Analysis: Normal sinus rhythm, first-degree AV block (prolonged AV conduction), right bundle branch block, old inferior wall myocardial infarction, right–left arm lead switch

There is a regular rhythm at a rate of 96 bpm. There is a P wave (+) before each QRS complex with a stable PR interval (0.28 sec). The P waves are positive in leads II, aVF, and V4-V6. However, they are negative in leads I and aVL (^), while they are positive in lead aVR. This is an unusual P-wave axis and suggests that there may be an ectopic atrial focus or that there is a right–left (R–L) arm lead switch. The QRS complexes have a widened duration (0.16 sec) and a morphology of a right bundle branch block (RSR′ morphology in lead V1 [←] and terminal broad S waves in leads V5-V6 [→]). However, the morphology in lead I is strange, as there is a deep QS complex (↑) as well as a terminal broad R wave (↓). Because there is a right bundle branch block morphology in the precordial leads, the QRS complex is the result of an R–L arm lead switch. If the leads were properly placed, lead I would have a normal R wave with a broad terminal S wave and lead aVR would have a normal Q wave. The lead switch also accounts for the negative P wave in lead I and the positive P wave in lead aVR. The axis appears to be indeterminate, between −90° and +/-180° (negative QRS complex in leads I and aVF). However,

since there is lead switch present, the QRS complex is not actually negative in lead I. Moreover, the QRS complexes in leads II and aVF have a QS morphology, which is characteristic for an old inferior wall myocardial infarction. This accounts for what looks like a left axis or left anterior fascicular block (negative QRS complex in leads II and aVF, not considering lead I). Hence the indeterminate axis in this patient is not indicative of a conduction problem; rather it is the result of R–L arm lead switch and an old inferior wall myocardial infarction. No fascicular or other conduction abnormalities are present. The R–L arm lead switch should be confirmed by repeating the ECG with the leads on the correct limbs. Otherwise, no other workup is necessary. The QT/QTc intervals are prolonged (400/510 msec) but are normal when the prolonged QRS complex duration is considered (320/405 msec).

R–L arm lead switch generally affects leads I and aVL (negative P wave, QRS complex, and T wave) and aVR (positive P wave, QRS complex, and T wave). Leads II, III, and aVF are usually not affected. ■

Notes

This ECG is from a 48-year-old man with advanced multivessel coronary disease and ischemic cardiomyopathy.

What portions of the cardiac conduction system have been affected by his disease?

What other abnormalities are depicted?

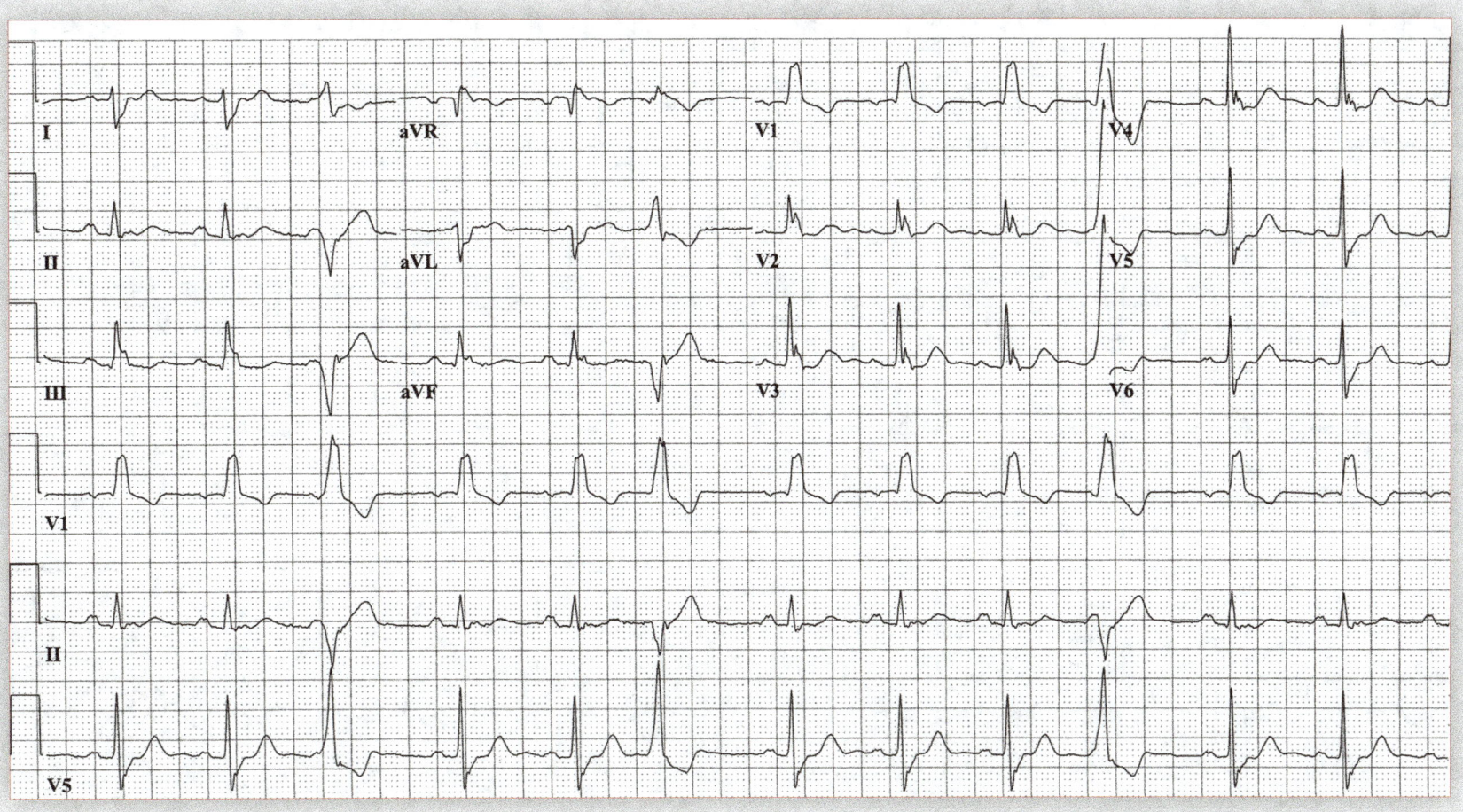

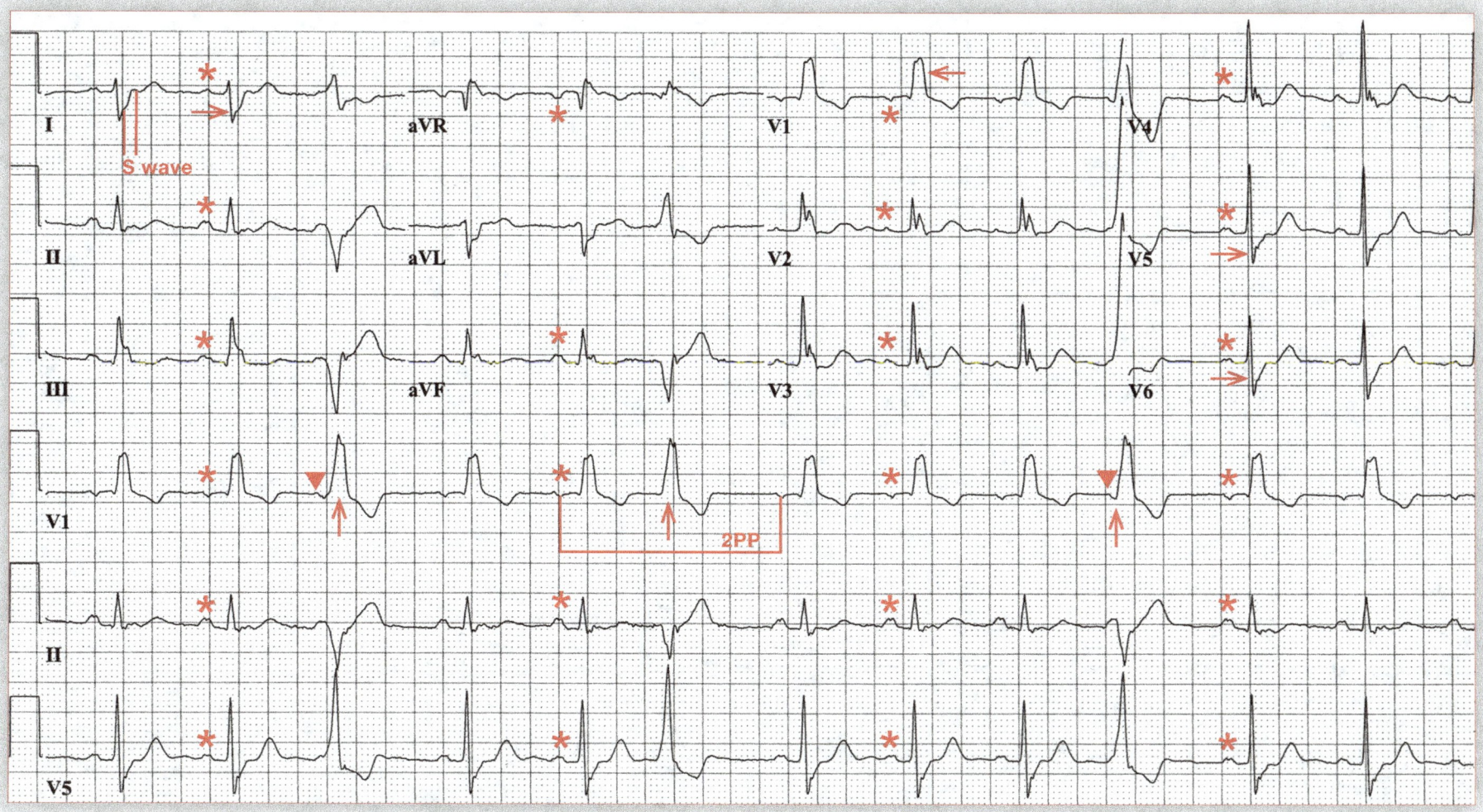

ECG 94 Analysis: Normal sinus rhythm, left posterior fascicular block, right bundle branch block, premature ventricular complexes

The ECG shows a regular rhythm at a rate of 80 bpm. There is a P wave (*) before each QRS complex with a stable PR interval (0.16 sec). The P wave is positive in leads I, II, aVF, and V4-V6. Hence, there is a normal sinus rhythm. The QRS complex duration is prolonged (0.16 sec), and there is a pattern of a right bundle branch block (RBBB; broad R wave in lead V1 [←] and broad terminal S wave in leads I and V5-V6 [→]). The QT/QTc intervals are prolonged (400/460 msec) but are normal when the prolonged QRS complex duration is considered (320/370 msec). The axis is rightward, between +90° and +180°. The QRS complex is negative in lead I (even when the S wave [‖] due to the RBBB is not considered) and positive in lead aVF. Hence there is a left posterior fascicular block. It should be remembered that with an RBBB there is a terminal broad S wave in lead I that may give the appearance of a negative QRS complex but actually represents delayed right ventricular activity and is not considered part of axis determination. The RBBB and left posterior fascicular block are indicative of bifascicular block.

In addition there are three complexes that are premature, are wider, and have a different morphology (↑). An on-time sinus P wave can be seen before the first and third of these premature complexes (▼); however, the PR interval is very short and hence there is not likely to be AV conduction. These premature complexes are followed by a full compensatory pause (*ie*, the PP interval around the premature complex [⊔] is twice the underlying sinus [PP] interval). These are premature ventricular complexes and since the morphology of all three is the same they are unifocal.

The presence of bifascicular block indicates more advanced conduction system disease. In this case, it is related to the presence of an ischemic cardiomyopathy. Bifascicular block due to left posterior fascicular block is less commonly seen than bifascicular block due to left anterior fascicular block; however, it has the same implications with regard to the development of complete heart block. While such patients are at increased risk for developing complete heart block, the incidence of this is low. In several studies, the incidence of progression to complete AV block was about 1% to 1.5% per year. Indeed, mortality in these patients, often due to arrhythmia, was related to the underlying heart disease and not to the development of complete heart block. There is no specific therapy for bifascicular block except for discontinuation or avoidance of drugs that may further impair cardiac conduction. Pacemakers are not indicated for asymptomatic patients. However, the insertion of a pacemaker is considered (class II indication) for patients with a bifascicular block associated with syncope that can be attributed to transient complete heart block, based on the history and the exclusion of other plausible causes of syncope (specifically ventricular tachycardia in a patient with coronary disease, an old myocardial infarction, and ischemic cardiomyopathy). ■

Notes

A 56-year-old man admitted for abdominal pain is diagnosed with acute cholecystitis. He is treated with intravenous fluids and antibiotics. An ECG is obtained and the resident calls the cardiology fellow for advice about what it shows.

What is the abnormality?

What diagnostic medication could be given to further evaluate this abnormality?

Is any therapy warranted?

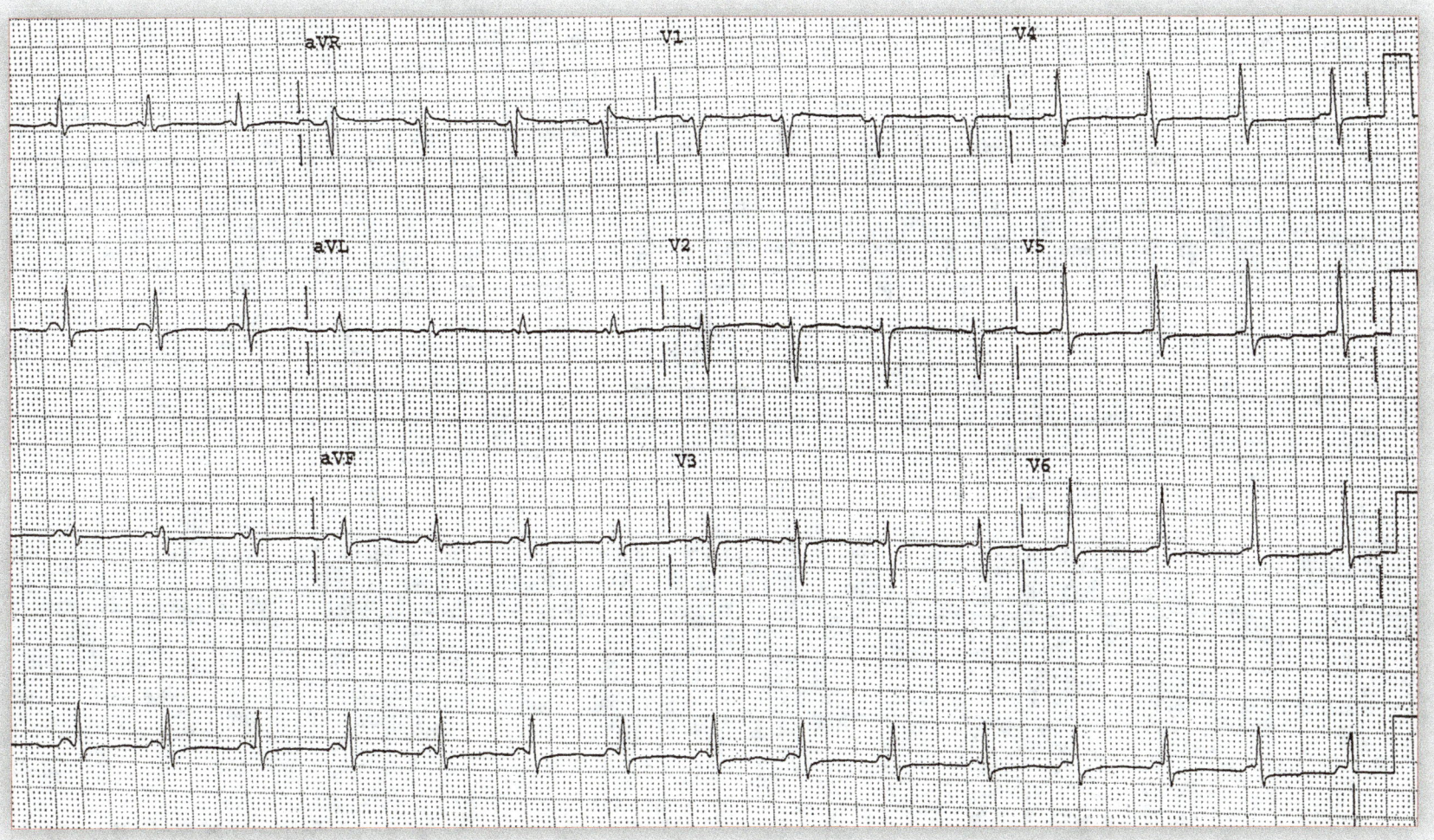

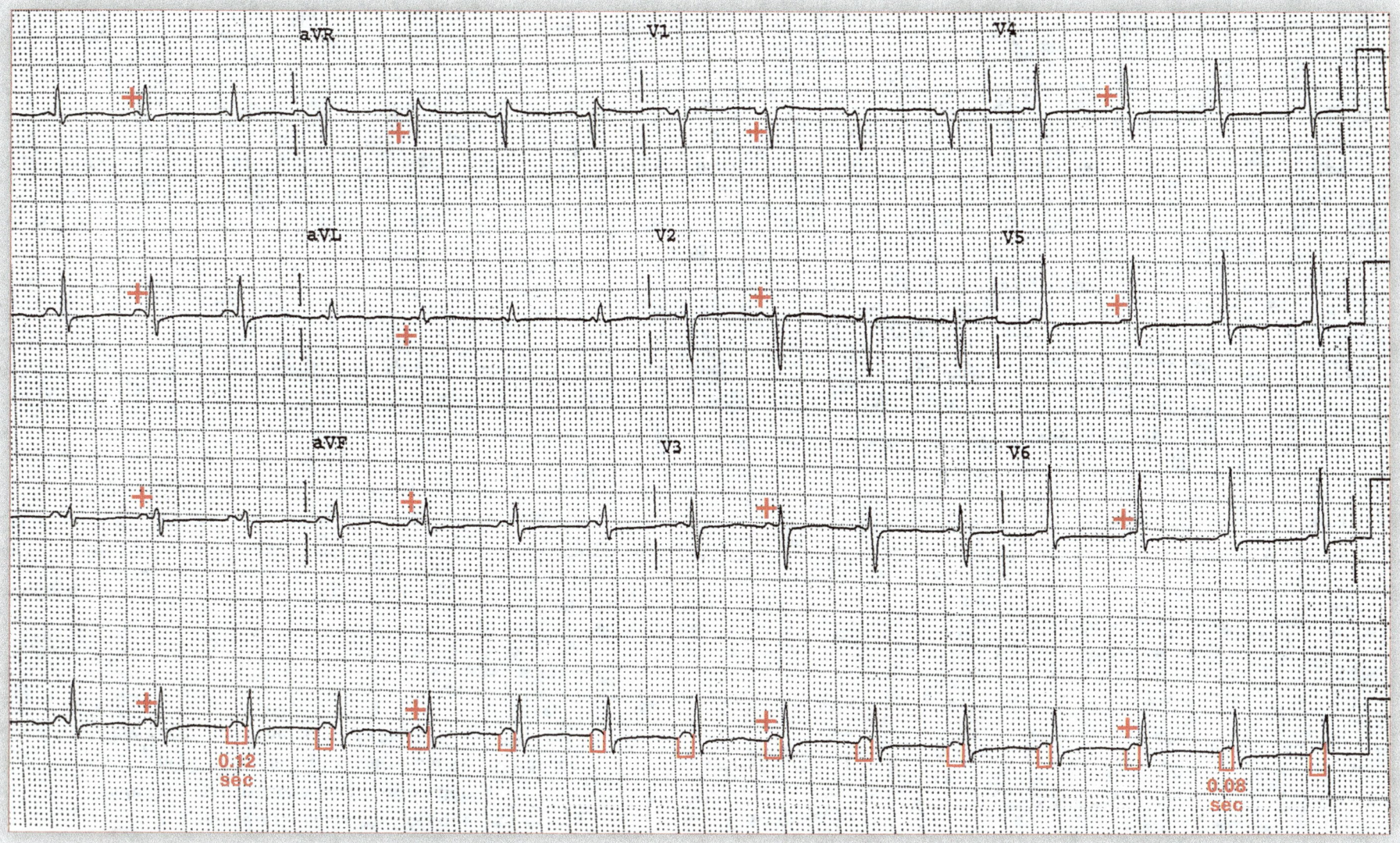

ECG 95 Analysis: Normal sinus rhythm, isorhythmic AV dissociation, junctional rhythm

There is a regular rhythm at a rate of 94 bpm. There is a P wave (+) before each QRS complex, and the P waves are positive in leads I, II, aVF, and V4-V6. Hence this is a normal sinus rhythm. The PR interval is very short, but it is not constant (⊔); the PR intervals are becoming progressively shorter (from 0.12 to 0.08 sec). Hence AV dissociation is present. The ventricular rate is also 94 bpm, and the QRS complex has a normal duration (0.08 sec) and morphology. The axis is normal, between 0° and +90°. Hence these are junctional complexes and this is a junctional rhythm.

With AV dissociation there is no relationship between the atrial and ventricular activity (*ie*, the P waves are dissociated from the QRS complexes). Hence there are variable PR intervals. There are two etiologies for AV dissociation. The first is complete heart block (third-degree AV block), in which the atrial rate is faster than the ventricular rate because there is an escape rhythm (junctional or ventricular).

The second is an accelerated lower pacemaker focus (junctional or ventricular), in which case the atrial rate is slower than the ventricular rate. When the two rates are identical, the etiology for AV dissociation is unclear; this is termed isorhythmic dissociation.

In general, isorhythmic dissociation is a benign condition and no specific therapy is needed because in this case there is a stable junctional rhythm. The etiology for the isorhythmic dissociation can be established if there is a change in either the atrial or ventricular rate and observing a difference between the two. This might happen spontaneously. If not, atropine might be effective as it will increase the sinus rate but will have no effect on the junctional rate. Hence, if there is capture and a stable PR interval with the faster atrial rate, the etiology is an accelerated junctional rhythm. If AV dissociation persists at the faster sinus rate, the diagnosis is complete heart block. ■

Notes

A 32-year-old man with HIV presents to his infectious disease physician with complaints of recurrent pre-syncope. The episodes are unheralded and worsen during exercise or exertion. He further notes some decrement in his functional capacity due to an indolent onset of exertional dyspnea. On exam, his vital signs are notable for a radial pulse of 38 bpm and his blood pressure is normal. The physical exam is notable for temporal wasting. His lung fields are clear. Jugular venous pressure is 8 cm H_2O. His cardiac exam reveals a diffuse point of maximal impulse that is displaced 2 cm laterally and a soft, blowing systolic apical murmur. Gallop sounds are not heard. His abdominal exam is unremarkable. His extremities show some wasting and fat redistribution. The physician obtains a surface 12-lead ECG.

What abnormalities are seen to explain the patient's symptoms?

What further testing is needed?

What therapy is indicated?

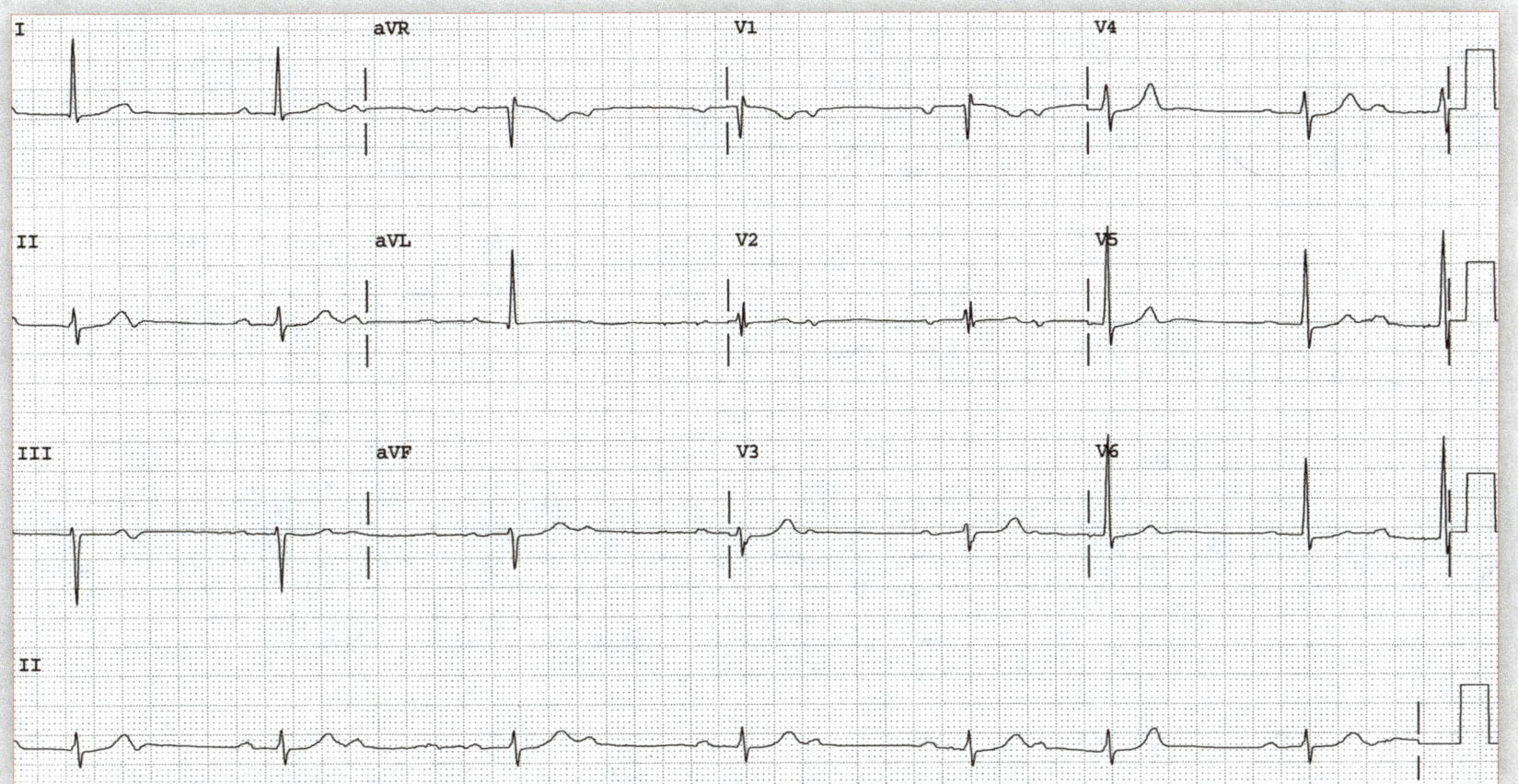

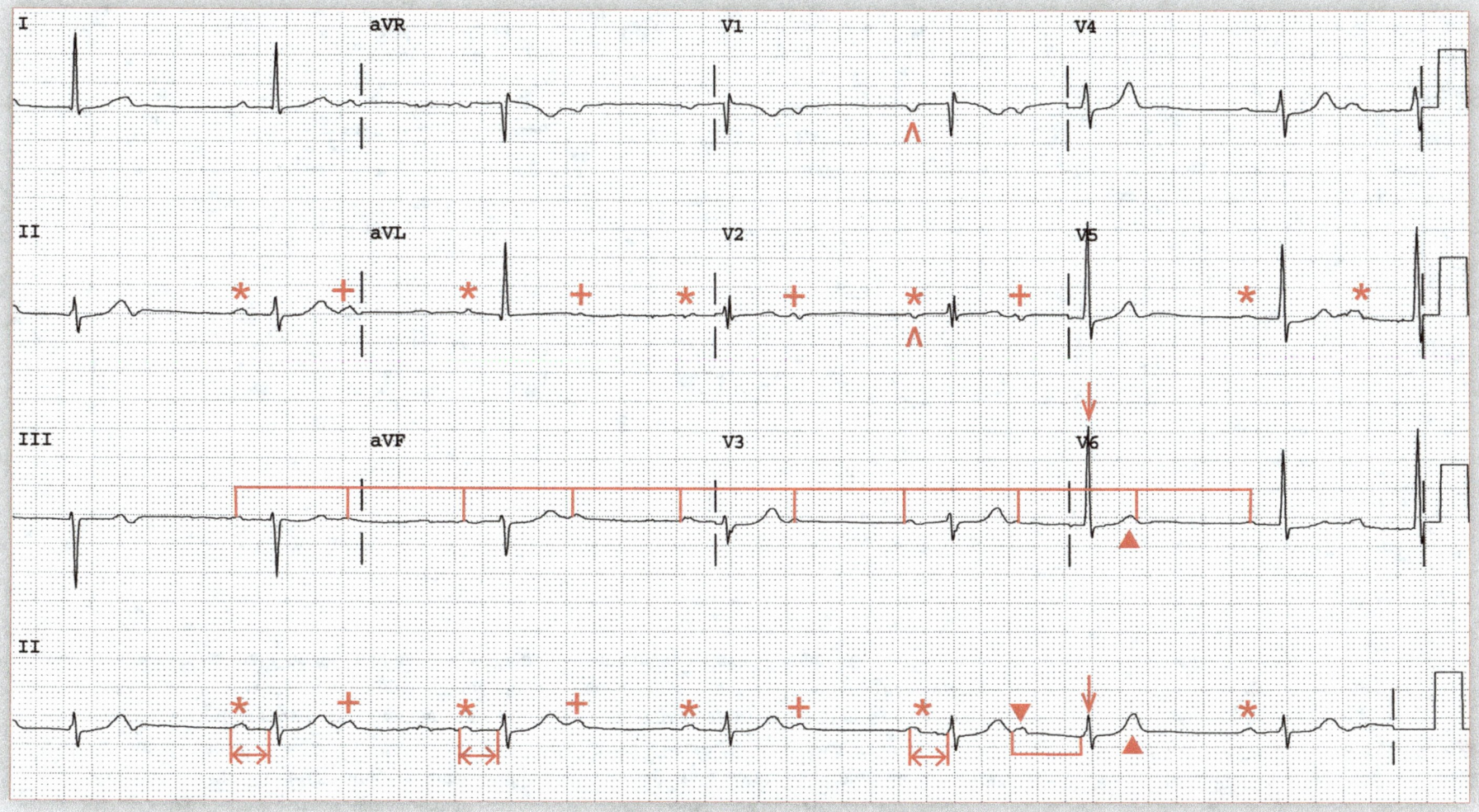

ECG 96 Analysis: Normal sinus rhythm, left atrial hypertrophy (abnormality), first-degree AV block (prolonged AV conduction), 2:1 and 3:2 Mobitz type I second-degree AV block

The initial portion of the ECG shows a regular rhythm at a rate of 38 bpm. There is a P wave (*) before each QRS complex with a stable PR interval (↔) of 0.30 second, defining first-degree AV block (prolonged AV conduction). A left atrial abnormality is present based on the negative P wave (^) in leads V1-V2. A second P wave (+) can be seen after the T wave. The PP interval is regular (⊓), and the atrial rate is 80 bpm. The P waves are positive in leads I, II, aVF, and V4-V6, defining a normal sinus rhythm. Hence initially there is a second-degree AV block with a pattern of 2:1 AV conduction. However, another pattern is seen at the end of the tracing. There is an early QRS complex (↓) with a PR interval (⊔) that is now prolonged to 0.48 second. The occurrence of an early QRS complex means that it is in response to the preceding P wave (▼). There is an on-time but nonconducted P wave (▲) following this early QRS complex (by measuring the PP interval [⊓] it can be seen that the P wave is on the T wave, altering its morphology). This represents second-degree AV block with a Wenckebach pattern and 3:2 conduction. Therefore, in this case the 2:1 AV conduction is the result of Wenckebach or Mobitz type I. With 2:1 AV block, the etiology (Mobitz type I or II) cannot be established unless there is a change in the conduction pattern (with two or more sequentially conducted P waves), as occurred in this case. The QRS duration is normal (0.08 sec) and there is a physiologic left axis, between 0° and –30° (positive QRS complex in leads I and II and negative QRS complex in lead aVF). The QT/QTc intervals are normal (420/334 msec).

HIV-associated cardiomyopathy is a well-described entity in patients with AIDS, particular in those with prolonged duration after the time of diagnosis. The prevalence of cardiomyopathy is approximately 10% in industrialized nations. Etiologies include direct effects of the HIV virus with associated myocarditis, opportunistic pathogen-associated myocarditis, and highly active antiretroviral therapy (HAART)–associated cardiomyopathy. This patient manifests signs on physical exam of a dilated left ventricle and systolic dysfunction. In that context, relatively benign AV block such as first-degree and second-degree Mobitz type I (Wenckebach) as seen in this patient can be symptomatic. Pacemaker implantation may be considered in these patients (whereas it is generally not indicated in patients who have normal left ventricular function). Initial evaluation and therapy should include echocardiographic assessment of left ventricular function, inpatient institution of medical therapy for systolic heart failure, and consideration of pacemaker implantation if his conduction abnormality persists and the pre-syncopal symptoms are not relieved by initiation of heart failure therapy. His antiretroviral medications should be reviewed for those known to cause left ventricular dysfunction, such as nucleoside reverse-transcriptase inhibitors. A complete review of his HIV status, viral load, and compliance/response to antiretroviral therapy is warranted. ■

A 56-year-old man is admitted to the hospital for pneumonia. While on telemetry, the nurse notices variation in the patient's surface ECG tracing. She obtains a 12-lead ECG.

What abnormalities are noted?

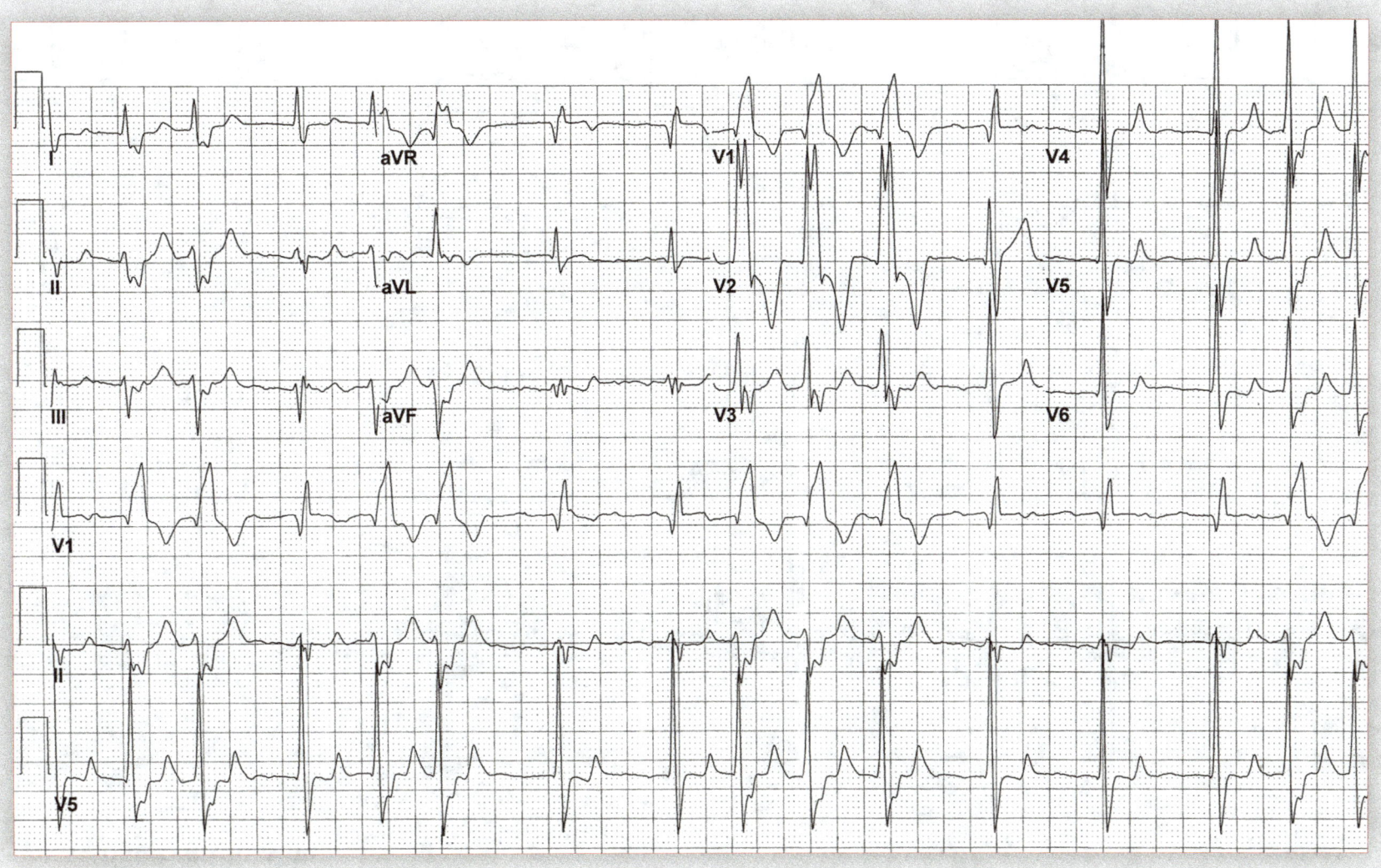

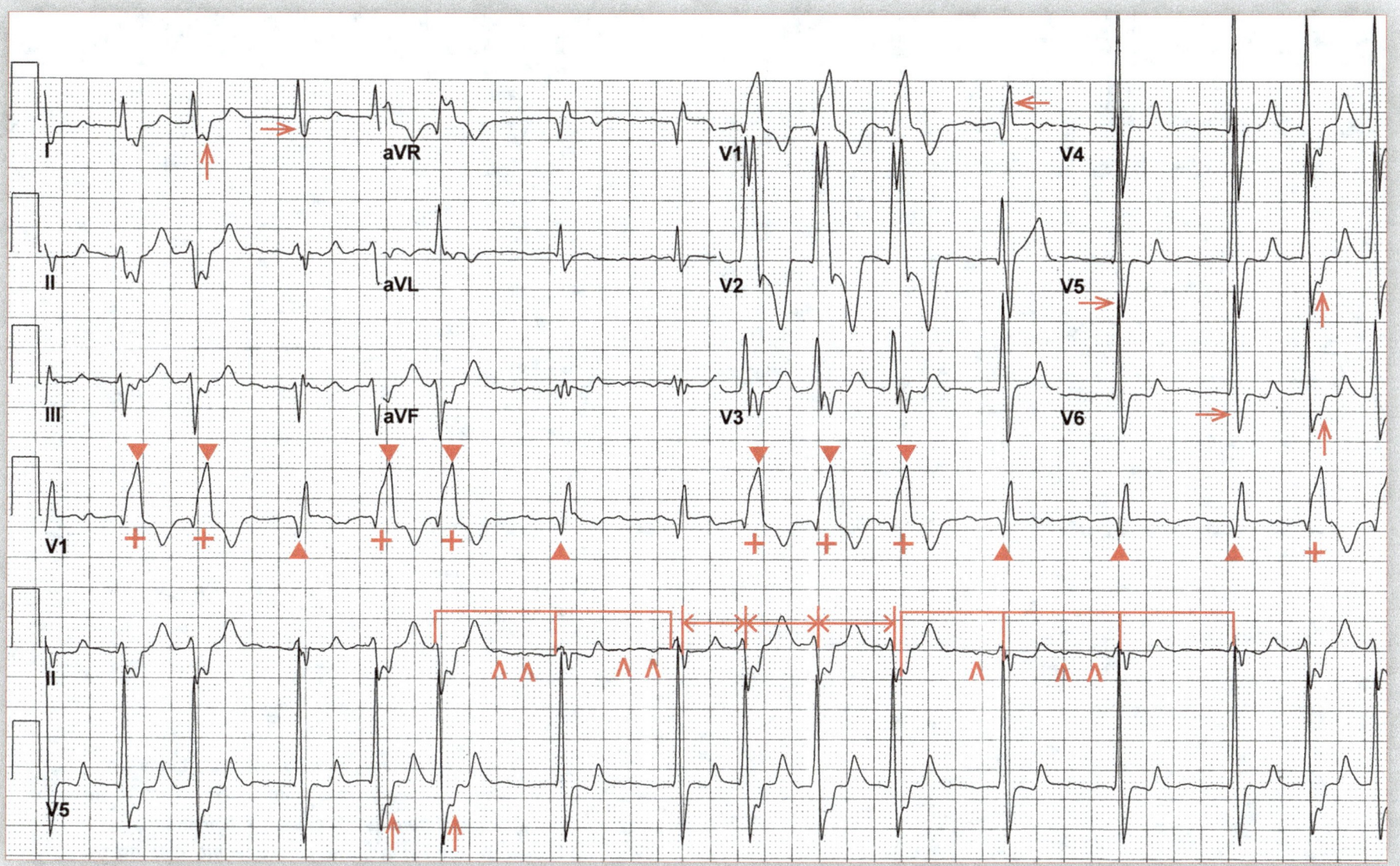

ECG 97 Analysis: Atrial fibrillation, left anterior fascicular block, rate-related right bundle branch block

The rhythm is irregularly irregular at an average rate of 78 bpm. There are no organized P waves, but there are occasional low-amplitude unorganized undulations of the baseline (^), best seen in the lead V1 rhythm strip. The rhythm is, therefore, atrial fibrillation. Two QRS complex morphologies are seen. The narrower complexes (▲) have a duration of 0.10 second and an axis between −30° and −90° (positive QRS complex in lead I and negative QRS complex in leads II and aVF with an rS morphology). This is a left anterior fascicular block. These complexes have a narrow R′ morphology in lead V1 (←) and an S wave in leads I and V5-V6 (→), suggesting a right ventricular conduction delay (although this morphology is often referred to as an incomplete right bundle branch block [RBBB]). The wider QRS complexes (+) have a duration of 0.16 second with a typical RBBB pattern (broad R wave in lead V1 [▼] and broad S wave in leads I and V5-V6 [↑]). Hence this is evidence for bifascicular disease (*ie*, RBBB and left anterior fascicular block). The RBBB occurs whenever the RR interval is shorter (↔), that is, with a faster ventricular rate. The RBBB is not present when the RR intervals are longer (⊓). Therefore, this is a rate-related RBBB. The QT/QTc intervals of the narrower QRS complex are normal (400/456 msec and 380/430 when corrected for the slightly prolonged QRS complex duration). The QT/QTc intervals for the complexes with an RBBB are the same (460/525 msec and 380/430 when corrected for the prolonged QRS complex duration).

Intermittent or rate-related RBBB is indicative of underlying conduction disease of the right bundle that becomes manifest only when the heart rate is faster. In this situation, the diseased bundle is unable to conduct impulses that are at rapid rates and hence block within the bundle develops. It is often the precursor of a permanent RBBB and has the same implications and prognosis of a persistent RBBB and a persistent bifascicular block. ■

Practice Case 98

A 55-year-old woman is admitted with transient syncope. The episode was unheralded and lasted a few seconds. She has otherwise been well, improving gradually after presenting 2 months ago with fatigue, weight loss, and tremor leading to the diagnosis of Graves' disease. She has been on anti-thyroid medication since her diagnosis, and her symptoms have largely resolved. On exam,

ECG 98A

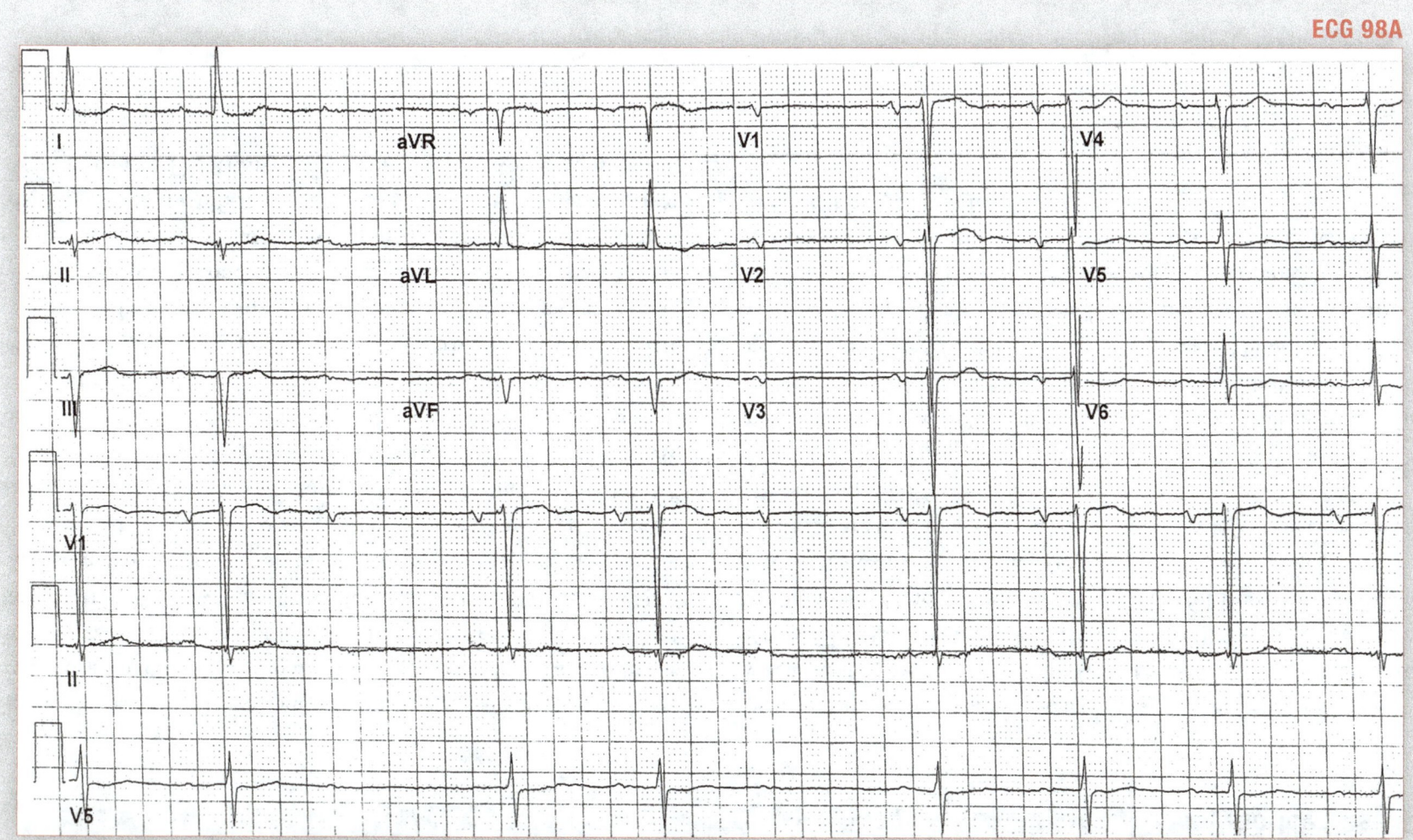

exophthalmos is noted. Her heart rate is 58 bpm. Her cardiac exam is notable for a fixed split S2. The remainder of her exam is normal. As part of her evaluation, an ECG is obtained (ECG 98A). The patient is placed on telemetry and on the following day the resident notices a change in her QRS complexes. On jugular venous pressure inspection, cannon A waves are now seen. A second ECG is obtained (ECG 98B).

What abnormality is evident on the initial ECG (98A)?

What is the likely cause of this abnormality?

What does ECG 98B show?

What therapy is indicated?

ECG 98B

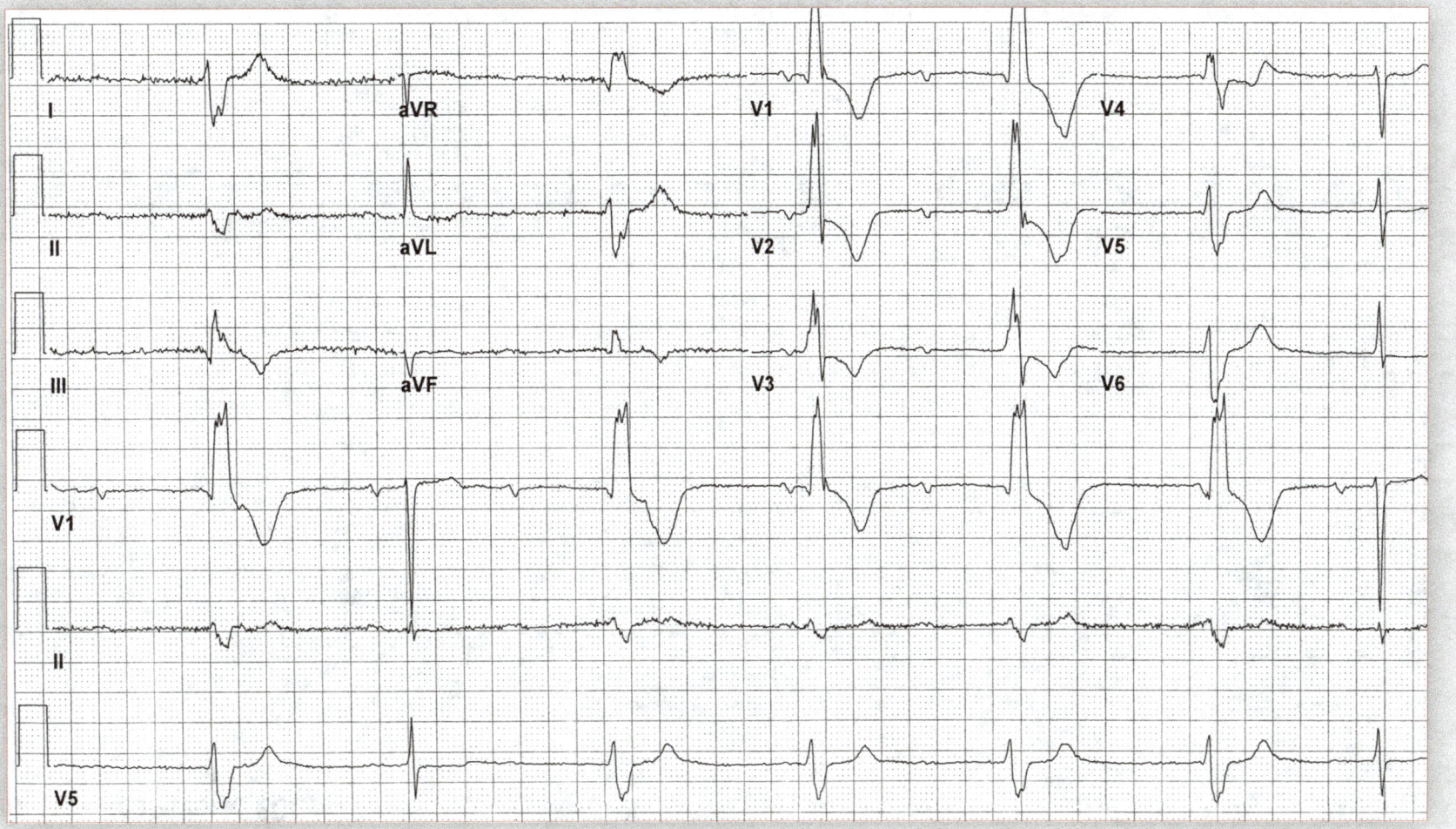

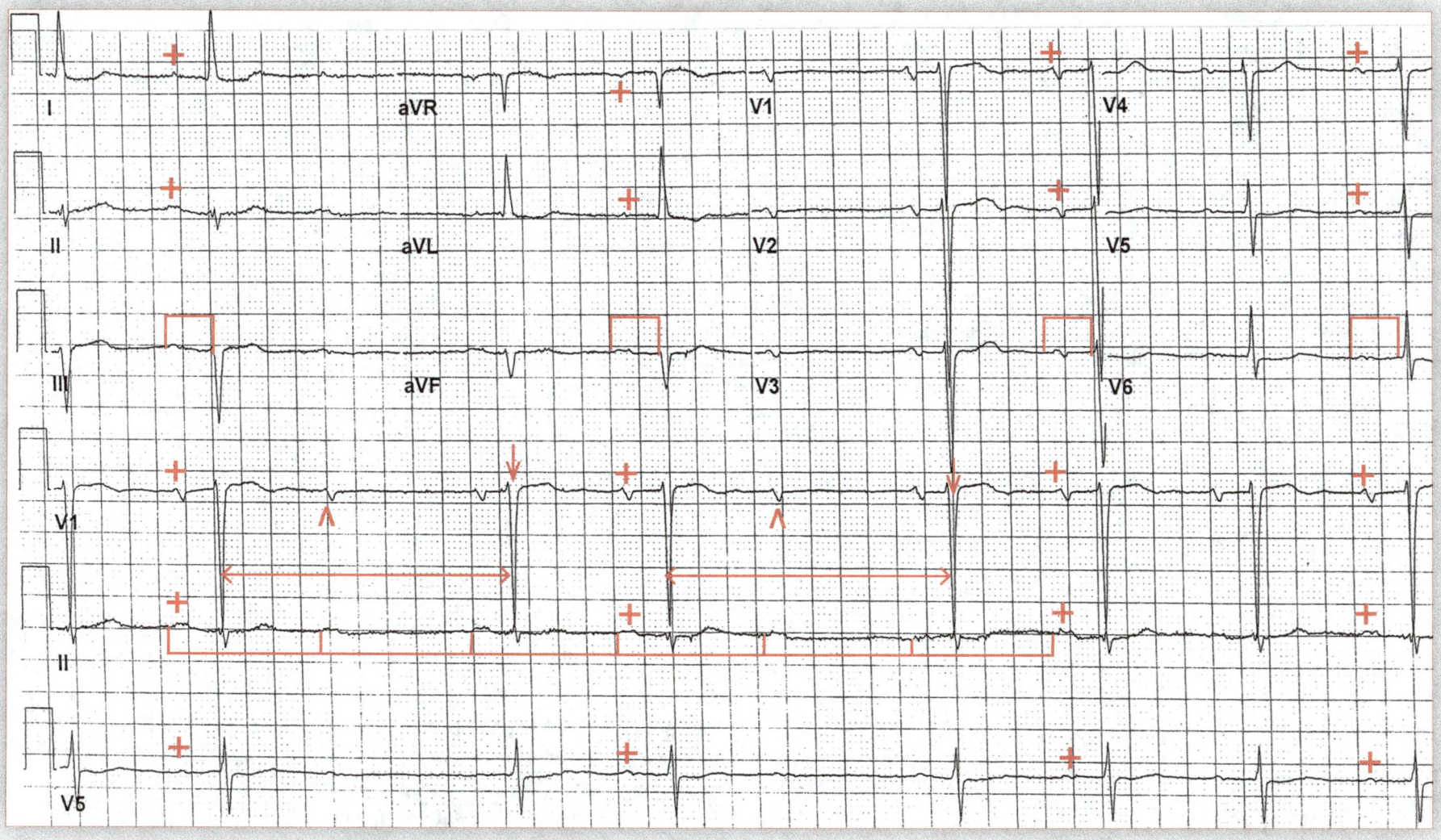

ECG 98A Analysis: Normal sinus rhythm, Mobitz type II
second-degree AV block, left anterior fascicular block

In **ECG 98A,** the rhythm is irregular as a result of two long pauses (↔) with the same duration (2.08 sec). The rhythm is, therefore, regularly irregular. The remaining RR intervals are all the same, at a rate of 58 bpm. The QRS complex duration is normal (0.08 sec) and there is a normal morphology. The axis is extremely leftward, between −30° and −90° (positive QRS complex in lead I and negative QRS complex in leads II and aVF with an rS morphology). This is a left anterior fascicular block. The QT/QTc intervals are normal (400/395 msec). There are P waves (+) before each QRS complex with a stable PR interval (0.28 sec) (⊓), except for a slightly shorter PR interval (0.24 sec)

before the third and fifth QRS complexes (↓). It is likely that the slightly shorter PR interval is the result of slight enhancement of AV conduction due to the longer RR interval (slower rate), which allows for more rapid AV conduction as the AV node has had more time for recovery. During each pause there is an on-time P wave (PP intervals are constant) (⊔) that does not have a QRS complex following it. Hence this is a second-degree AV block (*ie,* an occasional nonconducted P wave). As all of the PR intervals are constant (except for the PR interval after the long pause), this is a Mobitz type II second-degree AV block. The block is, therefore, within the His-Purkinje system. *continues*

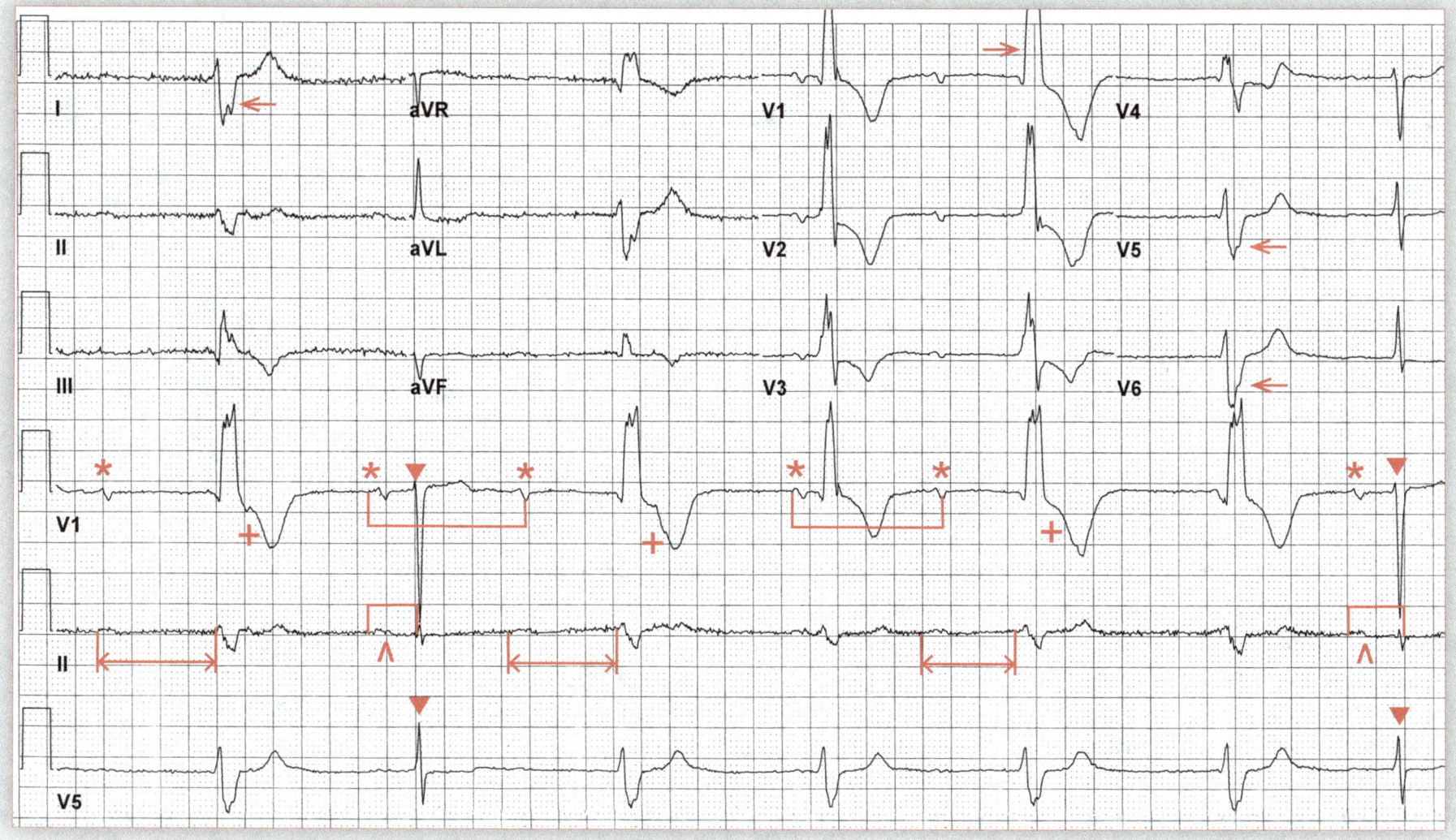

ECG 98B Analysis: Normal sinus rhythm, complete heart block,
escape ventricular rhythm, intermittent capture (intermittent AV conduction)

ECG 98B shows regular RR intervals at a rate of 44 bpm. However, the second and seventh QRS complexes (▼) are early. All the QRS complexes (except for the second and seventh) are wide (0.18 sec), and their morphology resembles that of a right bundle branch block (tall, broad R wave in lead V1 [→] and broad S wave in leads I and V5-V6 [←]). It is, however, not a typical right bundle branch block as there is a tall monophasic R wave in leads V1-V3. There are P waves (*) that have a regular PP interval (⊔) at a rate of 60 bpm. Some of the P waves are located within the ST segment (+) and are, therefore, less obvious. However, the P waves that are seen occur at a regular PP interval (⊔). The P waves are positive in leads I, II, aVF, and V4-V6 and hence there is an underlying normal sinus rhythm. The PR intervals are very variable (↔), and the P waves are dissociated from the QRS complexes. As the atrial rate is faster than the ventricular rate, there is complete (third-degree) AV block.

As indicated, the second and seventh QRS complexes (▼) have a normal duration (0.08 sec) and morphology. There is a P wave (^) before each, with the same PR interval (⊓) (0.28 sec). In addition, these two QRS complexes are early, indicating that they are the result of the P wave preceding them. Importantly, the two narrow QRS complexes have the same duration, morphology, and axis as the QRS complexes seen in **ECG 98A**. The PR interval associated with these QRS complexes is also identical to the PR intervals seen in **ECG 98A**. This is, therefore, complete AV block with an escape ventricular rhythm and intermittent capture. The captured complexes are identical to the conducted complexes seen in **ECG 98A**. The fact that the dissociated QRS complexes are wider and have a different morphology when compared with the captured complexes, which are narrow and have a normal duration and morphology, indicates that the dissociated complexes are ventricular in origin.

In this patient with Graves' disease, it would be important to check thyroid status as continued hyperthyroidism may be associated with complete AV block, although this usually occurs in patients with underlying conduction system disease. When the heart is "stressed" by the hyperthyroid state, complete AV block may become manifest. However, in this situation the sinus rate is likely to be more rapid than seen on these ECGs due to sympathomimetic effects seen with hyperthyroidism. Nevertheless, if hyperthyroidism was still present, with further therapy there would likely be resolution of the complete AV block. However, the presence of persistent complete AV block (in the absence of hyperthyroidism) associated with an escape ventricular rhythm is an indication for implantation of a permanent pacemaker. ■

Notes

An ECG from an asymptomatic 24-year-old woman is presented.

What notable findings are evident?

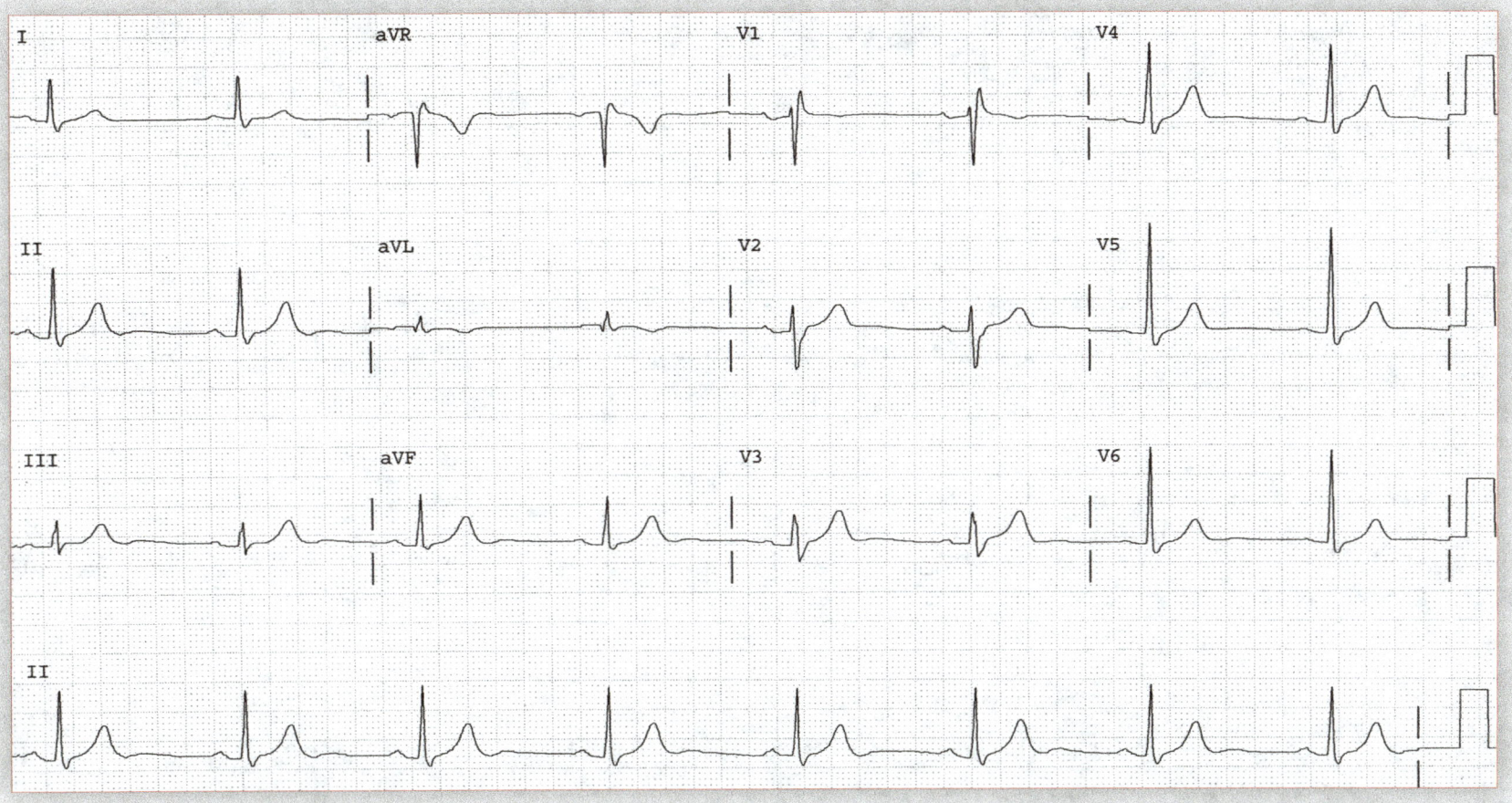

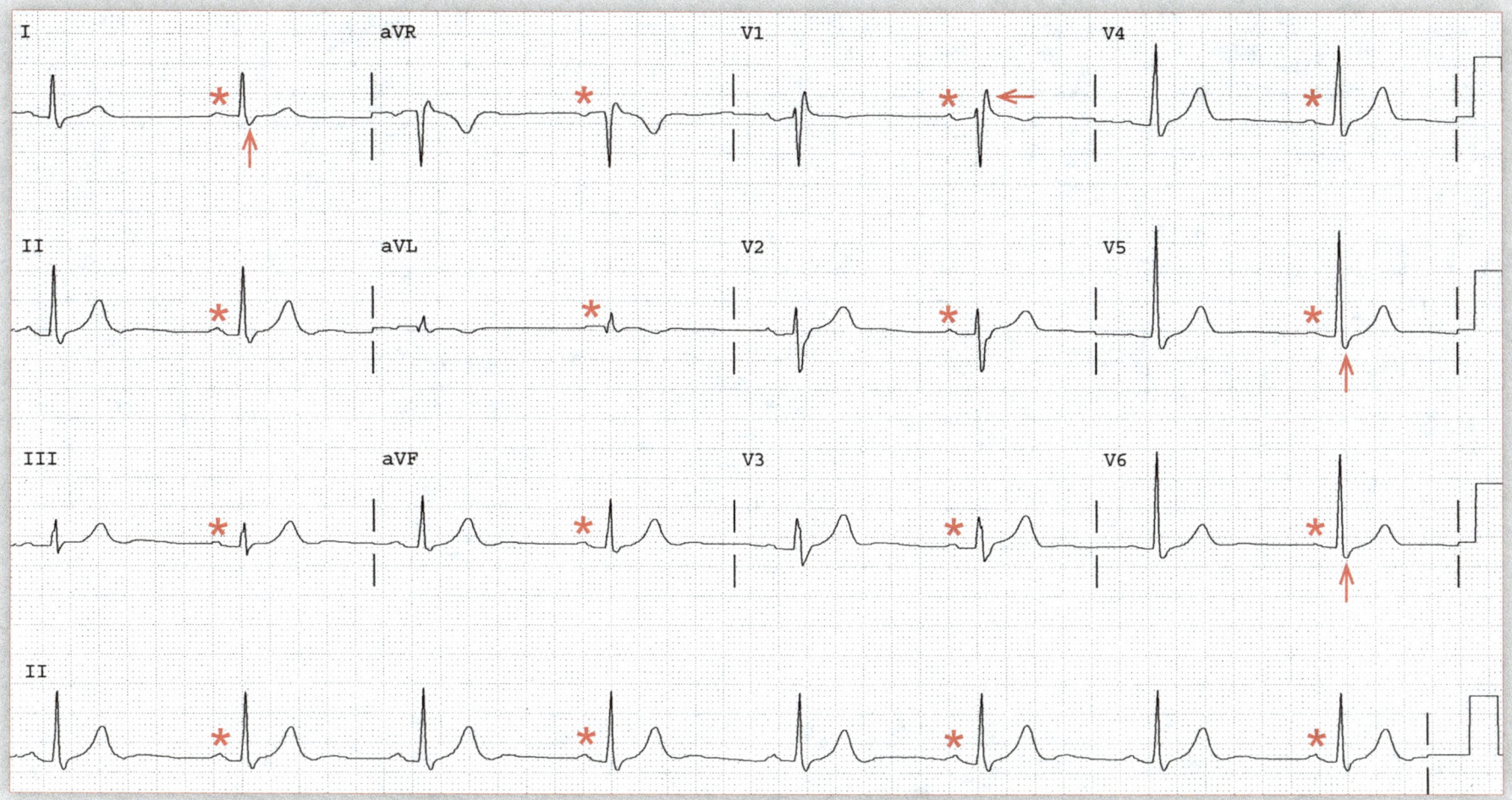

ECG 99 Analysis: Sinus bradycardia, intraventricular conduction delay to the right ventricle

The rhythm is regular at a rate of 46 bpm. There is a P wave (*) before each QRS complex with a stable PR interval (0.20 sec). The QRS duration is slightly prolonged (>0.10 but < 0.12 sec), and there is an RSR' complex in lead V1 (←) and a prominent S wave (↑) in leads I and V5-V6. Although the QRS complex morphology is that of a right bundle branch block (RBBB), the QRS complex duration is not wide enough for a bundle branch block. This has often been termed an incomplete RBBB, although it is actually a conduction delay to the right ventricle and is best termed an intraventricular conduction delay. The QT/QTc intervals are normal (440/385 msec).

The RSR' morphology seen in the early (right) precordial leads (ie, V1-V2) represents a spectrum of physiology ranging from normal delayed depolarization of the crista supraventricularis of the right ventricle to right intraventricular conduction delay to pathologic RBBB. The QRS complex width defines the diagnosis. If the QRS complex width is normal (ie, < 0.10 sec), the morphology is deemed a normal variant and is termed a crista pattern. If the QRS complex duration is slightly prolonged (0.10 to 0.12 sec), an intraventricular conduction delay to the right ventricle is present (this is often called an incomplete RBBB). If the QRS complex duration is longer than 0.12 second, the diagnosis is complete RBBB.

In this case, there is an intraventricular conduction delay to the right ventricle. The term incomplete RBBB, often applied to this pattern, is not accurate as the bundle manifests "all or none" conduction characteristics; that is, it either conducts (always at the same rate) or does not conduct. This is not of any clinical importance, although it may be associated with the development of a complete RBBB in the future. ■

Practice Case 100

A 76-year-old man with a history of coronary artery disease and a previous myocardial infarction (MI) is seen in the emergency department for complaints of intermittent fatigue and lightheadedness that have been occurring for the past week. He states that the symptoms occur episodically, unrelated to activity. Each episode lasts for about 30 minutes and then resolves spontaneously. Between the episodes he feels well. He came to the

ECG 100A

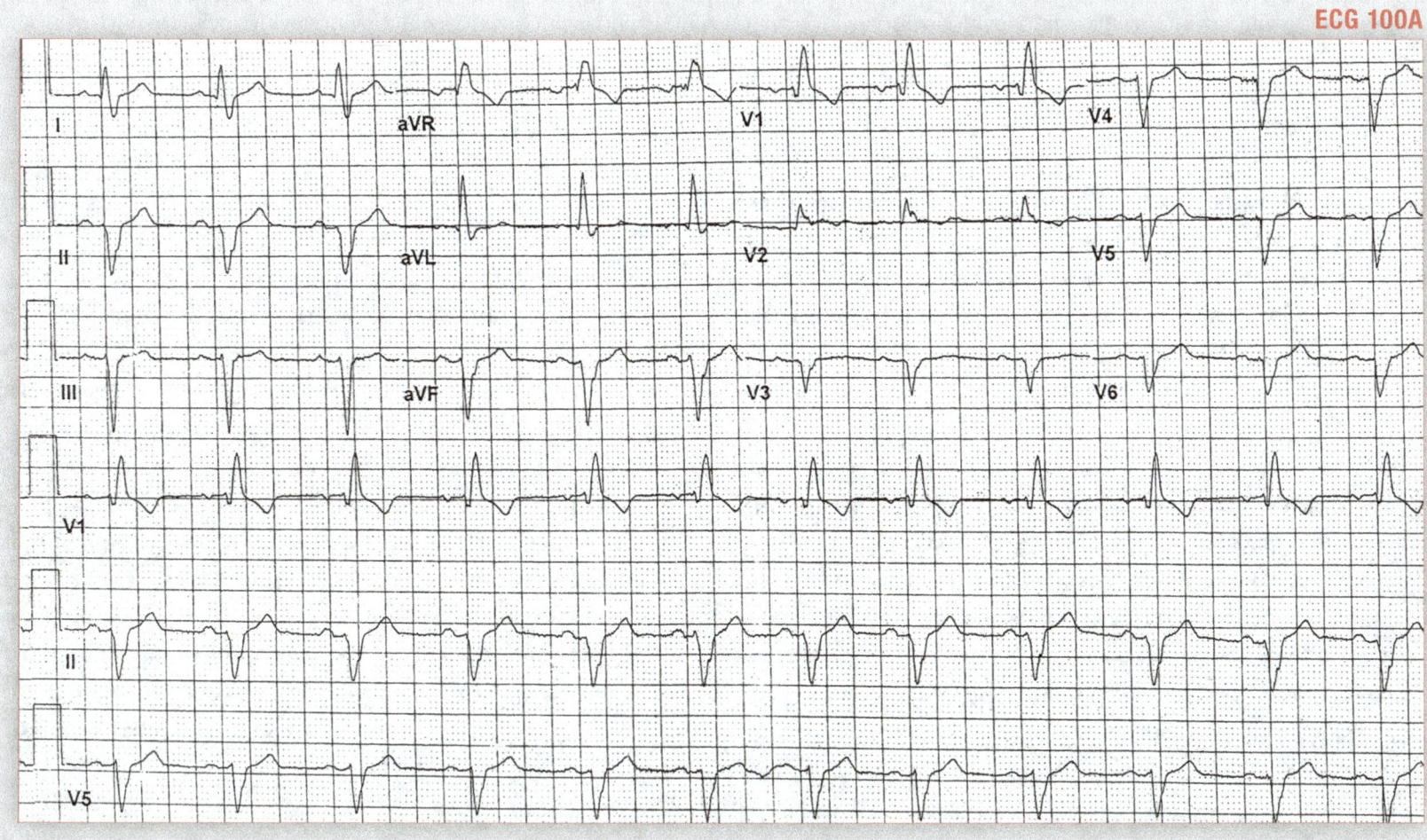

emergency department because of an episode that was of longer duration and associated with more severe lightheadedness. His physical exam is unremarkable, except for a blood pressure of 170/90 mm Hg. An ECG is obtained (ECG 100A). Because he lives alone, it was decided to admit him to a telemetry unit for observation. The following day he complained of lightheadedness, and on telemetry there was a change in his heart rate. An ECG was obtained (ECG 100B).

What abnormality is noted on the ECGs?

What is the etiology of the abnormality?

What treatment is indicated?

ECG 100B

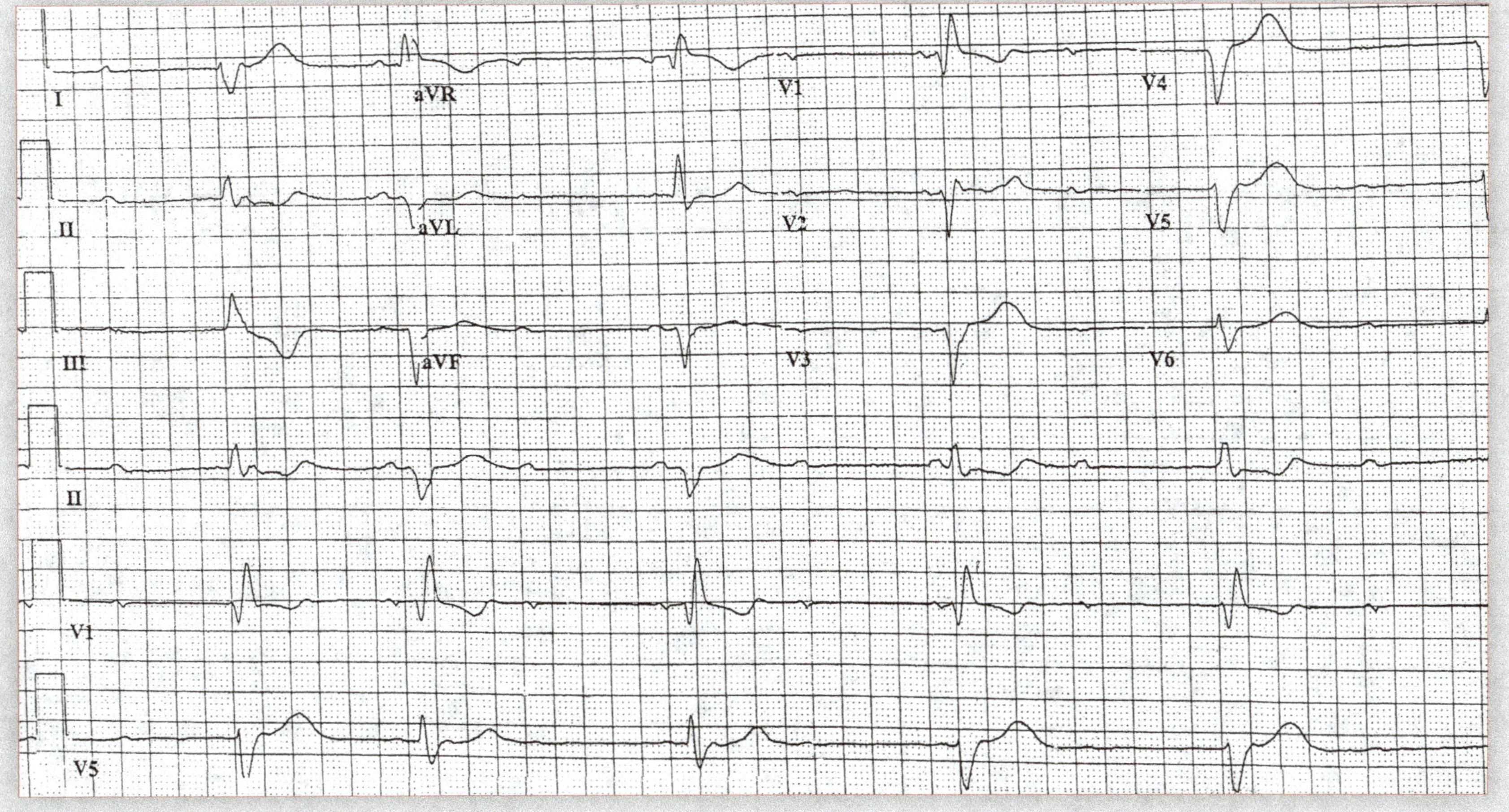

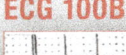

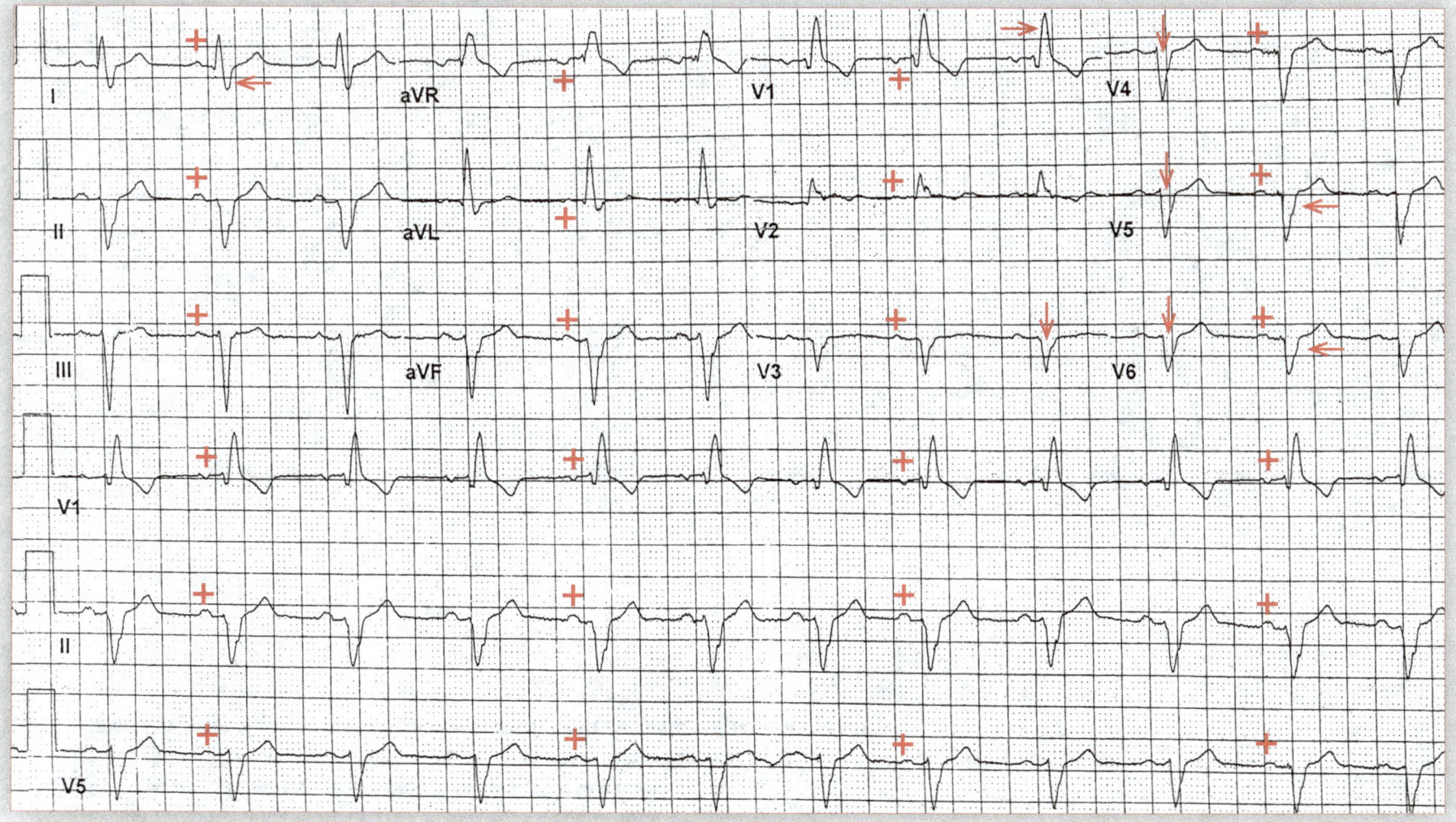

ECG 100A Analysis: Normal sinus rhythm, right bundle branch block (RBBB), left anterior fascicular block, old anterior wall MI

In **ECG 100A**, there is a regular rhythm at a rate of 76 bpm. There is a P wave (+) before each QRS complex with a stable PR interval (0.18 sec). The P wave is positive in leads I, II, aVF, and V4-V6. Hence this is a normal sinus rhythm. The QRS complex duration is increased (0.16 sec), and it has a morphology of a typical right bundle branch block (RBBB), with an RSR′ complex in lead V1 (→) and a broad terminal S wave in leads I and V5-V6 (←). The axis is extremely leftward, between −30° and −90° (positive QRS complex in lead I and negative QRS complex in leads II and aVF, with an rS morphology).

There are no Q waves in leads II and aVF; hence the extreme left axis is due to a left anterior fascicular block. There is a deep Q wave in lead V3 and probably in leads V4-V6 (↓), consistent with an old anterior wall myocardial infarction (MI). The QT/QTc intervals are slightly prolonged (400/450 msec) but are normal when the prolonged QRS complex duration is considered (320/360 msec). The presence of an RBBB and left anterior fascicular block indicates bifascicular disease.

continues

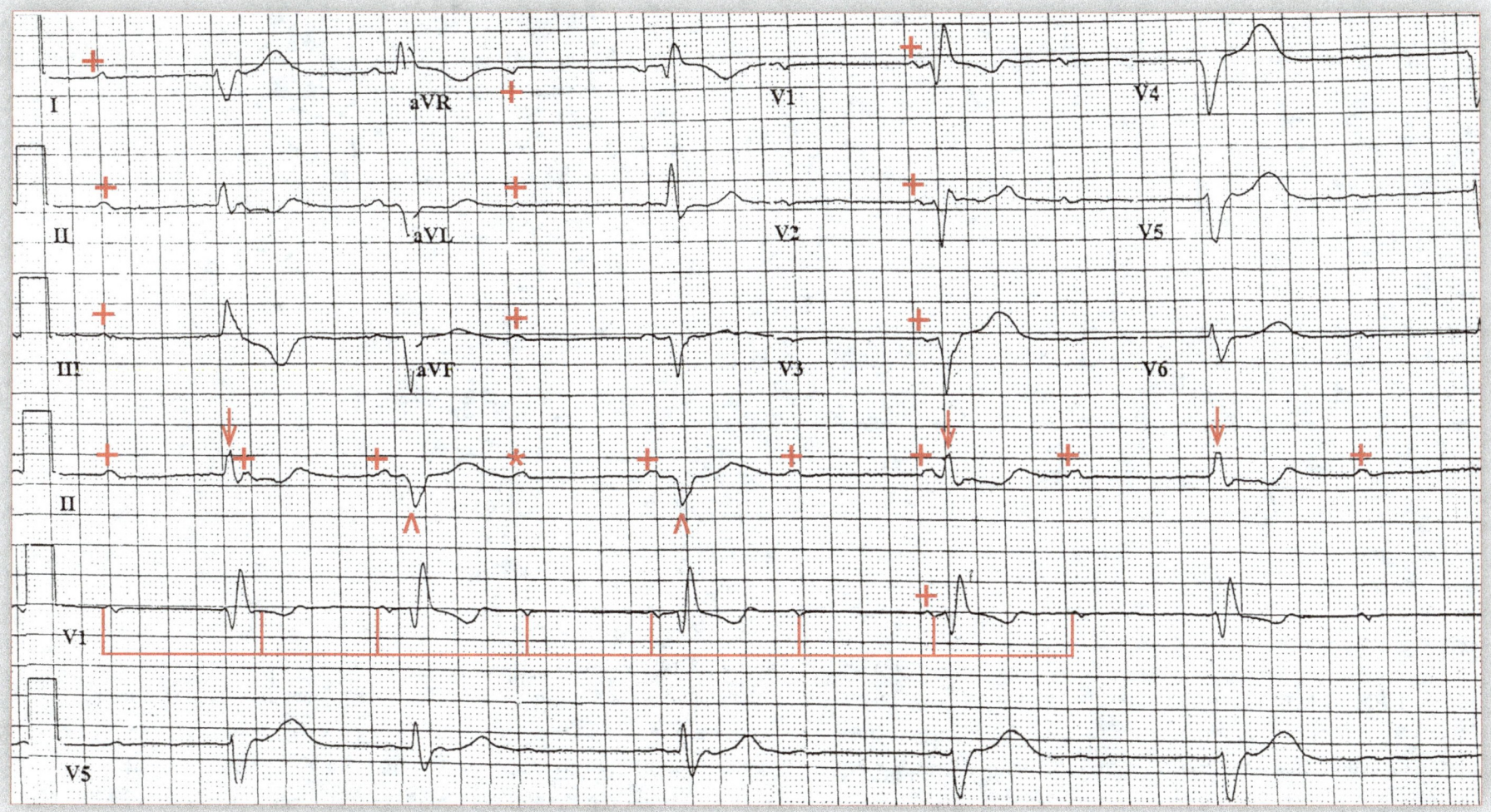

ECG 100B Analysis: Complete heart block, escape junctional rhythm with
RBBB and left posterior fascicular block, intermittent capture with Mobitz type I
2:1 AV block, trifascicular disease, old anterior wall MI

In **ECG 100B**, the rhythm is regular except for the second QRS complex, which is early (associated with a shorter RR interval). The rate is 32 bpm. P waves (+) are seen, and they occur with a regular interval (⊔) at a rate of 64 bpm. The PR intervals are variable, except for those associated with the second and third QRS complexes (^), both of which have the same PR interval (0.18 sec). This is the same as the PR interval seen in **ECG 100A**. Therefore, there is AV dissociation and, as the atrial rate is faster than the ventricular rate, complete heart block (third-degree AV block) is present. Complexes 2 and 3 (^) represent intermittent capture. All of the QRS complexes have a prolonged duration (0.16 sec) with an RBBB morphology, as noted in the lead V1 rhythm strip. The RBBB morphology is identical to the QRS morphology seen in **ECG 100A**. Similar to the QRS complexes in **ECG 100A**, there are also Q waves in leads V2-V5 due to an old anterior wall MI. The QT/QTc intervals are also the same.

However, there are changes in the QRS complex as seen in the lead II rhythm strip. This is primarily a result of a change in axis. Complexes 1, 4, and 5 (↓), which are dissociated, have an RBBB morphology and a QRS complex that is negative in lead I and positive in lead II. Although this QRS complex is not seen in lead aVF, the fact that it is negative in lead I and positive in lead II suggests that it is likely also positive in lead aVF and hence it has a right axis, a result

of a left posterior fascicular block. Complexes 2 and 3, which are conducted from the sinus P wave (*ie*, they are captured), also have an RBBB morphology, but they have a positive QRS complex in lead I and negative QRS complex in leads II and aVF, which is a left anterior fascicular block. These QRS complexes are identical in morphology and axis to those seen in **ECG 100A**. The rhythm is, therefore, sinus with complete heart block and intermittent capture. The escape rhythm is junctional as all of the QRS complexes have a typical RBBB morphology that is identical to what is seen in **ECG 100A**. However, there is alternating fascicular conduction, with the conducted complexes having a left anterior fascicular block that is identical to the QRS complexes in **ECG 100A** and the dissociated QRS complexes having a left posterior fascicular block. Therefore, while the escape rhythm is junctional, there is also evidence for trifascicular disease (*ie*, an RBBB with alternating left anterior and left posterior fascicular block).

It can be seen that there is a nonconducted P wave (*) between complexes 2 and 3, representing a brief period of second-degree AV block with a pattern of 2:1 AV conduction (2:1 AV block). Since the escape rhythm is junctional, the 2:1 AV block is a Mobitz type 1. As this patient is symptomatic and has evidence of AV nodal as well as His-Purkinje disease, placement of a permanent pacemaker is indicated. ■

A 72-year-old diabetic woman presents to her primary care physician 4 days after "a transient illness." When asked to elaborate, she states that several days ago she suffered a prolonged bout of indigestion with substernal burning resembling gastroesophageal reflux, intermittent sweats, fatigue, and mild shortness of breath. She assumed she had "caught a 24-hour stomach bug." For 2 days thereafter, she felt exhausted. Her symptoms have largely abated except for some lingering fatigue, which has brought her to her physician.

On exam, her heart rate is 72 bpm, and her blood pressure 148/88 mm Hg. There is no lymphadenopathy, and her head, ears, eyes, nose, and throat exam is normal. Her lungs are clear. Her jugular venous pressure is 7 cm H_2O with normal X and Y descents. Her cardiac exam is notable for an S4 gallop and a faint holosystolic murmur at the apex. Her abdominal, extremity, and neurologic exams are normal. An ECG is obtained.

What abnormality is noted?

Does it shed any light on her preceding illness?

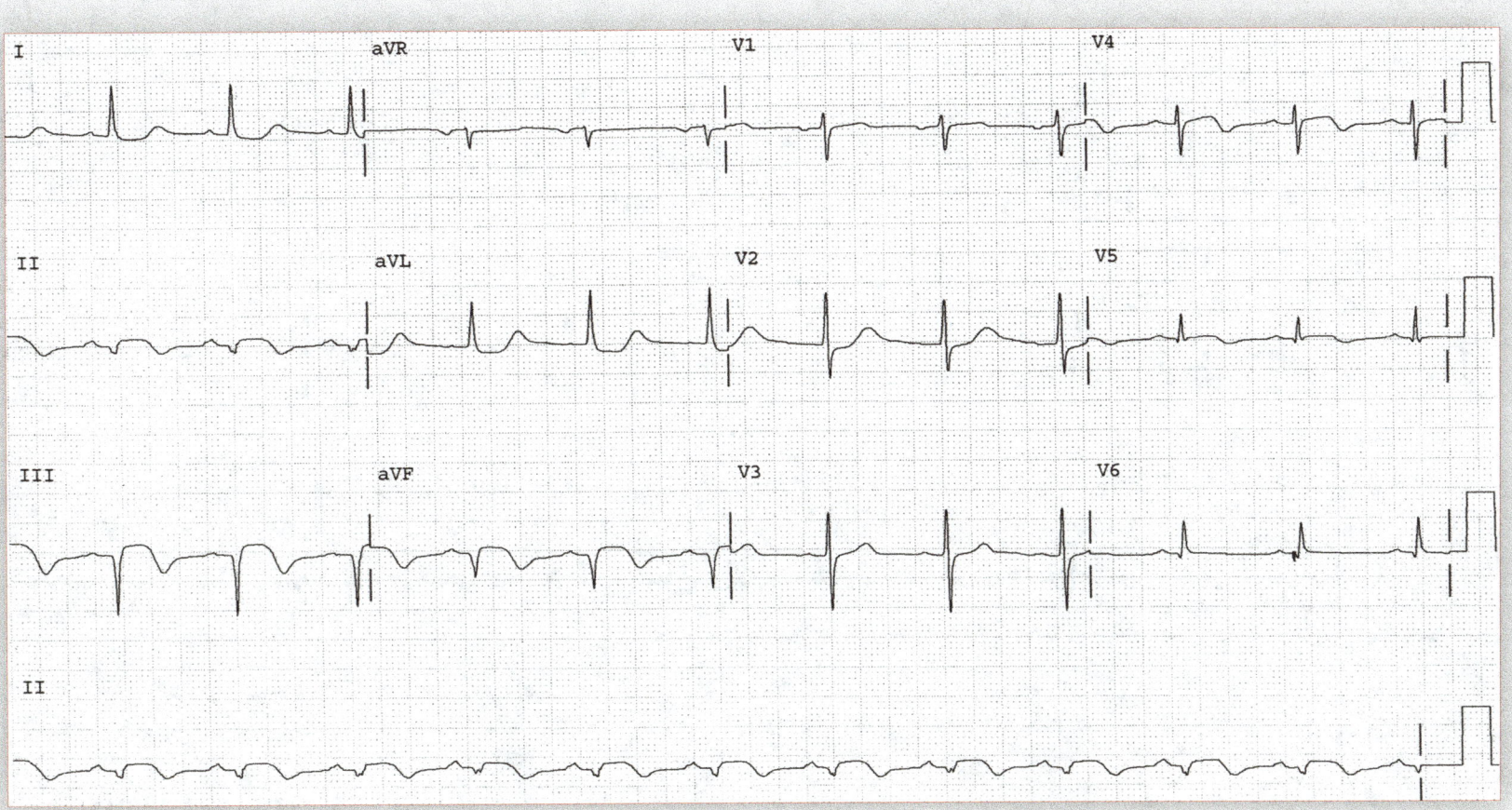

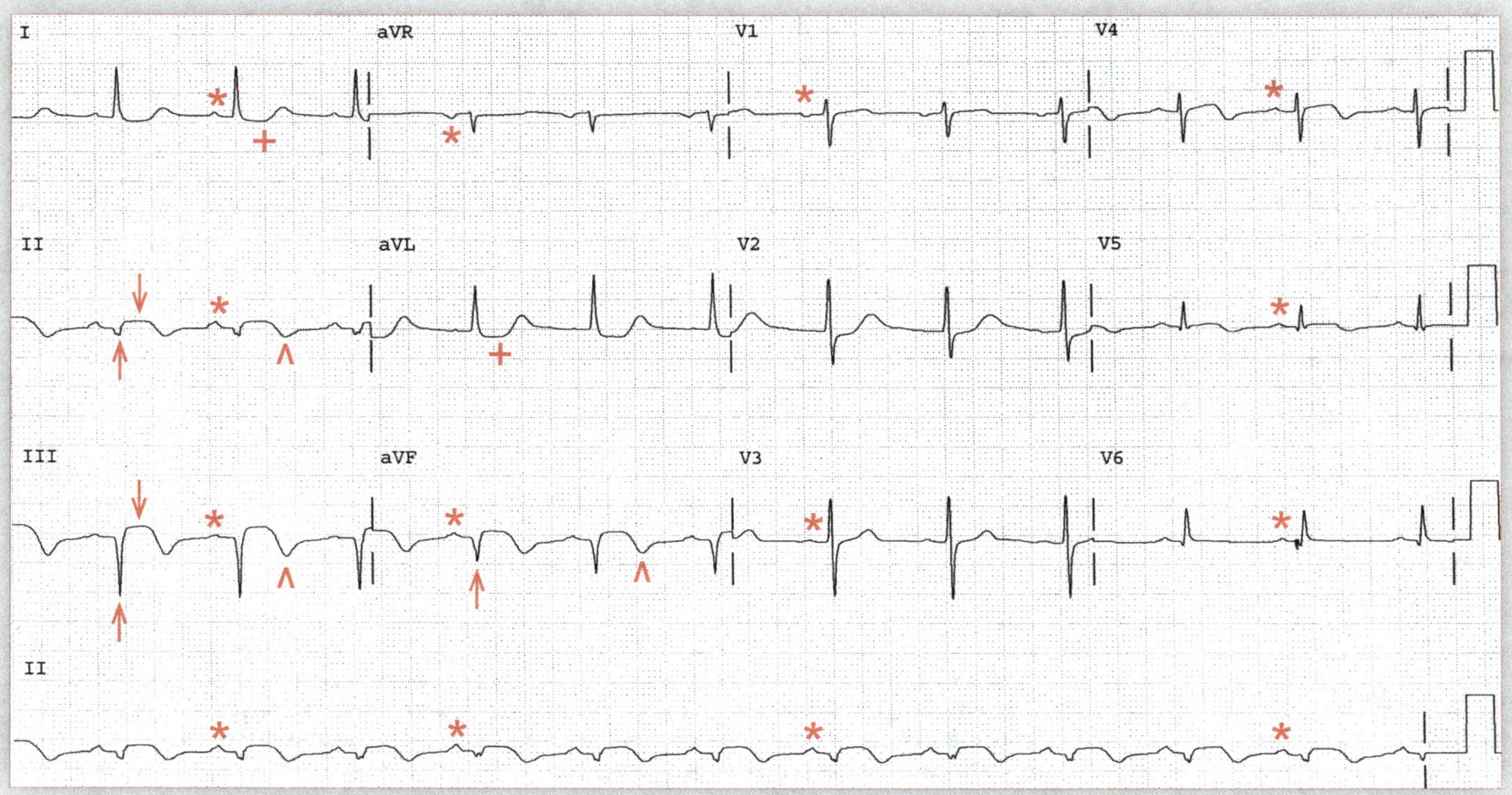

ECG 101 Analysis: Normal sinus rhythm, left axis, recent inferior wall myocardial infarction

There is a regular rhythm at a rate of 72 bpm. There is a P wave (*) before each QRS complex, with a stable PR interval (0.16 sec). The P waves are positive in leads I, II, aVF, and V4-V6. Hence this is a normal sinus rhythm. The axis is extremely leftward, between −30° and −90° (positive QRS complex in lead I and negative QRS complex in leads II and aVF). Although these are the criteria for a left anterior fascicular block, it can be seen that the initial waveform in leads II, III, and aVF is a Q wave (↑) and not an R wave (which is seen with a left anterior fascicular block). Hence the left axis in this case is the result of an inferior wall myocardial infarction (MI). There is slight ST-segment elevation (↓) in leads II, III, and aVF, and the T waves are inverted (^). In addition, there is slight ST-segment depression in leads I and aVL (+); these are reciprocal changes. These abnormalities indicate that the infarction is likely recent and reflect the ECG changes of an acute infarction that is still evolving. The QT/QTc intervals are normal (400/440 msec).

Her symptoms 4 days ago likely represented the onset of the ST-segment elevation MI. Although she had symptoms, they were misinterpreted as being gastrointestinal rather than cardiac in origin. This is not infrequent as an inferior wall MI often presents with substernal burning and fullness, symptoms that are often confused with a hiatal hernia or gastroesophageal reflux. In addition it has been reported that almost 50% of inferior wall MIs may be silent, without any recognizable symptoms. This may be especially frequent in a patient who has diabetes in whom there may be autonomic dysfunction. The anginal discomfort is a result of impulse transmission through unmyelinated fibers that travel along with the sympathetic nerves that innervate the heart and enter the spinal cord at the C7–T4 level. Hence neural transmission of anginal discomfort is interrupted in the presence of a diabetic autonomic neuropathy. These patients are said to have silent ischemia. However, it is actually painless or discomfortless ischemia; while they may not experience anginal discomfort, they will often have the other associated symptoms of ischemia, including shortness of breath, nausea, and diaphoresis.

Her physical exam also demonstrates a holosystolic murmur at the apex. Although it is not certain whether this murmur predated the MI, such murmurs, which are mitral in origin, are not uncommon with an inferior wall MI and are due to associated posteromedial papillary muscle dysfunction. An echocardiogram would be essential to further evaluate the murmur as well as left ventricular function and wall motion abnormalities. Routine post-MI therapy is indicated in this patient, including β-blocker, aspirin, statin, and possibly an angiotensin-converting enzyme inhibitor, depending on left ventricular function and the severity of the wall motion abnormality of the inferior segment of the left ventricle. ■

Notes

Index

Notes